STATE-OF-THE-ART SURVEYS ON FINITE ELEMENT TECHNOLOGY

sponsored by

THE APPLIED MECHANICS DIVISION

edited by

AHMED K. NOOR
GEORGE WASHINGTON UNIVERSITY CENTER
NASA LANGLEY RESEARCH CENTER
HAMPTON, VIRGINIA

WALTER D. PILKEY
UNIVERSITY OF VIRGINIA
CHARLOTTESVILLE, VIRGINIA

THE AMERICAN SOCIETY OF MECHANICAL ENGINEERS
United Engineering Center · 345 East 47th Street · New York, N.Y. 10017

Library of Congress Catalog Card Number 83-82420

FOREWORD

The finite element method represents one of the most significant developments in the history of computational methods. The use of modern finite element technology has transformed much of theoretical mechanics and abstract science into practical and essential tools for a multitude of technological developments which affect many facets of our life.

Finite element technology has emerged as a new discipline combining theoretical mechanics, approximation theory, numerical analysis, and computer science. It draws from developments made in each of the four disciplines and is nourished by them, but it also stands as a viable branch of knowledge in its own right. Today finite element technology can be used on any physical problem which can be stated in terms of differential, integral, or integro-differential equations.

The use of the finite element method may be traced back to antiquity. Early applications were in the field of geometry. In the pre-computer era, the finite element method was used in the analysis of naturally discrete systems such as structural frameworks and electrical networks. The modern version of the finite element method was first used in the approximation of a continuum by elements with multiple connecting points by Turner et al. (Ref. 1), Argyris (Ref. 2), and Clough (Ref. 3), who coined the name finite elements in 1960. Parallel developments were made in the mathematical physics literature by Courant (Ref. 4), in which the essence of triangular element was formulated, and by Prager and Synge (Ref. 5), in which the method of hypercircle was proposed.

The development of *modern* finite element technology spans a period of less than thirty years and may be divided into three stages. The first stage is characterized by development of simple two-dimensional and three-dimensional continuum elements, mostly for structural mechanics applications. The variational process for formulating the elemental matrices was introduced and all the elements developed were based on the stiffness (displacement) formulation.

In the second stage, the variational-based finite element approach was expanded to include multifield and generalized variational principles with relaxed continuity requirements. Weighted-residual finite element methods were introduced. The mathematical foundations of the finite element method received a great deal of attention during this stage. Efficient numerical algorithms for the solution of algebraic equations, and the extraction of eigenvalues were developed. Substructuring and modal synthesis techniques for handling large problems were introduced, and a number of general-purpose finite element program systems were released for public use. Also, the finite element method penetrated other areas of engineering and analysis such as heat transfer, fluid mechanics, electromagnetism, biomechanics, geomechanics, acoustics, aeromechanics, and fracture mechanics. Within each field to which finite element method has been applied, success on simpler problem classes has encouraged bolder applications (e.g., nonlinear and time-dependent (transient) response, and media interaction problems).

The third stage involved the development of special elements such as boundary-layer elements for viscous flow calculations, singular elements for fracture mechanics applications, and infinite elements for modeling unbounded domains. Other activities included establishment of the equivalence and similarities between various finite element formulations, application of finite element concepts to the discretization of boundary integral formulations, coupling of the finite element method with classical Rayleigh-Ritz and Bubnov-Galerkin techniques, and development of finite element algorithms which are suitable for new computer hardware (such as the array and vector processors and the microcomputers). Finite element mesh design, *a postriori* error estimates and adaptive refinement of the finite element model have received increasing attention in recent years. Strategies for mesh refinement and/or changing the order of the approximating polynomials in certain regions in order to achieve an optimal finite element solution have been proposed.

The success of the finite element method is mainly attributed to its generality, versatility and ability to analyze complex configurations. To-date there are approximately five hundred user-oriented finite element program systems and over two hundred pre- and postprocessing packages. There are over 20,000 finite element users worldwide who are estimated to spend about $500 million annually on finite element analysis. The number of publications on finite element technology has been increasing exponentially and the literature on the subject is nearly overwhelming. Therefore, there is a need to broaden the awareness among practicing engineers and research workers about the recent developments in various aspects of finite element technology. Although a number of survey papers have been written on the subject (see, for example, Refs. 6 and 7), there is a need for a state-of-the-art survey of the different aspects of finite element technology. This book is a modest attempt to fill this void. The intent of the book was to put the intense and diverse activities in finite element technology into proper perspective and to help broaden awareness of the state-of-the-art within the finite element users community and the research community. The book contains sixteen chapters which are written by leading experts in the field. The topics of these chapters were selected by the editors and are reviewed briefly here.

The first chapter describes the mathematical framework in which the finite element methods can be set in order for existence and uniqueness theorems to be applicable, and for error bounds to be computed. Only time-independent problems are considered. A knowledge of functional analysis (see, for example, Ref. 8) is prerequisite to understanding this chapter.

The basis functions for individual elements play a crucial role in finite element computation. A variety of basis functions are described in the second chapter of this book including polynomial and rational basis functions. Also, the use of subelement basis functions to generate macroelements is outlined and the concept of hierarchical basis functions is reviewed. The various considerations used in selecting the basis functions are outlined.

The use of a good finite element mesh is crucial for the efficient solution of practical problems. The mesh design is the subject of the third chapter. Guidelines are presented for selecting the element types, the grid arrangement and the mesh evolution strategy.

Chapters 4 and 5 deal with some of the recent developments in element technology. Special and singular elements for treating problems with singular derivatives of field variables are presented. Also, the variety of the multifield (mixed and hybrid) element models and formulations are reviewed.

The success of the finite element process is dependent on the skillful use of efficient numerical algorithms for handling the resulting large systems of algebraic equations. Chapters 6 and 7 deal with the various solution techniques for linear and nonlinear finite element equations.

The use of finite elements in automated (optimum) design of large systems requires the development of efficient repetitive analysis (reanalysis) techniques. Chapter 8 reviews the current methodology of reanalysis, modal syntheses, and dynamic design of large systems.

As with all approximate and numerical techniques, an error analysis is an essential part of the finite element solution process. Chapter 7 lists the various sources of errors in the finite element process and discusses the relative magnitudes, growth rates, estimates, and control of these different errors.

Finite element software is the subject of the succeeding three chapters. First, the status and trends in finite element software are given in Chapter 9; the various pre- and postprocessors and other programming aids are reviewed in Chapter 10. A description of the capabilities of some of the major finite element software systems is presented in Chapter 11.

Application of the finite element method to time-dependent problems is discussed in Chapter 12. The various temporal integration schemes are shown to be special cases of the weighted-residual finite element formulations. The use of explicit, implicit, and combined explicit-implicit techniques are reviewed.

The combined use of the finite element method and the classical Rayleigh-Ritz technique is reviewed in Chapter 14. The resulting hybrid technique is called the global-local finite element method. It is demonstrated that the hybrid technique combines the advantages of the two parent techniques and alleviates their major drawbacks. A number of practical applications are cited.

The use of the finite element method in conjunction with the boundary integral equation formulation to form the boundary element method is the subject of Chapter 15. The advantages of using the boundary element method are discussed and two approaches for applying the method are outlined.

Digital computers are the technological foundation of the finite element method. Considerable advances have been made in computer hardware, firmware and software. The major advances that are likely to impact finite element technology are reviewed and a scenario is given of future finite element systems in the last chapter, Chapter 16.

The book was originally planned to be published in late 1980; however, for various reasons, the publication date slipped until 1983. However, the majority of the chapters were revised to incorporate these developments, but a few do not include the developments that took place between 1981-1983.

The editors are indebted to the many individuals who contributed to this book; in particular, to members of the Committee of Computing in Applied Mechanics of ASME for their useful suggestions and encouragement. Special thanks go to the authors for the efforts they have made in preparing their manuscripts; to the reviewers of the various chapters for their careful reviews and useful suggestions; to Barbara Pilkey for her meticulous technical editing; and to Mrs. Mary Torian and Miss Cindy Ripley for their secretarial support in various phases of the project. It is our earnest hope that this effort to broaden awareness and to place in perspective the recent developments in finite element technology will serve the profession well.

Ahmed K. Noor
George Washington University Center
at NASA Langley Research Center
Hampton, Virginia

Walter D. Pilkey
University of Virginia
Charlottesville, Virginia

References

1 Turner, M. J., Clough, R. W., Martin, H. C., and Topp, L. J., "Stiffness and Deflection Analysis of Complex Structures," Journal of Aeronautical Sciences, Vol. 23, 1956, pp. 805-823.

2 Argyris, J. H., Energy Theorems and Structural Analysis, Butterworth, 1960 (reprinted from Aircraft Engineering, 1954-55).

3 Clough, R. W., The Finite Element in Plane Stress Analysis, Proceedings of the Second ASCE Conference on Electronic Computation, Pittsburgh, PA., September 1960.

4 Courant, R., "Variational Methods for Solution of Problems of Equilibrium and Vibration," Bulletin of the American Mathematical Society, Vol. 49, 1943, pp. 1-23.

5 Prager, W. and Synge, J. L., "Approximation in Elasticity Based on the Concept of Function Space," Quarterly Journal of Applied Mathematics, Vol. 5, 1947, pp. 241-269.

6 Zienkiewicz, O. C., "The Finite Element Method: From Intuition to Generality," Applied Mechanics Reviews, Vol. 23, No. 3, March 1970, pp. 249-256.

7 Hughes, T. J. R., "Some Current Trends in Finite Element Research," Applied Mechanics Reviews, Vol. 33, No. 11, November 1980, pp. 1467-1477.

8 Oden, J. T., Applied Functional Analysis: A First Course for Students of Mechanics and Engineering Science, Prentice Hall, 1979.

CONTENTS

LIST OF TEXTBOOKS AND MONOGRAPHS ON FINITE ELEMENT TECHNOLOGY

Since the publication of the first textbook on finite element method in 1967 (Zienkiewicz, O. C. and Cheung, Y. K., The Finite Element Method in Structural and Continuum Mechanics, McGraw-Hill, London), over one hundred and sixty monographs and conference proceedings have been published on the subject. For the benefit of the readers of this book, all of the English books and some of the foreign books that the editors are aware of are listed herein. Also included is a list of the conference proceedings devoted solely to finite elements. The references are divided into eleven categories as follows: fundamentals, mathematical foundations, structural and solid mechanics applications, fluid mechanics applications, other applied science and engineering applications, computer implementation and software systems, computational and modeling aspects, special topics, boundary element methods, bibliographies, and proceedings of symposia and conferences on finite element technology. The references in each of the first ten sections are arranged alphabetically, and in the last section they are arranged in chronological order.

I. FUNDAMENTALS

1.1 Bathe, K. J., Finite Element Procedures in Engineering Analysis, Prentice-Hall, Inc., Englewood Cliffs, New Jersey, 1981.

1.2 Becker, E. B., Carey, G. F., and Oden, J. T., Finite Elements: An Introduction, Vol. 1, Prentice-Hall, Inc., Englewood Cliffs, New Jersey, 1981.

1.3 Carey, G. F. and Oden, J. T., Finite Elements: A Second Course, Prentice-Hall, Inc., Englewood Cliffs, New Jersey, 1983.

1.4 Cheung, Y. K. and Yeo, M. F., A Practical Introduction to Finite Element Analysis, Pitman Publishing, London, 1979.

1.5 Cook, R. D., Concepts and Applications of Finite Element Analysis, second edition, John Wiley and Sons, New York, 1981.

1.6 Davies, A. J., The Finite Element Method: A First Approach, Clarendon Press, Oxford, 1980.

1.7 Desai, C. S. and Abel, J. F., Introduction to the Finite Element Method. A Numerical Method for Engineering Analysis, Van Nostrand Reinhold Company, New York, 1972.

1.8 Desai, C. S., Elementary Finite Element Method, Prentice-Hall, Inc., Englewood Cliffs, New Jersey, 1979.

1.9 Dhatt, G. and Touzot, G., Une presentation de la methode des elements finis, Maloine S. A. Editeur, Paris, 1981.

1.10 Fenner, R. T., Finite Element Methods for Engineers, Macmillan, London, 1975.

1.11 Gallagher, R. H., Finite Element Analysis - Fundamentals, Prentice-Hall, Inc., Englewood Cliffs, New Jersey, 1975.

1.12 Hinton, E. and Owen, D. R. J., An Introduction to Finite Element Computations, Pineridge Press, Swansea, United Kingdom, 1979.

1.13 Huebner, K. H. and Thornton, E. A., The Finite Element Method for Engineers, second edition, Wiley Interscience, New York, 1982.

1.14 Irons, B. and Ahmad, S., Techniques of Finite Elements, John Wiley and Sons, New York, 1980.

1.15 Irons, B. and Shrive, N., Finite Element Primer, John Wiley and Sons, New York, 1983.

1.16 Martin, H. C. and Carey, G. F., Introduction to Finite Element Analysis. Theory and Application, McGraw-Hill, New York, 1972.

1.17 Nath, B., Fundamentals of Finite Elements for Engineers, Athlone Press, London, 1974.

1.18 Norrie, D. H. and de Vries, G., An Introduction to the Finite Element Method, second edition, Academic Press, New York, 1978.

1.19 Oden, J. T., Finite Elements of Nonlinear Continua, McGraw-Hill, New York, 1972.

1.20 Owen, D. R. J. and Hinton, E., A Simple Guide to Finite Elements, Pineridge Press, Swansea, United Kingdom, 1980.

1.21 Rao, S. S., The Finite Element Method in Engineering, first edition, Pergamon Press, Elmsford, New York, 1982.

1.22 Segerlind, L. J., Applied Finite Element Analysis, John Wiley and Sons, New York, 1976.

1.23 Tong, P. and Rossettos, J. N., Finite Element Method - Basic Techniques and Implementation, The MIT Press, Cambridge, MA., 1977.

1.24 Zienkiewicz, O. C., The Finite Element Method, third edition, McGraw-Hill, New York, 1977.

1.25 Zienkiewicz, O. C., Introductory Lectures on the Finite Element Method, International Center for Mechanical Sciences, Udine, Italy, Springer-Verlag, 1978.

1.26 Zienkiewicz, O. C. and Morgan, K., Finite Elements and Approximation, Wiley Interscience, New York, 1982.

II. MATHEMATICAL FOUNDATIONS

2.1 Aziz, A. K. (ed.), The Mathematical Foundations of the Finite Element Method with Applications to Partial Differential Equations, Academic Press, New York, 1972.

2.2 Ciarlet, Ph., Kesavan, S., Ranjan, A., and Vanninathan, M., Lectures on the Finite Element Method/by Ph. Ciarlett; Notes by S. Kesavan, A. Ranjan and M. Vanninathan. Tata Institute of Fundamental Research, Bombay, India, 1975.

2.3 Ciarlet, P. G., The Finite Element Method for Elliptic Problems, North Holland Publ. Co., New York, 1978.

2.4 de Boor, C. (ed.), Mathematical Aspects of Finite Elements in Partial Differential Equations, Academic Press, New York, 1974.

2.5 Fairweather, G., Finite Element Galerkin Methods for Differential Equations, Marcel Dekker, Inc., New York, 1978.

2.6 Galligani, I. and Magenes, E. (eds.), Mathematical Aspects of Finite Element Methods, Lecture Notes in Mathematics, Vol. 606, Springer-Verlag, New York, 1977.

2.7 Mercier, B., Lectures on Topics in Finite Element Solution of Elliptic Problems, Springer-Verlag, 1979.

2.8 Mitchell, A. R. and Wait, R. A., The Finite Element Method in Partial Differential Equations, John Wiley and Sons, New York, 1977.

2.9 Nakazawa, S. and Kelly, D. W., Mathematics of Finite Elements - An Engineering Approach, Pineridge Press, Swansea, United Kingdom, 1983.

2.10 Oden, J. T. and Reddy, J. N., An Introduction to the Mathematical Theory of Finite Elements, John Wiley and Sons, New York, 1976.

2.11 Oden, J. T. (in collaboration with G. F. Carey), Finite Elements: Mathematical Aspects, Vol. 4, Prentice Hall, Inc., New York, 1982.

2.12 Strang, R. and Fix, G., An Analysis of the Finite Element Method, Prentice Hall, Inc., New York, 1973.

2.13 Wachspress, E. L., A Rational Finite Element Basis, Academic Press, New York, 1975.

2.14 Whiteman, J. R. (ed.), The Mathematics of Finite Elements and Applications, Academic Press, London, 1973.

2.15 Whiteman, J. R. (ed.), The Mathematics of Finite Elements and Applications, Vol. 2, Academic Press, London, 1977.

2.16 Whiteman, J. R. (ed.), The Mathematics of Finite Elements and Applications, Vol. 3, Academic Press, London, 1979.

2.17 Whiteman, J. R. (ed.), The Mathematics of Finite Elements and Applications, Vol. 4, Academic Press, London, 1982.

2.18 Vichnevetsky, R., Computer Methods for Partial Differential Equations, Vol. 1, Prentice-Hall, Inc., Englewood Cliffs, New Jersey, 1981.

III. STRUCTURAL AND SOLID MECHANICS APPLICATIONS

3.1 Ashwell, D. G. and Gallagher, R. H. (eds.), Finite Elements for Thin Shells and Curved Members, John Wiley and Sons, London, 1976.

3.2 Belytschko, T. and Marcal, P. V. (eds.), Finite Element Analysis of Transient Nonlinear Structural Behavior, AMD Vol. 14, American Society of Mechanical Engineers, 1975.

3.3 Bernadou, M. and Boisserie, J. M., The Finite Element Method in Thin Shell Theory: Application to Arch Dam Simulations, Birkhauser, Boston, 1982.

3.4 Brebbia, C. A. and Connor, J. J., Fundamentals of Finite Element Techniques for Structural Engineers, John Wiley and Sons, New York, 1974.

3.5 Bowes, W. H. and Russel, L. T., Stress Analysis by the Finite Element Method for Practicing Engineers, Lexington Books, Lexington, MA., 1975.

3.6 Cheung, Y. K., Finite Strip Method in Structural Analysis, Pergamon Press, Elmsford, New York, 1976.

3.7 Hinton, E. and Owen, D. R. J. (eds.), Finite Element Software for Plates and Shells, Pineridge Press, Swansea, United Kingdom, 1983.

3.8 Holand, I. and Bell, K. (eds.), Finite Element Methods in Stress Analysis, Lectures presented at the Technical University of Norway, Jan. 6-11, 1969; published by TAPIR.

3.9 Hughes, T. J. R., Pifko, A., and Jay, A. (eds.), Nonlinear Finite Element Analysis of Plates and Shells, presented at the Winter Annual Meeting of the American Society of Mechanical Engineering, Washington, D.C., Nov. 15-20, 1981, AMD Vol. 48, 1981.

3.10 Kamal, M. M. and Wolf, J. A. (eds.), Finite Element Applications in Vibration Problems, American Society of Mechanical Engineers, 1977.

3.11 Korneev, V. G., Finite Element Schemes of High Orders of Accuracy, (in Russian), Izdatel'stvo Leningradskogo Universiteta, Leningrad, U.S.S.R., 1977.

3.12 Morozov, E. M. and Nikishkov, G. P., The Finite Element Method in Fracture Mechanics (in Russian), Izdatel'stvo Nauka, Moscow, U.S.S.R., 1980.

3.13 Oden, J. T. and Carey, G. F. (compilers), Finite Elements: Special Problems in Solid Mechanics, Prentice-Hall, Inc., New York, 1983.

3.14 Owen, D. R. J. and Hinton, E., Finite Elements in Plasticity - Theory and Practice, Pineridge Press, Swansea, United Kingdom, 1981.

3.15 Przemieniecki, J. S., Theory of Matrix Structural Analysis, McGraw-Hill, New York, 1968.

3.16 Rockey, K. C., Evans, H. R., Griffiths, D. W., and Nethercot, D. A., The Finite Element Method - A Basic Introduction, second edition, Halsted Press, John Wiley and Sons, New York, 1980.

3.17 Robinson, J., An Integrated Theory of Finite Element Methods, Wiley Interscience, New York, 1973.

3.18 Robinson, J., Understanding Finite Element Stress Analysis, Robinson and Associates, Wimborne, England, 1981.

3.19 Rossmanith, H. P. (ed.), Finite Elemente in der Bruchmechanik, Springer-Verlag, Wien, 1982.

3.20 Schaeffer, H. G., MSC/NASTRAN - Static and Normal Mode Analysis, second edition, Schaeffer Analysis, Mont Vernon, New Hampshire, 1982.

3.21 Task Committee on Finite Element Analysis of Reinforced Concrete Structures, "State-of-the-Art Report on Finite Element Analysis of Reinforced Concrete," American Society of Civil Engineers, 1982.

3.22 Tottenham, H. and Brebbia, C. A. (eds.), Finite Element Techniques in Structural Mechanics, Lectures presented at Southampton University, England, April 1970.

3.23 Ural, O., Finite Element Method: Basic Concepts and Applications, Intext Educational Publishers, 1973.

IV. FLUID MECHANICS APPLICATIONS

4.1 Baker, A. J., Finite Element Computational Fluid Mechanics, McGraw-Hill, New York, 1983.

4.2 Connor, J. C. and Brebbia, C. A., Finite Element Techniques for Fluid Flow, Butterworth, London, 1976.

4.3 Chung, T. J., Finite Element Analysis in Fluid Dynamics, McGraw-Hill, New York, 1978.

4.4 Gallagher, R. H., Oden, J. T., Taylor, C., and Zienkiewicz, O. C. (eds.), Finite Elements in Fluids, Vols. 1 and 2, John Wiley and Sons, New York, 1975.

4.5 Gallagher, R. H., Zienkiewicz, O. C., Oden, J. T., Cecchi, M. M., and Taylor, C. (eds.), Finite Elements in Fluids, Vol. 3, John Wiley and Sons, New York, 1978.

4.6 Gallagher, R. H., Norrie, D. H., Oden, J. T., and Zienkiewicz, O. C. (eds.), Finite Elements in Fluids, Vol. 4, John Wiley and Sons, New York, 1982.

4.7 Hughes, T. J. R. (ed.), Finite Element Methods for Convection Dominated Flows, presented at the Winter Annual Meeting of the American Society of Mechanical Engineers, New York, Dec. 2-7, 1979; sponsored by Applied Mechanics Division, ASME, AMD Vol. 34, 1979.

4.8 Norrie, D. H. (ed.), Proceedings of the International Conference on Finite Elements in Flow Problems, Third, Banff, 1980.

4.9 Oden, J. T., Gallagher, R. H., Zienkiewicz, O. C., Kawahara, M. T., and Kawai, T. (eds.), Finite Elements in Fluids, Vol. 5, John Wiley and Sons, London, 1983.

4.10 Raviart, P. A., Finite Element Methods in Fluid Mechanics, Editions Eyrolles, Paris, Electricite de France, direction des etudes et recherches, 1981.

4.11 Taylor, C. and Hughes, T. G., Finite Element Programming of the Navier-Stokes Equations, Pineridge Press, Swansea, United Kingdom, 1981.

4.12 Thomasset, F., Implementation of Finite Element Methods for Navier-Stokes Equations, Springer-Verlag, New York, 1981.

V. OTHER APPLIED SCIENCE AND ENGINEERING APPLICATIONS

5.1 Chari, M. V. K. and Silvester, P. P., Finite Elements in Electrical and Magnetic Field Problems, John Wiley and Sons, New York, 1981.

5.2 Gallagher, R. H., Simon, B., Johnson, P., and Gross, J. (eds.), Finite Elements in Biomechanics, John Wiley and Sons, New York, 1982.

5.3 Gudehus, G. (ed.), Finite Elements in Geomechanics, John Wiley and Sons, New York, 1977.

5.4 Kamal, M. M. and Wolf, J. A. (eds.), "Finite Element Applications in Acoustics," presented at the Vibrations Conference of the Design Engineering Technical Conference, Hartford, Connecticut, Sept. 20-23, 1981, ASME.

5.5 Naylor, D. J. and Pande, G. N., Finite Elements in Geotechnical Engineering (with chapters contributed by B. Simpson and R. Tabb), Pineridge Press, Swansea, United Kingdom, 1981.

5.6 Pinder, G. F. and Gray, W. G., Finite Element Simulation in Surface and Subsurface Hydrology, Academic Press, New York, 1977.

5.7 Simon, B. R. (ed.), Finite Elements in Biomechanics, Proceedings of the International Conference held at the University of Arizona, Tucson, Feb. 18, 1980, Vol. 1, Pineridge Press, Swansea, United Kingdom, 1980.

5.8 Williams, M. M. R., Finite Element Methods in Radiation Physics, Pergamon Press, Elmsford, New York, 1982.

VI. COMPUTER IMPLEMENTATION AND SOFTWARE SYSTEMS

6.1 Akin, J. E., Application and Implementation of Finite Element Methods, Academic Press, London, 1982.

6.2 Hinton, E. and Owen, D. R. J., Finite Element Programming, Academic Press, New York, 1977.

6.3 Fredriksson, B. and Mackerle, J., Structural Mechanics: Finite Element Computer Programs - Surveys and Availability, Advanced Engineering Corporation, Linköping, Sweden, 1978.

6.4 Fredriksson, B. and Mackerle, J., Structural Mechanics: Pre- and Post-processor Programs - Surveys and Availability, Advanced Engineering Corporation, Linköping, Sweden, 1977.

6.5 Fredriksson, B. and Mackerle, J., Finite Element Review, Report AEC-L003, Advanced Engineering Corporation, Linköping, Sweden, 1978.

6.6 Fredriksson, B. and Mackerle, J., Stress Analysis Programs for Fracture Mechanics, Advanced Engineering Corporation, Linköping, Sweden, 1979.

6.7 Fredriksson, B. and Mackerle, J., Structural Mechanics Finite Element Computer Programs 1970-1980, Advanced Engineering Corporation, Linköping, Sweden, 1980.

6.8 Smith, I. M., Programming the Finite Element Method, John Wiley and Sons, New York, 1982.

6.9 Finite Element Systems Handbook, second edition, CML Publications, Computational Mechanics Center, Ashurst Lodge, Hampshire, England, 1983.

VII. COMPUTATIONAL AND MODELING ASPECTS

7.1 Conaway, J. H. (ed.), Finite Element Modeling, First Chautauqua on Finite Element Modeling, Harwichport, MA., Sept. 15-17, 1980, Wallace Press, Milford, New Hampshire, 1980.

7.2 Gloudeman, J. F. and Rosanoff, R. E. (eds.), Computational Aspects of the Finite Element Method, Bundesanstalt für Material prüfung, Berlin, 1979.

7.3 Oden, J. T. and Carey, G. F., Finite Elements: Computational Aspects, Vol. 3, Prentice Hall, New Jersey, 1983.

7.4 Shephard, M. S. and Gallagher, R. H. (eds.), Finite Element Grid Optimization, presented at the Third National Congress on Pressure Vessels and Piping, San Francisco, California, June 24-29, 1979, PVP-38, American Society of Mechanical Engineers, 1979.

VIII. SPECIAL TOPICS

8.1 Atluri, S. N., Gallagher, R. H., and Zienkiewicz, O. C. (eds.), Hybrid and Mixed Finite Element Methods, Wiley Interscience, New York, 1983.

8.2 Glowinski, R., Rodin, E. Y., and Zienkiewicz, O. C. (eds.), Energy Methods in Finite Element Analysis, John Wiley and Sons, New York, 1979.

8.3 Kardestuncer, H., Finite Element Methods Via Tensors, International Center for Mechanical Sciences, Udine, Italy, 1974.

8.4 Reddy, J. N. (ed.), Penalty-Finite Element Methods in Mechanics, presented at the Winter Annual Meeting of the American Society of Mechanical Engineers, Phoenix, Arizona, Nov. 14-19, 1982, AMD Vol. 51, 1982.

IX. BOUNDARY ELEMENT METHODS

9.1 Banerjee, P. K. and Butterfield, R. (eds.), Developments in Boundary Element Methods I, Applied Science Publishers, London, 1979.

9.2 Banerjee, P. K. and Shaw, R. P. (eds.), Developments in Boundary Element Methods II, Applied Science Publishers, London.

9.3 Brebbia, C. A., The Boundary Element Method for Engineers, John Wiley and Sons, New York, 1978.

9.4 Brebbia, C. A. and Walker, S., Boundary Element Techniques in Engineering, Butterworth, London, 1981.

9.5 Brebbia, C. A. (ed.), Progress in Boundary Element Methods, John Wiley and Sons, New York, 1982.

9.6 Banerjee, P. K. and Butterfield, R., Boundary Element Methods in Engineering Science, McGraw-Hill, New York, 1981.

9.7 Mukherjee, S., Boundary Element Methods in Creep and Fracture, Applied Science Publishers, England, 1982.

X. BIBLIOGRAPHIES AND HANDBOOKS

10.1 Norrie, D. and de Vries, G., Finite Element Bibliography, Plenum Press, New York, 1976.

10.2 Whiteman, J. R., A Bibliography for Finite Elements, Academic Press, London, 1975.

10.3 Kardestuncer, H. (ed.), Finite Element Handbook, McGraw-Hill, New York, 1984.

XI. PROCEEDINGS OF SYMPOSIA AND CONFERENCES ON FINITE ELEMENT TECHNOLOGY

11.1 de Veubeke, Fraeijs B. (ed.), Matrix Methods of Structural Analysis, Pergamon Press, Elmsford, New York, 1964.

11.2 Przemieniecki, J. S., et al. (eds.), Matrix Methods in Structural Mechanics - Proceedings of the First Conference, Wright Patterson Air Force Base, Ohio, AFFDL-TR-66-80, Oct. 26-28, 1965.

11.3 Berke, L., et al. (eds.), Proceedings of the Second Conference on Matrix Methods in Structural Mechanics, Wright Patterson Air Force Base, Ohio, AFFDL-TR-68-150, Oct. 15-17, 1968.

11.4 Rowan, W. H. and Hackett, R. M. (eds.), Proceedings of the Symposium on Application of Finite Element Methods in Civil Engineering, Nov. 13-14, 1969, Vanderbilt University, Tennessee.

11.5 Proceedings of the Symposium on Finite Element Techniques, Institut fur Statik und Dynamik der Luft und Raumfahrtkonstruktionen, Universitat Stuttgart, 1969.

11.6 Gallagher, R. H., Yamada, Y., and Oden, J. T. (eds.), Recent Advances in Matrix Methods in Structural Analysis and Design, Proceedings of the First Japan-U.S. Seminar on Matrix Methods in Structural Analysis and Design, Tokyo, Aug. 25-30, 1969, University of Alabama Press, 1970.

11.7 Proceedings of the Conference on the Application of the Finite Element Methods to Stress Analysis Problems in Nuclear Engineering, June 30-July 1, 1971, Ispra, Italy.

11.8 NASTRAN Users' Experiences, Survey of NASTRAN Applications in Static and Dynamic Structural Analysis Problems, Colloquium held at Hampton, Virginia, Sept. 13-15, 1971, NASA TM-X-2378.

11.9 Bader, R. M., et al. (eds.), Proceedings of the Third Conference on Matrix Methods in Structural Mechanics, Wright Patterson Air Force Base, Ohio, AFFDL-TR-71-160, Oct. 1971.

11.10 McCutcheon, J. O., Mirza, M. S., and Mufti, A. A. (eds.), Finite Element Method in Civil Engineering, Proceedings of the Specialty Conference held at McGill University, June 1-2, 1972, Montreal, Canada.

11.11 Oden, J. T., Clough, R. W., and Yamamoto, Y. (eds.), Advances in Computational Methods in Structural Mechanics and Design, Proceedings of the Second U.S.-Japan Seminar on Matrix Methods in Structural Analysis and Design, Aug. 1972, University of Alabama in Huntsville.

11.12 NASTRAN Users' Experiences, Application of NASTRAN to Static and Dynamic Structural Analysis, Second NASTRAN Users' Colloquium, Hampton, Virginia, Sept. 11-12, 1972, NASA TM-X-2637.

11.13 Oden, J. T. and Oliveira, E. R. A. (eds.), Lectures on Finite Element Methods in Continuum Mechanics, The University of Alabama in Huntsville, 1973.

11.14 NASTRAN Users' Experiences, Third NASTRAN Users' Colloquium, Hampton, Virginia, Sept. 11-12, 1973, NASA TM-X-2893.

11.15 Proceedings of the Workshop Meeting on Computational Aspects of the Finite Element Method, Sept. 17-18, 1973, University of Stuttgart, West Germany.

11.16 Pulmano, V. A. and Kabaila, A. P. (eds.), Proceedings of the 1974 International Conference on Finite Element Methods in Engineering, University of New South Wales, Australia, Aug. 28-30, 1974.

11.17 NASTRAN Users' Experiences, NASTRAN Users' Colloquium, Hampton, Virginia, Sept. 9-11, 1975, NASA TM-X-3278.

11.18 Proceedings of the International Conference on Finite Element Methods in Engineering, Dec. 6-7, 1974, Coimbatore, India; sponsored and organized by Coimbatore Institute of Technology, 1974.

11.19 Proceedings of the Conference on Computational Aspects of the Finite Element Method, Sept. 8-9, 1975, Imperial College, London.

11.20 Robinson, J. (ed.), Proceedings of the World Congress on Finite Element Methods in Structural Mechanics, Oct. 12-17, 1975, Bournemouth, Dorset, England.

11.21 Proceedings of the Workshop on Finite Elements, Rennes, France, May 3-5, 1976; sponsored by the Societe Mathematique de France. Workshop on Finite Elements, Rennes, France, 1976. Universite de Rennes and Institut National des Sciences Appliquees de Rennes, 1976.

11.22 NASTRAN Users' Experiences, NASTRAN Users' Colloquium, Moffett Field, California, Oct. 5-6, 1976, NASA TM-X-3428.

11.23 Bathe, K. J., Oden, J. T., and Wunderlich, W. (eds.), Formulations and Computational Algorithms in Finite Element Analysis, U.S.-Germany Symposium held at Massachusetts Institute of Technology, Cambridge, MA., Aug. 1976, MIT Press, 1977.

11.24 Sixth NASTRAN Users' Colloquium held at Cleveland, Ohio, Oct. 4-6, 1977, NASA CP-2018.

11.25 Pahl, P. J., Stein, E., et al. (eds.), Finite Element Method in Structural Design (in German), Proceedings of the Conference held at Hannover Technical University, April 1978, Verlag Von Wilhelm Ernst and Sohn, 1978.

11.26 Seventh NASTRAN Users' Colloquium held at Huntsville, Alabama, Oct. 4-6, 1978, NASA CP-2062.

11.27 Kardestuncer, H. and Bowley, W. W. (eds.), Proceedings of the Symposium on the Unification of Finite Elements - Finite Differences and Calculus of Variations, University of Connecticut, Storrs, 1978.

11.28 Robinson, J. (ed.), Finite Element Methods in the Commercial Environment, Vols. 1 and 2, Robinson and Associates, Dorset, England, 1978.

11.29 Abel, J. F., Kawai, T., and Shen, S. F. (eds.), Interdisciplinary Finite Element Analysis, Proceedings of the U.S.-Japan Seminar held at Cornell University, Aug. 7-11, 1978; sponsored by U.S. National Science Foundation and the Japan Society for Promotion of Science.

11.30 Eighth NASTRAN User's Colloquium held at Greenbelt, Maryland, Oct. 30-31, 1979, NASA CP-2131.

11.31 Bathe, K. J. (ed.), Nonlinear Finite Element Analysis and ADINA, Proceedings of the ADINA Conferences 1977, 1978 and 1979, Massachusetts Institute of Technology, Cambridge.

11.32 Proceedings of the International Conference on Engineering Applications of the Finite Element Method, May 1979, A.S. Computas, Hovik, Norway.

11.33 Kardestuncer, H. (ed.), Proceedings of the Symposia on the Unification of Finite Elements - Finite Differences and Calculus of Variations, University of Connecticut, Storrs, 1979, 1980 and 1982.

11.34 Kabaila, A. P. and Pulmano, V. A. (eds.), Finite Element Methods in Engineering, Proceedings of the Third International Conference in Australia on Finite Element Methods, held at the University of New South Wales, Sydney, Australia, July 2-6, 1979.

11.35 Pister, K. S., Reynolds, R. R., and William, K. J. (eds.), Proceedings of the International Conference on Finite Elements in Nonlinear Mechanics (FENOMECH '78), Aug. 30-Sept. 1, 1978, Institut fur Statik und Dynamik der Luft- und Raumfahrtkonstruktionen, Universitat Stuttgart, West Germany, 1979.

11.36 Ninth NASTRAN Users' Colloquium, Proceedings of a Colloquium held at John F. Kennedy Space Center, Florida, Oct. 22-23, 1980, NASA; National Technical Information Service, Springfield, Virginia, 1980, NASA CP-2151.

11.37 Brebbia, C. A. (ed.), New Developments in Boundary Element Methods, Proceedings of the Second International Seminar at Southampton University, March 1980.

11.38 Wang, S., Alonso, C., Brebbia, C., Gray, W., and Pinder, G. (eds.), Finite Elements in Water Resources, Proceedings of the Third International Conference held at the University of Mississippi, May 1980, CML Publications, Computational Mechanics Center, Ashurst Lodge, Hampshire, England.

11.39 Wunderlich, W., Stein, E., and Bathe, K. J. (eds.), Nonlinear Finite Element Analysis in Structural Mechanics, Proceedings of the Europe-U.S. Workshop, Ruhr Universitat Bochum, West Germany, July 28-31, 1980, Springer-Verlag, Berlin, 1981.

11.40 Abel, J. F., Kawai, T., and Shen, S. F. (eds.), Interdisciplinary Finite Element Analysis, Proceedings of the U.S.-Japan Seminar held at Cornell University, Aug. 7-11, 1978; published by Cornell University, Ithaca, New York, 1981.

11.41 Hughes, T. J. R., Gartling, D., and Spilker, R. L. (eds.), New Concepts in Finite Element Analysis, presented at the Applied Mechanics Conference, Boulder, Colorado, June 22-24, 1981, ASME AMD Vol. 44, 1981.

11.42 Brebbia, C. A. (ed.), Further Developments in Boundary Element Methods, Proceedings of the Third International Seminar, July 1981, CML Publications, Computational Mechanics Center, Ashurst Lodge, Hampshire, England.

11.43 St. Doltsinis, J., Straub, K., and Willam, K. J. (eds.), FEMOMECH '81, Proceedings of the Second International Conference on Finite Elements in Nonlinear Mechanics, Institut fur Statik und Dynamik der Luft-und Raumfahrtkonstruktionen, Universitat Stuttgart, West Germany, Aug. 25-28, 1981, North Holland Publishing Co., Amsterdam, The Netherlands, 1982.

11.44 Robinson, J. (ed.), New and Future Developments in Commercial Finite Element Methods, Robinson and Associates, Dorset, England, 1981.

11.45 Tenth NASTRAN Users' Colloquium held at New Orleans, Louisiana, May 13-14, 1982, NASA CP-2249.

11.46 Holz, P., Meissner, U., Brebbia, C. A., Pinder, G., and Gary, W. (eds.), Finite Elements in Water Resources, Vol. 4, Proceedings of the Fourth International Conference held in Hanover, June 1982, CML Publications, Computational Mechanics Center, Ashurst Lodge, Hampshire, England.

11.47 Brebbia, C. A. (ed.), Boundary Elements, Proceedings of the Fourth International Conference on Boundary Element Methods held at Southampton University, Sept. 1982, CML Publications, Computational Mechanics Center, Ashurst Lodge, Hampshire, England.

11.48 Proceedings of the Symposium on Finite Element Method, Beijing, China, Gordon and Breach Science Publishers, New York, 1982.

CHAPTER ONE

MATHEMATICAL THEORY OF FINITE ELEMENTS

F. Brezzi
Instituto di Matematica Applicata
Universita di Pavia
I.A.N. of the C. N. R. and Université Pierre
et Marie Curie, Paris

ABSTRACT

In this chapter we briefly describe the mathematical framework in which the finite element methods can be set in order to obtain existence and uniqueness proofs for the approximate problem and to compute error bounds. For simplicity, only time independent problems are treated. We emphasize abstract theorems which have the widest field of applications; nevertheless, each subject is correlated to a model problem and examples of applications can be found in the references. Some theorems in functional analysis are stated without proof, while most of the theorems dealing with the numerical approximation are presented with at least a sketch of the proof.

NOTATION

D = domain in R^n, ∂D = boundary of D,
$x = (x_1, \ldots, x_n)$ = current point in D,
for $\alpha = (\alpha_1, \ldots, \alpha_n)$ multi-integer ($\alpha_i \geq 0$)

$$|\alpha| = \sum_{i=1}^{n} \alpha_i \qquad D^\alpha f = \frac{\partial^{|\alpha|} f}{\partial x_1^{\alpha_1} \cdots \partial x_n^{\alpha_n}} .$$

For m integer ≥ 0

$$|f|_{m,D} = \Big(\sum_{|\alpha|=m} \int_D (D^\alpha f)^2 dx\Big)^{1/2} ,$$

$$\| f \|_{m,D} = \Big(\sum_{\ell=0}^{m} |f|^2_{\ell,D}\Big)^{1/2} ,$$

$$H^m(D) = \{f \mid \| f \|_{m,D} < +\infty\}$$

$H_o^1(D) = \{f \mid f \in H^1(D),\ f = 0 \text{ on } \partial D\}$,

$H^{-1}(D) = (H_o^1(D))' = \text{dual space of } H_o^1(D)$.

For a more precise definition of the spaces $H^s(D)$ we refer to [1] and [2].

VARIATIONAL FORMULATIONS

Let us consider the following model problem. We are given a smooth function $d(x) \geq 0$ in D and an $n \times n$ matrix $A(x)$ whose coefficients $A_{ij}(x)$ are smooth functions in D; we assume that A is symmetric, that is, $A_{ij} = A_{ji}$, and that there exists a constant $\alpha > 0$ such that

$$\sum_{i,j=1}^{n} A_{ij}(x)\, \xi_i \xi_j \geq \alpha \sum_{i=1}^{n} \xi_i^2 \qquad \forall\, x \in D \qquad \forall\, \xi \in R^n. \tag{1}$$

We are also given a function $f(x)$ in $L^2(D)$ and we consider the following problem:

Find $u(x)$ such that:
$$-\text{div}\,(A(x) \text{ grad } u(x)) + d(x)\, u(x) = f(x) \text{ in } D, \tag{2}$$
$u = 0$ on ∂D.

It can be proved that problem (2) has a unique solution $u(x)$ and that $u \in H^2(D)$.

More generally, if D, $A(x)$ and $d(x)$ are smooth enough, then the condition $f \in H^r(D)$, $r \geq 0$, will imply $u \in H^{r+2}(D)$. We refer to [1] for the proof and for more general results. Our purpose is to find different equivalent formulations of problem (2). For this purpose let $v(x)$ be a function in $H_o^1(D)$; multiplying the first equation of (2) by $v(x)$ and integrating over D we get

$$\int_D (-\text{div}(A(x) \text{ grad } u(x))v(x) + d(x)\, u(x)\, v(x))dx = \int_D f(x)\, v(x)dx ,$$

and using Green's formula:

$$\int_D ((A(x) \text{ grad } u(x)) \text{ grad } v(x) + d(x)\, u(x)\, v(x))dx = \int_D f(x)\, v(x)dx.$$

We set for u, v in $H_o^1(\Omega)$:

$$a(u,v) = \int_D ((A(x) \text{ grad } u(x) \text{ grad } v(x) + d(x)\, u(x)\, v(x))dx \tag{3}$$

$$(f,v) = \int_D f(x)\, v(x)dx.$$

It is clear that the solution $u(x)$ of (2) is also a solution of the following variational problem:

Find $u(x)$ in $H_o^1(D)$ such that:
$$a(u,v) = (f,v) \quad \forall\, v \in H_o^1(D). \tag{4}$$

Let us prove that the solution of (4) is unique; we check first that, for any v in $H_o^1(D)$, (1) implies:

$$a(v,v) = \int_D \Big(\sum_{i,j=1}^{n} A_{ij}(x) \frac{\partial v}{\partial x_i} \frac{\partial v}{\partial x_j} + dv^2\Big)dx \geq \alpha \int_D \Big(\sum_{i=1}^{n} \Big(\frac{\partial v}{\partial x_i}\Big)^2 dx = \alpha\, |v|_{1,D}^2 \tag{5}$$

Suppose now that $\bar{u}$ is another solution of (4); then we must have

$$a(u - \bar{u}, v) = 0 \qquad \forall\, v \in H_o^1(D). \tag{6}$$

Taking $v = u - \bar{u}$ in (6) and using (5) we get

$$|u - \bar{u}|^2_{1,D} = 0$$

and, therefore, $u - \bar{u}$ = constant. Since both u and $\bar{u}$ are in $H^1_o(D)$, they both vanish on ∂D, and we can conclude that $u = \bar{u}$.

This kind of result is a particular case of a well-known theorem in functional analysis: the Lax-Milgram theorem. In order to state the theorem we consider first a more general setting: we are given a real Hilbert space V ($H^1_o(D)$ in our example) and a mapping $a: V \times V \to R$ such that:

$$a(\sum_{i=1}^{2} \lambda_i v_i, \sum_{j=1}^{2} \mu_j w_j) = \sum_{i,j=1}^{2} \lambda_i \mu_j \, a(v_i, w_j), \quad \lambda_i \mu_j \in R, \; v_i, w_j \in V \tag{7}$$

(i.e., $a(u,v)$ is <u>bilinear</u>).

$\exists M > 0$ such that (8)

$$a(u,v) \leq M \, \| u \|_V \, \| v \|_V \quad u,v \in V$$

(i.e., $a(u,v)$ is <u>continuous</u>).

$\exists \alpha > 0$ such that (9)

$$a(v,v) \geq \alpha \, \| v \|^2_V \quad v \in V$$

(i.e., $a(u,v)$ is <u>V-elliptic</u>).

Finally, let F be an element of the dual space V', that is a linear mapping from V to R such that $|F(v)| \leq c \, \| v \|_V$ for some constant c independent of v (in our example $F(v) = (f,v)$[(1)]).

<u>THEOREM 1</u> (Lax-Milgram). <u>If V is a real Hilbert space, $a(u,v)$ a bilinear continuous V-elliptic form on $V \times V$ and $F \in V'$, then the problem</u>

Find u in V such that:
$$a(u,v) = F(v) \quad \forall v \in V, \tag{10}$$

<u>has a unique solution.</u>

<u>Proof</u>

For the proof we refer, for instance, to Ref. [3].

We end this section with a third equivalent formulation of problem (2). Let us consider the functional $J : V \to R$ defined by

$$J(v) = \frac{1}{2} a(v,v) - F(v).$$

If u is a solution of (2), or, in the abstract setting, of (10), then we have for all v in $V = H^1_o(D)$

$$\begin{aligned} J(v) - J(u) &= \frac{1}{2} a(v,v) - \frac{1}{2} a(u,u) - F(v-u) \\ &= \frac{1}{2} a(v-u, v-u) + a(u,v) - F(v) + F(u) \\ &= \frac{1}{2} a(v-u, v-u) + F(u) \\ &\geq F(u) = a(u,u) \geq 0 \end{aligned} \tag{11}$$

---

(1) In the following the notation (F,v) will also be used instead of $F(v)$.

and, therefore, u realizes the minimum of J over V. On the other hand, if $J(\bar{u}) = J(u)$ for some $\bar{u}$ in V, then proceeding as in (11) we have

$$0 = J(\bar{u}) - J(u) = \frac{1}{2} a(\bar{u} - u, \bar{u} - u) + a(u, u)$$

and using (5) again, we get $\bar{u} = u$. Therefore, u is the unique solution of the minimum problem:

$$\text{Find } u \text{ in } V \text{ such that:} \quad J(u) \leq J(v) \quad \forall\, v \in V = H_o^1(D) \tag{12}$$

We remark that the above argument can be applied in the abstract setting of the Lax-Milgram theorem provided $a(u,v) = a(v,u)$; that is, when $a(u,v)$ is symmetric (as it is in our model problem).

FINITE ELEMENT SUBSPACES

The finite element method is, from the mathematical point of view, a particular case of the so-called Ritz-Galerkin method. In particular, we can say that whereas the finite difference method is an approximation of the partial differential operator, the finite element method is essentially an approximation of the space (V in our setting) in which the solution is sought. Referring to our model problem in the form of (4) (or (10)), this amounts to choosing a (finite-dimensional) subspace V_h of $V = H_o^1(D)$ and considering the approximate problem:

$$\text{Find } u_h \text{ in } V_h \text{ such that:} \quad a(u_h, v) = F(v) \quad \forall\, v \in V_h. \tag{13}$$

Problem (13) is the general form of a Ritz-Galerkin approximation of (2). Particular choices of the spaces V_h give rise to the finite element method. We shall examine here some of those choices and, in particular, the simplest ones. Assume that for each value of the real parameter h (mesh size) we are given a decomposition of D as finite union of nonoverlapping triangles T, such that

a. Two distinct triangles T_1 and T_2 have a common side, or a common vertex, or empty intersection

b. The maximum side of each triangle has length smaller or equal to h

c. The maximum angle of each triangle is bounded by some $\nu_o < \pi$, independent of h.

For a given value of h, τ_h will indicate the set of all the triangles in which D is subdivided. For each integer $k \geq 1$, we can introduce the spaces

$$V_h^k = \{v \mid v \in C^o(\bar{D}),\ v_{|T} \in P_k \quad \forall\, T \in \tau_h\} \subset H^1(D) \tag{14}$$

where P_k denotes the set of polynomials of degree $\leq k$ in the two variables x_1, x_2. We also set

$$\overset{\circ}{V}{}_h^k = \{v \mid v \in V_h^k,\ v = 0 \ \text{ on } \partial D\} \subset H_o^1(D). \tag{15}$$

We shall also write V_h instead of $\overset{\circ}{V}{}_h^k$ if no confusion is possible. It can be proved that the spaces V_h^k have the following approximation property.

<u>THEOREM 2. There exists a constant</u> $c = c(k,\nu_o)$ <u>such that for any</u> v <u>in</u> $H^m(D)$, <u>$1 \leq m \leq k+1$ and for any</u> $h > 0$ <u>we have</u>

$$\inf_{w \in V_h^k} \| v-w \|_{r,D} \leq c\, h^{m-r} |v|_{m,D} \qquad r = 0,1. \tag{16}$$

<u>Proof</u>

The proof can be found, for instance, in Ref. [4].

Remark
Since the spaces V_h^k are finite-dimensional, the norms are equivalent on the finite element spaces. However, the constants of equivalence depend usually on h. For instance, let us assume that the family of decompositions τ_h is quasi-uniform, in the sense that there exists a constant $\gamma > 0$, independent of h, such that for each h and for each T in τ_h we have

$$\rho(T) \geq \gamma h$$

where $\rho(T)$ is the radius of the inscribed circle of T. Then one can prove (cf. e.g., [4]) that there exists a constant $c = c(k, \nu_o, \gamma)$ such that for each v in V_h^k

$$\| v \|_{1,D} \leq c h^{-1} \| v \|_{0,D} \tag{17}$$

More general inequalities of this type can be found in Ref. [4]. For a much more careful analysis of the approximation properties of the finite element subspaces we refer to A-26, [4], [5], [6] and the references contained therein. More recent results in this direction can be found in [7].

ABSTRACT ERROR ESTIMATES FOR LINEAR ELLIPTIC PROBLEMS

In this section we shall derive abstract bounds for the distance between the solution u of a problem of type (10) and the solution u_h of a general approximation of type (13). The main result is the following.

THEOREM 3. (Céa [8]). Let V be a real Hilbert space, a(u,v) a bilinear continuous V-elliptic form on V x V, and F an element of V'. For any closed subspace V_h of V the approximate problem (13) has a unique solution u_h and the distance between u_h and the solution u of (10) is bounded by:

$$\| u-u_h \|_V \leq \frac{M}{\alpha} \operatorname*{Inf}_{v \in V_h} \| u-v \|_V \tag{18}$$

where M and α are the constants which appear in (8) and (9), respectively.

Proof
Existence and uniqueness of u_h follow from Theorem 1. From (10) and (13) we have

$$a(u-u_h, v_h) = 0 \qquad \forall v_h \in V_h \subset V$$

and, therefore:

$$\alpha \| u-u_h \|_V^2 \leq a(u-u_h, u-u_h) = a(u-u_h, u-v_h) \leq M \| u-u_h \|_V \| u-v_h \|_V$$

For all v_h in V_h. The estimate (18) follows immediately.

Applying the above theorem to the finite element approximation of the model problem (2), we have that choosing $V_h = \overset{o}{V}{}_h^k$ we have the following error bound:

$$\| u-u_h \|_{1,D} \leq c h^k |u|_{k+1,D} \tag{19}$$

with constant c independent of u and h.

A generalization of Céa's theorem is obtained dealing with "nonconforming" or "delinquent" finite elements. This is a particular case of the "external approximations" studied by Céa in [8], and corresponds, in our framework, to a choice of V_h which does not satisfy the relationship $V_h \subset V$. Assume, to fix the ideas, that $V = H_o^1$ as in problem (4), and that V_h is chosen to be the space of piecewise linear functions which are continuous at the midpoint of each internal side. Differentiation across the interelement boundaries being no longer allowed, the bilinear form a(u,v) defined in (3) has to be replaced by

$$a_h(u,v) = \sum_{T \in \tau_h} \{\int_T ((A \text{ grad } u) \text{ grad } v + d\, uv)dx\} \tag{20}$$

It is clear that $a_h(u,v) = a(u,v)$ whenever u and v are smooth enough. In an abstract setting, we should state that we are given a bilinear continuous form $a_h(u,v)$ defined on $V_h \times V_h$ and V_h-elliptic. We could also assume that we are given a normed linear space υ, such that $V_h \subset \upsilon$ and $V \subset \upsilon$, and a bilinear continuous form $\tilde{a}(u,v)$ defined on $\upsilon \times \upsilon$ such that

$$\tilde{a}(u,v) = a(u,v) \qquad u,v \in V ,$$

$$\tilde{a}(u,v) = a_h(u,v) \qquad u,v \in V_h .$$

In our example υ could be chosen as

$$\upsilon = \prod_{T \in \tau_h} H^1(T) \quad ; \quad \| v \|_\upsilon^2 = \sum_{T \in \tau_h} \| v \|_{1,T}^2$$

while $\tilde{a}(u,v)$ can still be defined by the right-hand side of (20). We may also assume that an approximation $f_h \in V_h'$ of f is also given although, in the practical cases, $V_h \subset L^2(D)$ and $f \in L^2(D)$, so that (f,v_h) makes sense for $v_h \in V_h$ and, therefore, the choice $f_h \equiv f$ is allowed. In a general form, the approximate problem is

$$\text{Find } \bar{u}_h \text{ in } V_h \text{ such that} \qquad \tag{21}$$
$$a_h(\bar{u}_h, v_h) = (f_h, v_h) \qquad \forall\, v_h \in V_h.$$

An analogy of Céa's theorem still holds.

THEOREM 4. Suppose that there exists a norm $\| \ \|_h$ on V_h such that:

$$a_h(v_h,v_h) \geq \alpha \| v_h \|_h \qquad \forall\, v_h \in V_h$$

for some $\alpha > 0$ independent of h. Then we have for all v_h in V_h:

$$\| u_h - v_h \|_h \leq c \| v_h - u \|_h + \sup_{w_h \in V_h} (a_h(u,w_h) - (f_h,w_h)) \| w_h \|_h^{-1} . \tag{22}$$

Proof

We refer to [4] for the proof of (22). In our model case it is possible to show that

$$\sup_{w_h \in V_h} (a_h(u,w_h) - (f,w_h)) \| w_h \|_h^{-1} \leq c\, h \| u \|_{2,D}$$

where we took $f_h = f$ and $\| \ \|_h = \| \ \|_\upsilon$. In a general case the evaluation of the second term on the right-hand side of (22) involves some measure of the discontinuity of the functions in V_h across the interelement boundaries. A continuity test called the "patch-test" is often useful for that purpose. We refer to [4], [6] and [9]-[15] for more details on that matter.

MORE GENERAL ABSTRACT APPROXIMATIONS

We have seen that if $a(u,v)$ is symmetric and V-elliptic, problem (10) is equivalent to the minimum problem (12). In that case, the Lax-Milgram theorem provides simultaneously existence and uniqueness for the continuous problem (10) and for the approximate problem (13) assuming only that $V_h \subset V$. However, it may happen that the V-ellipticity of $a(u,v)$ fails but the existence and uniqueness of the solution of (10) still hold true. In fact, it can be shown (see, e.g., [16] and [17]) that for every given f in V', problem (10) has a unique solution if and only if

$$\operatorname*{Inf}_{v \in V} \ \operatorname*{Sup}_{w \in V} \ a(v,w) \ \| w \|^{-1} \ \| v \|^{-1} \geq \alpha_1 \tag{23}$$

$$\operatorname*{Inf}_{w \in V} \ \operatorname*{Sup}_{v \in V} \ a(v,w) \ \| v \|^{-1} \ \| w \|^{-1} \geq \alpha_2 \tag{24}$$

for some positive constants α_1, α_2. Unfortunately, conditions (23) and (24) do not imply the existence of a unique solution for the approximate problem (13) unless some additional condition is required for V_h. A similar situation is also found when a problem of type (10) is approximated by means of two subspaces $V_h \subset V$ and $W_h \subset V$ (of the same dimension) at the same time. To make this more explicit, suppose that we choose V_h first and look for an approximate solution u_h in V_h. If $v_h^{(1)}$, $v_h^{(2)}$, ..., $v_h^{(N+1)}$ is a basis in V_h, u_h will have the form

$$u_h(x) = \sum_{j=1}^{N} U_j \ v_h^{(j)}(x) \tag{25}$$

In order to determine the N unknowns U_1, ..., U_N, we need N linear conditions; for this we choose N linearly independent functions $w_h^{(1)}$, $w_h^{(2)}$, ..., $w_h^{(N)}$ in V (but not necessarily in V_h), and we write

$$a(u_h, w_h^{(i)}) = (f, w_h^{(i)}) \qquad i = 1,2, \ldots, N. \tag{26}$$

If the matrix $S_{ij} = a(v_h^{(j)}, w_h^{(i)})$ is nonsingular, then (26) has a unique solution.
If $W_h \equiv \text{span}\ \{w_h^{(1)}, \ldots, w_h^{(N)}\}$ is different from V_h, then the V-ellipticity of $a(u,v)$ will not be enough to ensure that (26) has a unique solution. Therefore, one cannot use the Céa theorem to get abstract error bounds. In those cases one may use the following general theorem which can also be useful when $W_h = V_h$ but $a(u,v)$ is not V-elliptic.

THEOREM 5. (Babuska [17]). *Let V be a Hilbert space and let $a(u,v)$ be a bilinear continuous form on $V \times V$. Let V_h and W_h be finite dimensional subspaces of V such that $\dim(V_h) = \dim(W_h)$ and*

$$\operatorname*{Inf}_{v \in V_h} \ \operatorname*{Sup}_{w \in W_h} \ \| v \|_V^{-1} \ \| w \|_V^{-1} \ a(v,w) \geq \alpha_1 > 0 \tag{27}$$

then for any given $f \in Y'$ problem

Find u_h in V_h such that:

$$a(u_h, w_h) = (f, w_h) \qquad \forall\, w_h \in W_h \tag{28}$$

has a unique solution. Moreover, if u is a solution of (10) we have

$$\| u-u_h \|_V \leq (1 + M\alpha_1^{-1}) \ \operatorname*{Inf}_{v \in V_h} \ \| u-v \|_V \tag{29}$$

where M is the continuity constant of $a(u,v)$ defined in (8).

Proof

It is easy to check that condition (27) implies that the matrix S_{ij} associated with the linear problem (28) is nonsingular, and therefore, (28) has a unique solution. In order to prove (29) we remark that for any $v \in V_h$ we have

$$\alpha_1 \| v-u_h \|_V \leq \operatorname*{Sup}_{w \in W_h} \ a(v-u_h, w) \ \| w \|_V^{-1}$$

$$= \operatorname*{Sup}_{w \in W_h} \ a(v-u, w) \ \| w \|_V^{-1} \leq M \ \| v-u \|_V$$

so that

$$\| u-u_h \|_V \leq \| u-v \| + \| v-u_h \|_V \leq (1+M\alpha_1^{-1}) \| u-v \|_V \qquad \forall\, v \in V_h$$

and (29) follows.

For a more general form of this theorem we refer to [17]. A very interesting application of the above result to advection diffusion problems can be found in [18], but the range of application is much broader (see, e.g., [19] and [20]).

Remark

It is interesting to point out the different use made in problem (28) of the two spaces V_h and W_h. The space V_h is the one in which the solution u_h is sought; it is often called the space of trial functions. The space W_h, instead, is used in order to require that u_h solve some discrete equations close to the original problem (10); for this reason W_h is also called the space of test functions. In many practical cases the choice $V_h=W_h$ is the simplest and most useful one. Nevertheless, there are cases (see, for instance, [18] and the references contained therein) in which a careful choice of $W_h \neq V_h$ provides, through some upwinding effect, a numerical stability that would be irrevocably lost with the obvious choice $W_h=V_h$.

Another typical case of linear variational problem in which we do not have V-ellipticity is the case of Lagrangian multipliers for linear constraints. Suppose that we are still given a bilinear continuous form $a(u,v)$ on $V \times V$ and an element f in V', and suppose that we must minimize the functional

$$J(v) = \frac{1}{2}\, a(v,v)-(f,v)$$

under the linear constraint $Bv=g$; here B could be, for instance, a linear continuous operator from V into the dual space M' of some Hilbert space M, and g a given element in M'. The Lagrange multipliers technique gives

$$\operatorname*{Inf}_{Bv=g} J(v) = \operatorname*{Inf}_{v\in V} \operatorname*{Sup}_{\varphi\in M} \{J(v) + (Bv-g,\varphi)\} \; ;$$

setting

$$\mathcal{L}(v,\varphi) = \{J(v) + (Bv-g,\varphi)\}$$

the Kuhn-Tucker conditions for $\mathcal{L}(v,\varphi)$ to be stationary at a point $(u,\psi) \in V \times M$ yield

$$\begin{aligned} a(u,v) + (Bv,\psi) &= (f,v) \qquad && \forall\, v\in V \,, \\ (Bu,\varphi) &= (g,\varphi) && \forall\, \varphi\in M \,. \end{aligned} \tag{30}$$

Problem (30) could be considered itself as a variational problem on the product space $V \times M$. However, since we are now dealing with a stationary point which is not a minimum but a saddle point, no ellipticity could be expected. Babuska's technique can be applied to this kind of problem (see, e.g., [19] and [20]). Nevertheless, the following theorem is more specific and allows us to deal with hypotheses directly made on $a(u,v)$ and B.

THEOREM 6. *Let* $K = \mathrm{Ker}(B)$ *be defined as*

$$K = \{v \mid v\in V,\ Bv = 0\}.$$

If $a(u,v)$ *is elliptic on* K *and* B *satisfies*

$$\operatorname*{Inf}_{\varphi\in M} \operatorname*{Sup}_{v\in V} \| v \|_V^{-1} \| \varphi \|_M^{-1} (Bv,\varphi) \geq \beta > 0 \tag{31}$$

then problem (30) *has a unique solution.*

Proof
The proof can be found in Ref. [21].

As far as the discretization is concerned we may suppose that we are given two finite-dimensional subspaces V_h and M_h of V and M, respectively, and we consider the approximate problem:

$$\begin{aligned}&\text{Find } (u_h,\psi_h) \text{ in } V_h \times M_h \text{ such that:}\\ &a(u_h,v_h) + (Bv_h,\psi_h) = (f,v_h) \quad \forall\, v_h \in V_h\,, \\ &(Bu_h,\varphi_h) = (g,\varphi_h) \quad \forall\, \varphi_h \in W_h\,.\end{aligned} \tag{32}$$

We have then the following abstract error estimate.

THEOREM 7. *Let us set*

$$K_h = \{v \mid v \in V_h\,,\ (Bv_h,\varphi_h) = 0 \quad \forall\ \varphi_h \in M_h\}.$$

If a(u,v) *and* B *satisfy*

$$a(v,v) \geq \bar{\alpha}\ \| v \|_V^2 \qquad \forall\ v \in K_h\,, \tag{33}$$

$$\operatorname*{Inf}_{\varphi \in M_h}\ \operatorname*{Sup}_{v \in V_h}\ \| v\|_V^{-1}\ \| \varphi \|_M^{-1} (Bv,\varphi) \geq \bar{\beta} > 0 \tag{34}$$

for some constants $\bar{\alpha}$, $\bar{\beta}$ *independent of* h, *then problem* (32) *has a unique solution and we have the following abstract error bound:*

$$\| u-u_h \|_V + \| \psi-\psi_h \|_M \leq \bar{\gamma}\ (\operatorname*{Inf}_{v \in V_h}\ \| u-v \|_V + \operatorname*{Inf}_{\varphi \in M_h}\ \| \psi-\varphi\|_M)$$

with $\bar{\gamma}$ = *constant independent of* h.

Proof
The proof can be found in [21]. For applications and for more general results we refer, for instance, to [22]-[33] and the references contained therein.

Remark
In the applications, the proof of (34) is usually the main difficulty. However, if the space V_h is made of discontinuous functions (i.e., independently assumed on each element), the condition (34) can be verified element by element or, better, once and for all on the master element; here it becomes a simple algebraic condition on a fixed small matrix, called "compatibility condition" or "rank condition" (see, e.g., [20], [22], [24] and [34]). If V_h is not made of discontinuous functions, one can try the application of the so-called "Fortin's trick": prove (31) first and then look for a linear operator Π_h: $V \to V_h$ such that:

$$\| \Pi_h\ v \|_V \leq c\ \| v \|_V \qquad \forall\ v \in V$$

$$(B(v-\Pi_h\ v),\varphi) = 0\ \forall \varphi \in M_h$$

Then (34) is simply proved since we get:

$$\begin{aligned}&\operatorname*{Inf}_{\varphi \in M_h}\ \operatorname*{Sup}_{v \in V_h}\ \| \varphi \|^{-1}\ \| v \|^{-1}\ (Bv,\varphi)\\ &\geq \operatorname*{Inf}_{\varphi \in M_h}\ \operatorname*{Sup}_{v \in V}\ \frac{1}{c}\ \| \varphi \|^{-1}\ \| \Pi_h\ v \|^{-1}\ (B\ \Pi_h,\ v,\varphi)\\ &\geq \frac{1}{c}\ \operatorname*{Inf}_{\varphi \in M_h}\ \operatorname*{Sup}_{v \in V}\ \| \varphi \|^{-1}\ \| v \|^{-1}\ (Bv,\varphi) \geq \frac{1}{c}\ \beta\ .\end{aligned}$$

For additional details see [35]. Other strategies can be found in [36] and [37].

FURTHER REMARKS ON THE LINEAR CASE AND PRACTICAL ASPECTS

The various abstract theorems stated above provide, at best, error bounds of the type

$$\| u-u_h \|_V \leq c \inf_{v \in V_h} \| u-v \|_V \tag{35}$$

where u and u_h are, respectively, the actual solution and the finite element solution, and V_h is the space of trial functions. Relation (35) has the following meaning: The finite element solution u_h is the best possible approximation one can have (in the norm of V: usually some kind of energy norm) for u among the trial functions V_h (except for the factor c that depends on the problem but not on V_h). In its turn, the right hand side of (35) can be evaluated using the mesh size h, the degree of the trial functions, the regularity of u, and some constant depending on the maximum angle in the decomposition. For instance, if V is a closed subspace of $H^1(D)$ and if $V_h = V_h^k$ as in (14) and (15), we have from (16) that

$$\| u-u_h \|_V \leq c \inf_{v \in V_h} \| u-v \|_V \leq c\, h^k \| u \|_{k+1,D} . \tag{36}$$

In general, from (35) and (36) we have an error estimate of the type

$$\| u-u_h \|_V \leq c\, h^s \| u \|_{s,D} \tag{37}$$

with s depending on the degree of the trial functions and on the regularity of u. An estimate of the type of (37) is often considered as the final goal by mathematicians, but it is not usually very meaningful for engineers, so that some additional remarks are needed.

1. In practical cases, estimates like (37) are in good agreement with the numerical experiments. In fact, in a full logarithmic scale (log h, log $\| u-u_h \|$) the computed errors lie almost on a straight line having a slope close to s (predicted by the theory).

2. When u is not very regular, an estimate like (37) provides a natural bound for the degree of polynomials to be used as trial functions. For instance, if the solution is expected to have "reasonable" values together with its derivatives up to the order 3, but with "wild" fourth derivatives, then quadratic polynomials may be used but the use of cubics will, in general, be a waste of effort (and money).

3. Inequalities such as (37) refer to the exact solution u_h of the discretized problem. Simple considerations in linear algebra (and numerical experiments) show that the computed solution u_h^* can move away from u_h when the total number of unknowns becomes too large. Therefore, for a large number of unknowns some procedure to check a posteriori the error bound in the solution of the linear system is worthwhile. For some recent and very interesting results in this field see [38]. See also Chapters 6 and 9 of this book.

4. Do not be too worried if the mesh size h is several miles. One can always use the light-year as unit! More seriously: everything depends on the expected behavior of the exact solution u; if it does not oscillate within several steps of length h, the approximate solution will usually be very good no matter how big h is. A change of scale and some calculus will show this very clearly. The matter is obviously much more delicate in nonlinear problems.

5. If one is interested in the behavior of the error with respect to the number of degrees of freedom, an estimate such as (37) shows that, for a regular u, polynomials of high degree are worth considering. Of course, their implementation may be more complicated, and the stiffness matrix may become ill-conditioned. Still, in many cases different directions as the "P-version" of

finite elements (see, e.g., [39]) or spectral methods (see, e.g., [40] and [41]) have considerable practical interest.

6. It is often useful to couple finite element methods with other procedures, such as boundary integrals (see Chapter 15 of this book). In such cases the abstract theorems quoted above do not apply. Error bounds for the coupling of finite elements and boundary integrals can be found in [42] and [43].

7. As stated, usually the norm $\| \ \|_V$ which appears in (37) is an "energy norm", that is, in mathematical terms, some kind of H^1 norm. It is often interesting to have also error estimates in some other norms, like the L^2 - norm, the L^∞-norm, or the $W^{1,\infty}$ norm. In the case of L^2 norm, one can apply the following argument, called "Aubin-Nitsche trick". Let us consider, for simplicity, the model problem (2) and its approximation (13). It is easy to see that the auxiliary problem

$$\begin{aligned}&\text{Find } \psi \in V \text{ such that}\\ &a(\psi,v) = (u-u_h,v) \qquad \forall\, v \in V\end{aligned}$$

has a unique solution ψ and that

$$\| \psi \|_{H^2(D)} \leq c \; \| u-u_h \|_{L^2(D)} \quad .$$

Therefore, one has for every ψ_h in V_h

$$\begin{aligned}\| u-u_h \|^2_{L^2(D)} &= (u-u_h,\, u-u_h) = a(u-u_h,\psi)\\ &= a(u-u_h,\, \psi-\psi_h) \leq M \, \| u-u_h \|_V \;\; \| \psi-\psi_h \|_V \quad ,\end{aligned}$$

so that

$$\| u-u_h \|^2_{L^2(D)} \leq c \; \| u-u_h \|_V \inf_{\psi_h \in V_h} \| \psi-\psi_h \|_V$$

If the space V_h is such that

$$\inf_{\psi_h \in V_h} \| \psi-\psi_h \|_V \leq c\; h \; \| \psi \|_{H^2(D)}$$

(as it is given by (16) for $V_h = V_h^k$, $k \geq 1$), then we get

$$\| u-u_h \|_{L^2(D)} \leq c\; h \; \| u-u_h \|_V$$

which is again of optimal type. The situation is entirely different in the case of L^∞ estimates, which are much more complicated. We refer to [44], [45] and, in particular, to [46] for this type of result.

8. In our model problem we assumed homogeneous Dirichlet boundary conditions. For more general boundary conditions we refer to [4], [5] and [6]. We also assumed that D was a polygon, otherwise, isoparametric finite elements have to be used in order to get optimal error bounds. As essential references see [4] and [47].

9. Fourth-order problems do not, in general, bring major additional difficulties from the point of view of basic ideas (except for the lack of a maximum principle). On the other hand, it usually gives rise to a number of little technical difficulties. It is especially on that kind of problem that such variants as nonconforming or non-standard finite elements can be helpful. See, for instance, [22] and [26] and the references contained therein.

NONLINEAR PROBLEMS

As we have seen, the approximation of linear elliptic problems can be carried out by rather general instruments. This is not the case for nonlinear problems which essentially lack, up to now, a general theory from both theoretical and numerical point of view. We shall deal here with three particular cases of nonlinear problems; variational inequalities, monotone operators, and compact perturbations. Within each case, some particular "model problem" will be chosen.

Variational Inequalities

Let us consider again the function

$$J(v) = \frac{1}{2} a(v,v) - (f,v)$$

with $a(u,v)$, for instance, given by (3). Assume that we are given a function ψ that is smooth in D and such that $\psi \leq 0$ on ∂D. We set

$$K = \{v \mid v \in H_0^1(D), \quad v \geq \psi \quad \text{a.e. in } D\} \tag{38}$$

We note that condition $\psi \leq 0$ on ∂D implies that K is non-empty. K is, moreover, a closed convex subset of $H_0^1(D)$. As a model problem we shall take the following one:

$$\begin{aligned} &\text{Find } u \in K \text{ such that:} \\ &J(u) \leq J(v) \qquad \forall\, v \in K. \end{aligned} \tag{39}$$

A possible physical interpretation of (39) is almost evident; we minimize some kind of potential energy under unilateral constraints. Problems of the form (39) have been studied intensively in recent years from the mathematical point of view (see Refs. [48], [49], and [50]). We have seen that when $K = H_0^1(D) = V$ the problem of minimizing J is equivalent to the variational equation (4). The situation is quite similar in this case, although variational inequalities have to be considered instead of variational equations.

PROPOSITION. The solution u of (39) is the unique solution of the following variational inequality:

$$\begin{aligned} &\text{Find } u \in K \text{ such that} \\ &a(u,v-u) \geq (f,v-u) \qquad \forall\, v \in K \end{aligned} \tag{40}$$

Proof

Since K is convex, for any $v \in K$ and $\lambda \in [0, 1]$ the function $w(\lambda) = \lambda v + (1-\lambda)u$ belongs to K. From (39), $J(w(o)) = J(u) \leq J(w(\lambda))$ for $\lambda \in [0, 1]$. Hence, the function $F(\lambda):[0, 1] \to R$ defined by $F(\lambda) = J(w(\lambda))$ has a minimum for $\lambda = 0$ and, therefore, $F'(o) \geq 0$. A simple computation shows that $F'(0)=a(u,v-u)-(f,v-u)$ and, therefore, u is a solution of (40). In order to show the uniqueness, suppose that (40) has another solution $\bar{u}$.

Then we must have

$$a(\bar{u}, u-\bar{u}) \geq (f, u-\bar{u})$$

and letting $v = \bar{u}$ in (40)

$$a(u,\bar{u}-u) \geq (f,\bar{u}-u)$$

we have

$$a(\bar{u}-u,u-\bar{u}) \geq 0$$

and from (5) we get $u = \bar{u}$.

As in the case of linear problems, existence and uniqueness of the solution of a problem such as (40) can be obtained by means of a general abstract theorem.

THEOREM 8. (Lions-Stampacchia) Let V be a real Hilbert space, a(u,v) a bilinear continuous form on V x V which is V-elliptic, and K be a closed convex subset of V. Then for any given f in V' the problem:

$$\text{Find } u \in K \text{ such that} \quad a(u,v-u) \geq (f,v-u) \quad \forall\, v \in K \tag{41}$$

has a unique solution.

Proof
For the proof and more details we refer to Ref. [51].

The following abstract approximation theorem can be considered as the natural extension of Céa's theorem.

THEOREM 9. ([52]) Using the hypotheses of Theorem 8, assume that we are given a finite-dimensional subspace $V_h \subset V$ and a closed convex subset K_h in V_h. Let $u_h \in K_h$ be the unique solution of

$$a(u_h,v-u_h) \geq (f,v-u_h) \quad \forall\, v \in K_h \; ; \tag{42}$$

then we have for each u in V and for each v_h in K_h

$$\| u-u_h \|_V^2 \leq \frac{1}{\alpha} (M \| u-u_h \|_V \; \| u-v_h \|_V + a(u,v_h-u_h) - (f,v_h-u_h)) \tag{43}$$

Proof
We have

$$\alpha \| u-u_h \|^2 \leq a(u-u_h,u-u_h) = a(u-u_h,u-v_h) + a(u-u_h,v_h-u_h)$$

$$\leq M \| u-u_h \| \; \| u-v_h \| + a(u,v_h-u_h) - (f,v_h-u_h).$$

and Eq. (43) follows.

Inequality (43) is, perhaps, not very eloquent, but, it is, in the writer's opinion, the best starting point for deriving error estimates in the applications. As an example, let us go back to our model problem (39) or, equivalently, to its variational formulation (40). Theorem 7 tells us that there exists a unique solution u to our problem. Moreover, it can be shown ([49]) that if $\psi \in H^2(D)$, then u also belongs to $H^2(D)$, and, moreover, we have the "complementarity relationships":

$$\begin{aligned} &\mathcal{A}u \geq f && \text{a.e. in } D, \\ &u \geq \psi && \text{in } D, \\ &(\mathcal{A}u-f)(u-\psi) = 0 && \text{a.e. in } D \end{aligned} \tag{44}$$

where $\mathcal{A}u = -\text{div}(A(x) \text{ grad } u) + d(x)u$ as in (2). Let now $V_h = \overset{o}{V}{}_h^1$ be the set of continuous, piecewise linear, trial functions and consider the approximate convex

$$K_h = \{v | v \in V_h \; , \quad v \geq \psi \text{ at the nodes}\}$$

(nodes = vertices of the triangulation). In general, $K_h \not\subset K$. Since K_h is a closed convex subset of V_h, Theorem 7 yields the existence and uniqueness to the solution of (42) in our concrete situation. Use (43) in order to establish error bounds. To this end, we define first the piecewise linear interpolants u^I, ψ^I of u and ψ, respectively, and we note that obviously $u^I \in K_h$ so that we can take $u^I = v_h$ in (43) and get

$$\| u-u_h \|_V^2 \leq \frac{M}{\alpha} c \; h \; \| u \|_{2,D} \; \| u-u_h \|_V + \frac{1}{\alpha} (\mathcal{A}u-f,u^I-u_h) \tag{45}$$

From relationships (44) we have

$$(Au-f,u^I-u_h) = (Au-f,u^I-u + u-\psi + \psi-\psi^I + \psi^I-u_h)$$

$$= (Au-f,u^I-u + \psi-\psi^I) + (Au-f,\psi^I-u_h)$$

Since $u_h \in K_h$, $u_h \geq \psi^I$. From (44) we have:

$$(Au-f,\psi^I-u_h) \leq 0$$

so that

$$(Au-f,u^I-u_h) \leq (Au-f,(u-\psi)^I - (u-\psi)) \leq c\ h\ (\| u \|_{2,D} + \| \psi \|_{2,D})$$

Finally, (45) gives

$$\| u-u_h \|_V \leq c\ h\ (\| u \|_{2,D} + \| \psi \|_{2,D})$$

which is the original estimate of Falk [53] but with the simpler proof of [52]. The advantage of the abstract estimate (43) over other similar ones ([4] and [53]) is that (43) allows the use of the complementarity relations (44), which, as here, lead to a considerable simplification of the proof. Also note that, in general, the solution of an obstacle problem of the type of Eqs. (38) and (39) is not very smooth. For very smooth data one can prove that the second derivatives of u are bounded ([54]) but they will never be continuous. Therefore, the use of a piecewise cubic approximation is usually worthless. For piecewise quadratics, the following error bound has been proved:

$$\| u-u_h \|_V \leq c(\varepsilon)\ h^{3/2-\varepsilon} \quad \text{for all } \varepsilon > 0 ;$$

(see [51]). Additional results on the approximation of variational inequalities can be found in Refs. [55]-[59] and in the references contained therein.

Remark
The numerical solution of complementarity systems similar to Eq. (42) has been studied widely in recent years. Essential references can be found in Refs. [55], [59], and [60].

Variational Inequalities and Free Boundary Problems

A revolutionary point of view has developed during the last ten years in connection with obstacle problems similar to Eqs. (38) and (39). In order to explain this, suppose, for simplicity, that in our model problem (38) and (39) we have $\psi = 0$ and let us define the set

$$D_N = \{x | x \in D, \quad u(x) > \psi(x) \equiv 0\} \tag{46}$$

Since the solution u is a priori unknown, the set D_N itself will be a priori unknown. Formulae (44) yield

$$Au = f \quad \text{in } D_N \tag{47}$$

$$u = 0 \quad \text{on } \partial D_N \tag{48}$$

and since u is C^1 in D and $u \equiv 0$ in $D-D_N$, we must have

$$\frac{\partial u}{\partial n} = 0 \quad \text{on } \partial D_N \cap D \tag{49}$$

The subdomain D_N being itself unknown, problem (47), (48) and (49) may be regarded as a classical free boundary problem. Needless to say, the real practical interest goes the opposite direction; for a given free boundary problem (for instance,

(47), (48) and (49)), the best thing to do is to transform it, whenever it is possible, into a variational inequality of type (38) and (39) on the fixed domain D, which can then be solved without difficulty (while the problem in the form (47)-(49) is much more difficult to deal with). This passage from a free boundary problem back to a variational inequality on a fixed domain is quite simple in the particular case (47)-(49). Unfortunately, this is not always the case, although some special tricks such as the "Baiocchi's transform" (cf. e.g., [50], [61], and [62]) can be helpful in achieving the task. This way of dealing with free boundary problems allows a very elegant and effective treatment of various problems, such as filtration of fluids through porous media, Stefan's problem on ice melting, and a number of others. In particular, from the numerical point of view, the advantage of solving a free boundary problem on a fixed domain is impressive saving of computer time (and money). The recent literature on the subject is vast; we refer to [50], [59] and [63] for an extensive list of references.

Remark

A generalization of problems similar to (41) can be obtained allowing a dependence of the convex K on the solution u itself. Suppose that we are given a map $v \to K(v)$ from V into the set of closed convex subsets of V. With the hypotheses of Theorem 8, one can consider the problem:

$$\begin{aligned}&\text{Find } u \in V \text{ such that:}\\ &u \in K(u),\\ &a(u,v-u) \geq (f,v-u) \qquad \forall v \in K(u)\end{aligned} \tag{50}$$

This kind of problem is much more difficult than (41) from both theoretical and numerical points of view. We refer to [64] for mathematical results, examples of applications, and references. The study of error bounds for the finite element approximation of problems like (50) has been carried out only for isolated cases; see, e.g., [65], [66] and [67].

Nonlinear Equations with Monotone Operators

An operator B from a Hilbert space V into its dual V' is said to be monotone if, for any u,v in V, we have $(B(u)-B(v),u-v) > 0$. It is easy to see that if V is a space of functions $D \to R$ and if $B(v) = f(v)$ for some function $f : R \to R$, then B is monotone if the function f is nondecreasing. The following extension of the Lax-Milgram theorem can be proved (cf., e.g., [68] and [69] for a much more general setting).

THEOREM 10. *Let V be a Hilbert space, a(u,v) a bilinear continuous form on V x V which is V-elliptic and let B be a continuous monotone operator from V into V'. Then the problem:*

$$\begin{aligned}&\text{Find } u \in V \text{ such that}\\ &a(u,v) + (B(u),v) = 0 \qquad \forall v \in V\end{aligned} \tag{51}$$

has a unique solution.

As a model problem we can take:

$$\begin{aligned}&Au + u^3 - \lambda u = f \qquad \text{in } D \subset R^2\\ &u = 0 \qquad \text{on } \partial D\end{aligned} \tag{52}$$

with $Au = -\mathrm{div}(A(x)\mathrm{grad}\ u) + d(x)u$ as in (2), $f \in L^2(D)$ and $\lambda \leq 0$. It is easy to check that the operator $B : v \to v^3 - \lambda v - f$ is monotone for $\lambda \leq 0$; it is also continuous from $V = H_0^1(D)$ into $L^2(D)$ and, therefore, into V'. Therefore, Theorem 10 can be applied and we prove the existence and uniqueness of the solution of (52).

For a given finite dimensional subspace V_h of V, we may now consider the discretized problem:

Find $u_h \in V_h$ such that

$$a(u_h,v) + (u_h^3-\lambda u_h-f,v) = 0 \qquad \forall\, v \in V_h \tag{53}$$

Since V_h is itself a Hilbert space, Theorem 10 also provides existence and uniqueness for the solution u_h of (53). In order to get error bounds we can use the following abstract theorem.

THEOREM 11. _With the hypotheses of Theorem 10, assume that we are given a finite dimensional subspace_ V_h _of_ V. _Then the discretized problem_

Find $u_h \in V_h$ such that

$$a(u_h,v) + (B(u_h),v) = 0 \qquad \forall\, v \in V_h \tag{54}$$

has a unique solution and we have for all $v_h \in V_h$:

$$\| u-u_h \|_V^2 \le c \; \| u-u_h \|_V \; \| u-v_h \|_V + (B(u_h)-B(u),v_h-u); \tag{55}$$

$$\| u-u_h \|_V^2 \le c \; \| u-u_h \|_V \; \| u-v_h \|_V + (B(v_h)-B(u),v_h-u_h) \tag{56}$$

for some constant c _independent of_ V_h.

Proof

We have

$$\alpha \; \| u-u_h \|_V^2 \le a(u-u_h,u-u_h) = a(u-u_h,u-v_h) + a(u-u_h,v_h-u_h) \tag{57}$$

$$\begin{aligned} a(u-u_h,v_h-u_h) &= (B(u_h)-B(u),v_h-u_h) = (B(u_h)-B(u),v_h-u) \\ &+ (B(u_h)-B(u),u-u_h) \le (B(u_h)-B(u),v_h-u); \end{aligned} \tag{58}$$

$$\begin{aligned} a(u-u_h,v_h-u_h) &= (B(u_h)-B(u),v_h-u_h) = (B(u_h)-B(u),v_h-u) \\ &+ (B(u_h)-B(u),u-u_h) \le (B(u_h)-B(u),v_h-u) \end{aligned} \tag{59}$$

Finally, (57) and (58) give (55) while (57) and (59) give (56).

As an example, let us consider problem (53) with a piecewise linear approximation. It is clear that the continuous solution u of (52) belongs to $H^2(D)$. Therefore, we can take $v_h = u^I$ (piecewise linear interpolation of u) in (56) and have

$$\| u-u_h \|_V^2 \le c \; (h \; \| u \|_{2,D} + \| B(u^I)-B(u) \|_{0,D}) \; \| u-u_h \|_V$$

However,

$$\| B(u^I)-B(u) \|_{0,D} \le \| u^I-u \|_{0,D} \; \| (u^I)^2 + u^I u + u^2-\lambda \|_{0,D} \le c \; h^2 \; \| u \|_{2,D} \tag{60}$$

so that

$$\| u-u_h \|_V \le c \; h \; \| u \|_{2,D}$$

As a matter of fact, the abstract estimate (55) could be used as well. Note that $B(u_h)$ is bounded in $L^2(D)$, and then taking $v_h = u^I$ in (55) again:

$$\begin{aligned} \| u-u_h \|_V^2 &\le c \; h \; \| u-u_h \|_V \; \| u \|_{2,D} + (\| B(u) \|_{0,D} \\ &+ \| B(u_h) \|_{0,D}) \cdot c \; h^2 \; \| u \|_{2,D} \end{aligned}$$

which again leads to (60).

In general, either (55) or (56) will be easier to deal with depending on the particular problem. More general results and applications can be found in Refs. [52] and [70]. For additional references see also Refs. [4] and [55].

Compact Perturbations

Let us consider again problem (52) as a model problem, but suppose now $\lambda > 0$; the operator $B(v) = v^3-\lambda v-f$ is no longer monotone and, hence, Theorem 10 does not apply. In fact, it can be proved (see Ref. [71]) that taking $f = 0$ for simplicity, for some values of $\lambda > 0$ at least four different nonzero solutions coexist with the trivial one $u = 0$.

A similar situation often occurs in several problems as, for instance, stationary problems in hydraulics, in nonlinear mechanics, in chemistry, and so on. As an abstract formalism to deal with this kind of problem we shall use the following. We are given:

a. a real Hilbert space V;

b. a continuous bilinear form $a(u,v)$ from $V \times V$ into R, which is V-elliptic;

c. an operator $B(\lambda,u)$ from $R \times V$ into a Hilbert space $W \subset V'$.

We shall also assume that:

d. the injection of W in V' is compact (that is, every sequence g_n which is bounded in W contains a subsequence which converges strongly in V');

e. the mapping $(\lambda,u) \to B(\lambda,u)$ is r times continuously differentiable ($r \geq 4$) and the rth derivative $D^rB(\lambda,u)$ is bounded on the bounded subsets of $R \times V$.

Regarding our model problem it is easy to check that from Sobolev imbedding theorems (see, e.g., [21]), if a function v belongs to $H^1(D)$ $(D \subset R^2)$, then $v \in L^p(D)$ for every $p < +\infty$. Hence, we can take, for instance, $W = L^2(D)$ in (63). Hypothesis (e) is also satisfied with $r = \infty$. Finally, it is well known that, if D is a bounded domain, the injection of $H^{\alpha+\beta}(D)$ into $H^{\alpha}(D)$ is compact for any $\alpha \in R$ and $\beta > 0$ (see [1] and [2], for instance). Since in our case $W = L^2(D) = H^0(D) \subset H^{-1}(D) = (H^1_0(D))' = V'$, hypothesis (d) also holds true. We point out that the present abstract setting (a-e) also apply to other more complicated (and more interesting) problems, like the two-dimensional stationary Navier-Stokes equations or the von Karman equations for plates (although, in those cases, a little bit more of functional analysis is needed; see [29], [72], and [73] for such proofs).

In the abstract setting of (a) to (e) we consider the abstract problem:

$$\begin{aligned}&\text{Find } (\lambda,u) \text{ in } R \times V \text{ such that}\\ &a(u,v) + (B(\lambda,u)v) = 0 \qquad \forall\, v \in V\end{aligned} \tag{61}$$

which can also be written:

$$F(\lambda,u) \equiv u+T\,B(\lambda,u) = 0 \tag{62}$$

where $T \in \mathcal{L}(V',V)$ is defined in the following way: for each $p \in V'$, we define as Tp the unique solution of the problem:

$$\begin{aligned}&Tp \in V,\\ &a(Tp,v) = (p,v) \qquad \text{for all } v \in V\end{aligned} \tag{63}$$

In our model problem $T = A^{-1}$.

The operator TB is compact from $R \times V$ into V, so that, for fixed λ, the operator $I + TB$ can be regarded as a compact perturbation of the identity (which justifies the title of the subheading).

The abstract setting does not guarantee that problem (61) has a solution and, whenever a solution exists, uniqueness cannot be expected in the general case. Hence, we shall assume here that a solution exists, and see how such solution can be approximated by means of finite element discretization.

For a given finite-dimensional subspace $V_h \subset V$ we may introduce the discretized problem:

$$\text{Find } (\lambda,u_h) \text{ in } R \times V_h \text{ such that:} \qquad a(u_h,v_h) + (B(\lambda,u_h)v_h) = 0 \qquad \forall\, v \in V_h \tag{64}$$

or equivalently

$$F_h(\lambda,u_h) \equiv u_h + T_h\, B(\lambda,u_h) = 0 \tag{65}$$

with T_h: $p \in V' \to T_h\, p \in V_h$ defined as the unique solution of

$$T_h\, p \in V_h \qquad a(T_h\, p,v_h) = (p,v_h) \qquad \forall\, v_h \in V_h \tag{66}$$

We recall now the notion of Fréchet derivative of a mapping G: $V_1 \to V_2$ (V_i being Banach spaces) at a point $\bar{x} \in V_1$. The Fréchet derivative of G at $\bar{x}$ is defined (if it exists) as the unique linear continuous operator $DG(\bar{x})$ from V_1 into V_2 such that:

$$\| G(\bar{x}+x) - G(\bar{x}) - DG(\bar{x})\, x \|_{V_2} \le o(\| x \|_{V_1}) \quad \text{for all } x \in V_1. \tag{67}$$

If the space V_1 is a product space, as in our case, $V_1 = R \times V$, one can also take partial derivatives with respect to one of the variables, "freezing" all other variables as is usually done in elementary calculus. For instance, in our model case $B(\lambda,u) = u^3-\lambda u + f$, it is easy to see that the total and partial Fréchet derivatives of B at $\bar{\lambda},\bar{u}$ are:

$$DB(\bar{\lambda},\bar{u}) \;:\; (\lambda,u) \to 3\bar{u}^2\cdot u-\lambda\bar{u}-\bar{\lambda}u \qquad (\in \mathcal{L}(R \times V,V))$$

$$D_uB(\bar{\lambda},\bar{u}) \;:\; u \to 3\bar{u}^2\cdot u-\bar{\lambda}u \qquad (\in \mathcal{L}(V,V))$$

$$D_\lambda B(\bar{\lambda},\bar{u}) \;:\; \lambda \to -\lambda\bar{u} \qquad (\in \mathcal{L}(R,V))$$

For a short and elementary but very clear discussion of Fréchet derivatives and other tools that we shall use in the sequel, we refer to Ref. [74].

The following abstract lemma plays a crucial role in the study of finite element approximation of problems of the type (62). Assume that X, Y and Z are real Banach spaces and $\phi(x,y)$ is a C^r mapping ($r \ge 2$) from $X \times Y$ into Z, with rth derivatives bounded on all bounded subsets of $X \times Y$, and assume that (x_o,y_o) $(x_o,y_o) \in X \times Y$ is a solution of $\phi(x_o,y_o) = 0$, such that $D_y\, \phi(x_o,y_o)$ is an isomorphism from Y onto Z. Then we can apply the implicit function theorem (see, e.g., [74], [75] or [76] for more details) and get the existence of a neighborhood U of x_o and a mapping $g : U \to Y$ r times continuously differentiable such that

$$\Phi(x,g(x)) = 0 \qquad \text{identically in U} \tag{68}$$

Suppose now that we are given a sequence Φ_h of C^r mappings from $X \times Y$ into Z such that Φ_h converges uniformly to Φ on all the bounded subsets of $U \times Y$ together with all the derivatives up to the order r. Then we have the following results:

LEMMA 1. With the above hypotheses, there exists $h_o > 0$ and for all $h \le h_o$ a C^r mapping g_h from U into Y such that:

$$\Phi_h(x,g_h(x)) = 0 \qquad \text{identically in U;} \tag{69}$$

moreover, we have:

$$\| g(x)-g_h(x) \|_Y \le c\, \| \Phi_h(x,g(x)) \|_Z \qquad x \in U \tag{70}$$

with c *constant independent of* x *and* h.

Proof
For the proof we refer to Refs. [73] and [77].

Remark
In fact, an estimate more precise than (70) can be proved:

$$\| D^m(g(x)-g_h(x)) \|_{\mathscr{L}_m(X,Y)} \leq c \sum_{\ell=0}^{m} \| D^\ell (\phi_h(x,g(x))) \|_{\mathscr{L}_\ell(X,Z)} \tag{71}$$

for $m = 0, 1, \ldots, r-1$.

Moreover, if $x = x(t)$, $|t| \leq t_o$ is a curve in U with parameter t, we can prove

$$\left\| \frac{d^m}{dt^m} (g(x(t))-g_h(x(t))) \right\|_{\mathscr{L}_m(R,Y)} \leq c \sum_{\ell=0}^{m} \left\| \frac{d^\ell}{dt^\ell} \phi_h(x(t),g(x(t))) \right\|_{\mathscr{L}_\ell(R,Z)} . \tag{72}$$

A direct application of Lemma 1 to problems (62) and (65) gives the following theorem.

THEOREM 12. *Assume that for each* v *in* V *we have*

$$\lim_{h \to 0} \ \operatorname{Inf}_{v_h \in V_h} \| v-v_h \|_V = 0 \tag{73}$$

Then if (λ_o,u_o) *is a solution of* (62) *such that* $D_u F(\lambda_o,u_o)$ *is an isomorphism of* V *onto itself, there exist a neighborhood* $N = N_\lambda \times N_u$ *of* (λ_o,u_o) *and an* $h_o > 0$ *such that both problems* (62) *and* (65) *for* $h \leq h_o$ *have a unique branch of solutions* $u = u(\lambda)$ *and* $u_h = u_h(\lambda)$, *respectively, in* N, *i.e.,*

$$F(\lambda,u(\lambda)) \equiv 0 \quad ; \quad F_h(\lambda,u_h(\lambda)) = 0 \qquad \lambda \in N_\lambda$$

moreover we have:

$$\| u_h(\lambda)-u(\lambda) \|_V \leq c \operatorname{Inf}_{v \in V_h} \| u(\lambda)-v \|_V \qquad \lambda \in N_\lambda \tag{74}$$

with c *constant independent of* λ *and* h.

Proof (sketch)
We remark first that the mapping F_h defined in (65) can be considered as a mapping from R x V (instead of R x V_h) into V. As a matter of fact, problem (65) itself can be considered in the whole V for, if $\tilde{u}$ is a solution of $F_h(\lambda,\tilde{u}) = 0$, then $\tilde{u} = -T_h B(\lambda,\tilde{u})$ and, therefore, $u \in V_h$ automatically. Lemma 1 then gives

$$\begin{aligned} \| u_h(\lambda)-u(\lambda) \|_V &\leq c \| F_h(\lambda,u(\lambda)) \|_V = c \| F_h(\lambda,u(\lambda))-F(\lambda,u(\lambda)) \|_V \\ &= c \| (T_h-T) B(\lambda,u(\lambda)) \|_V \end{aligned} \tag{75}$$

On the other hand, the abstract estimate (18) for linear problems applied to (63) and (66) with $p = B(\lambda,u(\lambda))$ gives

$$\| (T_h-T) B(\lambda,u(\lambda)) \|_V \leq \frac{M}{\alpha} \operatorname{Inf}_{v \in V_h} \| TB(\lambda,u(\lambda))-v \|_V \tag{76}$$

and since $TB(\lambda,u(\lambda)) = -u(\lambda)$ we have (74) from (75) and (76). For the details of the proof we refer to [73] and [77].

If, for instance, we have $V = H^1(D)$ or $V = H^1_o(D)$ (as in our model problem) and in (64) we choose $V_h = V^k_h$, or $V_h = \overset{o}{V}{}^k_h$, respectively, (see definitions (14) and (15)), then (73) is easily satisfied and the estimate (74) becomes

$$\| u_h(\lambda)-u(\lambda) \|_V \leq c\, h^k \, \| u(\lambda) \|_{k+1,D} \quad \lambda \in N_\lambda, \tag{77}$$

that is, an optimal error bound as in the linear case. We also remark that using (71) we could prove optimal error bounds for the distance between the derivatives $\frac{du_h}{d\lambda}$ and $\frac{du}{d\lambda}$.

Considerable research has been devoted in recent years to the study of the behavior of the solutions of (62) and (65) in a neighborhood of a critical point (λ_o,u_o), that is, a point (λ_o,u_o) which is a solution of (62) but such that $D_u(\lambda_o,u_o)$ is not an isomorphism of V onto V. Such points are of great practical interest since it is there that solutions may appear or disappear or change in stability. For a theoretical study we refer to Refs. [75], [78], [79] and the references contained therein. From the numerical point of view we quote among the essential references [77], [80]-[83] and [84]. In particular, in [77] and [84] optimal error bounds are obtained in the general framework (a to e) for the particular cases of "normal limit points" and "simple bifurcation points." A normal limit point is a point (λ_o,u_o) where the (multivalued) application $\lambda \to u(\lambda)$ implicitly defined by (62) has a tangent orthogonal to the λ axis. With some minor further assumptions we may have that for $\lambda > \lambda_o$ (resp. $\lambda < \lambda_o$) there are two different solutions $u_1(\lambda)$ and $u_2(\lambda)$ close to u_o while for $\lambda < \lambda_o$ (resp. $\lambda > \lambda_o$) there are no solutions close to u_o. In such cases it is proved in [77] that the approximate problem (65) shows a similar behavior and is possible to parametrize the branches of continuous and discrete solutions in such a way that an optimal error bound in the form of (74) still holds. Moreover, the branch of approximate solutions also shows a critical point (λ_h^c,u_h^c) and the distance $\lambda_h^c-\lambda_o$ can be estimated with a "double order of convergence," that is, for example, in the case of (77) we have

$$|\lambda_h^c-\lambda_o| \leq c\, h^{2k} \ ;$$

we refer to [77] for all the details.

On the other hand, a simple bifurcation point is a point (λ_o,u_o) in which two different branches of solutions of (62) intersect transversely. If one of the two branches is the trivial one $(\lambda,0)$, then the approximate problem (65) also has a simple bifurcation point $(\lambda_h^o,0)$, and the distance $\lambda_h^o-\lambda_o$ has a double order of convergence; moreover, the nontrivial branches of continuous and approximate solutions can be parametrized in such a way that an optimal error bound of type (74) still holds. In a general case, that is, for instance, for the so-called secondary bifurcation, the set of solutions of the approximate problem is C^r-diffeomorphic to a hyperbola (usually nondegenerate) but the distance between the set φ of solutions of (62) in a neighborhood N of (λ_o,u_o) and the set φ_h of solutions of (65) in N is still bounded with the optimal order. For instance, in the case of (52) we have

$$\mathcal{D}(\varphi \ , \ \varphi_h) \leq c\, h^k$$

where the distance $\mathcal{D}$ between two sets R,S is defined by

$$\mathcal{D}(R,S) = \max \left(\sup_{x\in R} \ \inf_{y\in S} \ \| x-y \|, \ \sup_{y\in S} \ \inf_{x\in R} \ \| y-x \|\right) .$$

For a more detailed analysis we refer to Ref. [84]. Some cases of multiple bifurcation are analyzed in Refs. [85] and [86].

Remark

Concerning the numerical computation of the approximate solutions in a neighborhood of a critical point we refer, for instance, to Refs. [86]-[89] and the references contained therein.

REFERENCES

1 Lions, J. L., and Magenes, E., Non-homogeneous Boundary Value Problems and Applications, Vol. 1, Springer-Verlag, 1972.

2 Adams, R. A., Sobolev Spaces, Academic Press, New York, 1975.

3 Yoshida, K., Functional Analysis, Academic Press, New York, 1965.

4 Ciarlet, P. G., The Finite Element Method for Elliptic Problems, North Holland Publ., Amsterdam, 1978.

5 Babuska, I., and Aziz, A. K., "Survey Lectures on the Mathematical Foundations of the Finite Element Method," The Mathematical Foundations of the Finite Element Method with Applications to Partial Differential Equations, ed. by A. K. Aziz, Academic Press, 1972, pp. 1-359.

6 Strang, G., and Fix, G. J., An Analysis of the Finite Element Method, Prentice Hall, Englewood Cliffs, 1973.

7 Bramble, J. H., and Scott, R., "Simultaneous Approximation in Scales of Banach Spaces," Mathematics of Computation, Vol. 32, No. 144, Oct. 1978, pp. 947-954.

8 Céa, J., "Approximation Variationnelle des Problèmes aux Limites," Ann. Inst. Fourier (Grenoble), Vol. 14, fasc. 2, 1964, pp. 345-444.

9 Strang, G., "Variational Crimes in the Finite Element Method," The Mathematical Foundations of the Finite Element Method with Applications to Partial Differential Equations, ed. by A. K. Aziz, Academic Press, 1972, pp. 689-710.

10 Nitsche, J. A., "Convergence of Nonconforming Methods," Mathematical Aspects of Finite Elements in Partial Differential Equations, ed. by Carl de Boor, Academic Press, 1974, pp. 15-53.

11 Lascaux, P. M., and Lesaint, P., "Some Nonconforming Finite Elements for the Plate Bending Problem," R.A.I.R.O., R1, 1975, pp. 9-53.

12 Céa, J., "Approximation Variationnelle; Convergence des Éléments Finis; un Test," Journées Elements Finis, Université de Rennes (Rennes), 1976.

13 Stummel, F., "The Generalized Patch Test," SIAM Journal of Numerical Analysis, Vol. 16, No. 3, June 1979, pp. 449-471.

14 Raviart, P. A., and Thomas, J. M., "Primal Hybrid Finite Element Methods for Second Order Elliptic Equations," Mathematics of Computation, Vol. 31, No. 138, April 1977, pp. 391-413.

15 Quarteroni, A., "Primal Hybrid Finite Element Methods for Fourth-Order Elliptic Equations," Calcolo, Vol. 16, No. 1, 1979, pp. 21-59.

16 Necas, J., Les Methodes Directes en Theorie des Equations Elliptiques, Masson et Cie, Editeurs, Paris, 1967.

17 Babuska, I., "Error-Bounds for Finite Element Method," Numerische Mathematik, Vol. 16, No. 4, 1971, pp. 322-333.

18 Griffiths, D. F., and Lorenz, J., "An Analysis of the Petrov-Galerkin Finite Element Method," Computer Methods in Applied Mechanics and Engineering, Vol. 14, No. 1, April 1978, pp. 39-64.

19 Oden, J. T., and Lee, J. K., "Dual Mixed-Hybrid Finite Element Method for Second Order Elliptic Problems," in Mathematical Aspects of Finite Element Methods, Lecture Notes in Mathematics, No. 606, ed. by I. Galligani and E. Magenes, Springer-Verlag, Berlin, 1977, pp. 275-291.

20 Babuska, I., Oden, J. T., and Lee, J. K., "Mixed-Hybrid Finite Element Approximations of Second-Order Elliptic Boundary-Value Problems," Computer Methods in Applied Mechanics and Engineering, Vol. 11, No. 2, May 1977, pp. 175-206.

21 Brezzi, F., "On the Existence, Uniqueness and Approximation of Saddle-Point Problems Arising From Lagrangian Multipliers," R.A.I.R.O., Vol. 8, No. R-2, 1974, pp. 129-151.

22 Brezzi, F., and Marini, L. D., "On the Numerical Solution of Plate Bending Problems by Hybrid Methods," R.A.I.R.O., Vol. 9, No. R-3, 1975, pp. 5-50.

23 Bercovier, M., Regularisation Duale des Problemes Variationnelles Mixtes. Application aux Elements Finis Mixtes et Extension a Quelques Problemes Nonlineaires, Doctoral thesis, Universite de Rouen, 1976.

24 Thomas, J. M., Sur l'analyse Numerique des Methodes d'elements Finis Hybrides et Mixtes, Doctoral Thesis, Universite Pierre et Marie Curie, Paris, 1977.

25 Raviart, P. A., and Thomas, J. M., "Dual Finite Element Models for Second Order Elliptic Problems," in Energy Methods in Finite Element Analysis, ed. by R. Glowinski, E. Y. Rodin and O. C. Zienkiewicz, John Wiley and Sons, 1979, pp. 175-192.

26 Brezzi, F., "Nonstandard Finite Elements for Fourth Order Elliptic Problems," in Energy Methods in Finite Element Analysis, ed. by R. Glowinski, E. Y. Rodin and O. C. Zienkiewicz, John Wiley and Sons, 1979, pp. 193-212.

27 Glowinski, R., and Pironneau, O., "Numerical Methods for the First Biharmonic Equation and for the Two-Dimensional Stokes Problem," SIAM Review, Vol. 21, No. 2, April 1979, pp. 167-212.

28 Rannacher, R., "On Nonconforming and Mixed Finite Element Method for Plate Bending Problems. The Linear Case," R.A.I.R.O., Vol. 13, No. 4, 1979, pp. 369-387.

29 Girault, V., and Raviart, P. A., Finite Element Approximation of the Navier-Stokes Equations, Lecture Notes in Mathematics, Vol. 749, Springer-Verlag, Berlin, 1979.

30 Scapolla, T., "A Mixed Finite Element Method for the Biharmonic Problem," R.A.I.R.O., Vol. 14, No. 1, 1980, pp. 55-79.

31 Falk, R., and Osborn, J., Error Estimates for Mixed Methods - for the Approximation Solution of Elliptic Boundary Value Problems, MRC Technical Summary Report 1936, University of Wisconsin, 1979.

32 Fix, G. J., Gunzburger, M. D., and Nicolaides, R. A., "Theory and Applications of Mixed Finite Element Methods," in Constructive Approaches to Mathematical Models, ed. by C. V. Coffman and G. J. Fix, Academic Press, 1979, pp. 375-393.

33 Babuska, I., Osborn, J., and Pitkaranta, J., Analysis of Mixed Methods Using Mesh Dependent Norms, MRC Technical Summary Report 2003, University of Wisconsin, 1979.

34 Brezzi, F., "Sur une Methode Hybride Pour l'approximation du Probleme de la Torsion d'une Barre Elastique," Ist. Lombardo Accad. Sci. Lett. Rend., A-108, 1974, pp. 274-300.

35 Fortin, M., "An Analysis of the Convergence of Mixed Finite Element Methods," R.A.I.R.O., Vol. 11, No. 4, 1977, pp. 341-354.

36 Bercovier, M., and Pironneau, O., "Error Estimates for Finite Element Method Solution of the Stokes Problem in the Primitive Variable," Numerische Mathematik, Vol. 33, 1979, pp. 211-224.

37 Johnson, C., and Pitkaranta, J., Analysis of Some Mixed Finite Element Methods Related to Reduced Integration, Chalmers Institute of Technology, Goteborg, 1980.

38 Golub, G. H., Dalquist, G., and Nash, S., "Bounds for the Error in Linear Systems," Proc. Workshop on Semi-Infinite Programming, Bad Honnef, West Germany, Aug. 30-Sept. 1, 1978.

39 Babuska, I., Szabo, B. A., and Katz, I. N., The P-Version of the Finite Element Method, Report WU/CCM-79/1, Washington University, St. Louis, 1979.

40 Gottlieb, D., and Orszag, S. A., Numerical Analysis of Spectral Methods: Theory and Applications, CBMS Regional Conference Series in Applied Mathematics, No. 26, SIAM, Philadelphia, 1977.

41 Canuto, C., and Quarteroni, A., "Proprietes d'approximation dans les Espaces de Sobolev de Systemes de Polynomes Orthogonaux," C.R. Acad. Sci. Paris Ser. A-B, Vol. 290, No. 19, 1980, pp. A925-A928.

42 Brezzi, F., and Johnson, C., "On the Coupling of Boundary Integral and Finite Element Methods," Calcolo, Vol. 16, No. 2, 1979, pp. 189-201.

43 Johnson, C., and Nedelec, J. C., "On the Coupling of Boundary Integral and Finite Element Methods," Mathematics of Computation, Vol. 35, No. 152, October 1980, pp. 1063-1079.

44 Ciarlet, P. G., and Raviart, P. A., "Maximum Principle and Uniform Convergence for the Finite Element Method," Computer Methods in Applied Mechanics and Engineering, Vol. 2, 1973, pp. 17-31.

45 Scott, R., "Optimal L^∞ Estimates for the Finite Element Method on Irregular Meshes," Mathematics of Computation, Vol. 30, No. 136, October 1976, pp. 681-697.

46 Nitsche, J. A., "L^∞ Convergence of Finite Element Approximation," Journées Eléments Finis, Université de Rennes, 1975.

47 Ciarlet, P. G., and Raviart, P. A., "The Combined Effect of Curved Boundaries and Numerical Integration in Isoparametric Finite Element Methods," in The Mathematical Foundations of the Finite Element Method with Applications to Partial Differential Equations," ed. by A. K. Aziz, Academic Press, 1972, pp. 409-474.

48 Duvaut, G., and Lions, J. L., Les Inequations en Mecanique et en Physique, Dunod, Paris, 1972.

49 Brezis, H., "Problemes Unilateraux," J. de Math. Pures et Appliquees, Vol. 51, 1972, pp. 1-168.

50 Baiocchi, C., and Capelo, A. C. S., Disequazioni Variationali e Quasi-variazionali. Applicazioni a Problemi di Frontiera Libera, Quaderni dell'Unione Matematica Italiana, No. 4,7, Pitagora (Bologna), 1978. English version to appear in Wiley.

51 Lions, J. L., and Stampacchia, G., "Variational Inequalities," Comm. Pure Appl. Math., Vol. 20, 1967, pp. 493-519.

52 Brezzi, F., Hager, W. W., and Raviart, P. A., "Error Estimates for the Finite Element Solution of Variational Inequalities, Parts I and II," Numerische Mathematik, Vol. 28, No. 4, 1977, pp. 431-443; and Vol. 31, 1978/79, No. 1, pp. 1-16.

53 Falk, R. S., "Error Estimates for the Approximation of a Class of Variational Inequalities," Mathematics of Computation, Vol. 28, No. 128, October 1974, pp. 963-971.

54 Brezis, H., and Kinderlehrer, D., "The Smoothness of Solutions to Nonlinear Variational Inequalities," Indiana University Mathematics Journal, Vol. 23, 1973/74, pp. 831-844.

55 Glowinski, R., Lions, J. L., and Tremolieres, R., Analyse Numerique des Inequations Variationnelles, (two volumes), Dunod, 1976.

56 Mercier, B., Sur la Theorie et l'analyse Numerique de Problemes de Plasticite, Doctoral Thesis, Universite Pierre et Marie Curie, Paris, 1977.

57 Glowinski, R., "Finite Elements and Variational Inequalities," in The Mathematics of Finite Elements and Approximations III, edited by J. R. Whiteman, Academic Press, 1979, pp. 135-171.

58 Glowinski, R., Lectures on Numerical Methods for Nonlinear Variational Problems, Springer-Verlag, Berlin, 1980.

59 Magenes, E. (Ed.), Free Boundary Problems, Proceedings of a Seminar Held in Pavia, Sept.-Oct. 1979 (two volumes), ed. Tecnoprint, Bologna, 1980.

60 Cottle, R. W., Golub, G. H., and Sacker, R. S., "On the Solution of Large, Structured Linear Complementarity Problems: the Block Partitioned Case," Applied Mathematics and Optimization, Vol. 4, No. 4, 1977/78, pp. 347-364.

61 Magenes, E., "Topics in Parabolic Equations. Some Typical Free Boundary Problems," in Boundary Value Problems for Linear Evolution Partial Differential Equations, edited by H. G. Garnir, Reidel Publishing Co., Dordrecht, Holland, 1977, pp. 239-312.

62 Baiocchi, C., Comincioli, V., Magenes, E., and Pozzi, G. A., "Free Boundary Problems in the Theory of Fluid Flow Through Porous Media: Existence and Uniqueness Theorems," Ann. Mat. Pura Appl., (4)97, 1973, pp. 1-82.

63 Oden, J. T., and Kikuchi, N., Theory of Variational Inequalities, TICOM Report 79-4, University of Texas at Austin, 1979.

64 Bensoussan, A., and Lions, J. L., "Applications des in Equations Variationnelles en Contr ole Stochastique," in Studies in Mathematics and Its Applications, Vol. 12, Elsevier North Holland Publishing Co., 1982, pp. 559-564.

65 Cortey Dumont, P., Doctoral Thesis, Universite de Besancon, 1977.

66 Loinger, E., "On Finite Element Approach to Quasi-Variational Inequalities," Calcolo, Vol. 17, No. 3, 1980, pp. 197-209.

67 Cortey Dumont, P., "Approximation Numerique d'une Inequation Quasi-Variationnelle Liee a des Problemes de Gestion de Stock," R.A.I.R.O., Vol. 14, No. 4, 1980, pp. 335-346.

68 Brezis, H., Operateurs Maximaux Monotones et Semi-Groupes de Contractions Dans Les Espaces de Hilbert, North Holland Mathematics Studies, No. 5, North Holland Publishing Co., 1973.

69 Lions, J. L., Quelques Methodes de Resolution des Problemes Aux Limites Nonlineaires, Dunod; Gauthier-Villars, Paris, 1969.

70 Noor, M. A., and Whiteman, J. R., "Error Bounds for Finite Element Solutions of Mildly Nonlinear Elliptic Boundary Value Problems," Numerische Mathematik, Vol. 26, 1976, pp. 107-116.

71 Ambrosetti, A., and Mancini, G., "Sharp Nonuniqueness Results for Some Nonlinear Problems," Nonlinear Anal., Vol. 3, No. 5, 1979, pp. 635-645.

72 Brezzi, F., "Finite Element Approximations of the von Karman Equations," R.A.I.R.O., Vol. 12, No. 4, 1978, pp. 303-312.

73 Brezzi, F., Rappaz, J., and Raviart, P. A., "Finite Dimensional Approximation of Nonlinear Problems, Part I, Branches of Nonsingular Solutions," Numerische Mathematik, Vol. 36, No. 1, 1980, pp. 1-25.

74 Crandall, M. G., "An Introduction to Constructive Aspects of Bifurcation and the Implicit Function Theorem," in Applications of Bifurcation Theory, ed. by P. H. Rabinowitz, Academic Press, 1977, pp. 1-35.

75 Nirenberg, L., Topics in Nonlinear Functional Analysis, New York University, 1974.

76 Berger, M., Nonlinearity and Functional Analysis: Lectures on Nonlinear Problems in Mathematical Analysis, Academic Press, New York, 1977.

77 Brezzi, F., Rappaz, J., and Raviart, P. A., "Finite Dimensional Approximation of Nonlinear Problems, Part II, Limit Points," Numerische Mathematik, Vol. 37, No. 1, pp. 1-29.

78 Sattinger, D. H., Topics in Stability and Bifurcation Theory (Lecture Notes in Mathematics, 309), Springer Verlag, Berlin, 1973.

79 Prodi, G., and Ambrosetti, A., "Analisi Nonlineare," Quaderni Sc. Norm. Sup. Pisa, I (Pisa), 1973.

80 Kikuchi, F., An Iterative Finite Element Scheme for Bifurcation Analysis of Semilinear Elliptic Equations, Tokyo University Institute of Space and Aeronautical Science Report No. ISAS-542, 1976.

81 Kikuchi, F., "Finite Element Approximations to Bifurcation Problems of Turning Point Type," in Computing Methods in Applied Sciences and Engineering (Proc. Third International Symposium, Versailles, 1977), I, pp. 252-266, Lecture Notes in Mathematics, 704, Springer Verlag, Berlin, 1979.

82 Fujii, H., and Yamaguti, H., "Structure of Singularities and Its Numerical Realization in Nonlinear Elasticity," Journal of Mathematics, Kyoto University, Vol. 20, No. 3, 1980, pp. 489-590.

83 Fujii, H., "Numerical Pattern Formation and Group Theory," in Computing Methods in Applied Sciences and Engineering, edited by R. Glowinski and J. L. Lions, North Holland, 1980, pp. 63-81.

84 Brezzi, F., Rappaz, J., Raviart, P. A., "Finite Dimensional Approximation of Nonlinear Problems, Part III, Simple Bifurcation Points," Numerische Mathematik, Vol. 38, No. 1, 1981, pp. 1-30.

85 Rappaz, J., and Raugel, G., Finite Dimensional Approximation of Bifurcation Problems at a Multiple Eigenvalue, Report No. 71, Centre de Mathematiques Appliquees, Ecole Polytechnique, Palaiseau (Paris), 1981.

86 Keller, H. B., "Numerical Solution of Bifurcation and Nonlinear Eigenvalue Problems," in Applications of Bifurcation Theory, edited by P. H. Rabinowitz, Academic Press, 1977, pp. 359-384.

87 Langford, W. F., "Numerical Solution of Bifurcation Problems for Ordinary Differential Equations," Numerical Mathematics, Vol. 28, No. 2, 1977, pp. 171-190.

88 Rheinboldt, W. C., "Numerical Methods for a Class of Finite Dimensional Bifurcation Problems," SIAM Journal Numer. Anal., Vol. 15, No. 1, February 1978, pp. 1-11.

89 Keller, H. B., "Global Homotopies and Newton Methods," in Recent Advances in Numerical Analysis, edited by C. de Boor and G. H. Golub, Academic Press, New York, 1978.

CHAPTER TWO

BASIS FUNCTIONS AND EVALUATION OF ELEMENT CHARACTERISTICS

E. L. Wachspress
General Electric Company
Schenectady, New York

ABSTRACT

Definition of a basis for polynomial approximation over each element of a partitioned region is fundamental to any finite element computation. Triangles and rectangles for which polynomial basis functions are available are widely used. Polynomial bases in isoparametric coordinates allow use of three- and four-sided elements having straight or curved sides. Rational basis functions can be constructed for the much wider class of "well-set algebraic elements." Theory for generating rational bases draws heavily on classical algebraic geometry. Other devices discussed include blending, macroelements, adaptive and hierarchical refinement, nonconforming elements, and the significance of conjugate bases in the fitting of discontinuous functions. An attempt is made not only to expose methods in current use but also to indicate research frontiers and thereby to motivate continued analysis of diverse elements.

INTRODUCTION

For finite element computation, one defines a space of finite dimension from which an approximate solution to a problem of interest is drawn. The approximation space is generated from element basis functions. Properties of the element "part" or "wedge" bases defined only over the element determine the character of the finite element approximation space. The approximation over a collection of elements may be expanded in terms of nodal "pyramid" functions which are composites of element wedge functions.

If, for example, node i is on the interface of elements m and m' only, the pyramid function $P_i(\underline{x})$ is defined as equal to wedge $N_{im}(\underline{x})$ associated with node i in element m for $\underline{x}$ in m and equal to wedge $N_{im'}(\underline{x})$ for $\underline{x}$ in element m'. $P_i(\underline{x})$, is zero elsewhere. Then if the expansion of $u(\underline{x})$ contains the component $a_i P_i(\underline{x})$, the approximations in elements m and m', respectively, contain components $a_i N_{im}(\underline{x})$ and $a_i N_{im'}(\underline{x})$. The wedge basis functions N combine to form the pyramids P.

In this chapter significant properties of element basis functions will be discussed, and some of the more ubiquitous elements will be described. Polynomial bases and polynomial approximation within elements play a central role in finite element analysis, and the next four sections deal with polynomial bases in both physical and isoparametric coordinates.

Polynomial bases are available only for a restricted class of elements, and one of the frontiers in finite element analysis is the development of methods for treating more general element geometry. In this chapter discussion of more sophisticated elements is concerned more with current research than with engineering practice. Construction of rational basis functions over "algebraic elements" gives insight into fundamental aspects of finite element computation and suggests means for improving standard techniques. For example, modifications of blending functions to achieve a higher degree of approximation within elements are disclosed in a later section of this chapter.

Use of patchwork approximation within an element is discussed. Adaptive refinement refers to mesh subdivision or approximation-space expansion within elements to improve accuracy. "Hierarchic" bases, introduced to improve efficiency of basis expansion, are reviewed briefly near the end of the chapter.

An element is said to be nonconforming when the approximation space admits functions not contained in the space associated with the functional used for obtaining the discrete equations. Motivation for use of nonconforming elements is sketched, along with theoretical justification for success of such elements.

Conjugate basis functions introduced by Oden [B-2] for least squares smoothing of discontinuous functions derived from finite element approximations are discussed briefly in the final section of the chapter.

This chapter is mostly devoted to discussion of Lagrangian basis functions that achieve C^0 continuity over the collection of elements. Although there is some mention of C^1 elements, spline approximation to achieve C^p with p greater than one is not discussed because such elements have limited usefulness and are restricted to problems for which very smooth solutions are demanded. Singular functions and other special basis functions are discussed in Chapter 4. These functions have restricted application but lead to large gains in accuracy when used properly. Orthogonal polynomials are more appropriate as basis functions for global approximation. They have gained new importance from the global-local methods (Chapter 15). Trigonometric and exponential bases generally have poor approximation properties for finite element computation and are not recommended.

The survey by Carey in [B-3] is a particularly good reference for material relating to finite element basis function theory and application.

THE ROLE OF BASIS FUNCTIONS IN FINITE ELEMENT COMPUTATION

Basis functions are of fundamental importance in the finite element method. The mathematical theory discussed in Chapter 1 draws heavily on properties of patchwork finite element approximation spaces. The approximation in each element of each function to be estimated is of the form

$$\tilde{u}(\underline{x}) = \sum_{i=1}^{I_m} a_{im} N_{im}(\underline{x}) \tag{1}$$

for $\underline{x}$ in element m

"Best" values for the free parameters a_{im} are computed by solving [Chapters 7, 8] a system of equations usually obtained from a stationarity principle applied to a suitable functional.

The basis (or interpolation) functions $N_{im}(\underline{x})$ must satisfy conditions that depend on the governing equations, boundary conditions, and stationarity principle. For example, functionals associated with second order partial differential equations often admit trial functions that are continuous but do not necessarily have continuous first derivatives. On the other hand, functionals commonly used for solving fourth order systems require trial functions that have continuous first derivatives. Finite-element geometry for which convenient C^1 approximation spaces are known is very limited. Alternative functionals can be developed to remove derivative continuity constraints [Chapter 5], but other numerical problems may arise with these modified functionals.

If particular non-smooth behavior of the solution is known to occur in an element, special basis functions with that behavior may be introduced in that element to improve the local approximation. Alternatively, element geometry may be chosen so that standard basis functions for the element exhibit known unusual behavior . For example, singular behavior at crack tips is sometimes simulated by use of elements for which conventional basis functions are singular at the crack tips. (A detailed discussion of special and singular basis functions is given in Chapter 4.)

The basis functions are the building blocks of the approximation spaces. They must be chosen to yield a prescribed degree of approximation within the elements while retaining the appropriate order of continuity across element interfaces. The basis functions must satisfy all boundary and continuity conditions not incorporated in the functional.

Functional form of basis functions depends on element geometry and required interelement continuity. Once elements and bases have been chosen, discrete equations must be developed. Discretization usually requires evaluation of integrals over the elements of products of basis functions and their derivatives of various orders. Simple algebraic expressions for the basis functions facilitate computation.

When the parameters a_{im} in Eq. 1 are function values at nodes, the interpolation is said to be "Lagrangian". A specific point, $\underline{x}_{im}$, is associated with node i of element m, and the basis functions are chosen so that

$$N_{im}(\underline{x}_{jm}) = \delta_{ij} = \begin{cases} 1 \text{ when } i = j \\ 0 \text{ when } i \neq j \end{cases} \qquad (2)$$

This is the "discrete orthonormality" property.

When the parameters include nodal values and derivative, the interpolation is said to be of the "Hermite" type. The normalization in Eq. 2 may be generalized. For example, if a_{km} is the x_1-derivative of the function at node j, then

$$N_{km}(\underline{x}_{im}) = \frac{\partial N_{km}(\underline{x}_{im})}{\partial x_p} = 0 \qquad \text{for all i, } (p \neq 1)$$

$$\text{and} \qquad \frac{\partial N_{km}(\underline{x}_{im})}{\partial x_1} = \delta_{ij} \qquad (3)$$

The concept of basis function "support" must be explored. Support refers to the boundary beyond which the basis function is identically zero. Finite element discrete systems are characterized by sparse matrices. This sparsity is achieved through use of basis functions with "small support." For C^o approximation, it is customary to choose a basis function that is nonzero only on elements containing the node associated with the function. Higher order continuity can be achieved in rare cases with such functions. There is another class of elements for which higher order continuity is achieved by extending the support and imposing additional basis function conditions along the support. For C^1 continuity one may demand zero normal derivative of the basis function along the support.

The class of elements for which suitable basis functions are known becomes more restricted as function properties are made more demanding. Severest restrictions relate to order of continuity at element interfaces. Fortunately, many problems of practical concern may be solved with C^o approximation spaces.

For a given element geometry, properties required of the basis functions do not often define unique functions. One must select a particular basis, and the choice depends on desired as well as required characteristics. Suppose the error in terms of a prescribed norm is minimized with basis N_r when the approximation is $\tilde{u}_r$: $||\tilde{u}_r - u|| = \min_{\{a_{im}\}} ||u(N_r) - u||$. A "best" basis is one for which $||\tilde{u}_r - u||$ takes on the lowest possible value for a given partitioning. The basis that achieves this best approximation need not be unique. Even when it is possible to establish the existence of a unique best basis, such functions may not be suitable for computation. They may be difficult to evaluate, and derivation of associated finite element equations may be intractable or more time-consuming than warranted by the anticipated increase in accuracy. Polynomial bases are often best from a numerical standpoint. One must strike a balance between closeness of the approximation space to the exact solution and computational efficiency. Just how this is accomplished is part of the art of finite element computation. An arsenal of basis function alternatives is described in this chapter. The user must choose his own weapon.

PROPERTIES OF BASIS FUNCTIONS

Order of Continuity

Except for special singular elements and macroelements within which patchwork bases are used, elements are defined with "regular" wedge basis functions. The term regular here denotes bounded value and derivatives of all order interior to the element. Order of continuity of the composite approximation is then determined by behavior at element interfaces. The more common applications are with C° approximation, in which case the approximations on any element interface must be the same when approached from either side.

Analysis is facilitated by first establishing a degree of variation on the interface and then ascertaining the corresponding degrees of freedom. A polynomial of degree n in $\underline{x}$ (where $\underline{x}$ denotes the r-dimensional coordinate space with components $x_1, x_2, \ldots, x_r$) over the complex field $\mathbb{K}$ is of the form

$$P_n(\underline{x}) = \sum_{o \leq s_1 + s_2 \ldots + s_r \leq n} c_{s_1, s_2, \ldots, s_r} x_1^{s_1} x_2^{s_2} \ldots x_r^{s_r} \qquad (4)$$

where the coefficients are in $\mathbb{K}$ and there is at least one nonzero coefficient for which the sum of the s_i is equal to n. Consider for illustrative purposes a line interface of a two-dimensional network. The degree of variation is defined as the maximum degree of polynomial in x and y needed to yield the approximation values with no error along the interface. Suppose degree-two variation is established. Then there is a set of a_i for each approximation such that

$$\tilde{u}(x,y) = a_0 + a_1 x + a_2 y + a_3 x^2 + a_4 y^2 + a_5 xy \qquad (5)$$

On the interface line, either one of the coordinates is constant or there is a linear relationship between x and y. Hence, on the interface there is a coordinate t (equal to one of x and y) and a triplet (b_0, b_1, b_2) determined from the a_i for which

$$\tilde{u}(x,y) = b_0 + b_1 t + b_2 t^2 \quad \text{mod (interface)} \qquad (6)$$

Thus, there are three degrees of freedom for degree-two approximation on a straight line.

A curve is irreducible if it cannot be represented as the union of component curves. In defining the boundary of an element in finite element computation, one always chooses irreducible curves for boundary segments between adjacent vertices. Suppose an element interface is a segment of an irreducible conic. Then there is a quadratic relationship coupling the coordinates on this interface. One of xy, x^2, and y^2 may be eliminated from Eq. 5 in terms of other components for evaluating $\tilde{u}$ on the interface. Suppose xy appears in the equation of the conic interface and that xy is eliminated. Then there are coefficients c_i such that

$$\tilde{u}(x,y) = c_0 + c_1 x + c_2 y + c_3 x^2 + c_4 y^2 \quad \text{mod (conic interface)} \qquad (7)$$

and it is seen that there are five degrees of freedom for quadratic (degree-two) variation on a conic side.

To achieve continuity across a line on which there is degree-two variation, one may fix values at three nodes on the line. These are usually the vertices and a node near the midpoint (Fig. 1a). On a conic side, values may be fixed at five nodes (Fig. 1b).

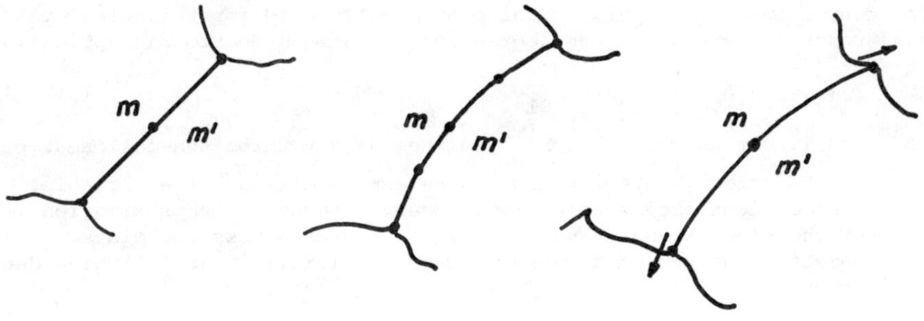

Fig. 1 Degrees of freedom on a line and a conic

One alternative shown in Fig. 1c is fitting the values and tangential derivatives at vertices and value at a side node.

To achieve C^1 continuity, one must also consider the variation of the normal derivative along the interface. The most common C^1 element is a rectangle with bicubic basis functions. Value, gradient (two first derivatives) and the mixed second derivative are fit at each of the four vertices. A cubic has four degrees of freedom on a line. Values and tangetial derivatives at the endpoints of each side assure continuity across the line. Normal derivatives and tangential derivatives of the normal derivatives (mixed derivatives) at these vertices assure continuity of the normal derivative across the side.

The ease with which C^1 approximation is attained with bicubic bases over rectangles should not be misconstrued. The only other C^1 element in common use is the triangle with quintic bases and 21 or 18 degrees of freedom, depending on the method used. A C^1 macrotriangle with a cubic basis is described in Section 2.8. It is important to note that C^1 approximation is not easily achieved and that higher order continuity requires more than just fitting higher derivatives at nodes. Of course, C^n approximation with $n > 1$ is even more difficult to achieve.

The C^1 discussion has centered primarily on approximation in two space dimensions. The situation is much more tractable in one dimension. Now Hermite interpolation at vertices yields higher order continuity. On the other hand, as the number of dimensions of the coordinate space grows the degree of difficulty increases. Three-dimensional C^0 approximation is achieved without great difficulty for a wide assortment of elements. The bicubic C^1 rectangle does not generalize to a tricubic C^1 parallelepiped. Tetrahedral elements are common in three dimensions, and both C^0 and C^1 [A-4] approximations are in use for these elements.

Degree of Approximation

Approximation over an element is of degree k if the interpolation functions provide a basis for all polynomials of degree less than k + 1 but not of degree k + 1. Let the subscripts on polynomials hereafter denote the maximum allowable degrees. Thus, degree k approximation with basis N^{im} over element m requires the existence of a set of a_{im} for any P_k such that

$$P_k(\underline{x}) - \sum_i a_{im} N^{im}(\underline{x}) = 0 \qquad \text{for all } \underline{x} \text{ in element } m \tag{8}$$

Superscripts are used here to denote the basis functions in order not to confuse identification with degree. The basis functions are not necessarily polynomials.

The remainder of this discussion is restricted to approximation in the plane for convenience. Analysis is quite straightforward for triangles with polynomial bases. There are three degrees of freedom in degree one approximation:

$$P_1(x,y) = a_{00} + a_{10}x + a_{01}y \tag{9}$$

If the N^{im} are linear and $P_1 - \sum_i a_i N^{im}_1$ vanishes at any three non-collinear points in m, then the N^{im} are a basis for degree one approximation. The triangle vertices are an obvious choice as element nodes. Degree one approximation is achieved over the element and C^o continuity is assured across the sides.

A fundamental theorem of algebra is used implicitly in establishing degree of approximation:

Theorem 2.1. Let Q be a polynomial in x and y that is a product of distinct irreducible factors and let P be a polynomial not identically zero. Then if P vanishes everywhere on the curve of Q (set of points on which Q = 0), Q must be a factor of P. This theorem is proved in higher algebra texts.

In the triangle analysis, it was observed that the polynomial of degree one, $R(x,y) \equiv P_1(x,y) - \sum_i a_i N_1^{im}(x,y)$, vanished at three non-collinear points. Consideration of the degrees of freedom on any of the lines joining any two of these points assures vanishing of R on any of these lines. The product of these lines is a cubic and R is of maximal degree one. Hence, by the theorem, R must be identically zero. Note that if the three points were collinear, then Q would be a line and R could be the linear form that vanishes on the line. Degree-one approximation would not follow if the points were collinear. This illustrates the importance of choosing independent data points. This will be considered in greater depth subsequently.

Analysis of degree-two approximation with quadratic basis functions over a triangle is similar. There are six degrees of freedom in the general quadratic. Three nodes are introduced at side midpoints. The difference polynomial, R, is of maximal degree two and vanishes on the triangle perimeter which is of order three. Again, R must be the zero polynomial.

For degree-three approximation on a triangle, introduction of two nodes on each side is adequate to assure interelement continuity and the vanishing of R on the triangle sides. But now R is of maximal degree three and need not be the zero polynomial to vanish on the triangle perimeter. An interior node may be introduced for degree-three approximation.

Less trivial arguments apply to more complex elements, and these will be given when specific elements are discussed. A particularly relevant field of mathematics is that of algebraic geometry, a field unfortunately foreign to most practitioners.

POLYNOMIAL BASES IN GLOBAL COORDINATES

C^o Approximation Over Triangles and Tetrahedra

Basis functions for triangles have already been discussed to illustrate concepts relating to degree of approximation over elements. The triangle is well suited for finite element computation. Polynomial bases are easily generated for any desired degree of approximation. Referring to Fig. 2, one denotes the linear form that vanishes

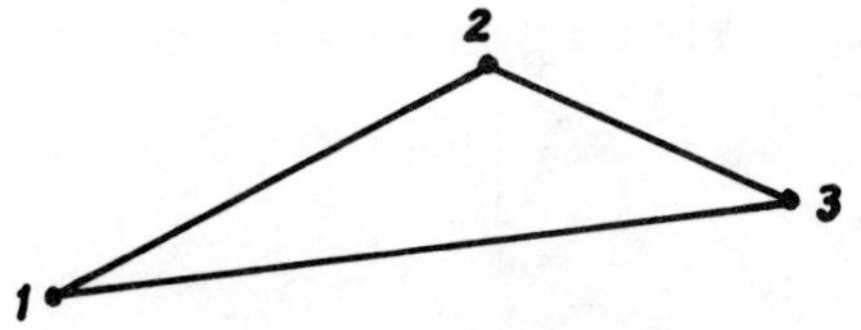

Fig. 2 A triangle

on the line determined by points p and q, normalized to unity at point s, by $(p;q)_s$. A degree one basis for the triangle is

$$N_1(x,y) = (2;3)_1, \quad N_2(x,y) = (3;1)_2, \quad N_3(x,y) = (1;2)_3 \tag{10}$$

The function $u(x,y) = \sum_{i=1}^{3} u_i N_i(x,y)$ is linear and takes on vertex values u_i. These basis functions are the areal (normalized barycentric) coordinates which may be defined alternatively by

$$\begin{vmatrix} N_1 \equiv r \\ N_2 \equiv q \\ N_3 \equiv p \end{vmatrix} = \begin{vmatrix} 1 & 1 & 1 \\ x_1 & x_2 & x_3 \\ y_1 & y_2 & y_3 \end{vmatrix}^{-1} \begin{vmatrix} 1 \\ x \\ y \end{vmatrix} \tag{11}$$

The absolute value of the determinant of the 3x3 matrix is twice the area of the triangle. Hence, the inverse exists when the three vertices are not collinear.

Areal coordinates provide a geometric representation that facilitates finite element computation. Since the transformation in (11) is linear, any degree of approximation achieved in areal coordinates carries over to the global (x,y) coordinates. A degree two basis is given in Fig. 2.3 for a six-node triangle with midside nodes 4, 5, and 6.

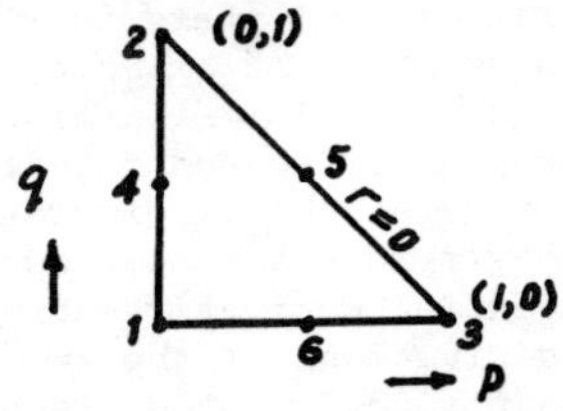

$$N_1 = r(2r - 1) \qquad N_2 = q(2q - 1)$$

$$N_3 = p(2p - 1) \qquad N_4 = 4\,rq$$

$$N_5 = 4\,pq \qquad N_6 = 4\,pr$$

$$(p + q + r = 1)$$

Fig. 3 The six-node triangle

The basis functions are quadratic in the local (areal) coordinates and are therefore also quadratic in the global (x,y) coordinates. Theorem 2.1 guides selection of nodes for higher degree approximation. One interior node and four nodes on each side (including vertices) are required for degree-three. Three non-collinear interior nodes and five nodes on each side are required for degree-four Lagrangian approximation.

Generalization to tetrahedra is straightforward. Volumetric coordinates are defined by

$$\begin{vmatrix} s \\ r \\ q \\ p \end{vmatrix} = \begin{vmatrix} 1 & 1 & 1 & 1 \\ x_1 & x_2 & x_3 & x_4 \\ y_1 & y_2 & y_3 & y_4 \\ z_1 & z_2 & z_3 & z_4 \end{vmatrix}^{-1} \begin{vmatrix} 1 \\ x \\ y \\ z \end{vmatrix} \tag{12}$$

The matrix is nonsingular when the volume of the tetrahedron determined by the four vertices is nonzero (that is, the points are not coplanar). Node placement for triangle and tetrahedron approximation is indicated in Table 1.

Table 1 Node Placement for Approximation Over A Collection of Triangles or Tetrahedra.

Degree of approximation	Triangle: Three vertices for all k — side nodes (excluding vertices) per side	interior nodes	total nodes	Tetrahedron: Four vertices for all k — edge nodes (excluding vertices) per edge	face nodes (excluding edges) per face	interior nodes	total nodes
1	0	0	3	0	0	0	4
2	1	0	6	1	0	0	10
3	2	1	10	2	1	0	20
4	3	3	15	3	3	1	35
k	${}_{k-1}C_1$	${}_{k-1}C_2$	${}_{k+2}C_2$	${}_{k-1}C_1$	${}_{k-1}C_2$	${}_{k-1}C_3$	${}_{k+3}C_3$

Hermite interpolation involves fitting of derivatives as well as values. Although derivatives must be introduced for C^1 approximation, there is widespread use of Hermite interpolation that achieves only C^0. For example, one may fit values and first derivatives at triangle vertices and value at an interior point with ten cubic basis functions. The interior node is needed for degree three approximation and can be eliminated from the finite element discrete equations by static condensation [Ch. 7]. Continuity across triangle edges is achieved with or without this node. Value and tangential derivatives are common to elements sharing a vertex and these values and derivatives at the two vertices of a side determine unique cubic variation along that side. That C^1 is not achieved in general follows from the fact that the normal derivative variation along a side is quadratic and its value is fit only at the vertices. In general, there is a jump in the quadratic component of the normal derivative on the side. This is amplified later in the chapter.

C^0 Bases for Rectangles, Parallelograms and Parallelepipeds

Rectangles are treated in much the same manner as triangles. Basis functions for degree-one approximation over the rectangle in Fig. 4a are

$$N_1(x,y) = (2;3)_1(3;4)_1, \qquad N_2(x,y) = (3;4)_2(4;1)_2$$
$$N_3(x,y) = (4;1)_3(1;2)_3, \qquad N_4(x,y) = (1;2)_4(2;3)_4 \tag{13}$$

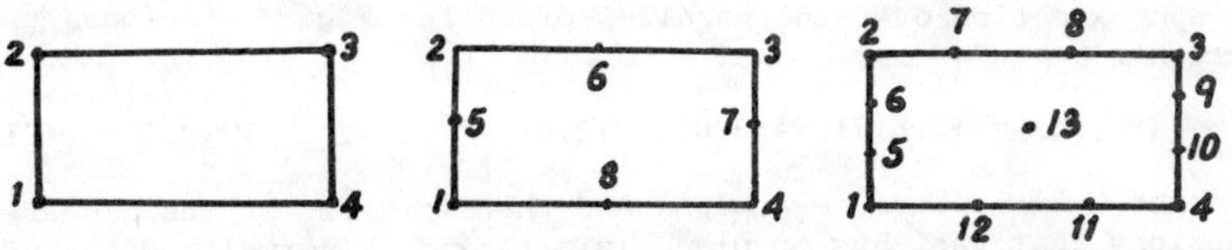

a. Degree one b. Degree two c. Degree three

Fig. 4 Nodes for Lagrangian approximation over a rectangle

Although these functions are bilinear, each either vanishes or is linear on each side of the rectangle. This follows from the fact that a linear form that vanishes on line (p;q) is constant on any line parallel to (p;q). For example, $(2;3)_1$ is equal to unity all along side (1;4). The symbol (p;q) denotes either the line determined by p and q or a linear form that vanishes on the line. When necessary, the meaning is clarified by the prefix "side" or "line" or "linear form." N_1 satisfies

$$\begin{aligned} N_1(x,y) &\equiv (3;4)_1 \bmod (1;4) \\ &\equiv (2;3)_1 \bmod (1;2) \end{aligned} \tag{14}$$

(The first congruence in (14) is read "$N_1(x,y)$ is congruent on side (1;4) to linear form $(3;4)_1$".)

The interpolant of U(x;y) is

$$u(x,y) = \sum_{i=1}^{4} U_i N_i(x,y) \tag{15}$$

Let U be linear in x and y. Consider the deviation

$$D(x,y) = U(X,y) - u(x,y) = U(x,y) - \sum_{i=1}^{4} U_i N_i(x,y) \tag{16}$$

Both U and u are linear on each side of the rectangle. D vanishes at the vertices. Therefore, D must vanish on the entire perimeter which is an irreducible curve of order four. D is of maximal degree two. By Theorem 2.1, D must be the zero polynomial. Degree one approximation is thus demonstrated.

The eight nodes in Fig. 4b yield degree-two with basis functions of the type

$$\begin{aligned} N_1(x,y) &= (2;3)_1(3;4)_1(5;8)_1 && \text{at vertices, and} \\ N_5(x,y) &= (2;3)_5(3;4)_5(4;1)_5 && \text{at side nodes} \end{aligned} \tag{17}$$

These trilinear functions vanish or are bilinear on each rectangle side.

For degree-three approximation, one may introduce another eight side nodes and an interior node. The basis functions are quartic and vanishing of a quartic on the perimeter does not guarantee vanishing everywhere. Hence, an interior node may be needed for degree-three approximation (though not for continuous approximation with cubic variation permitted on sides.) Degree-three approximation may be achieved without the interior node by clever choice of basis functions for the eight-node element [B-1]. This is the degree-three "serendipity" element [B-6].

The analysis applies to parallelograms. Parallel opposite sides are essential for reduction of degree of variation of basis functions on the perimeter.

Hermite interpolation may be used. One may replace the side nodes in the degree-three basis by derivative conditions at vertices. Just as for the triangle, this yields only C^o approximation.

Generalization to three dimensions is straightforward. A suitable basis for degree-one approximation over the parallelepiped in Fig. 5 includes trilinear basis functions:

$$N_1(x,y,z) = (5;6;7)_1(4;3;8)_1(2;3;6)_1 \tag{18}$$

Note that three points determine a plane and that $(p;q;r)_1$ is the linear form in three dimensions that vanishes on plane $(p;q;r)$ and is normalized to unity at node 1.

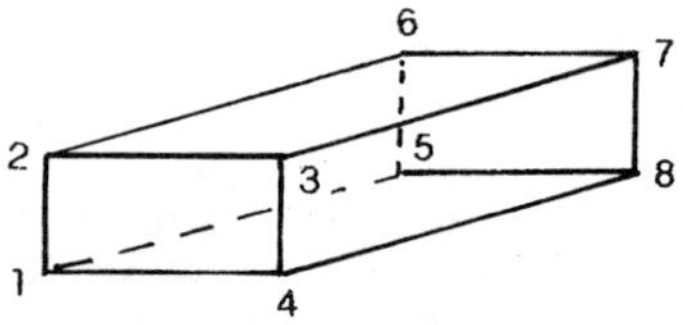

Fig. 5 Degree-one approximation over a parallelepiped

Higher degree approximation is achieved by introduction of more nodes: twelve edge nodes for degree-two, another twelve edge nodes plus six face nodes for degree-three, and more edge, face and interior nodes for higher degree approximation.

Isoparametric Elements

Isoparametric elements in common use are triangles and squares in two dimensions and tetrahedra and cubes in three dimensions. Generalizations will be examined in this chapter. This section will be concerned primarily with three- and four-sided elements in two dimensions. The six-node isoparametric triangle provides a convenient introduction (Fig. 6).

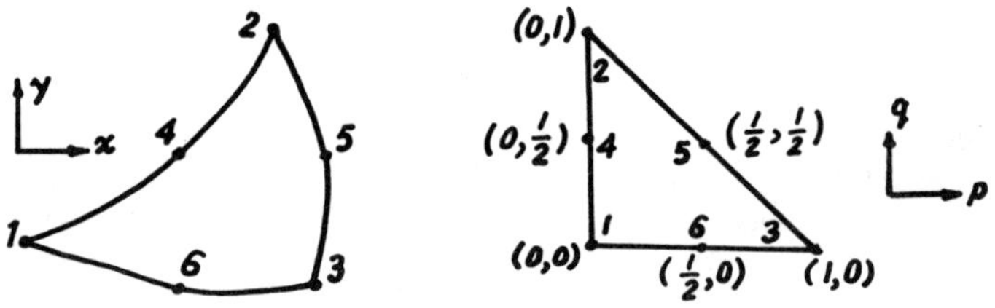

a. Global (x,y) coordinates b. Local (p,q) coordinates

Fig. 6 A triangle with curved sides

The triangle with curved sides in Fig. 6a is to be approximated by an isoparametric element. One first selects six nodes, three of which are vertices and three of which are nodes approximately centered on the sides. One now considers the straight-sided isosceles right-triangle in Fig. 6b with the indicated six nodes. The degree-two basis in p,q coordinates for this triangle is used to map the six nodes in the p,q plane into the six selected nodes of the curved triangle in the x,y plane. The mapping from p,q to x,y is:

$$x = \sum_{i=1}^{6} x_i N_i(p,q), \qquad y = \sum_{i=1}^{6} y_i N_i(p,q) \tag{19}$$

where the N_i are the degree-two basis functions (see Fig. 3).

Only the coordinates of the six nodes enter into this mapping. Thus, the straight sides of the p,q triangle do not map into the curved sides of the actual element in general. Each side of the curved triangle is approximated by an "isoparametric parabola" determined uniquely by the three nodes on the side.

Such elements are often used to model curved region boundaries, in which case only one side is curved. (When the three nodes on a side are collinear, the isoparametric parabola reduces to a straight line.) The region boundary is thus represented by piecewise isoparametric parabolas.

A key feature of isoparametrics is use of the mapping functions as basis functions. Thus, $N_1(x,y)$ is not usually given in explicit form:

$$N_i[x(p,q),\ y\ (p,q)] = N_i(p,q) \tag{20}$$

where

$$(p,q) \rightarrow (x,y) \text{ with } (19)$$

Equations (19) and the identity

$$\sum_i N_i(p,q) = 1 \tag{21}$$

guarantee a degree-one basis in the x,y plane. The mapping is not generally linear so that the degree-two basis in local coordinate space (p,q) does not yield a degree-two basis in the x,y plane.

The isoparametric parabola into which a side is mapped depends only on the coordinates of the three nodes on the side. This ensures that the parabola is common to elements sharing these nodes. The isoparametric triangulation covers the region of interest with no overlap. The approximation is quadratic in the local coordinates on each side. Continuity is achieved since the quadratic variation is uniquely determined by the three nodal values on the side.

The same technique is used to map a square in local coordinates into a four-sided element defined by eight or nine nodes (Fig. 7). The ninth node does not affect the boundary definition, and the degree of freedom associated with this node may be eliminated by static condensation [Ch. 7].

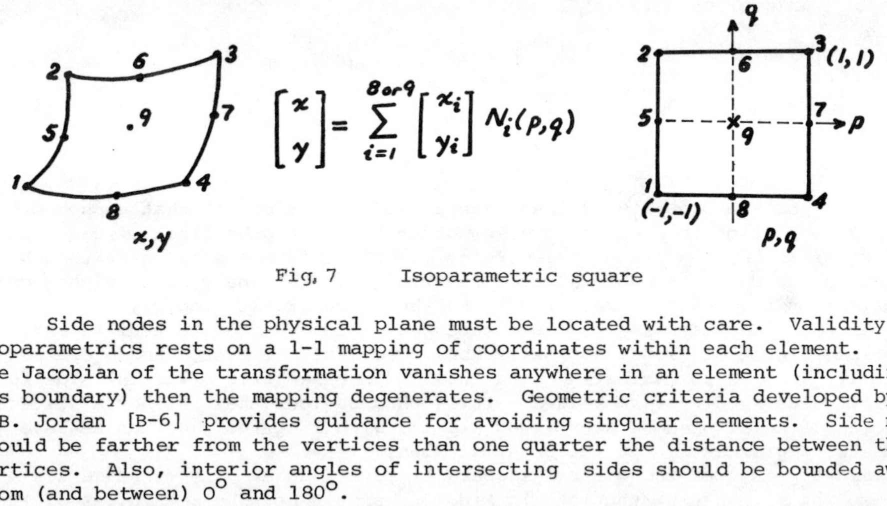

Fig. 7 Isoparametric square

Side nodes in the physical plane must be located with care. Validity of isoparametrics rests on a 1-1 mapping of coordinates within each element. If the Jacobian of the transformation vanishes anywhere in an element (including its boundary) then the mapping degenerates. Geometric criteria developed by W.B. Jordan [B-6] provides guidance for avoiding singular elements. Side nodes should be farther from the vertices than one quarter the distance between the vertices. Also, interior angles of intersecting sides should be bounded away from (and between) 0° and 180°.

Three-dimensional isoparametric elements are generated with degree-two bases for regular tetrahedra and cubes. The twenty-node brick is a popular element. Criteria for avoiding singular Jacobians are less well established in three dimensions. One should deviate as little as possible from cubes and regular tetrahedra. Side nodes should be centered on edges.

A "serendipity" element has only boundary nodes with just enough of them to guarantee interelement continuity with prescribed boundary variation. In two dimensions, a "Lagrangian" element includes in addition to the boundary nodes all interior nodes at intersections of lines connecting boundary nodes of like p or q. All elements achieve degree-one approximation in local (p,q) and global (x,y) coordinates. Lagrangian elements achieve higher degree local approximation. Members of these families are shown (in the isoparametric coordinate plane) in Fig. 8. with additional Lagrangian nodes indicated by ⊗.

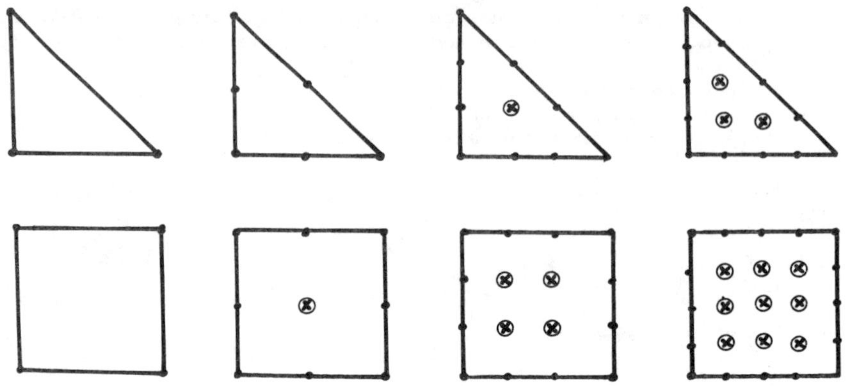

Fig. 8 Serendipity and Lagrangian elements

Basis functions for the six node triangle are given in Fig. 3. The basis functions for the eight-node isoparametric square are:

$$
\begin{aligned}
N_1(p,q) &= -\tfrac{1}{4}(1-q)(1-p)(1+p+q) \\
N_2(p,q) &= -\tfrac{1}{4}(1+q)(1-p)(1+p-q) \\
N_3(p,q) &= -\tfrac{1}{4}(1+q)(1+p)(1-p-q) \\
N_4(p,q) &= -\tfrac{1}{4}(1-q)(1+p)(1-p+q) \\
N_5(p,q) &= \tfrac{1}{2}(1-p)(1-q^2) \\
N_6(p,q) &= \tfrac{1}{2}(1+q)(1-p^2) \\
N_7(p,q) &= \tfrac{1}{2}(1+p)(1-q^2) \\
N_8(p,q) &= \tfrac{1}{2}(1-q)(1-p^2)
\end{aligned} \qquad (22)
$$

An important property of these cubic basis functions is that each has quadratic variation in p on lines of constant q and in q on lines of constant p. Any linear combination of these functions has this property, even though the combination need not be a biquadratic function. In the analysis of higher order approximation this will be referred to as the "biquadratic property."

Higher order isoparametric elements can be constructed to achieve any prescribed degree of <u>global</u> approximation. One must, however, choose elements carefully. Degree-two variation on a curved (isoparametric parabola) side is uniquely determined by five values. It is thus obvious that neither a six-node triangle nor an eight-node four-sided element with a curved side can achieve degree-two approximation in the physical plane.

First, consider the general isoparametric triangle. The standard six-node mapping with basis functions in Fig. 3 should be used regardless of the desired degree of approximation. Then to achieve degree-k global approximation one should construct the degree-2k element in the p,q plane. The x,y values of added nodes should be determined from the six-node mapping. The procedure is illustrated for degree-two approximation:

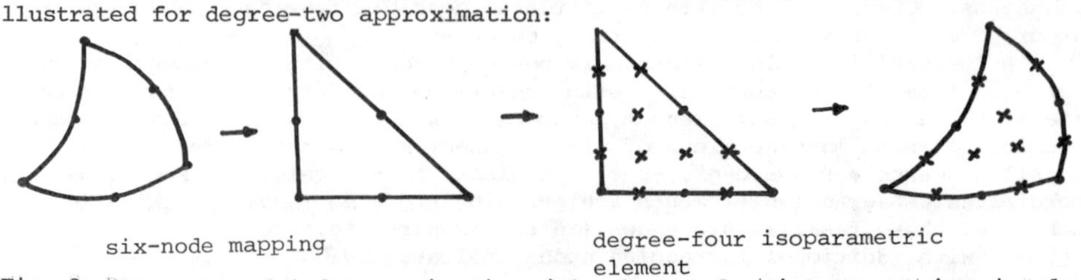

Fig. 9 Degree-two global approximation with a degree-four isoparametric triangle.

The mapping yields x and y quadratic in p and q. Any polynomial of maximal degree two in x and y is mapped into a polynomial of maximal degree four in p and q. The 15-node degree-four isoparametric element interpolates polynomials through degree four with no error. The interior-node degrees of freedom may be removed by static condensation.

Fewer nodes are needed if only one or two sides are curved. For a triangle with only one curved side, the element in Fig. 10 achieves degree two in the physical plane.

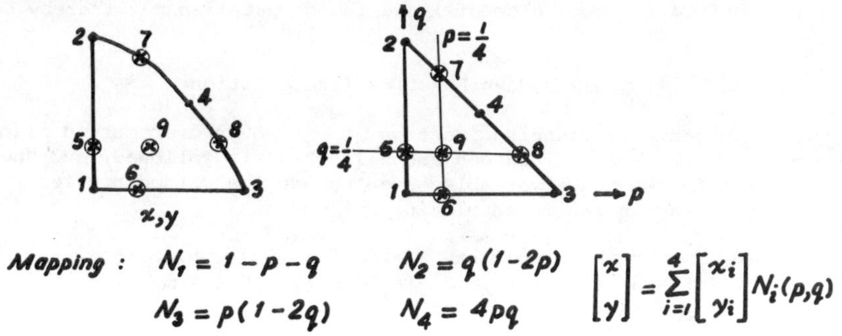

Fig. 10 Degree-two triangle with one curved side

⊗ in p,q determines location of ⊗ in x,y

The isoparametric basis is:

$$
\begin{aligned}
N_1(p,q) &= (1 - p - q)(1 - 4p)(1 - 4q) \\
N_2(p,q) &= \frac{1}{3}q(4q - 1)(1 - 4p)(1 - 2p) \\
N_3(p,q) &= N_2(q,p) \\
N_4(p,q) &= 4pq(4p - 1)(4q - 1) \\
N_5(p,q) &= \frac{16}{3}q(1 - p - q)(1 - 4p) \\
N_6(p,q) &= N_5(q,p) \\
N_7(p,q) &= \frac{16}{3}pq(4q - 1)(1 - 2p) \\
N_8(p,q) &= N_7(q,p) \\
N_9(p,q) &= 32pq(1 - p - q)
\end{aligned}
\tag{23}
$$

The interpolation error for a quadratic function of x and y is at most quartic in p and q and has the "biquadratic property". The error vanishes on the perimeter and on the lines $p = \frac{1}{4}$ and $q = \frac{1}{4}$. By Theorem 2.1, the error is the zero polynomial. Degree-two global approximation has been demonstrated. The interior degree of freedom may be removed by static condensation.

Higher degree approximation is achieved in similar fashion for four-sided elements. The simplest case is that of the convex straight-sided quadrilateral. The four-node degree-one mapping with the bilinear basis functions:

$$
\begin{aligned}
N_1(p,q) &= \tfrac{1}{4}(1 - p)(1 - q) \qquad & N_2(p,q) &= \tfrac{1}{4}(1 - p)(1 + q) \\
N_3(p,q) &= \tfrac{1}{4}(1 + p)(1 + q) \qquad & N_4(p,q) &= \tfrac{1}{4}(1 + p)(1 - q)
\end{aligned}
\tag{24}
$$

determines the location in the physical plane of nodes 5-9 in the degree-two Lagrangian element. (The side nodes 5-8 are at the side midpoints and the coordinates of the interior node are the averages of the vertex coordinates.) The (at most) quartic error in degree-two interpolation has the biquadratic property and hence must vanish identically.

For the general four-sided element, the eight-node or nine-node mapping yields x and y with the biquadratic property in p and q. Then the 25-node degree-four isoparametric square in Fig. 8 has a biquartic basis. Physical coordinates of the added 16 or 17 nodes are determined from the mapping. Application of Theorem 2.1 establishes degree-two approximation in x,y. The interior nodes may be eliminated by static condensation. The element may be chosen so that the interior nodes are at Gaussian quadrature points (three-by-three quadrature is often appropriate for such elements) and the computation may thereby be simplified.

Blending Function Interpolation

In this section, blending function interpolation over curved elements is discussed. The approach of Gordon and Hall [A-5] is followed, and the analysis is restricted to two space variables even though the method applies to any number of variables. Lagrangian interpolation polynomials

$$\phi_i(s) = \prod_{j\neq i} (s - s_j) \Big/ \prod_{j\neq i} (s_i - s_j), \quad 0 \le i \le m \qquad (25)$$

$$0 = s_o < s_1 < \ldots < s_m = h$$

$$\psi_j(t) = \prod_{i\neq j} (t - t_i) \Big/ \prod_{i\neq j} (t_j - t_i), \quad 0 \le j \le n \qquad (26)$$

$$0 = t_o < t_1 < \ldots < t_n = h$$

are used as blending functions. Let f(s,t) be defined on the square $[0 \le s \le h,\ 0 \le t \le h]$, and define the projectors

$$P_s[f] = \sum_{i=o}^{m} f(s_i,t)\ \phi_i(s); \qquad P_t[f] = \sum_{j=o}^{n} f(s,t_j)\ \psi_j(t) \qquad (27)$$

$$P_{st}[f] = P_s[f] + P_t[f] - P_s[P_t[f]]$$

It can be shown [A-5] that the interpolant $P_{st}[f]$ is equal to f along lines s_i and lines t_j. This is called "transfinite bivariate Lagrangian interpolation" by Gordon and Hall. The simplest useful interpolation is with the linear blending functions:

$$\phi_0(s) = 1 - s/h,\ \phi_1(s) = s/h,\ \psi_0(t) = 1 - t/h,\ \psi_1(t) = t/h \qquad (28)$$

in which case the interpolation is "transfinite bilinear Lagrangian."

The square may be mapped onto a curved element with parametrized boundary curves on each of its sides:

$$\begin{aligned} x &= f_1(s,t_j), \quad y = f_2(s,t_j) \qquad \text{for } j = 0,n \\ x &= f_1(s_i,t), \quad y = f_2(s_i,t) \qquad \text{for } i = 0,m \end{aligned} \qquad (29)$$

(When the f are rational functions of s and t, these are rational algebraic curves. Theory for constructing basis functions directly in the x,y coordinates for elements bounded by such curves is given later in this chapter.

A discrete form of blending interpolation may be used. Let

$$\bar{P}_t[f(s_i,t)] = \sum_{j=0}^{\bar{n}} f(s_i,\bar{t}_j)\ \bar{\psi}_j(t), \quad 0 = \bar{t}_0 < \bar{t}_1 \ldots < \bar{t}_{\bar{n}} = h. \qquad (30)$$

Then

$$\bar{P}_t P_s[f] = \sum_{i=o}^{m} \sum_{j=o}^{\bar{n}} f(s_i,\bar{t}_j)\phi_i(s)\bar{\psi}_j(t) \qquad (31)$$

is a discrete approximation to $P_s[f]$ that uses values of f only at points $(s_i, \bar{t}_j)$. In particular, if the $\bar{\psi}_j$ are the quadratic interpolation polynomials $(\bar{n} = 2)$, then curve f is approximated by the isoparametric parabola. Moreover, the mapping

$$\tilde{f}(m,n,\bar{m},\bar{n}) = (\bar{P}_t P_s + \bar{P}_s P_t - P_s P_t)\ [f] \qquad (32)$$

is a discrete approximation of transfinite bivariate Lagrangian interpolation. A family of approximations may be generated in this manner.

When the discrete aproximation in Eq. (32) is used, the barred and unbarred sets of s_i and t_j need not be related. If, however, one seeks an interpolatory formula, then a natural condition is that the barred sets, $\{\bar{s}_i\}$ and $\{\bar{t}_j\}$, contain the unbarred sets, $\{s_i\}$ and $\{t_j\}$, respectively. This ensures that $\tilde{f} = f$ at the $(\bar{m} + 1)(\bar{n} + 1) - (\bar{m} - m)(\bar{n} - n)$ points

$$\begin{array}{lll} (s_i,\bar{t}_j), & 0 \le i \le m, & 0 \le j \le \bar{n} \\ (\bar{s}_i,t_j), & i \in \{k \mid \bar{s}_k \notin \{s_i\}\}, & 0 \le j \le n. \end{array} \qquad (33)$$

The element mapping and the function approximation may be based on the same interpolation formulas just as in the isoparametric method. This is not essential. One may map a known boundary curve accurately while using a low order discrete function approximation on that boundary.

Basis functions are, in general, of some chosen degree in the s,t coordinates. The mapping relating s,t to x,y is generally nonlinear, so the degree of approximation in the global (x,y) coordinates is usually not greater than one. Discretization error bounds depend on the Jacobian of the mapping over the element.

In any event, the mapping and function approximation on any element boundary is made consistent for two elements sharing a boundary segment. This ensures continuity across the interface.

Degree-one approximation is attained when the interpolation and mapping are the same (isoparametric method) and may not be achieved when they differ. The degree of approximation often plays a key role in determining convergence characteristics of finite element computation so that the more general blending technique must be used with care. This is discussed further in the next section.

RATIONAL BASES FOR ALGEBRAIC ELEMENTS

Construction of Rational Bases

Polynomial basis functions that achieve continuous patchwork approximation exist for a limited set of element geometries. In two dimensions this includes triangles, parallelograms, and some obscure shapes of little practical interest. Polynomials in isoparametric coordinates provide a generalization for approximation over a wider class of three- and four-sided elements. If one extends the class of basis functions from polynomials to rational functions, then the class of allowable element geometries is broadened considerably. The extended class of elements is that of "well-set algebraic" elements, which will now be defined for two-space.

The closed boundary of an <u>algebraic element</u> is a specified set of segments of simple (irreducible) algebraic curves, each containing only simple points of its curve, with each segment defining a <u>side</u> of the element and adjacent segments meeting at <u>vertices</u>. The element is <u>well-set</u> if the vertices are ordinary intersection points of adjacent curves (that is, the curves do not have a common tangent at a vertex) and if the curve on which a boundary segment lies contains no point, other than that segment, on the boundary of or interior to the element. A curve is rational if it has a rational parametrization. Theory for construction of basis functions is more definitive when each boundary component is a rational curve. It will be assumed in the ensuing discussion that all boundary components are rational curves.

A simple introduction to the role of rational functions is provided by construction of a degree-one basis for a convex quadrilateral (Fig. 11) It was observed at the end of the section on polynomial bases in global coordinates

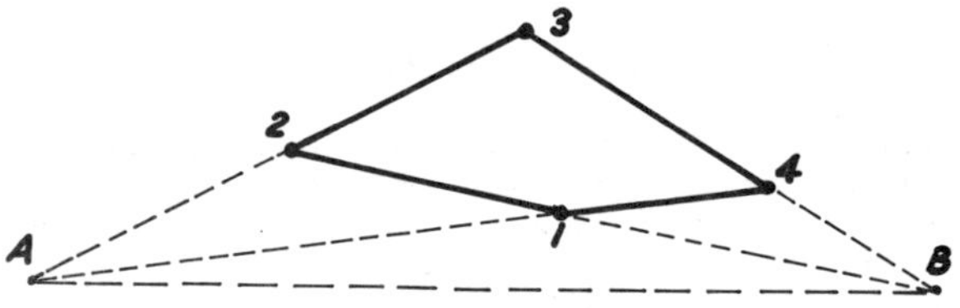

Fig. 11. A convex quadrilateral

that parallel opposite sides were essential in order that the bilinear form (2;3)(3;4) have linear variation on sides (1;4) and (1;2). In Fig. 11, line (A;B) is the exterior diagonal of the quadrilateral. For any convex quadrilateral, (A;B) is nonzero over the quadrilateral. A convex quadrilateral is a well-set algebraic element. The "well-set" condition is a generalization for the class of algebraic elements of "convexity" for polygonal elements.

Consider the rational basis function candidate:

$$N_1(x,y) = (2;3)_1(3;4)_1/(A;B)_1 \tag{34}$$

It will first be shown that N_1 varies linearly on sides (1;4) and(1;2). These are the sides on which N_1 has nonzero values and are called the "adjacent" sides of node-1.

Let $L_1(x,y)$, $L_2(x,y)$ and $L_3(x,y)$ be linear forms such that the lines on which $L_s(x,y) = 0$ are distinct. A necessry and sufficient condition for the existence of nonzero constants a, b, c such that

$$a\,L_1(x,y) + b\,L_2(x,y) + c\,L_3(x,y) = 0$$

is that the three lines be concurrent. (All lines of the same slope meet at a common point at infinity. This is made more precise in the projective plane where the "line at infinity" is mapped into the visible "absolute line".)

In Fig. 11, lines (2;3), (1;4) and (A;B) are concurrent (at point A). Therefore; one may write

$$a\,(2;3)_1 + b(1;4) + c\,(A;B)_1 = 0$$

and since $(2;3)_1 = (A;B)_1 = 1$ at node-1, $c = -a$. Thus,

$$(2;3)_1 = (-b/a)\,(1;4) + (A;B)_1$$

It follows that

$$N_1(x,y) = (2;3)_1(3;4)_1/(A;B)_1 = (3;4)_1 \bmod (1;4)$$

Similar reasoning with lines (1;2), (3;4) and (A;B) yields

$$N_1(x,y) = (2;3)_1 \bmod (1;2)$$

The other three basis function candidates for degree-one approximation are:

$$N_2(x,y) = (3;4)_2(4;1)_2/(A;B)_2$$

$$N_3(x,y) = (4;1)_3(1;2)_3/(A;B)_3$$

$$N_4(x,y) = (1;2)_4(2;3)_4/(A;B)_4 \qquad (35)$$

Let $L(x,y)$ be of maximal degree one. Then the interpolation error in approximating L with these basis functions is

$$D(x,y) = L(x,y) - \sum_{i=1}^{4} L(x_i,y_i)N_i(x,y) = \frac{[L(x,y)\ (A;B)_1 + P_2(x,y)]}{(A;B)_1} \qquad (36)$$

where P_2 is a polynomial of maximal degree two which depends on L. Since the basis functions are linear on each side, D must vanish over the perimeter of the quadrilateral. The perimeter is a curve of order four with simple components. By Theorem 2.1, polynomial $(A;B)_1D(x,y)$, of maximal degree two, must be the zero polynomial. This establishes degree-one approximation, and the basis function candidates are validated.

To achieve degree-two approximation, one introduces a node on each side (Fig. 12) and uses basis functions exemplified by

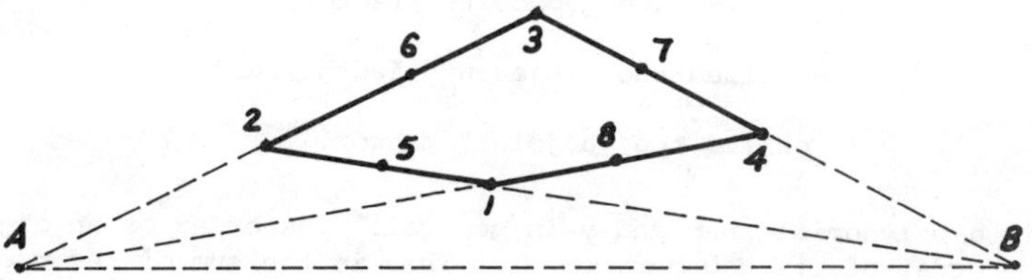

Fig. 12. Degree-two quadrilateral approximation

$$N_1(x,y) = (2;3)_1(3;4)_1(5;8)_1/(A;B)_1$$

$$N_5(x,y) = (2;3)_5(3;4)_5(4;1)_5/(A;B)_5 \qquad (37)$$

Each basis function now has either quadratic variation or vanishes on a side. The interpolation error for any quadratic $Q(x,y)$ vanishes on the perimeter. The previous argument with $(A;B)D(x,y)$ now a polynomial of maximal degree three suffices to prove that $D(x,y)$ is zero over the quadrilateral (where the basis functions are well-defined).

For degree-three and higher degrees of approximation, more nodes must be introduced on the boundary. Additional interior nodes are also needed. This is described in detail in [B-5].

Two aspects of the construction warrant emphasis. First the denominator common to all basis functions for a given element is defined precisely by the element boundary curve and is bounded away from zero over the element. Second, even though the basis functions are rational they provide a basis for polynomial approximation.

The quadrilateral construction generalizes in several directions. Mathematical foundations are provided by some sophisticated results drawn from the field of mathematics known as algebraic-geometry. This theory resolves difficulties associated with multiple points of curves and with complicated structure at intersection points of curves. Application of algebraic-geometry to construction of finite element basis functions is developed in detail in [B-5].

An example of the need for refinement of simple concepts is provided by Bezout's theorem in which it is asserted that there are st elements in the intersection set of a curve of order s with a curve of order t. How does one allow for the fact that two parallel lines do not intersect? The curve $y - x^2$ intersects the line $y = 0$ at the origin only, even though $st = 2$ in this case. It would seem at first glance that two circles meet in zero, one or two points. But Bezout says they always meet in four points. One must learn how to count intersection points. The set of points common to curves F and G in a generalized sense is called the "divisor of F on G" (or of G on F). The key theorem for basis function construction is a derivative of analysis by Max Noether over a hundred years ago:

<u>Theorem 2.2</u> Let polynomials P and S have no common component and let T be an irreducible curve. Then $P \equiv S \bmod T$ if and only if the divisors of P and S on T are identical. (The symbol $P \equiv S$ here denotes existence of a constant b for which $P - bS = 0$ at all points on curve T).

Rational basis functions may be constructed to achieve any prescribed degree of approximation over any given well-set algebraic element in two or three space variables. The construction developed in [B-5] is too complex to be described here, and just a few of the salient features will be exposed. Theorem 2.2 will be applied to verify desired properties of the basis functions for an example. Only two-dimensional elements will be considered here.

Each basis function is of the form

$$N_i(x,y) = k_i \frac{P^i R^i}{Q} \tag{38}$$

where k_i normalizes N_i to unity at (x_i, y_i),

P^i is called the "opposite" factor,

R^i is called the "adjacent" factor, and

Q is called the "adjoint" factor.

Each factor is a polynomial in x and y in general. The order of an algebraic element is the order of its boundary curve. This is the sum of the orders of the sides. The order of a straight-sided quadrilateral is, for example, four. The multiple points of the boundary curve of order m determine a unique adjoint curve of maximal order $m - 3$. The polynomial of least degree that vanishes everywhere on this curve is the adjoint factor common to all basis functions for the element. The opposite factor is the polynomial of least degree that vanishes over all boundary components which do not contain node i. The adjacent factor depends on several things and is best described for a specific example. The key properties which determine the unique rational basis for a given element are:

1. Each basis function is a rational function of x and y,

2. The functions are chosen so that $N_i(x_j, y_j) = \delta_{ij} \begin{array}{l} = 1 \text{ if } i = j \\ = 0 \text{ if } i \neq j, \end{array}$ (6.6)

3. N_i either vanishes or has degree k variation on each side for degree k approximation over the element, and

4. For any polynomial F of maximal degree k,

$$F(x,y) - \sum_i F(x_i; y_i) N_i(x,y) = 0 \tag{39}$$

over the element.

The element in Fig. 13 is of order five. The construction increases in complexity as the orders of the side components increase. An element with only linear sides is a convex polygon. An element with only linear and conic sides but having at least one conic side is called a "polycon."

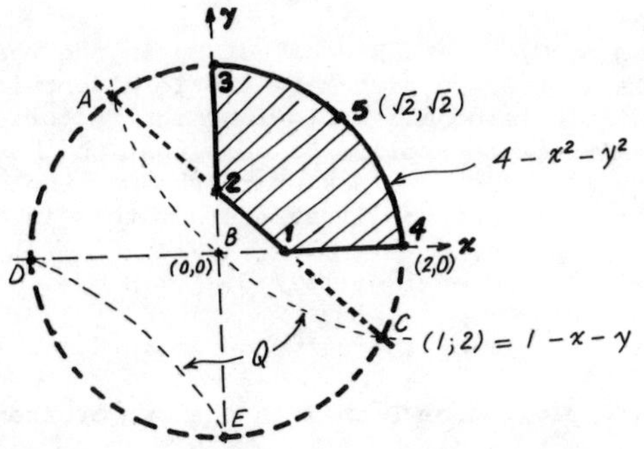

Fig. 13. A four-sided polycon of order five

In general, the adjoint Q is determined by the multiple points of the element boundary. Let p range over all nonvertex multiple points of the boundary and let r_p be the multiplicity at p. (The concept of "neighborhoods" is introduced for nonordinary multiple points at which intersecting branches of the boundary curve have common tangents. For this discussion, it is convenient to assume that all boundary multiple points are ordinary.) The adjoint is the <u>unique</u> curve of maximal order m - 3, where m is the order of the element, that has multiplicity r - 1 at p. In Fig. 13, points A, B, C, D, and E determine a unique conic on which

$$Q = x^2 + y^2 + 4xy + 2x + 2y \tag{40}$$

vanishes.

For degree-one approximation over the element there is a node at each vertex and on the conic side. The adjacent factors for nodes 1, 2 and 5 are unity. The basis functions for these nodes are:

$$\begin{aligned} N_1(x,y) &= x(4 - x^2 - y^2)/Q(x,y) \\ N_2(x,y) &= x(4 - x^2 - y^2)/Q(x,y) \\ N_5(x,y) &= 2xy(x + y - 1)(1 + \sqrt{2})/Q(x,y) \end{aligned} \tag{41}$$

The adjacent factors for nodes 3 and 4 are (5;E) and (5;D), respectively. The basis functions for these nodes are

$$\begin{aligned} N_3(x,y) &= y(y + x - 1)[y + 1 - (1 + 1/\sqrt{2})x]/Q(x,y) \\ N_4(x,y) &= x(y + x - 1)[x + 1 - (1 + 1/\sqrt{2})y]/Q(x,y) \end{aligned} \tag{42}$$

The only polycon adjacent-factor construction not illustrated by this element is for a vertex node at the intersection of two conic sides. The adjacent factor in that case is a quadratic form that vanishes on the conic determined by the two side-nodes on the conic sides that meet at the vertex and the three nonvertex intersections of those sides (Fig. 14).

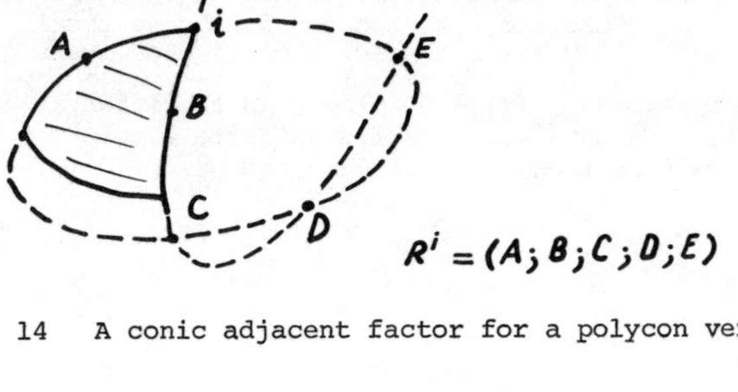

Fig. 14 A conic adjacent factor for a polycon vertex

Note that two of C, D, and E need not be in the real plane. Coallescing of multiple points is treated with more subtle algebraic-geometry concepts. In any case, coefficients of all basis function factors are always real.

Theorem 2.2 may now be applied to show that the basis functions in Eqs. (41) and (42) vary linearly on sides where they are not identically zero. Function N_3 will be examined to illustrate how this is done. Let

$$P = (1;4)(1;2)(5;E), \quad S = (4;5)Q, \text{ and}$$

$$T \text{ be the curve on which } 4 - x^2 - y^2 = 0$$

in Theorem 2. The divisor of P on T is the sum of the divisors of its components:

$$\begin{aligned} P\circ T &= (1;4)\circ T + (1;2)\circ T + (5;E)\circ T \\ &= \{D, 4, A, C, 5, E\} \end{aligned}$$

The divisor of S on T is

$$\begin{aligned} S\circ T &= (4;5)\circ T + Q\circ T \\ &= \{4, 5, A, C, D, E\} \end{aligned}$$

Thus, $P\circ T = S\circ T$ and by Theorem 2, $P \equiv S \bmod T$. Since N_3 is normalized to unity at node 3:

$$N_3 = k_3(1;4)(1;2)(5;E)/Q = (4;5)_3 \bmod (4 - x^2 - y^2)$$

Now let T be the y-axis and let X be any point not on T. Then $P\circ T = \{B, 2, E\}$ and $S = (2;X)Q$ has the divisor $S\circ T = \{2, B, E\}$. Therefore, $N_3 = (2;X)_3 \bmod X$.

Having demonstrated linearity of the basis functions on the sides in this fashion, one verifies that degree-one approximation is achieved by noting that the deviation of the linear interpolant times Q is a polynomial of maximal degree three that vanishes on the perimeter which is a curve of order five with no multiple components. By Theorem 1, the deviation must vanish over the entire element.

Polynomial bases are desirable. Values, derivatives, and indefinite integrals of polynomials are easily obtained. Integration over complex geometric configurations is problematic, and one often resorts to approximate numerical quadrature. Rational functions share many of the beneficial properties of polynomials with the notable exception of easy evaluation of integrals. Rational bases arise, however, for element geometry requiring numerical quadrature in any case.

There are certain geometries for which integrals required over the elements are easily evaluated in closed form. These elements will be considered in the next subsection.

The construction of rational basis functions provides insight which suggests modifications to isoparametric and blending function techniques to enhance their effectiveness.

A Practicable Algebraic Element

There is a class of algebraic elements for which numerical application is quite practicable. Consider a region bounded by vertical lines $x = a$ and $x = b$ and by the curves $y - Q_1(x) = 0$ and $y - Q_2(x) = 0$, where Q_1 and Q_2 are polynomials in x for which $Q_1(x) - Q_2(x) \neq 0$ in the interval [a, b]. This region may be partitioned into elements for a finite element computation with each element of the type shown in Fig. 15. Let $Q(x) = Q_2(x) - Q_1(x)$ and define

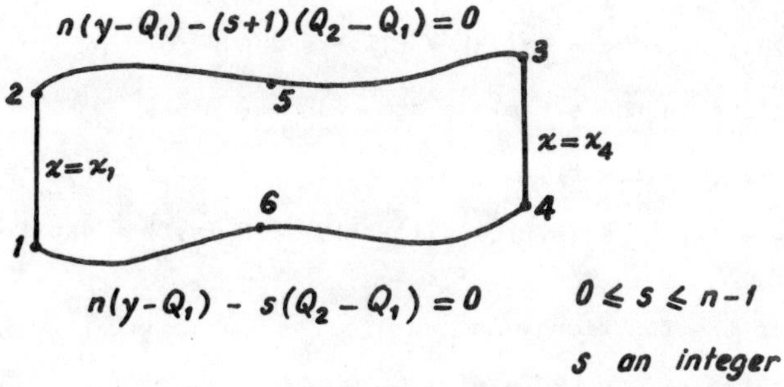

Fig. 15. A general element of the partitioned region

$y' = y - Q_1(x)$. Then the basis functions for degree-one approximation are all of the form

$$N_i(x,y') = (ny' - gQ)P^i(x)/Q(x)\ , \quad g = s,\ s+1 \tag{43}$$

where Q is common to all basis functions for all elements in the partition and P^i is a polynomial of the same degree as Q which varies over the nodes and elements. Integrals usually required for finite element discretization are easily evaluated (analytically) over these elements with these rational basis functions.

Consider, for example, an element with $Q_1 = 0$ and $Q_2 = 1 + x/4 - x^3/48$. Side nodes (nodes 5 and 6 in Fig. 15) may be chosen at $x = 1/2(x_1 + x_4)$. The basis function for node 5 is then

$$N_5(x,y) = \frac{8(x - x_1)(x_4 - x)(x + x_1 + x_4)(ny - sQ(x))}{3(x_1 + x_4)(x_4 - x_1)^2\ Q(x)} \tag{44}$$

Note that the factor $(x + x_1 + x_4)$ is the adjacent factor and that basis functions constructed in this manner yield degree-one approximation over the element.

A comparison with blending functions is most revealing. The algebra is simplified if one considers the element in Fig. 16, but the results apply in general. The transfinite blending element of Gordon and Hall (Ref. [A-5] and the previous section) relates this element to a unit square. The straightforward blending approximation yields only degree zero approximation over the element. More sophisticated third-order isoparametric blending would yield degree-one approximation. Any prescribed degree of approximation can be attained directly in the global coordinates with rational basis functions. This is illustrated by detailed study of the element shown in Fig. 16.

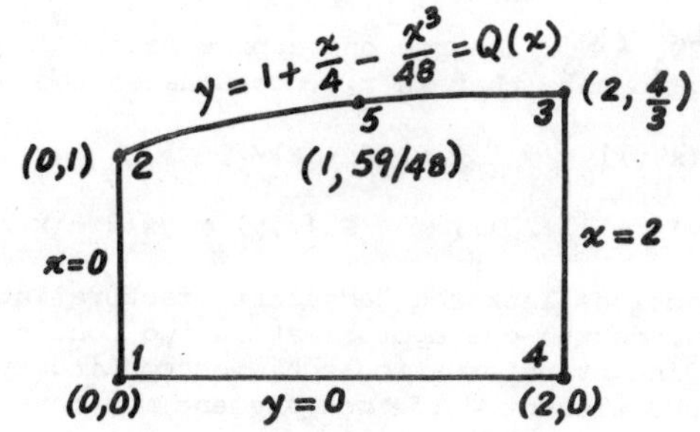

Fig. 16. A specific element

A transfinite bilinear Lagrangian mapping that transforms the unit square in (s,t) coordinates into this element is

$$x = 2s \qquad y = tQ(2s) = t(1 + s/2 - s^3/6) \tag{45}$$

The basis functions in the s,t plane are

$$N_1(s,t) = (1 - s)(1 - t), \qquad N_2(s,t) = t(1 - 2s)(1 - s)$$
$$N_3(s,t) = st(2s - 1), \quad N_4(s,t) = s(1 - t), \quad N_5(s,t) = 4st(1 - s) \tag{46}$$

The expansion of the function y is

$$y \sim \sum_{i=1}^{5} y_i N_i(s,t) = N_2 + \frac{4}{3} N_3 + \frac{59}{48} N_5$$
$$= t(1 - 2s)(1 - s) + \frac{4}{3} st(2s - 1) + \frac{59}{12} st(1 - s)$$
$$= t(1 + \frac{7}{12} s - \frac{s^2}{4})$$
$$= y \frac{(1 + \frac{7}{12} s - \frac{s^2}{4})}{(1 + \frac{s}{2} - \frac{s^3}{6})} = y \frac{(1 + \frac{7}{24} x - \frac{x^2}{16})}{1 + \frac{x}{4} - \frac{x^3}{48}} \tag{47}$$

The approximation has no error at the nodes, but degree one is not attained with this approximation.

The rational basis functions for this element are

$$N_2(x,y) = y(2 - x)\ (1 - x)\ (3 + x)/6Q(x)$$
$$N_3(x,y) = yx(x^2 - 1)/6Q(x) \tag{48}$$
$$N_5(x,y) = yx(4 - x^2)/3Q(x)$$

and now

$$y \sim N_2 + \frac{4}{3} N_3 + \frac{59}{48} N_5$$
$$= \frac{y}{Q} [\frac{(2 - x)(1 - x)(3 + x)}{6} + \frac{2}{9} x(x^2 - 1) + \frac{59}{3 \cdot 48} x(4 - x^2)] \tag{49}$$
$$= \frac{y}{Q} [1 + \frac{x}{4} - \frac{x^3}{48}] = y$$

Similarly, $x = 2N_3 + 2N_4 + N_5$. Degree one approximation is attained.

It is interesting to note that in x,y coordinates the blending bases are

$$N_2[s(x,y),t(x,y)] = y(1 - x)(2 - x)/2Q(x)$$
$$N_3(x,y) = yx(x - 1)/2Q(x) \qquad N_5(x,y) = yx(2 - x)/Q(x) \tag{50}$$

The blending basis functions lack the "adjacent" factors introduced in the rational bases to achieve degree-one approximation and continuity along element interfaces. The blending transformation achieves continuity but not degree-one approximation within the element. The new element may thus be considered as a corrected blending-function element.

The rational basis may be expressed in s,t coordinates as:

$$N_1(s,t) = (1-t)(1-s)$$
$$N_2(s,t) = t(1-s)(1-2s)(3+2s)/3$$
$$N_3(s,t) = st(4s^2-1)/3 \qquad (51)$$
$$N_4(s,t) = s(1-t)$$
$$N_5(x,t) = 8ts(1-s^2)/3$$

For this particular element, the rational functions indicate how one may modify the blending functions to achieve degree-one approximation. It is not true in general that rational basis functions can be expressed as polynomials in transformed coordinates obtained by the blending function approach. This is always possible for elements of the type shown in Fig. 15.

GENERALIZED ISOPARAMETRICS

The "higher order transformation" method introduced by McLeod [A-7] is applicable to a variety of geometries and will be described here for the simple case of degree-two approximation over a three-sided element having only one curved side. As in the standard isoparametric method, the curved side is approximated by a parabolic arc via the mapping

$$\begin{vmatrix} x \\ y \end{vmatrix} = \sum_{i=1}^{6} \begin{vmatrix} x_i \\ y_i \end{vmatrix} N_i(p,q) \qquad (52)$$

with isoparametric basis functions N_i given in Fig. 3. There are five degrees of freedom in the general quadratic on a conic. To ensure continuity across a parabolic side, one must introduce two additional side nodes. These are nodes 7 and 8 in Fig. 17.

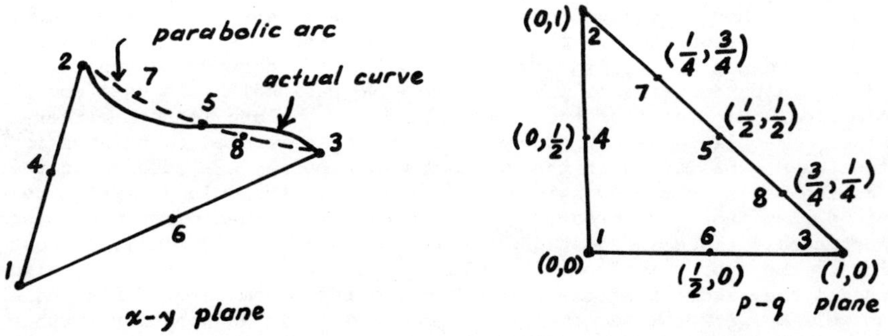

Fig. 17 A three-sided element with one curved side

Let $C_i(x,y)$, $i = 1, 2, \ldots, 6$, be a quadratic basis for Lagrangian interpolation over nodes 1 - 6. These six nodes do not all lie on any conic. Hence, the basis is uniquely determined by the discrete orthonormality conditions

$$C_i(x_j,y_j) = \delta_{ij};\ i = 1, 2, \ldots, 6$$

Having chosen nodes 7 and 8 in the p,q plane, one may locate these points in the x,y plane with the aid of Eq. (51) and obtain the linear forms $(5;8)_7$ and $(5;7)_8$ in x and y. Basis functions for nodes 7 and 8 may then be defined as

$$N_7(p, q, x, y) = 16pq(5;8)_7/3$$
$$N_8(p, q, x, y) = 16pq(5;7)_8/3 \qquad (53)$$

Degree-two approximation may now be achieved by replacing the six conventional N_i by

$$N_i(p, q, x, y) = C_i(x, y) - C_i(x_7,y_7)N_7(p,q,x,y) - C_i(x_8,y_8)N_8(p,q,x,y) \; ; \qquad (54)$$

$$i = 1, 2, \ldots, 6$$

The N_i are quadratic in p and q. Hence, Eq. (52) yields x and y as quadratics in p and q. The basis functions N_i are thus quartic in p,q. Since N_7 and N_8 vanish on the straight sides, the interpolant with this basis is at most quadratic in x and y on the straight sides. Interelement continuity is assured. The degree-two basis, $C_i(x,y)$, is contained in the N_i basis so that degree-two approximation is achieved.

McLeod applied this approach to elements with isoparametric transformations of higher order to obtain curves other than parabolas in p,q space, to approximation of degree greater than two, and to elements with more than four sides. For the latter, rational isoparametric bases were required. The algebra becomes more abstruse as the element becomes more complex.

There is some arbitrariness in choice of basis functions. A basis for degree-k approximation is of dimension (k+1)(k+2)/2. The number of nodes required for interelement continuity with degree-k variation on each side is greater than this (say n nodes). One chooses any [n - (k+1)(k+2)/2] of these nodes and defines associated basis functions as was done in Eq. (53), and one then generates the remaining basis functions from the degree-k Lagrangian interpolation basis as was done in Eq. (54).

The isoparametric mapping in (52) can be generalized to yield higher order curves in the x,y plane. For example, nodes 7 and 8 in Fig. 17 may be placed on the actual curve when the six basis functions in (51) are replaced by eight functions with an isoparametric cubic instead of a parabolic arc. Mitchell [A-8] indicated advantages of cubics for approximating element boundaries.

Isoparametric elements may have more than four sides. The key to isoparametrics is the identification of a basis in the p,q plane. The advantage of the isoparametric method is derived primarily from the existence of simple accurate quadrature formulas in the p,q plane. An element with n sides may be generated from a regular n-gon in the p,q plane. The most straightforward generalization of conventional isoparametrics is with a degree-two rational basis used for the transformation. Each side of the element in the x,y plane is then either straight or parabolic. Higher order curves may be generated by using a more sophisticated p,q basis. When the transformation basis is also used as the approximation basis, the conventional isoparametric methodology carries over to the n-sided elements. The presence of rational rather than polynomial bases is hardly noticeable since integrations are not performed analytically in most applications. The approximation is only of degree one, in general. Guidelines for bounding the Jacobian of the transformation away from zero within the element are less well known for more complex elements. This is an area for further research.

One may introduce the isoparametric mapping only for evaluation of integrals over elements. Rational basis functions may be constructed to achieve any desired degree of approximation directly in the x,y plane. The inverse isoparametric mapping is not needed for most computations. One sets quadrature points in the p,q plane first and then determines the corresponding x,y points. Values for integrands are then evaluated at these points. Frequently, the computer time used to set up finite element equations is not a significant portion of the total time. Complexity of incorporating sophisticated elements in a program limits utility of these elements. However, once an element is developed, gains in computational efficiency may be realized.

MACROELEMENTS

One may partition an element into sub-elements and express each element basis function in terms of the subelement bases. The result is a set of patchwork basis functions for the composite macroelement. Consider, for example, the macro-quadrilateral in Fig. 18. Let $N_i(x,y)$ for $i = 1, 2, 3, \ldots, 8$ be a basis for degree-two approximation over the quadrilateral. This basis could contain functions of a complicated form, but suppose values for N_i may be computed at nodes $s = 1, 2, \ldots, 13$ of the macroelement. Let $N_{sn}(x,y)$ denote the standard degree-two basis function for node s of triangle n, where s runs over the six nodes of the triangle. It can be shown that the patchwork basis

$$M_i(x,y) = \sum_{s(n)} N_i(x_s,y_s)N_{sn}(x,y) \quad , \quad x,y \text{ in } n, \quad n = 1, 2, 3, 4 \tag{55}$$

is a basis for degree-two approximation over the quadrilateral in Fig. 18.

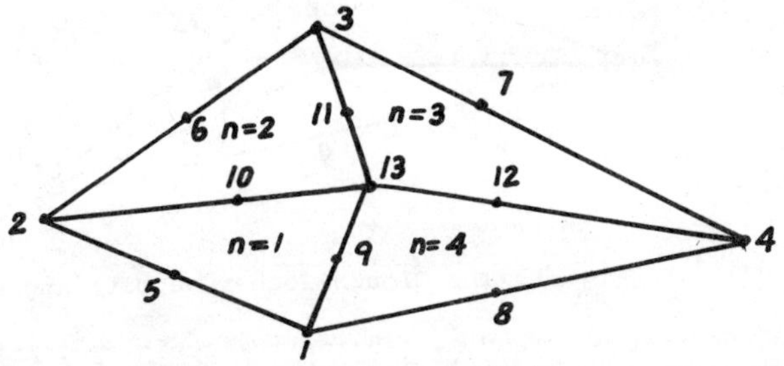

Fig. 18 A macroquadrilateral

For each triangle n and any given polynomial P of maximal degree two:

$$\begin{aligned}\sum_{i=1}^{8} P(x_i,y_i)M_i(x,y) &= \sum_{i=1}^{8} P(x_i,y_i)\sum_{s(n)} N_i(x_s,y_s)N_{sn}(x,y) \\ &= \sum_{s(n)}\Big[\sum_{i=1}^{8} P(x_i,y_i)N_i(x_s,y_s)\Big]N_{sn}(x,y) \\ &= \sum_{s(n)} P(x_s,y_s)N_{sn}(x,y) = P(x,y)\end{aligned} \tag{56}$$

This kind of approximation may have application, but for common finite element computation it is preferable not to restrict basis function values at interior nodes through definition of N_i for the macroelement. One may consider instead the four triangles as standard elements and eliminate the degrees of freedom at nodes 9 through 13 by static condensation, thereby arriving at the equivalent of a macroquadrilateral for the solution stage of the algorithm.

The relationship between this static condensation and choice of N_i at the outset is brought into focus by the following analysis. One distinguishes between two approximations made in finite element computation: the first is restriction of permitted function variation on element boundaries and the second is the number of degrees of freedom of the approximation within each element. For each well-posed finite element computation there is a "best" (in some sense usually related to a norm) approximation subject to the first (element boundary) constraint only. A particular set of "optimum" basis functions, dependent on the problem being solved, yields this best solution. Choice of a set of N_i for a macroelement restricts the degrees of freedom within the element and leads to a second approximation with properties dependent upon the shape of the N_i. The method of static condensation, on the other hand, yields the "best" patchwork approximation (within the element partitioning constraint imposed) to the optimum macroelement basis. As the interior degrees of freedom of the macroelement are increased with the variation on the boundary of fixed degree, the finite element equations obtained by static condensation approach the equation one would obtain with the optimum macroelement basis [B-5]. This basis is not usually known or of a form suitable for computation.

An entirely different motivation for use of macroelements is the desire to achieve higher order of continuity with fewer degrees of freedom in each element. The Clough-Tocher macrotriangle is a popular element for obtaining C^1 continuity with a triangular grid. In the second section it was noted that quintics are needed for C^1 approximation over a triangular grid, but that a patchwork cubic approximation is known. The element in Fig. 19 has

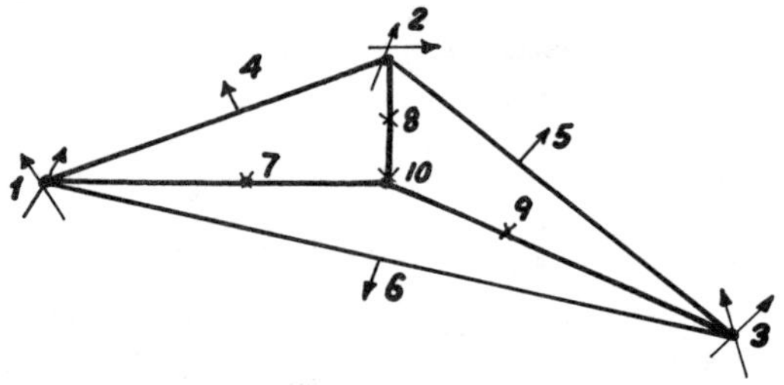

Fig. 19 The Clough-Tocher macrotriangle

a total of 30 degrees of freedom, ten for the cubic approximation in each triangle. Twenty-one of these degrees of freedom are used to fit values and first derivatives at the vertices, and normal derivatives at midpoints of the macroelement sides (nodes 4, 5, and 6). The interior degrees of freedom are constrained to yield C^1 continuity. At node 10, value and gradient are equated for the three subtriangles. This accounts for six degrees of freedom. Normal derivatives of adjacent triangles are equated at nodes 7, 8, and 9. This accounts for the remaining three degrees of freedom. The cubic variation on each subelement side is fixed by value and tangential derivatives at vertices. The quadratic normal derivative variation on each of these sides is fixed by values at vertices and midpoints. This macrotriangle cannot be considered a composite of triangular subelements with interior degrees of freedom removed by static condensation. The interior degrees of freedom are constrained by the continuity conditions. Use of the full cubic within each subelement would yield only C^0 continuity.

ADAPTIVE REFINEMENT AND HIERARCHIC BASES

Adaptive refinement has been approached in two ways. One may introduce a finer grid in a region over which observed discretization error is unacceptable [A-2], or one may increase the degree of approximation within some of the existing elements in this region [A-3]. Each approach requires new considerations regarding basis functions.

Mesh refinement is facilitated by use of nodes with restricted variation. In Fig. 20, element C has been subdivided into nine subelements. To maintain continuity across element interface (1;2), one may restrict variation at nodes 3 and 4. For equal spacing and nodal values u_i,

$$u_3 = (2u_1 + u_2)/3 \quad \text{and} \quad u_4 = (u_1 + 2u_2)/3 \tag{57}$$

retains linearity of the approximation along the side. This is often easier to implement than the introduction of transitional elements like B in Fig. 21.

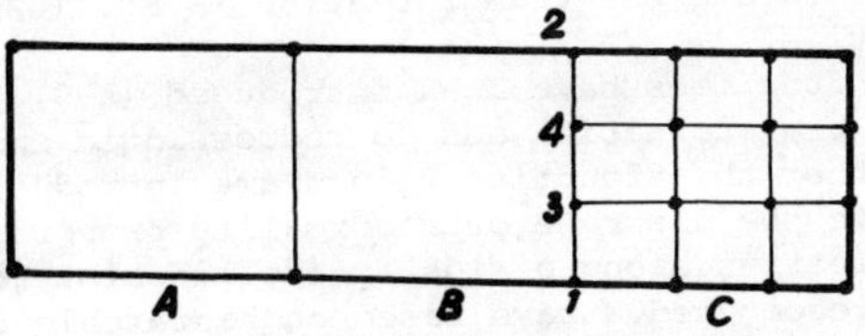

Fig. 20 Local refinement with restricted nodes

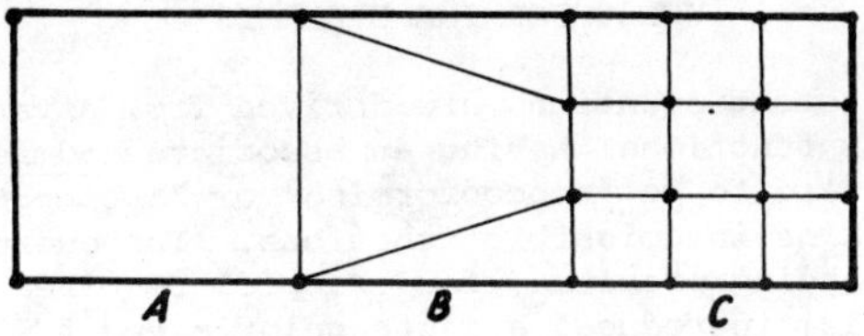

Fig. 21. Local refinement with transition elements

Similar interfacing is required when the degree of approximation is increased locally in the "p-version" of finite element computation [A-3]. Conventional degree-one and degree-two basis functions for rectangles are given in Eqs. (13) and (17). For example:

$$N_1^{(1)} = (2;3)_1(3;4)_1$$
$$N_1^{(2)} = (2;3)_1(3;4)_1(5;8)_1 \qquad (58)$$
$$N_5^{(2)} = (2;3)_5(3;4)_5(4;1)_5$$

If a computation with a degree-one basis is to be refined to degree-two over this element, one may retain the degree-one basis and append the degree-two side-node functions (for nodes 5-8). Appropriate linear combinations of these hybrid basis functions yield the standard degree-two basis. For example,

$$N_1^{(2)} = N_1^{(1)} - \frac{1}{2}(N_5^{(2)} + N_8^{(2)}) \qquad (59)$$

Although this reduces arithmetic for the refinement, the discrete orthogonality property, $N_i(x_j,y_j) = \delta_{ij}$, is lost.

Let matrix M be defined by

$$\underline{N}^{(1,2)} = M\underline{N}^{(2)} \qquad (60)$$

where the elements of $\underline{N}^{(2)}$ and $\underline{N}^{(1,2)}$ are the conventional and the hybrid basis functions, respectively. For example, $m_{11} = 1$, $m_{15} = m_{18} = \frac{1}{2}$, and the remaining elements in row one of M are zero. One may first generate stiffness matrix $B^{(1)}$ for degree-one approximation. This has presumably been done prior to the refinement. One next borders this matrix with the contribution from the appended side node bases:

$$B^{(1,2)} = \begin{bmatrix} B^{(1)} & B_{12} \\ B_{21} & B_{22} \end{bmatrix} \qquad (61)$$

The contribution for degree-two approximation with the standard basis functions is then obtained by a similarity transformation with M:

$$B^{(2)} = M^T B^{(1,2)} M \qquad (62)$$

Matrix M is easily obtained and the transformation in Eq. (62) requires relatively little computer time.

"Hierarchic" basis functions have been introduced [A-9] to eliminate the need for the similarity transformation and to reduce logic and arithmetic of refinement. Parameters other than function values are introduced at each level of approximation to preserve the discrete orthonormality property (Eq. (2)). For example, the second derivative along a side at its midpoint replaces the value at the midside node. Precomputed arrays based on hierarchic families permit convenient use of elements of different degrees in the same mesh with automatic matching at interfaces [A-10].

NONCONFORMING ELEMENTS

Discrete finite element equations are derived from a variational principle applied to a particular functional having an associated admissible trial function space. An element is said to be "nonconforming" or "incompatible" when the approximation space contains inadmissible functions. The energy functional commonly used for plate bending problems, for example, requires continuous trial functions. Wilson [A-12] introduced a rectangular element with two "nodeless" functions added to the usual four degree-one basis functions. These nodeless functions permitted discontinuous quadratic variation along element interfaces. In the notation of Fig. 4a, Wilson's added functions are:

$$N_5 = (1;4)(2;3) \qquad \text{and} \qquad N_6 = (1;2)(3;4) \tag{63}$$

To obtain a C^1 basis for the solution of problems like the biharmonic that require C^1 trial functions, one may use one of the elements previously discussed in the sections on properties of functions and macroelements. Alternatively, one may resort to a nonconforming element. A common practice with triangular elements is to fit values and gradients at vertices, thereby allowing discontinuous quadratic variation of normal derivatives along interfaces. Such elements have been used successfully, although "variational crime" [B-4] may not pay.

Several means have been devised to circumvent nonconformity. The functional may be generalized to admit a wider class of trial functions (Chap. 5 and 15). This results in additional contributions to the discrete equations from the discontinuities formerly ignored. A supplementary basis may be introduced to remove the discontinuity. For example, rational basis functions have been used to eliminate discontinuous normal derivatives across triangle interfaces.

a. Nonconforming C^1 element

b. Conforming C^1 element

Free parameters are nodal values and gradients (and perhaps centroid value).

Fig. 22. Nonconforming and conforming C^1 triangle elements

The ten-parameter (if one includes the value at the centroid) element in Fig. 22a almost achieves C^1 with degree-three approximation over the element. Unfortunately, the quadratic variation of the normal derivative along each side is not tied down uniquely by its vertex values. Supplementary rational basis functions are introduced (Fig. 22b) to tie down the normal derivatives at side midpoints. The function at node 5, for example, must have zero value on the perimeter, zero normal derivative all along sides (1;2) and (1;3), and quadratic variation of the normal derivative along (2;3). Let Q denote the quadratic that vanishes on the circle containing the triangle vertices (the circumscribed circle). Then the rational basis function associated with node 5 is:

$$N_5 = \frac{(1;2)^2(1;3)^2(2;3)}{Q} \tag{64}$$

The algebraic geometry theory (Theorem 2) facilitates proof that this function is appropriate. The only property that is not obvious is the quadratic variation of the normal derivative on side (2;3). This is verified by considering the intersections of the various factors with line (2;3):

$$\frac{\partial N_5}{\partial N} \equiv \frac{(1;2)^2(1;3)^2}{Q} \mod (2;3) \tag{65}$$

The intersection sets are:

$$\begin{aligned}(1;2)^2 \circ (2;3) &= \{2, 2\}\\ (1;3)^2 \circ (2;3) &= \{3, 3\}\\ Q \circ (2;3) &= \{2, 3\}\end{aligned} \tag{66}$$

Therefore,

$$(1;2)^2(1;3)^2 \equiv Q^2 \mod (2;3) \tag{67}$$

by Theorem 2. It follows that

$$\frac{(1;2)^2(1;3)^2}{Q} \equiv Q \mod (2;3) \tag{68}$$

and it has been shown that the normal derivative of N_5 along side (2;3) has quadratic variation.

The nonconforming element is more widely used than the conforming element with rational bases. It is not clear that the error reduction gained by the added functions justifies the increased work.

Theoretical justification for nonconforming elements has been attempted. One of the more successful indicators of merit is the "patch test." An element passes the patch test if there is no error in computed values in an element over which the true solution is linear. This presupposes the existence of an underlying degree-one basis. One should be suspicious of any element that does not pass the patch test. On the other hand, passing the test does not guarantee a satisfactory element. An attempt to generalize Wilson's element to convex quadrilaterals [A-11] led to mediocre results even when the added nodeless basis functions were chosen so that the patch test would be passed. Comparable results were obtained through use of "reduced quadrature" with the standard Wilson basis in isoparametric coordinates.

FITTING OF DERIVED FUNCTIONS

Let $u(\underline{x})$ be the finite element approximation to the solution of a problem obtained with nodal basis N_i:

$$u(\underline{x}) = u^i N_i(\underline{x}) \tag{69}$$

where repeated indices are summed over. Suppose one wishes to approximate a function of u with the same basis. The approximation

$$f(u) = [f(u)]^i N_i(\underline{x}) \tag{70}$$

is adequate when f has the same order continuity as u, but may not be feasible otherwise. A common example is when the N_i provide a basis for C^0 approximation and f is a derivative of u. Derivatives of the finite element approximation are not defined at element interfaces. This section is concerned with fitting of piecewise continuous derived functions that are well defined within elements but not on their boundaries. A derivative denoted by u' will be used henceforth to be representative of such a derived function.

Average values computed at i in the elements sharing node i may be used as the nodal value in Eq. (70). This is often adequate but is not generally applicable. Relative size and importance of adjacent elements is not taken into account.

Global least squares fitting of derived functions has met with some measure of success. A norm $|| \quad ||$ is induced by an inner product that may include an importance weighting factor (density function)

$$(a,b) = \int a(\underline{x})\ b(\underline{x})\ r(\underline{x})\ \underline{dx} \quad , \quad r(\underline{x}) \geq 0$$

$$||c(\underline{x})|| = (c,c)^{\frac{1}{2}} \tag{71}$$

If the approximation to u' is $w(\underline{x})$, then one seeks nodal values w^i to minimize

$$||w^i N_i(\underline{x}) - \underline{u}^i N_i'(\underline{x})|| \tag{72}$$

Matrix notation is convenient. Let

$$\underline{u}^T = (u^1,\ u^2,\ ,,,) \ ; \ \underline{w}^T = (w^1,\ w^2,\ \ldots)$$

$$g_{ij} = (N_i,\ N_j) \quad ; \quad h_{ij} = (N_i,\ N_j')$$

$$G = [g_{ij}] \quad ; \quad H = [h_{ij}]$$

Then Eq. (72) is minimized when

$$\underline{w} = G^{-1}H\ \underline{u} \tag{73}$$

(Note that G^{-1} exists since the N_i are linearly independent. Matrix G is, in general, positive definite.)

The elements of G^{-1} are denoted by g^{ij}. To solve for $\underline{w}$ one does not need to compute the g^{ij} (G^{-1} is not sparse). One needs only to solve for $\underline{w}$, the sparse system

$$G\ \underline{w} = H\ \underline{u} \tag{74}$$

The motivation for including this section in a chapter on basis functions is the existence of the "conjugate basis" defined by Oden [B-2] to provide insight into this least squares smoothing procedure. The nodal conjugate basis functions are defined by

$$N^i(\underline{x}) = g^{ij}N_j(\underline{x}) \tag{75}$$

These functions are, in general, nonzero over almost the whole region of interest. Oden demonstrated that the nodal values w^i for global smoothing of discontinuous functions like u' are the projections of these functions on the conjugate basis functions:

$$w^i = (N^i,\ u') \tag{76}$$

The proof is quite straightforward. From Eq. (73):

$$w^i = g^{ij}(N_j, N_k') u^k \tag{77}$$

By substituting Eq. (75) into Eq. (77) one obtains:

$$w^i = (N^i, N_k') u^k = (N^i, u') \tag{78}$$

The existence and significance of Oden's conjugate base is of theoretical interest even though the basis may not be used directly. Numerical difficulties have been experienced with this global least squares smoothing of derived functions.

Local least squares fitting [A-6] is a viable alternative. The fit is now confined to each element. The wedge (element) basis functions N_i appear in the norm minimization problem over element e:

$$\min_{w_e^i} \left|\left| w_e^i N_i(\underline{x}) - u^i N_i'^e(\underline{x}) \right|\right|_e \tag{79}$$

Interpolatory approximation characteristics of finite element methods seem to yield better estimates of derivatives interior to elements than near their boundaries. Experience indicates that quadrature points are better suited for sampling derived functions than are nodal points. Quadrature points are introduced through the discrete density function

$$r(\underline{x}) = w_q \, \delta \, (\underline{x} - \underline{x}_q) \tag{80}$$

where w_q is the quadrature weight at point q, and δ is the Dirac function that converts the integral to a summation. When isoparametrics are used, w_q may contain the Jacobian of the transformation as well as the quadrature weight for the local coordinate integration. The resulting approximation is not continuous and must be averaged at element interfaces. This averaging is more universally acceptable than direct averaging of u'. Numerical comparisons are given in [A-6].

CONCLUDING REMARKS

A variety of basis functions has been described. These functions play a crucial role in finite element computation. Although other bases are used along with those discussed here, construction of the various alternatives and their properties are governed largely by considerations dealt with in this chapter. An attempt has been made here not only to expose techniques now in use for solving problems but to indicate areas of current research and to motivate continued analysis of diverse elements.

REFERENCES

A. Journal Articles

1 Apprato, D., Arcangeli, R. et Gout, J. L., "Sur les elements finis rationnels de Wachspress," Numer. Math., Vol. 32, 1979, pp. 247-270.

2 Babuska, I., and Rheinboldt, W. C., "Reliable Error Estimation and Mesh Adaptation for the Finite Element Method," Univ. of Maryland Technical Note BN-910, 1979.

3 Babuska, I., Szabo, B. A., and Katz, I. N., "The P-version of the Finite Element Method," Washington Univ. (St. Louis) Center for Computational Mechanics Report WU/CCM-79/1, 1979.

4 Deleze, M., Goel, J. -J., and Meyenhofer, B., "Finite Elements of Cl-class on a Tetrahedron," I. J. N. M. E., Vol. 12, 1978, pp. 787-793.

5 Gordon, W. J., and Hall, C. A., "Transfinite Element Methods," Numer. Math., Vol. 21, 1973, pp. 109-129.

6 Hinton, E., and Campbell, J. S., "Local and Global Smoothing of Discontinuous Finite Element Functions using a Least Squares Method," I. J. N. M. E., Vol. 8, 1974, pp. 109-129.

7 McLeod, R. J. Y., "High Order Transformation Methods for Curved Finite Elements," J. Inst. Maths. Appl., Vol. 21, 1978, pp. 419-428.

8 Mitchell, A. R., "Advantages of Cubics for Approximating Element Boundaries," Comp. and Math. with Appl., special issue on Curved Finite Elements, Vol. 5, No. 4, 1979, pp. 321-328.

9 Peano, A. G., "Hierarchies of Conforming Finite Elements for Plane Elasticity and Plate Bending," Comp. and Maths. with Appl., Vol. 2, 1976, pp. 211-224.

10 Rossow, M. P., and Katz, I. N., "Hierarchal Finite Elements and Precomputed Arrays," I. J. N. M. E., Vol. 12, 1978, pp. 977-999.

11 Wachspress, E. L., "Incompatible Quadrilateral Basis Functions," I. J. N. M. E., Vol. 12, 1978, pp. 585-595.

12 Wilson, E. L., Taylor, R. L., Doherty, W. P., and Ghaboussi, J., "Incompatible Displacement Models," in Numerical and Computer Methods in Structural Mechanics, Academic Press, 1973, pp. 43-57.

B. Books, Monographs, and Proceedings

1 Ciarlet, P. G., The Finite Element for Elliptic Problems, Elsevier, North Holland, 1978.

2 Oden, J. T., Finite Elements of Nonlinear Continua, McGraw-Hill Book Co., 1972.

3 Pulmano, V. A. and Kabaila, A. P. (editors), Proceedings of the 1974 International Conference on Finite Element Methods in Engineering, University of New South Wales, August 28-30, 1974.

4 Strang, G., and Fix, G., An Analysis of the Finite Element Method, John Wiley and Sons, New York, 1976.

5 Wachspress, E. L., A Rational Finite Element Basis, Academic Press, 1975.

6 Zienkiewicz, O. C., The Finite Element Method, Third Edition, McGraw-Hill Book Co., 1977.

CHAPTER THREE

PRINCIPLES FOR DESIGN OF FINITE ELEMENT MESHES

R.J. Melosh and S. Utku
Civil Engineering Department
Duke University
Durham, North Carolina

ABSTRACT

A good finite element mesh yields behavior predictions of the desired accuracy much more efficiently than a bad one. Computer time can be reduced by factors of ten or more since the analysis with the good mesh requires fewer degrees of freedom, precludes the need for special calculations to control manipulation errors, and yields disciplined measures of discretization error.

This chapter examines finite element technology and processes which bear on designing good meshes. The technology includes data relating solution accuracy and run time to nodal siting, element type, and grid refinement. The processes include algorithms which determine the number of nodes and types of elements and algorithms which allocate nodes and element types.

Conclusions contain guidelines for choosing the element types and grid arrangements.

INTRODUCTION

The goal of mesh design is to select the number and location of finite element nodes and element types so that the associated analyses will be accurate enough. For the "best" mesh, accuracy is attained using least resources for the design and analysis processes.

The best mesh is characterized by economy, simplicity and discipline. Because it involves fewer degrees of freedom and lower degree element types, this mesh requires less calculations for the analysis (1). Since the mesh avoids disparate nodal spacing and extreme element geometrics, extra calculations to control the manipulation errors associated with these irregularities are avoided (2,3). Since the grid is fine enough to furnish reliable measures of discretization error (4,5), excessively fine meshes are excluded.

Data on meshing abound in the literature. Much of this data has as its primary value the building of credibility of the accuracy of proposed element models as a function of grid refinement. Of more direct interest are the citations that appear in the bibliography at the end of this chapter. This bibliography, compiled by Dave Turcke (and updated for this chapter) is the most complete bibliography of papers on finite element meshing known to the authors.

Notable among previous work are the studies of Ebner, Case and Mason, Mallett, and Key (6). These studies expose the complexity of mesh designing and provide some guidelines covering problems of idealization and discretization.

Research studies of nodal arrangement and refinement provide a narrower and deeper understanding of the mesh design problem. The importance, theorems, and pragmatics of optimum nodal siting have been researched by McNeice (4), Turcke (7), Carroll (8), Babuska (9) and others. The importance, theorems, and sensors for focused grid refinements have been the fruit of investigations by Melosh (10), Babuska (11), Szabo (12), Shephard(13), and others. Study of a design strategy in which both element type and grid refinement are treated as design variables is a recent development (1), suggesting that mesh design technology is still evolving.

This chapter reviews principles of good mesh design using results of an extensive study of the torsion problem. Thereby, it provides a context within which observations of all researchers can be placed. It addresses errors in replacing the continuum by discrete elements in linear finite element analysis. (Research in meshing for nonlinear problems is just beginning and will involve more extensive study.)

The chapter proceeds from definitions through mesh refinement strategy. The next section defines the mesh design problem and terminology. Subsequent sections introduce the principles of mesh arrangement and evolution. The last section cites generalizations for mesh designing.

Throughout the chapter, mesh design principles are set off in subparagraphs and embraced by quotation marks. Proven principles are underlined. Principles which are confirmed, without exception, by numerical experiments are not underlined.

The authors wish to express their appreciation to Dr. Ivo Babuska for the suggestions that he made that helped to strengthen this chapter.

THE MESH DESIGN PROBLEM

This section provides a statement of the design problem and definitions which abbreviate subsequent discussions.

Given the mathematical idealization of an engineering system; given the subset of finite element models that may be used in the analysis; then, the mesh design problem is to establish an acceptable discretization. The discretization is particularized by selecting the number of nodes and elements and the arrangement of nodes and element types so the associated analysis produces response predictions of adequate accuracy.

For a structural system, the idealization is established by selection of mathematical models of the geometry, material behavior, and boundary conditions. The subset of element types may include any of the large number of element types described in the literature. For a membrane, for example, available shapes include triangular, quadrilateral, and pentagonal, and behavior variables include displacements and displacement derivatives as generalized coordinates. For structures, typical responses of interest are deflections, stresses, stiffnesses, vibration modes and stability limits.

We may visualize the design as a point in the three-dimensional design space of Figure 1. The primary coordinates of the point are the number of nodes and the element type (or types). These are primary in the sense that varying either coordinate independently is sufficient to develop an acceptable mesh for most grids an analyst might select. The secondary coordinate is mesh arrangement: the siting of nodes and the disposition of element types. Varying mesh arrangement impacts upon analysis efficiency.

Constraints on mesh designs consist of limitations on computer resources and arrangements. Resource constraints are important: they may make it impossible to find an acceptable mesh. In examining design principles, however, they can be ignored. Mesh arrangement constraints limit nodal spacing and element shapes. (The elements must fill the space. Extreme element geometrics must be avoided. Relatively closely-spaced nodes are inadmissible. Symmetric structures must have symmetric meshes, etc.) These constraints can be viewed as limiting the design point to particular surfaces in the design space.

Among all meshes which are acceptable, we seek the mesh which minimizes the resources required for the design and analysis processes. This complicates

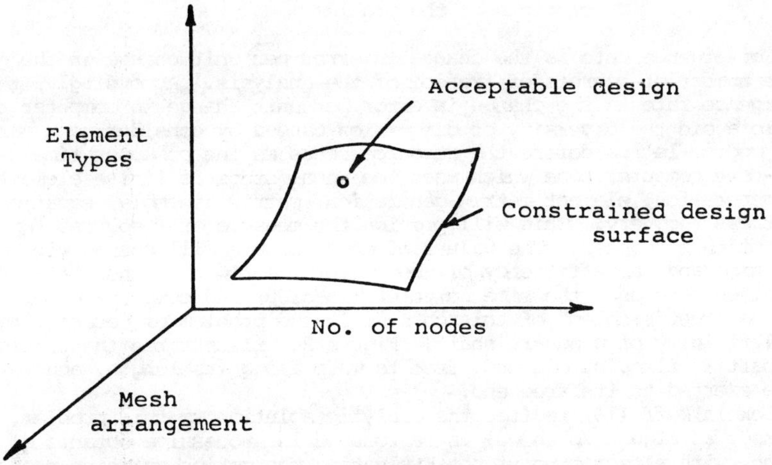

Fig. 1 Mesh design space

Design Variables

Nodal	Element Type	Arrangement
displacement components	trial functions	nodal spacing
displacement continuity	nodal pattern	element shape
displacement B.C. models	formulation basis	connectivity of nodes
equivalent loads models	strain-disp. model	allocation of element types
	material behavior constraints	allocation of B.C. models

discussion of mathematical error bounds and convergence rates with discussion of actual accuracy, effective convergence rates and the efficiency of design and solution algorithms and software.

We define accuracy by

$$d = -\log_{10}[(J_e - J_n)/J_e] \quad (1)$$

Where d is the number of digits of accuracy of the solution
J is the solution strain energy, and
e and n are subscripts denoting the exact and numerical solutions of the problem

Convergence rate is the change in error per unit change in the grid interval or the number of degrees of freedom of the analysis. Accordingly, the effective convergence rate is the change in error per unit change in computer time.

To avoid the diversity of discussion caused by considering a variety of computer codes, let us define the resource needs as the computer time required by an in-core computer code which uses the usual steps of finite element analysis: mesh generation, element matrix generation, matrix assembly, equation solution, and stress recovery. This will provide the measure of resources for all comparisons of this chapter. The values of this measure will change with computer cycle time and the efficiency of the computer software. Thus, all experimental data given here used the same computer (IBM5100) and computer code.

The "test problem" of this chapter is the problem of determining the torsional rigidity of a square shaft. Figure 2a illustrates the configuration. The shaft is fixed at one end, free to warp along its length, and twisted by a torque exerted at its free end.

Sokolnikoff (14) recites the analytic solution to this problem. The warping response, as Figure 2b shows, is reproduced in successive octants of the cross section, with alternating sign. Evaluating the series solution produces the torsional rigidity constant 2.249232.

For the numerical analyses, finite element models are formulated in terms of the warping values at the nodes (15). All models are constructed so the finite element analysis constitutes a Ritz analysis of the shaft. Thus, all numerical solutions underestimate the torsional constant.

Each analysis uses one of four element types for all elements of the mesh. These element types are designated by the degree of the warping function. Thus, the "linear element" (simplex element) assumes warping modeled by all terms of a polynomial through those linear in the x, y coordinates of the cross section (15). The "hyperbolic element" warping function includes, in addition, the xy term. The "superquadratic element" uses a polynomial which is complete through all second degree terms and includes some of the third degree. The "reduced integration element" uses the superquadratic function, but performs numerical integrations of strain energy density using only four Gauss points.

Figure 2c shows a typical analysis grid. Since all analyses are rectangular grid modules, special boundary conditions are introduced at the blackened nodes to imply antisymmetric response across the octant radial lines. Since all elements which cross the diagonals of the square shaft must be square to imply antisymmetric warping responses, all grid intervals along the x axis match those along y and all grids are NxN grids where N is the number of grid intervals along an axis.

We consider four types of meshes: optimum, regular, focused and undisciplined.

In an optimum mesh, the nodal coordinates are selected so that the coordinates and solution satisfy the equations:

$$\underset{\sim}{K}\,\underset{\sim}{w} - \underset{\sim}{t} = 0 \quad (2)$$

$$\left.\begin{aligned} \frac{1}{2}\,\underset{\sim}{w}^T \frac{\partial K}{\partial x_j}\,\underset{\sim}{w} - \frac{\partial \underset{\sim}{t}}{\partial x_j}\,\underset{\sim}{w} &= 0 \\ \frac{1}{2}\,\underset{\sim}{w}^T \frac{\partial K}{\partial y_j}\,\underset{\sim}{w} - \frac{\partial \underset{\sim}{t}}{\partial y_j}\,\underset{\sim}{w} &= 0 \end{aligned}\right\} \quad (3)$$

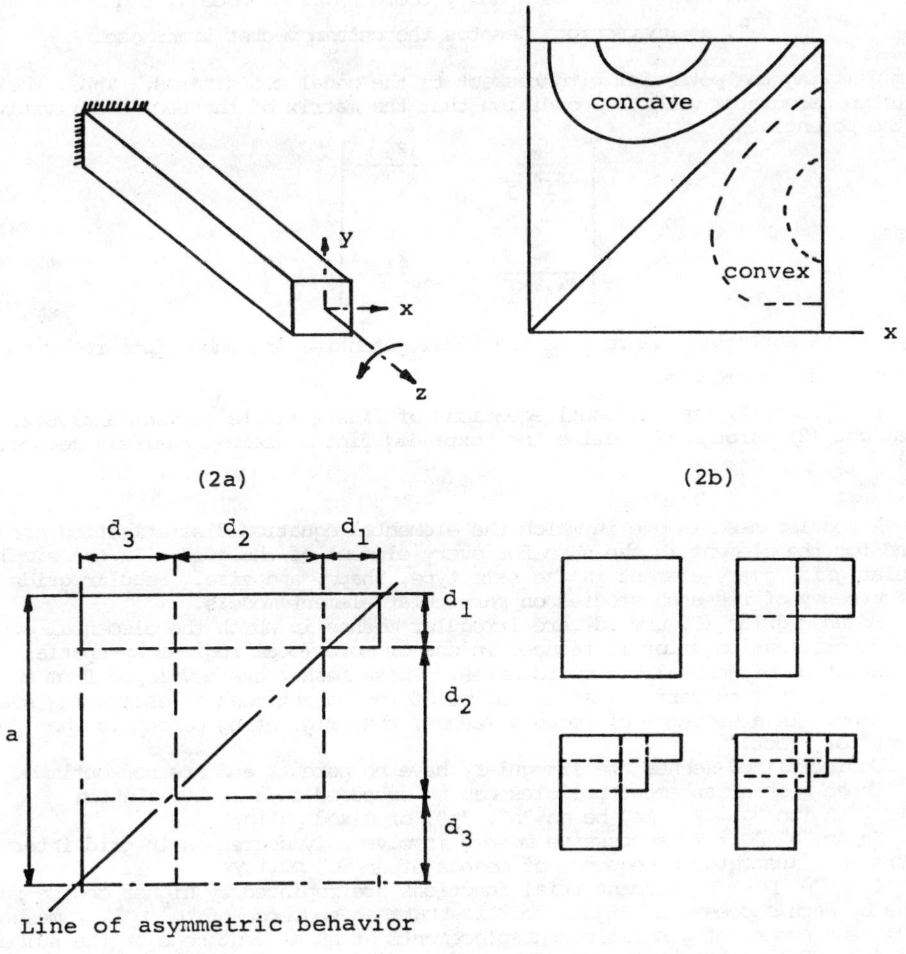

Fig. 2. Modeling characteristics

(2a) Square shaft in torsion
(2b) Warping function contours
(2c) Grid design parameters
(2d) A focused grid sequence

where

$\underset{\sim}{K}$ is the system stiffness matrix,

$\underset{\sim}{w}$ is the vector of warping values,

$\underset{\sim}{t}$ is the vector of equivalent loads,

x_j and y_j are the x and y coordinates of node j, and

T, a superscript, denotes the column vector transpose.

by minimizing the potential with respect to the nodal coordinates. Thus, the solution associates with the condition that the matrix of the second derivatives of the potential

$$\begin{bmatrix} \dfrac{\partial^2 \pi}{\partial x_i \partial x_j} & \dfrac{\partial^2 \pi}{\partial x_i \partial w_j} \\ \\ \dfrac{\partial^2 \pi}{\partial w_j \partial x_i} & \dfrac{\partial^2 \pi}{\partial w_i \partial w_j} \end{bmatrix} \tag{4}$$

is positive definite, where π is the total potential and subscripts refer to generic nodal variables.

Equations (2) are the usual equations of linear finite element analysis. Equations (2) through (4) define the "extended finite element analysis method." (16).

A regular mesh is one in which the elemental equation discretization error bound for the element is the same for every element of the grid. In the simplest regular grid, every element is the same type, shape, and size. Regular grids are the currency of research studies on particular element models.

Focused grids (Figure 2d) are irregular meshes in which the elemental equation discretization error is reduced in one or more local regions by spatial concentration of generalized coordinates. These meshes are developed from a parent mesh by considering inefficiencies of the parent mesh in estimating system responses. In a sequence of focused meshes, the originating parent is the "root parent" or "root."

Undisciplined meshes are irregular, have no parent, and are non-optimum.

These mesh arrangement policies can be embedded in a mesh evolution policy. The policy may be an "h", "p", or mixed policy.

In an "h" policy successive meshes involve only decreases in grid intervals. Figure 3a illustrates a sequence of meshes of an "h" policy.

In a "p" policy, element trial functions are replaced by higher degree functions by each successor. Figure 3b illustrates a sequence of "p" policy meshes. Either the number of generalized displacements at an element node or the number of nodes per element are increased to reduce discretization error.

A mixed policy involves changes in grid size and trial function degree in successive meshes.

We shall see that the effective rate of convergence when a mixed mesh development policy is used is better than that of either an "h" or "p" policy.

SELECTION OF MESH ARRANGEMENT

Mesh arrangement decisions include where to locate nodes and each type of element. This section examines the relation between those decisions and analyses accuracy and efficiency. It includes design principles for optimum grid arrangements.

Accuracy versus Grid Arrangement

Figure 4 shows results of a sequence of optimum grid solutions of the test

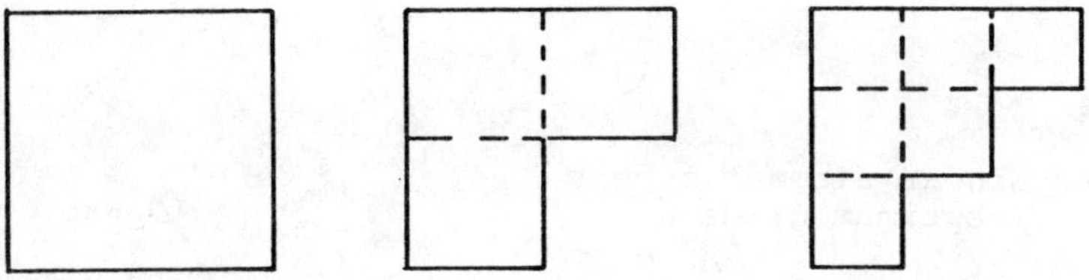

(3a)

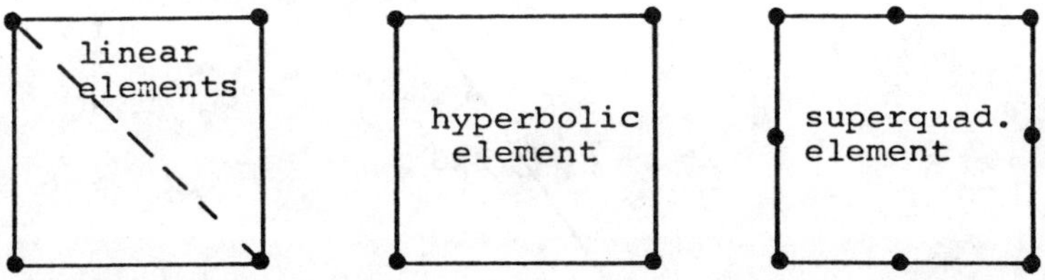

(3b)

(3c)

Fig. 3 Mesh evolution sequences

(3a) "h" convergence grid sequence
(3b) "p" convergence mesh sequence
(3c) Mixed convergence mesh sequence

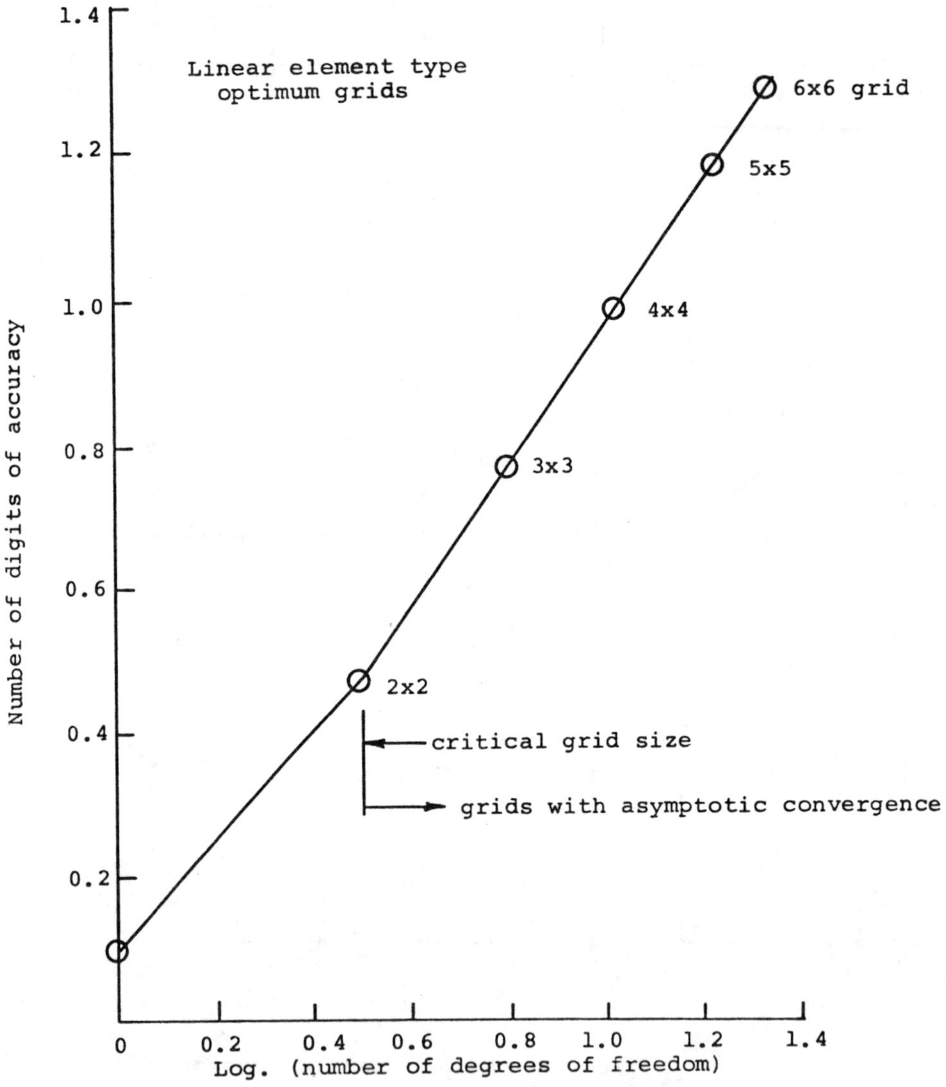

Fig. 4 Accuracy of the optimum grid sequence

problem using the linear element. The ordinate of the curve is the logarithm of the number of active degrees of freedom in the analysis. The abscissa is the number of digits of accuracy in the estimate of strain energy. Thus, the scales are log-log scales.

Studies leading to this curve illustrate the following principles of grid arrangement:

1. "The extended element method leads to uniquely defined nodal siting whenever the potential is sensitive to nodal positions."

Babuska (9) proves this hypothesis is a theorem for the two-point boundary value problem. The search for the optimum grid in the test problem suggests the proof is extendible to torsion. The fact that torsion, membrane, and three-dimensional stress problems involve La Place's equation indicates that a theorem may be developed for a broad class of problems in linear elastostatics.

This hypotheses means that the total potential is a convex function of the nodal coordinates and the unknowns. This fact justifies limiting the search for an optimum grid to finding a single optimum. (It also suggests the advantage of using a search algorithm such as Fletcher-Reeves (17) to implement search for the optimum.)

2. "The sequence of optimum grid solutions provides a monotonically convergent sequence in the energy norm."

This statement follows from statement 1 and the fact that elements fulfill requirements for monotonic convergence (18, 19). It is reflected in the fact that the curve of Figure 4 is single-valued with respect to the parameters.

This statement insures that analysis of a finer grid cannot yield a worse estimate of strain energy. Pragmatically, this means that results of two successively finer grids can yield measures of the discretization error in the analysis.

3. "There is a critical number of degrees of freedom above which convergence is a power of the interval size."

This rate of convergence is a consequence of the use of polynomial trial functions complete up to some degree of the polynomial. Since about 98 percent of available element models are based on polynomials, this theorem can be regarded as a practical generalization. The existence of critical level of refinement was observed first by Babuska (20).

This theorem reflects in Figure 4. The sequence of solutions defines a straight-line when the grid is finer than 1 x 1.

Figure 5 shows the envelope which embraces all possible grid arrangements of the test problem using the linear element. The ordinate of this curve, and of most of the rest of the curves of this chapter, is the logarithm of the computer time (in seconds) to perform the finite element analysis.

The upper branch of the envelope represents data for the optimum grid solutions of Figure 4. The points on this branch do not include the calculation time to find the optimum arrangement. As Turcke and Carroll note (1, 16,), the extended finite element method requires solving a set of nonlinear simultaneous equations even for the engineering system which behaves linearly. In general, solving Eqs. (3) penalizes the calculations, for solving (2) alone, by a factor of more than $\propto C^3$, where $\propto$ is the constant and C is the total number of free nodal coordinates. Turcke (21) notes a case in which optimization of a particular grid penalized the analysis time by a factor of forty. In the torsion studies of this chapter almost 85 percent of the computer resources were used in just locating the optimum grids (to two digits of accuracy).

Babuska (9) cites a theorum defining the quadratic character of the design surface in the neighborhood of the optimum grid. He indicates that the curvature is low, lending mathematical rationale to the Carroll principle:

4. "The practical goal of grid arrangement optimization is a set of near optimum values of the nodal coordinates."

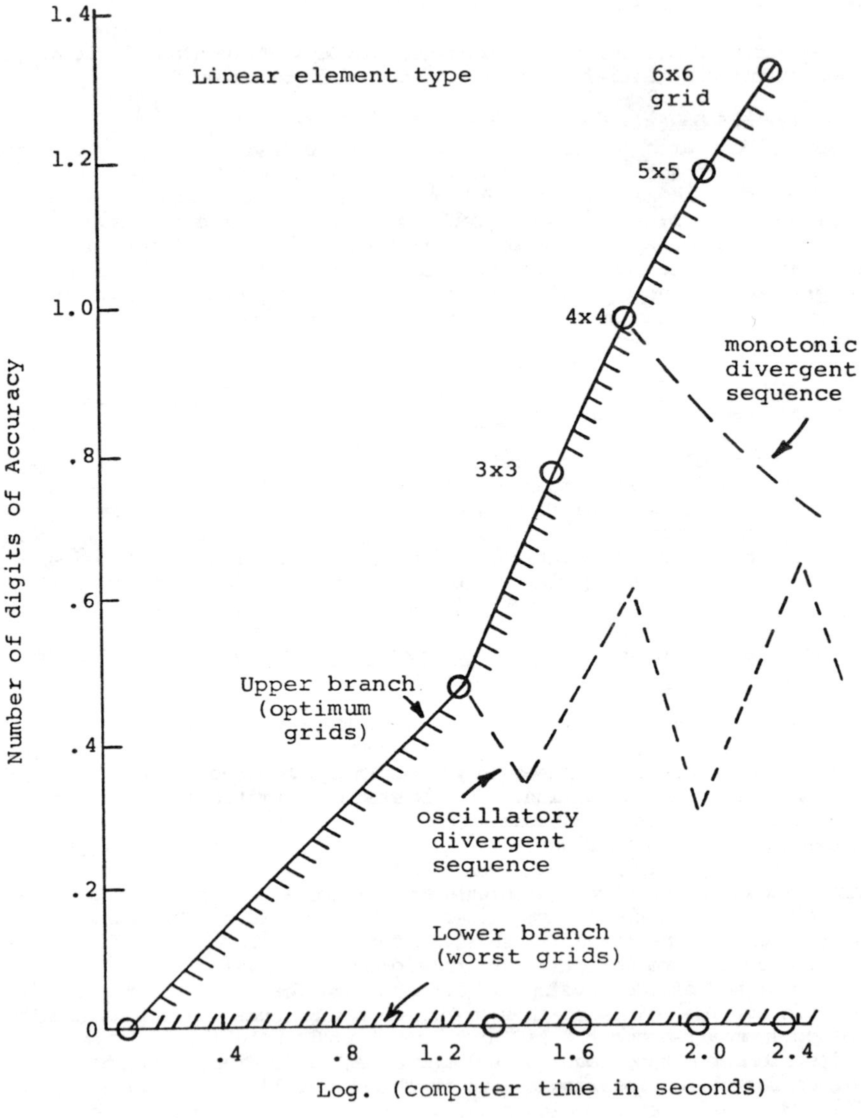

Fig. 5 Linear element: grid arrangement envelope

The lower branch of the envelope of Figure 5 defines analysis results for a sequence of meshes associated with worst grid arrangements. Worse grids involve nodes which are so close together that constraint equations must be introduced to eliminate computer manipulation errors.

When this is done, the analysis accuracy is the accuracy of the coarsest possible grid. Calculation times are slightly increased over those of comparable optimum grid arrangements in imposing kinematic constraints.

The sequence of worst grid arrangements is easily identified. For all practical purposes each grid is uniquely identified. The sequence provides a monotonic sequence of results in the energy norm. Since the effective rate of convergence is zero, the set is of interest only in defining the lower branch of the envelope.

Studying the envelope leads to two additional principles:

5. "The optimum grid associates with least computer time to attain a particular accuracy in the energy norm."

This principle follows from Eq. (3) and the fact that the number of calculations for an analysis is independent of the location of the nodes. Recalling that the data of Figure 5 excludes the computer time to find the optimum, we observe that Principle 5 identifies optimum grid results as ideal limiting results.

It follows from this principle and the existence of a worst grid that the advantage of optimizing grid arrangement can be measured by the number of digits of accuracy difference between results of analyses of these grids.

6. "Fixing the grid arrangement parameter is essential in guaranteeing convergence in finite element analysis."

Proof of this statement is by exception. The dotted curves of Figure 5 show that oscillating divergence and monotonic divergence can occur for the simplex element by particular choices of successive grid arrangements. Thus even though the element model can satisfy completeness requirements, convergence to the exact solution does not occur.

In the introduction of this chapter it was noted that grid arrangement primarily impacts upon solution efficiency. Principle 6 indicates that implicit in this conclusion is the assumption that an adequate grid arrangement policy is used. We shall see that optimum, regular, and focused arrangement policies are adequate.

Principle 6 reflects the fact that the envelope of Figure 5 enlarges as calculation time approaches infinity. Another consequence of this fact is that meshes of a particular element type which yield the same accuracy can differ in calculation time by orders of magnitude depending upon grid arrangements.

Accuracy Versus Element Type

Figure 6 shows grid arrangement envelopes for linear and superquadratic element analyses of the test problem. Comparing these envelopes leads to the following conclusions:

7. "A lower degree element type has the potential for meeting low accuracy requirements more efficiently than a higher degree, when accuracy is sensitive to element type."

In terms of Figure 6, this principle means a disjoint region must exist in the neighborhood of the junctures of the upper and lower branches of the grid arrangement envelopes.

Proof of this principle depends on two considerations. First, the higher degree element model contains the behavior states of the lower as a subset. Therefore, its juncture point must lie above that of the lower degree when accuracy is element type sensitive. Second, the higher degree element based analysis must involve more computer than the lower for the same grid. Therefore,

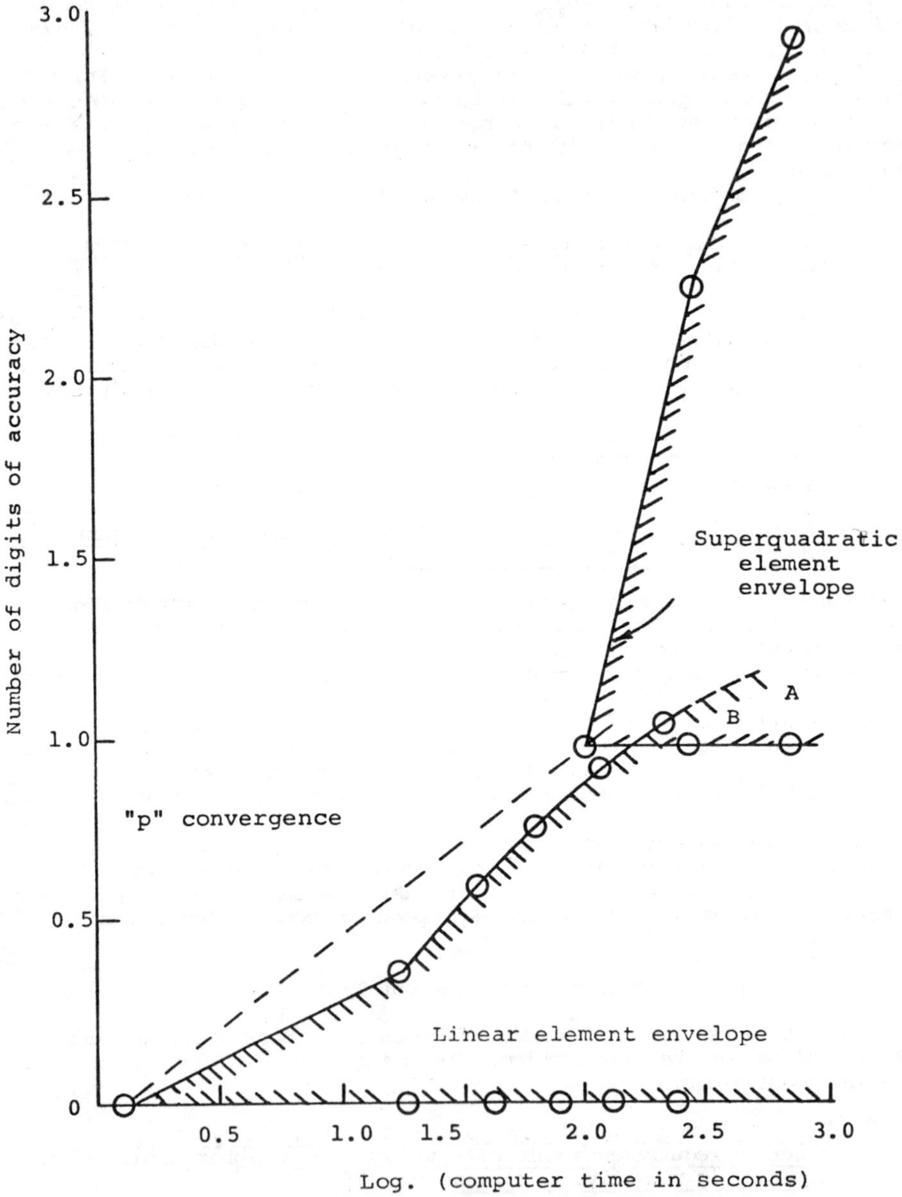

Fig. 6 Grid arrangement envelopes

the higher degree juncture point must fall to the right of the lower on plots like that of Figure 6. Accordingly, there exist accuracy levels, and grid arrangements and refinements for which the lower degree element is better.

8. "A higher degree element type has the potential for meeting high accuracy requirements more efficiently than a lower degree, when accuracy is sensitive to element type."

In terms of Figure 6, this principle asserts that a disjoint region of higher degree solutions must exist above the optimum solution branch of the lower degree.

The principle is a consequence of three considerations. First, the fact that each branch of the envelopes must exhibit monotonic convergence and is therefore single-valued in the computer time and accuracy coordinates. Second, the fact that, disregarding manipulation error, the upper branch of the grid arrangement envelope extends to infinity in the number of digits of accuracy that can be attained. Third, that the convergence rate (slope) along the upper branch must decrease monotonically (because the convergence becomes exponential and the number of calculation increases from a linear up to a cubic function of the number of degrees of freedom in the analysis as the grid is refined) with the higher degree element associating with a higher effective convergence rate.

These arguments also lead to the conclusion that the grid arrangement envelopes of a higher and lower degree element share an intersection. Thus, the priciple:

9. "Analyses using lower degree elements can produce higher accuracy and more efficient analyses than lower, and conversely, when different grid arrangements are used for each."

This principle is illustrated by the A and B analysis points in Figure 6. Here the A analysis is based on the hyperbolic torsion model and B on the superquadratic.

Principles 7 through 9 can serve to improve the perspective on the selection of element type. Without qualifying observations with a specification of grid arrangement, the claim that a higher degree element is always more efficient than a lower is invalid. The better element type to use depends on the grid arrangement to be used, the analysis accuracy required, characteristics of the implementing computer code, and the problem of interest.

A similar comparison between envelopes of the superquadratic and reduced integration superquadratic furnishes additional principles. Figure 7 shows these grid arrangement envelopes.

10. "Reduced integration elements of Type A have the potential for meeting high accuracy requirements more efficiently than fully-integrated ones, when accuracy is sensitive to this element distinction."

11. "Analysis using fully-integrated elements can produce higher accuracy more efficiently than when reduced integration elements of Type A are used and conversely, when different grid arrangements are used for each."

The proof of these statements follows the arguments supporting Principle 8 and 9. However, principles must be qualified by limiting the reduced integration elements to be of Type A, i.e., to be guaranteed to produce estimates of strain energy which are greater than or equal to the exact value.

Unfortunately, a number of reduced integration elements available to the analyst are not of Type A, are only of Type A for limited geometries, or have not been examined with respect to this characteristic. The authors believe use of these elements in production analyses should await further research.

On the other hand, use of a reduced integration element of Type A is advisable compared with its fully-integrated counterpart. Principle 10 and lack of a principle like Principle 7 recommend this guideline.

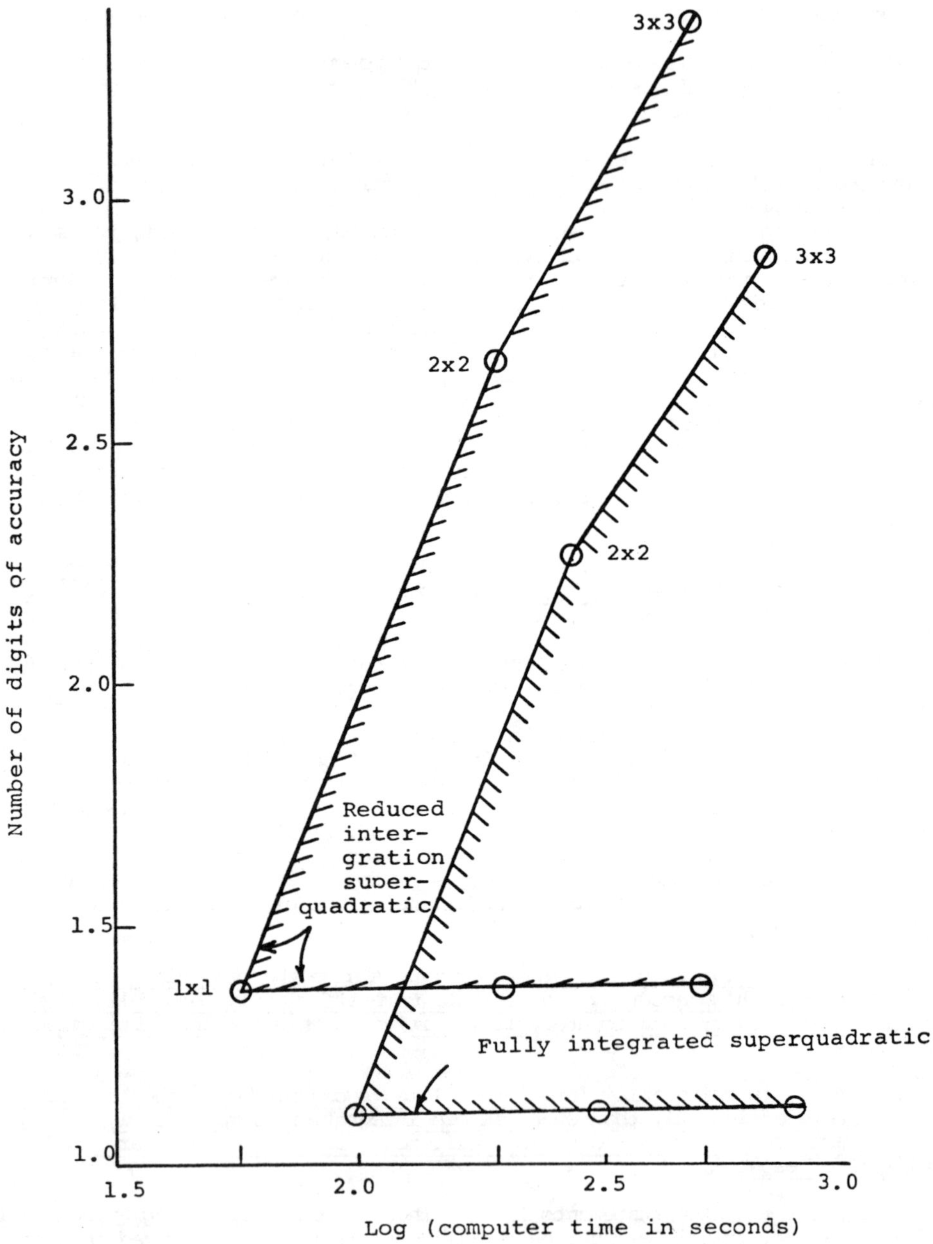

Fig. 7 Superquadratic elements: grid arrangement envelopes

Use of Optimized Grids

The properties of optimized grids make them suitable for a variety of research uses.

In this section, element types have been compared using the monotonic convergence property and the fact that optimized grids have maximum efficiency, we can neglect computer search time. Thus, results of all grid arrangements have been bounded and studied.

Because optimum grids are ideal and unique, it is suggested that they be used by the analyst for comparing the accuracy versus computer time relations of competing element types. This approach will make experimental data more problem independent and eliminate grid arrangement capriciousness.

One of the unanswered questions of finite element modeling is how large the element aspect ratio may be for a particular element type. (A heated controversy ensued when this question was posed by Ebner at the New Orleans National ASCE Conference (6).) Because the decision affects manipulation and discretization errors, the answer depends on the precision of calculations as well as element type.

The data of Table 1 suggests an approach to answering this question using numerical experiments. If grid arrangements are optimum for a particular element type for a variety of problems and typical computer arithmetic modes, a worst aspect ratio can be determined. For example, test problem experiments indicate that a maximum a/b ratio for the linear, hyperbolic, and superquadratic elements will be less than four. The data of Table 1 also demonstrate that the optimum grid changes with element type.

Table 1

Characteristics of Optimum Grids

Grid Size	Linear Element x_i or y_i values	Max. a/b*	Superquadratic Element x_i or y_i values	Max. a/b*
1 x 1	0., 1.	1.00	0., 1.	1.00
2 x 2	0., .64, 1.	1.78	0., .67, 1.	2.03
3 x 3	0., .42, .83, 1.	2.76	0., .40, .74, 1.	1.54

The next section uses optimum grids to define an ideal sequence of meshes for comparing mesh evolution strategies.

SELECTION OF THE MESH EVOLUTION STRATEGY

A mesh evolution strategy is a set of rules by which meshes are redesigned to arrive at an acceptable mesh. In this section, we evaluate the effectiveness of existing strategies.

Mesh Evolution

The common process of mesh evolution involves the following tasks:

1. Perform a finite element analyses of the system using a relatively coarse mesh and the favored element type.

2. Evaluate the quality of the solution to determine if the mesh is acceptable.

3. Accept the solution, or, if unacceptable, repeat tasks 1 and 2 using a refined mesh.

Thus, mesh evolution requires sensors which estimate the accuracy and efficiency associated with a given mesh and criteria for mesh redesign.

The goal of mesh evolution is the minimum computer time to identify an acceptable mesh and perform its finite element analyses. Thus, it is desirable that the process define where, how, and by how much a given mesh should be changed so it will nearly be a best mesh.

Current technology partially supports this goal. It includes sensors to identify accuracy and efficiency of a given mesh and some experience with indicated mesh changes on solution accuracy. Though these two aspects of mesh evolution are intertwined in research papers, the next sub-sections will discuss them separately.

Mesh Quality Sensors

Mesh quality sensors must lead to estimates of analyses discretization error, and, when accuracy is inadequate, define regions of the mesh which require refinement. They must be reliable-indicating mesh changes only when and where required. It is desirable that their evaluation require little computer time-hopefully a small fraction of the analysis time.

Babuska (22) indicates that sensors exist satisfying these requirements. In addition, sensors can be defined such that the error associated with the estimator is a function of the indicated error squared.

Table 2 lists many of the sensors suggested by researchers. The reference noted by each details the basis for the sensor and shows one or more simple elastostatic applications of the measure.

Researchers have demonstrated the value of such sensors in a variety of applications. Turcke shows use of isoenergetics for a variety of geometries and boundary conditions (30). Carroll (16, 31) and Shephard (13) show applications for point loads, singular element models, and inhomogeneous materials. Carroll (31) illustrates use for predictions of vibration and buckling modes. Shephard (13) deals with a semi-infinite region and the important problem of multiple loadings.

Table 3 cites the type, element model transportability, consistency with Ritz analysis, and relative computer time to evaluate the sensors of Table 2.

The type of sensor is indicated to be either accuracy or efficiency. An accuracy sensor produces zero values when the exact solution is attained. High local values recommend mesh refinements, though not necessarily in the region indicated. Efficiency sensors flag regions where discretization error is high. When the grid arrangement is optimum, these produce the same value for every region. The value may have little relation to solution accuracy.

Inconsistency with Ritz analysis implies some unreliability of the sensor in current production applications. Since most existing codes control discretionization error in the energy norm, a sensor which is independent of this norm can indicate local mesh improvements which do not lead to solution improvements.

The relative computer times to evaluate the norm vary from less than one percent (SED) to up to about ten percent of analysis time. The time column in Table 3 indicates the relative time with lower numbers flagging lower computer time.

Most of the sensors are not element transportable. This means that the interpretation of results could vary with each element type and, in any event, special logic would be needed for each element type in the computer code.

Table 2

Discretization Error Sensors

Sensor	Source	Basis
Isoenergetic contours	Oliveria (23)	Theorem that for optimum mesh, nodal boundaries lie on isoenergetic contours
Residual norm	Carey (24) Babuska (5)	Calculation of the bound on the norm of the residual of the differential equation addressed
Forward differences	Melosh, Killian (10) Peano (25)	Direct estimation of the change in potential due to each local change in mesh refinement
Optimization residuals	Carroll (16)	Nodal residuals of the condition that the potential be stationary w.r.t. nodal coordinates
Stress imbalance	Killian (26) Szabo (27)	Determination of the norm of interior and interelement violation of microscopic equilibrium
SED values	Melosh, Marcal (28)	Evaluation of the relative contribution of constant strain states to the total strain energy of response
Potential integral	Molmari, Viviani (29)	Determination of nodal coordinates to minimize metric weighted by estimate of potential

Table 3

Characteristics of Error Sensors

Sensor	Type	Consistency with Ritz	Relative Computer Time	Element Transportability
Isoenergetic contours	efficiency	yes	3	no
Residual norm	accuracy	no	4	no
Forward differences	accuracy	yes	8	no
Optimization residuals	efficiency	yes	9	yes
Stress imbalance	accuracy	no	3	no
SED values	efficiency	yes	1	yes
Energy integral	efficiency	no	5	no

Mesh Evolution Policies

Besides the constraints of mesh design, mesh refinement is usually constrained by additional conditions (10, 16, 27). These supplements establish policies on the following questions:

A. Will the grid interval be reduced, the element degree increased or both?

B. Will refinement allow the introduction of irregular elements?

C. Will the refinement be global or local?

The next paragraphs summarize principles which bear on these questions.

The Pony Express Policy

Recent literature demonstrates superior convergence rates using "p" refinement rather than the venerable "h" refinement. The literature leads to the conclusion that:

12. "The asymptotic convergence rate of a "p" refinement policy is twice that of a "h" strategy."

Babuska (32) proves the statement under the assumption that the grid interval is reduced everywhere in "h" meshing and every element is increased in degree for "p" meshing.

The data of Figure 6 illustrates the benefits of "p" meshing for the test problem. The upper branch of the grid envelopes show results from "h" sequences. The two juncture points represent results of a "p" sequence. Only the slopes in "h" sequences near the juncture points are higher than the effective "p" convergence indicated by the dotted line.

Figure 8 shows results of optimum grid analyses using linear, hyperbolic, and superquadratic element types.

The continuous curve is the result of a "pony express" policy of mesh refinement. In this strategy, analyses are performed with a particular element type (the pony) with increasingly finer grids, until the effective convergence degrades efficiency so much that the next higher degree element type becomes a better choice. Then, the element type (new pony) and grid are changed together.

The importance of this policy resides in the principle that:

13. "A pony express policy is the best policy for mesh refinement."

Since this policy can produce either "h" or "p" meshes, convergence of its analysis results cannot be inferior to either. Though implementation of this policy may double the analysis computer time, because there are two competing meshes at any stage, it avoids the large computer time penalties that can arise with a pure "h" or "p" strategy as seen in Figure 6.

The Regular Mesh Policy

Using a regular mesh policy, all grids would be regular or regular in subregions. The policy is advantageous because it caters to reducing computer time by replicating rather than generating element matrices.

Figure 9 facilitates assessing this policy. The figure shows pony express policy results using optimum grids and pony express curves from regular grids. The lower curve disregards replication computer time savings. The middle curve includes them. The upper curve includes them and exploits extrapolatability of regular grid sequences.

Examining this data, we conclude that:

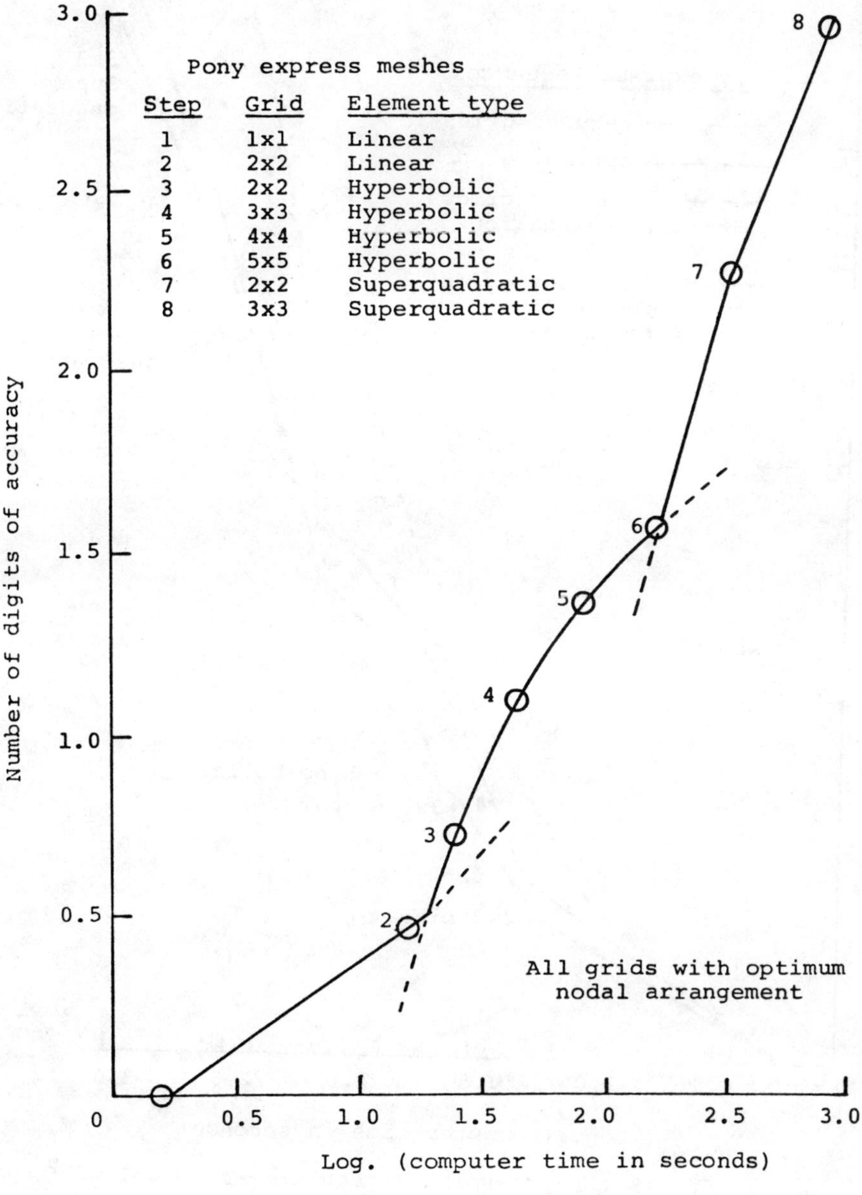

Fig. 8 Pony express optimum meshes

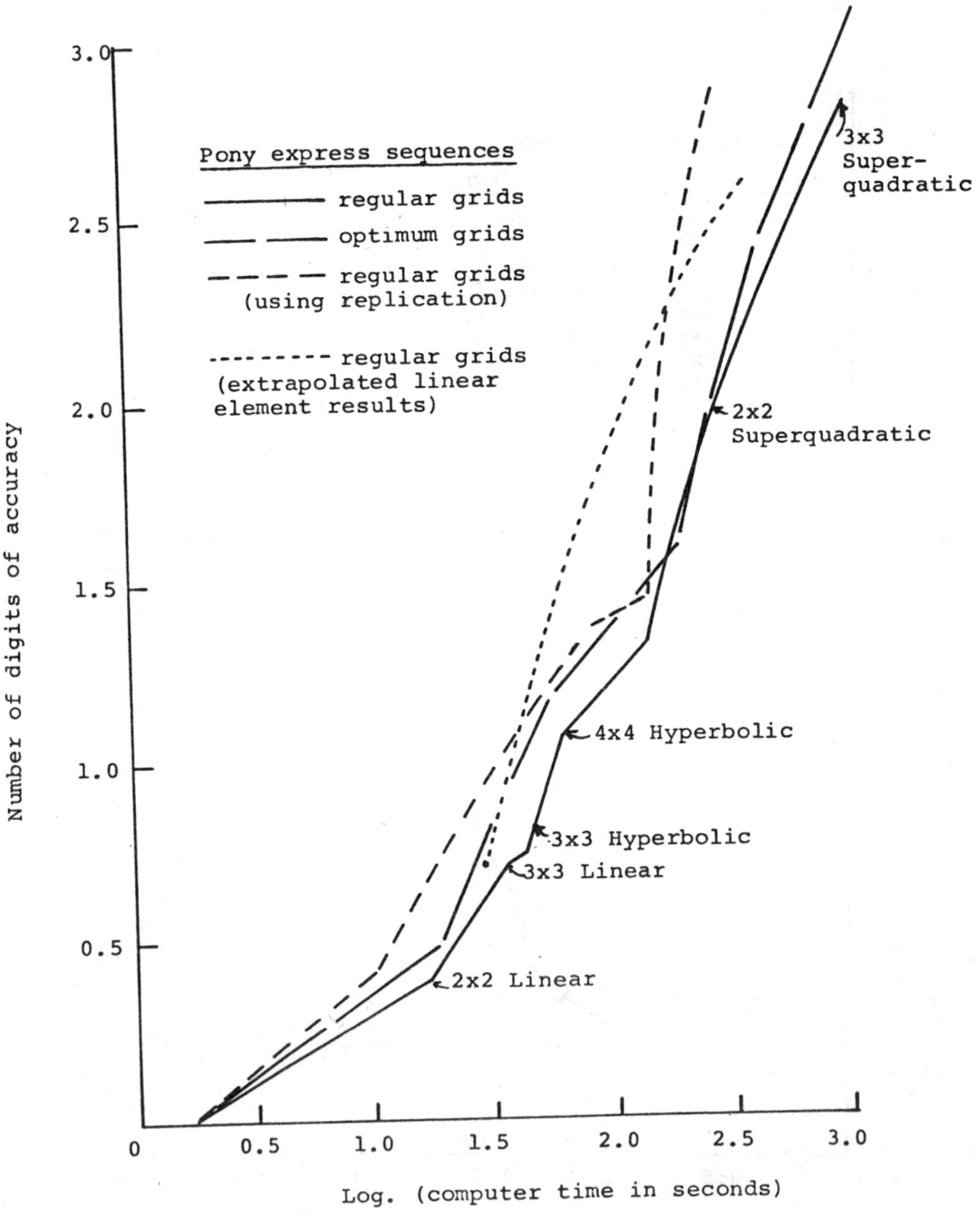

Fig. 9 Regular and irregular mesh results

14. "The sequence of regular grids produces a monotonically convergent sequence of the energy norm."

This is a theorem when each mesh includes the model of its predecessor as a subset. In general, however, it would require some qualifications on the problem characteristics (i. e., the relation between solution smoothness and the element degree). We observe that it is true for the torsion test problem by inspecting Figure 9.

15. "The sequence of regular grids produces a convergent sequence of the energy norm with error a power of the interval size for polynomial trial function elements."

This theorem on "h" convergence of regular grids is proven in the finite element context by Babuska (9). He also suggests that the convergence rate is independent of the problem.

One of the practical uses of Principle 15 is extrapolation of analysis results. The theorem points to use of Richardson's extrapolation. The importance of this powerful device is reflected in the upper (dotted) curve of Figure 9. The computer time plotted is the time required to perform the two finite element analyses that furnish the extrapolated result.

The efficiency of extrapolation analysis is dramatically better than the results produced by any single analysis. Since it is far better than direct use of optimum meshes (which results are neither amenable to extrapolation nor replication) we conclude that:

16. "Extrapolation can provide compelling reasons for use of regular meshes."

The compulsion is a consequence of the high efficiency of analysis and the few calculations required for extrapolation. The torsion analysis experiments indicate that when more than two analyses are required to attain the desired accuracy, extrapolation makes regular meshes more efficient than development of the results by any mesh. This conclusion is valid even if the "wrong" element has been chosen to attain the accuracy desired.

The generality of Principle 16 reflects the need for further research in extrapolation. The idea was shown to be effective for finite element analyses in 1958 but, based on its use in current production analyses, is still not considered viable for practical use.

Comparing the middle regular grid curve of Figure 9 with the lower curve leads to the conclusion that:

17. "Analysis economics associated with replication of element matrices become decreasingly important as the grid interval diminishes."

This conclusion is a consequence of the fact that as the grid gets finer, the number of calculations is increasingly dominated by the equation solving process.

The conclusion is manifest in experiments on the test problem. As Figure 9 shows, regular grids are more efficient than optimum for simplex element grids up to 6 x 6. However, the relatively small advantage of the regular meshes over the irregular meshes (in this case optimum grid), does not justify their use except when the ratio of the number of replicated elements to degrees of freedom is high and the number of degrees of freedom is small.

The Focused Mesh Policy

Figure 10 provides data for comparing pony express results for focused and optimum grids using the linear, hyperbolic and superquadratic element types.

The lowest curve in the figure shows results for focused mesh when the same implementing computer code is used as for the optimum grids. These results

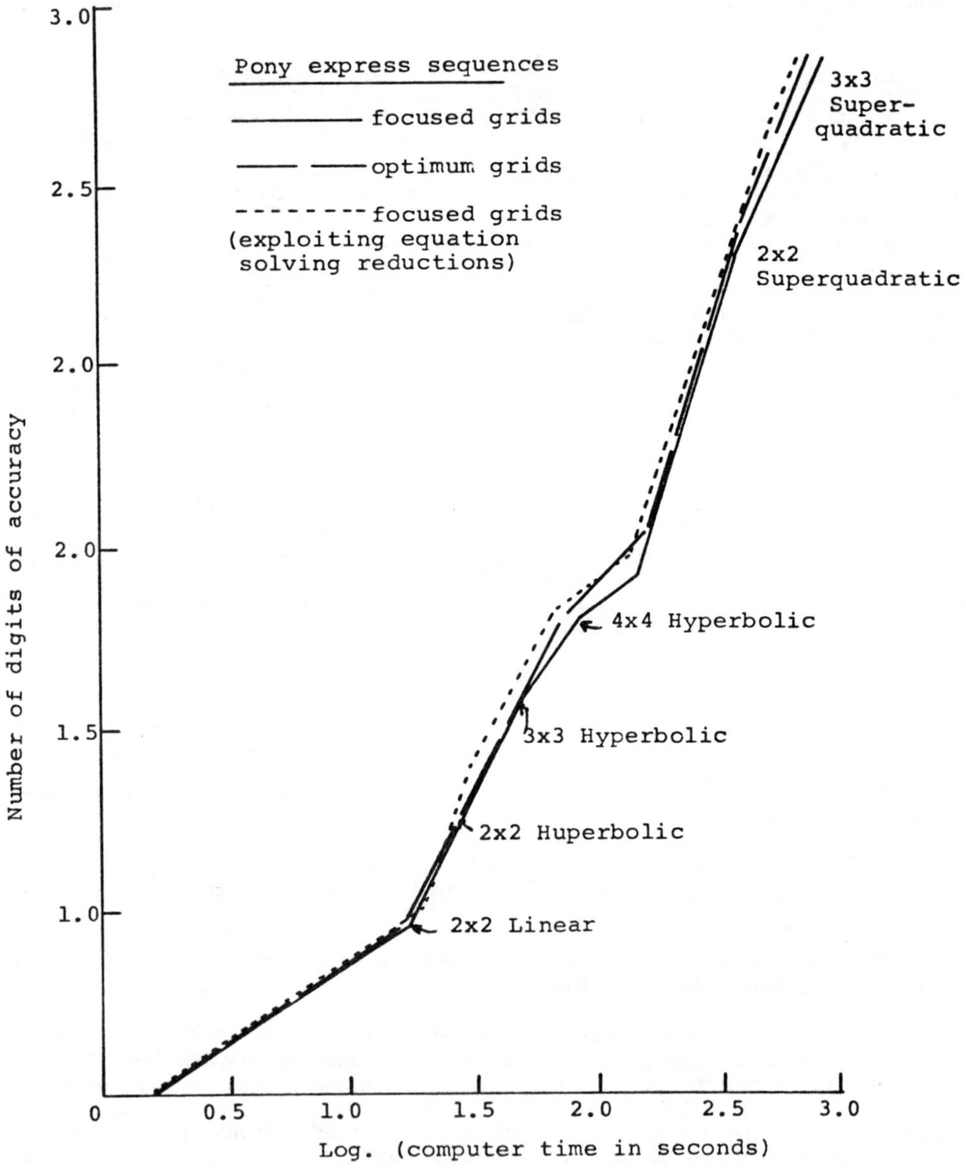

Fig. 10 Global and focused refinement results

illustrate that:

18. "The sequence of focused grids produces a monotonically convergent sequence of the energy norm."

Proof of this statement follows from the definition of the pony express policy and the fact that the element types used in analyses satisfy the sufficiency requirements of monotonicity (18, 19).

19. "The focusing policy results in grids which are near optimum arrangements."

As Figure 10 shows, when a focused grid is very close to the optimum grid curve, the rate of convergence tends to be less than the optimum and conversely. Thereby, the sequence of focused grid seeks the optimum grid configuration without violating Principles 5 and 18.

Statement 19 is confirmed for each of the element types of this study as well as the pony express policy.

The dotted curve of Figure 10 describes the accuracy-calculation time relation when the finite element analyses process is modified to exploit the fact that local subdivision changes only a small part of the system stiffness matrix. As a consequence, superposition can be used to reduce the number of calculations into solving the simultaneous equations (33).

The dotted curve illustrates the principle that:

20. "The analysis economics of a focused grid policy become increasingly important as grid refinement increases."

This statement is a consequence of the monotonically rising importance in calculation time of the number of equations as the number of equilibrium equations increases.

Because of this principle and principles 18 and 19, there must exist a grid size smaller than which the calculation time is less for the focused than for optimum grids (still ignoring optimum grid search time). Figure 9 shows that this occurs with the linear element when the grid size is greater than 1 x 1.

Comparing the data in Figures 9 and 10, we conclude that the focused grid policy will result in more efficient meshes than regular or optimum, exploiting calculation economics, whenever extrapolation is inadmissible, many degrees of freedom are needed to idealize the system accurately, or when accuracy requirements are low.

CONCLUSIONS

Based on the state-of-the art, as condensed into statements 1-20, we highlight the following generalization on mesh design:

1. The pony express policy, in which both grid size and element type are changeable during mesh refinement, is the ideal mesh evolution policy. It cannot be inferior to either an "h" or "p" policy and avoids the inordinate penalties that may associate with either of these.

2. The most efficient element model to use for a particular analysis varies with accuracy requirements, number of degrees of freedom, and computer implementation. Usually, higher degree elements should be selected when accuracy requirements are high and low degree, when low. Reduced integration elements, whenever they are guaranteed to be of Type A, should be preferred over the corresponding fully integrated element.

3. The most efficient grid arrangement varies with the analysis purpose,

computer code, and accuracy required. Generally, optimized grids should be used for studies of element characteristics, focused grids for production analyses of complex systems, and a regular grid when extrapolation can be exploited. Use of successive grids which lack the discipline of an optimum, focused or regular arrangement can lead to an acceptable mesh design. However, it could also incur exorbitant time penalties to attain the required accuracy or lead to oscillatory or divergent sequence of analysis results.

Considerable research has been completed on the problem of mesh designing. Much is known about optimum grids, adaptive grid development, and their relation to particular element types and problems. The rush of recent additions to the literature and the wealth of unanswered questions suggest the technology is still in an era of rapid change.

REFERENCES

1 Melosh, R. J., "Design Principles for Finite Element Meshing," NASA-ICASE Symposium on Mathematical Modeling, Langley Research Center, Hampton, Virginia, Oct. 24, 1979.

2 Melosh, R. J., "Manipulation Errors in Computer Solution of Critical Size Structural Equations," NASA CR-1784, National Aeronautics and Space Administration, Washington, D.C., June 1971.

3 Melosh, R. J., "Characteristics of Manipulation Errors in Solving Load-Deflection Equations," On General Purpose Finite Element Computer Programs, ASME, New York, 1970, pp. 123-242.

4 McNeice, G. M. and Marcal, P. V., "Optimization of Finite Element Grids Based on Minimum Potential Energy," Transaction 7, Brown University, Providence, Rhode Island, 1971.

5 Babuska, I. and Rheinboldt, W. C., "A Posteriori Error Estimates for the Finite Element Method," International Journal for Numerical Methods in Engineering, Vol. 12, 1978, pp. 1597-1615.

6 "Guidelines for Finite Element Idealization," edited by A. Ebner, ASCE National Convention, Preprint 2504, New Orleans, April 1975.

7 Turcke, D. J. and McNeice, G. M., "A Variational Approach to Grid Optimization in the Finite Element Method," Conference on Variational Methods in Engineering, Southampton University, England, Sept. 1972.

8 Carroll, W. E. and Barker, R. M., "A Theorem for Optimum Finite Element Idealization," International Journal of Solids and Structures, Vol. 9, 1973, pp. 883-895.

9 Babuska, I. and Rheinboldt, W. C., "Analysis of Optimal Finite Element Meshes in R^1," Mathematics of Computations, Vol. 33, No. 146, April 1978, pp. 435-463.

10 Melosh, R. J. and Killian, D. E., "Finite Element Analysis to Attain A Prespecified Accuracy," Proceedings of the Second National Congress on Computing in Structures, Washington, 1976.

11 Babuska, I., "The Self-Adaptive Approach in the Finite Element Method," The Mathematics of Finite Element Applications II, Academic Press, 1976, pp. 125-142.

12 Szabo, B. A. and Mehta, A. K., "P-Convergent Finite Element Approximations in Fracture Mechanics," International Journal for Numerical Methods in Engineering, Vol. 12, 1978, pp. 551-560.

13 Shephard, M. S., "Finite Element Grid Optimization with Interactive Graphics," Ph.D. Thesis, Department of Structural Engineering, Cornell University, June 1979.

14 Solonikoff, I. S., Mathematical Theory of Elasticity, McGraw-Hill Book Company, New York, 1956.

15 Herrmann, L. R., "Elastic Torsion Analysis of Irregular Shapes," Proceedings American Society of Civil Engineers Conference, Vol. 91, EM6, 1965, pp. 11-19.

16 Carroll, W. E., "Inclusive Criteria for Optimum Grid Generation in the Discrete Analysis Technique," Computers and Structures, Vol. 6, 1976, pp. 333-337.

17 Fletcher, R. and Reeves, C. M., "Function Minimization by Conjugate Gradients," Computer Journal, Vol. 7, No. 2, July 1964, pp. 149-154.

18 Melosh, R. J., "Basis for Derivation of Matrices for the Direct Stiffness Method," AIAA Journal, Vol. 1, July 1963, pp. 1631-1657.

19 Melosh, R. J. and Lobitz, D. W., "On a Numerical Sufficiency Test for Monotonic Convergence of Finite Element Models," AIAA Journal, Vol. 13, No. 5, May 1975, pp. 675-678.

20 Babuska, I. and Rheinboldt, W. C., "Reliable Error Estimation and Mesh Adaptation for the Finite Element Method," Note Bulletin 910, University of Maryland, April 1979.

21 Turcke, D. J., "Optimum Mesh Configuration in the Finite Element Method," Ph.D. Thesis, Department of Civil Engineering, University of Waterloo, Canada, July 1974.

22 Babuska, I., Miller, A., and Vogelius, M., "Mathematical Problems of Discrete Modeling and A-Posteriori Reliability Estimates," Symposium on Mathematical Modeling in Structural Engineering, NASA-Langley Research Center and George Washington University, Hampton, Virginia, October 1979.

23 de Arandes, O., "Optimization of Finite Element Solutions," Proceedings of the Third Conference on Matrix Methods in Structural Mechanics, AFFDL-TR-71-160, Wright-Patterson Air Force Base, Ohio, Dec. 1973, pp. 423-446.

24 Carey, G. F. and Humphrey, D. L., "Residuals, Adaptive Refinement and Nonlinear Iterations for Finite Element Computations," Finite Element Grid Optimization, ed. by M. Shephard and R. Gallagher, ASME Publication PVP-38, 1979.

25 Peano, A., Riccioni, R., Pasini, A., and Sardella, L., "Adaptive Approximation in Finite Element Structural Analysis," Trends in Computerized Structural Analysis and Synthesis, ed. by A. K. Noor and H. G. McComb, Jr., Pergamon Press, 1978, pp. 333-342.

26 Killian, D. E., "Selective Refinement of a Finite Element Mesh for Improved Accuracy," M.S. Thesis, Virginia Polytechnic Institute and State University, Blacksburg, Virginia, 1975.

27 Szabo, B. A., Busu, P. K., and Rossow, M. F., "Adaptive Finite Element Analysis Based on P-Convergence," NASA Conference Publication 2059, 2059, 1978, pp. 43-50.

28 Melosh, R. J., Marcal, P. V., "An Energy Basic for Mesh Refinement of Structural Continua," International Journal for Numerical Methods in Engineering, Vol. 11, Aug. 1977, pp. 1083-1091.

29 Molmari, G., Viviani, A., "Grid Iteration for Finite Element Grid Optimization," Finite Element Grid Optimization, ed. by M. S. Shephard and R. H. Gallagher, ASME Publication PVP-38, New York, 1979.

30 Turcke, D. J., "Finite Element Mesh Configurations Using Isoenergetics and Equalized Energy Levels," NASA CP-2059, 1978, pp. 89-99.

31 Carroll, W. E., "Recent Development Dealing with Optimum Finite Element Analysis Techniques," Finite Element Grid Optimization, ed. by M. Shephard and R. Gallagher, ASME Publication PVP-38, New York, 1979.

32 Sobieszczanski, J., "Matrix Algorithm for Structural Modification Based Upon the Parallel Element Concept," AIAA Journal, Vol. 7, No. 11, Nov. 1969, pp. 2132-2139.

BIBLIOGRAPHY

1 Babuska, I., "The Self-Adaptive Approach to the Finite Element Method," in the Mathematics of Finite Elements and Applications, II, Academic Press, 1976, pp. 125-142.

2 Babuska, I., Kellog, R. B., Pitkaranta, J., "Direct and Inverse Error Estimates for Finite Elements with Mesh Refinement," Transaction 907, Institute for Physical Sciences and Technology, University of Maryland, 1979.

3 Babuska, I., Rheinboldt, W. C., "Error Estimates for Adaptive Finite Element Computations," Transaction 854, University of Maryland, May, 1977.

4 Babuska, I., Rheinboldt, W., "Computational Aspects of Finite Element Analysis," in Mathematical Software - III, edited by Rice, J., Academic Press, Inc., New York, 1977, pp. 225-255.

5 Babuska, I., Rheinboldt, W., "Analysis of Optimal Finite Element Meshes in R^1," Bulletin 869, University of Maryland, 1977.

6 Babuska, I., Rheinboldt, W., "Mathematical Problems of Computational Decisions for the Finite Element Method," in Mathematical Aspects of Finite Element Methods, edited by Galligani, I., Magenes, E., Lecture Notes in Mathematics, Vol. 606, Springer Verlag, Germany, 1977, pp. 1-26.

7 Babuska, I., Rheinboldt, W. C., "A-Posteriori Error Estimates for the Finite Element Method," Int. Journal Numerical Methods Engineering, Vol. 12, 1978, pp. 1597-1615.

8 Babuska, I., Rheinboldt, W. C., "On a System for Adaptive Parallel Finite Element Computations," Proceedings 1978 Annual Conference of ACM, Vol. 1, Washington, D. C., Dec. 1978, pp. 480-489.

9 Babuska, I., Rheinboldt, W. C., "On the Reliability and Optimality of the Finite Element Method," Trends in Computerized Structural Analysis and Synthesis, edited by Noor, A. K., McComb, H. C., Pergamon Press, 1978, pp. 87-94.

10 Babuska, I., Rheinboldt, W. C., "Reliable Error Estimation and Mesh Adaptation for the Finite Element Method," Bulletin 910, University of Maryland, April 1979.

11 Babuska, I., Rheinboldt, W., Mesztengi, C., "Self-Adaptive Refinements in the Finite Element Method," Transaction 375, Dept. of Computer Science, University of Maryland, 1975.

12 Babuska, I., Szabo, B. A., Katz, I. N., "The P-Version of the Finite Element Method," Center for Computational Mechanics Report WU/CCN-79/1, Washington University, May 1979.

13 Babuska, I., Miller, A., Vogelius, M., "Mathematical Problems of Discrete Modeling and A-Posteriori Reliability Estimates," Symposium on Mathematical Modeling in Structural Engineering, NASA-Langley and George Washington University, Hampton, October 1979.

14 Brandt, A., "Multi-level Adaptive Solutions of Boundary-Value Problems," Mathematics of Computation, Vol. 31, No. 138, April 1977, pp. 333-390.

15 Carey, G. F., Finlayson, B. A., "Orthogonal Collocation on Finite Elements," Chemical Engineering Science, Vol. 30, 1975, pp. 587-596.

16 Carey, G. F., "An Analysis of Finite Element Equations and Mesh Subdivision," Computer Methods in Applied Mechanics and Engineering, Vol. 9, 1976, pp. 165-179.

17 Carey, G. F., "A Mesh-Refinement Scheme for Finite Element Computations," Computer Methods in Applied Mechanics and Engineering, Vol. 7, 1976, pp. 93-105.

18 Carey, G. F., "Adaptive Refinement and Nonlinear Fluid Problems," Computer Methods in Applied Mechanics and Engineering, Vols. 17-18, 1979, pp. 541-560.

19 Carey, G. F., Humphrey, D. I., "Residuals Adaptive Refinement and Nonlinear Iterations for Finite Element Computations," in Finite Element Grid Optimization, edited by Shephard, M., Gallagher, R., ASME Publication PVP-38, New York, 1979.

20 Carroll, W. E., "On Optimum Idealizations in Discrete Element Analysis," Ph.D. Thesis, Virginia Polytechnic Institute and State University, Blacksburg, Virginia, 1971.

21 Carroll, W. E., "Ramifications of Optimum Idealization Geometry in Discrete Element Analysis," Proceedings World Congress on Finite Element in Structural Mechanics, Bournemouth, England, 1975.

22 Carroll, W. E., "Inclusive Criteria for Optimum Grid Generation of the Discrete Analysis Technique," Computers and Structures, Vol. 7, 1976, pp. 335-337.

23 Carroll, W. E., "Application of Near Optimum Mesh Generation Technique to Conforming and Non-Conforming Finite Element Solutions," Symposium on Applications of Computer Methods in Engineering, University of Southern California, August 1977.

24 Carroll, W. E., "Recent Developments Dealing with Optimum Finite Element Analysis Techniques," in Finite Element Grid Optimization, edited by Shephard, M., Gallagher, R., ASME Publication PVP-38, New York, 1979.

25 Carroll, W. E., "User Oriented Mesh Refinements in the Discrete Element Analysis Technique," Proceedings 2nd Int. Conference on Vehicle Structural Mechanics, SAE, Southfield, MI, April 1977.

26 Carroll, W. E., "On the Reformulation of the Finite Element Method," Int. Symposium on Innovative Numerical Analysis in Applied Engineering Science, Versailles, France, May 1977.

27 Carroll, W. E., Barker, R. M., "A Theorem for Optimum Finite Element Idealization," Int. Journal Solids and Structures, Vol. 9, Nov. 7, 1973, pp. 883-894.

28 Case, W. R., Mason, J. B., "NASTRAN Finite Element Idealization Study," Guidelines for Finite Element Idealization, ASCE National Structural Engineering Convention, New Orleans, April 1975.

29 Chan, P., and Turcke, D. J., "An Algorithm to Plot Isostatics," (In preparation).

30 deBoor, C., "Good Approximation by Splines with Variable Knots II," Conference on Numerical Solution of Differential Equations," Lecture Notes in Mathematics, Springer-Verlag, Vol. 363, 1973, pp. 12-20.

31 deBoor, C., Rice, J. R., "An Adaptive Algorithm for Multivariate Approximation Giving Optimal Convergence Rantes," MRC Report 1773, University of Wisconsin, 1977.

32 Delfino, B., et al, "A Contribution to High-Precision Numerical Computation of Laplacian Fields," International Conference on Numerical Methods in Electrical and Magnetic Field Problems, Santa Margherita, Italy, June 1-4, 1976.

33 Denny, V. E., Landis, R. B., "A New Method for Solving Two-Point Boundary Value Problems Using Optimal Node Distributions," Journal Computational Physics, Vol. 9, 1972, pp. 120-137.

34 Durocher, L. L., Stango, R. J., "Grid Selection and Refinement Procedures in Finite Element Analysis," ASME Publication 78-DE-21, 1978.

35 Felippa, C. A., "Optimization of Finite Element Grids by Direct Energy Search," Appl. Math. Modelling, Vol. I, Sept. 1976, pp. 93-96.

36 Felippa, C. A., "Numerical Experiments in Finite Element Grid Optimization by Direct Energy Search," Appl. Math. Modelling, June 1977, pp. 239-244.

37 Fried, I., "A Gradient Computational Procedure for the Solution of Large Problems Arising from the Finite Element Discretization Method," Int. Journal Num. Meth. Eng., Vol. 2, 1970, pp. 477-494.

38 Fried, I., and Yank, S. K., "Best Finite Element Distribution Around a Singularity," AIAA Journal, Vol. 10, No. 9, September 1972.

39 Gallagher, R. H., and Greenberg, D. P., "Computer Graphics in Structural Engineering Research," Interactive Computer Graphics in Engineering, ASME Special Publications, Jan. 1977.

40 Guerra, F. M., Becker, E. B., "Finite Element Analysis for the Adaptive Method of Rezoning," TICOM Report 78-13, Texas Institute for Computational Mechanics, University of Texas at Austin, 1978.

41 "Guidelines for Finite Element Idealization," edited by Ebner, A., ASCE National Convention, Preprint 2504, New Orleans, April 1975.

42 Haber, R., Shephard, M., Abel, J. F., Gallagher, R. H., Greenberg, D. P., "A Generalized Graphic Preprocessor for Two-Dimensional Finite Element Analysis," ACM SIGGRAPH '78 Proceedings, Aug. 1978, pp. 323-329.

43 Katz, I. R., Peano, A. G., and Szabo, B. A., "Nodal Variables for Arbitrary Order Conformity Finite Elements," Tech. Report DOT-03-30108-5, Washington University, St. Louis, Mo., June 1975.

44 Killian, D. E., "Selective Refinement of a Finite Element Mesh for Improved Accuracy," Master's Thesis, Engineering Mechanics Dept., Virginia Polytechnic Institute and State University, Blacksburg, Va., 1975.

45 Masur, E. F.,"Some Remarks on the Optimal Choice of Finite Element Grids," Computer Methods Applied Mechanics and Eng., Vol. 14, 1978, pp. 237-248.

46 Melosh, R. J., Killian, D. E., "Finite Element Analysis to Attain Pre-specified Accuracy," 2nd Nat. Symposium on Computerized Structural Analysis and Design, George Washington University, March 1974.

47 Melosh, R. J., Marcal, P. V., "An Energy Basis for Mesh Refinement of Structural Continua," International Journal for Numerical Methods in Engineering, Vol. 11, No. 7, 1977, pp. 1083-1092.

48 Melosh, R. J., "Design Principles for Finite Element Meshing," NASA-ICASE Symposium on Mathematical Modeling, Langley Research Center, Hampton, Oct. 24, 1979.

49 McNeice, G. M., Marcal, P. V., "Optimization of Finite Element Grids Based on Minimum Potential Energy," Transactions of ASME Journal of Engineering for Industry, Vol. 95, No. 1, 1978, pp. 186-190.

50 Molinari, E., Viviani, A., "Grid and Matrix Optimization Procedures in Finite Element Methods," Proceedings of 1974 IEEE Winter Power Meeting, Jan. 29, 1976.

51 Molinari, G., Viviani, A., "Grid Iteration for Finite Element Grid Optimization," in Finite Element Grid Optimization, edited by Shephard, M., Gallagher, R., ASME Publication PVP-38, New York, 1979.

52 Nitsche, J. A., Schatz, A. H., "Interior Estimates for Ritz-Galerkin Methods," Mathematical Com., Vol. 28, 1974, pp. 937-948.

53 Oliveria, E. R. A., "Optimization of Finite Element Solutions," Proceedings of the Third Conference on Matrix Methods in Structural Mechanics, Wright-Patterson Air Force Base, Ohio, Oct. 1972.

54 Peano, A., Riccioni, R., "Automated Discretization Error Control in Finite Element Analysis," World Congress on Finite Elements, Oct. 1978.

55 Peano, A., Riccioni, R., Pasini, A., Sardella, L., "Adaptive Approximation in Finite Element Structural Analysis," Trends in Computerized Structural Analysis and Synthesis, edited by Noor, A. K., McComb, H. G., Pergamon Press, 1978, pp. 333-342.

56 Peano, A., Riccioni, R., Pasini, A., Sardella, L., "Self-Adaptive Convergence at the Crack Tip of a Dam Buttress," Proceedings Int. Conference on Numerical Methods in Fracture Mechanics," Swansea, Wales, Jan. 1978.

57 Peano, A., Riccioni, R., Pasini, A., Sardella, L., "Adaptive Approximations in Finite Element Structural Analysis," Computers and Structures, Vol. 10, 1979, pp. 333-342.

58 Pederson, P., "Some Properties of Linear Strain Triangles and Optimal, Finite Element Models," International Journal on Numerical Mathematical Engineering, Vol. 7, No. 4, 1973, pp. 415-431.

59 Peregra, V., Sewell, E. G., "Mesh Selection for Discrete Solutions of Boundary-Value Problems in Ordinary Differential Equations," Numerische Mathematik, Vol. 23, 1975, pp. 261-268.

60 Phillips, G. M., "Error Estimates for Best Approximation," Approximation Theory, edited by Talbot, A., Academic Press, London, 1970, pp. 1-8.

61 Prager, W., "A Note on the Optimal Choice of Finite Element Grids," Computational Methods Applied Mechanics and Engineering, Vol. 6, 1975, pp. 363-366.

62 Rheinboldt, W., "Numerical Continuation Methods for Finite Element Applications," in Formulations and Computational Algorithms in Finite Element Analysis, edited by Boothe, J., Oden, J. T., and Wunderlich, W., MIT Press, Cambridge, Mass., 1977, pp. 599-631.

63 Rheinboldt, W., Mesztengi, C., "On a Data Structure for Adaptive Finite Element Mesh Refinements," Transaction 660, University of Maryland, 1979.

64 Rheinboldt, W., "Solution Fields of Nonlinear Equations and Continuation Methods," ICMA-79-04, University of Pittsburg, March 1979.

65 Rossow, M. P., and Katz, I. R., "Hierarchal Finite Elements and Pre-computed Arrays," International Journal Num. Meth. Eng., Vol. 12, No. 6, 1978, pp. 977-1000.

66 Russell, R. B., "A Comparison of Collocation and Finite Difference for Two-Point Boundary Value Problems," SIAM Journal of Numerical Analysis, Vol. 14, 1977, pp. 19-39.

67 Sezuchi, Y., Tomita, Y., Hashimoto, S., "Optimal Finite Element Discretization Based on Two Factor Decision Criteria of Potential Energy and Condition

Number," Applications of Computer Methods in Engineering, University of Southern California, Los Angeles, August 1977.

68 Sewell, G., "An Adaptive Computer Program for the Solution of DIV (P (X,Y) Grad. U) - P (X,Y,U) on a Polygonal Region," The Mathematics of Finite Elements and Applications II, Academic Press, 1976.

69 Shephard, M. S., "Finite Element Grid Optimization with Interactive Computer Graphics," Ph.D. Thesis, Dept. of Structural Engineering, Cornell University, Jan. 1979.

70 Shephard, M. S., Gallagher, R. H., Abel, J. F., "Experience with Interactive Computer Graphics for the Synthesis of Optimal Finite Element Mesher," in Finite Element Grid Optimization, edited by Shephard, M., and Gallagher, R. H., ASME Publication PVP-38, New York, 1979.

71 Shephard, M. S., Gallagher, R. H., Abel, J. F., "Finite Element Solutions to Point-Load Problems," Journal of Engineering Mechanics, ASCE, Vol. 107, No. EM5, Oct. 1981, pp. 839-850.

72 Shephard, M. S., Gallagher, R. H., Abel, J. F., "The Synthesis of Near-Optimum Finite Element Meshes with Interactive Computer Graphics," International Journal for Numerical Methods in Engineering, Vol. 15, 1980, pp. 1021-1039.

73 Szabo, B. A., Mehta, A. K., "P-Convergent Finite Element Approximations in Fracture Mechanics," International Journal Numerical Methods in Engineering, Vol. 12, 1978, pp. 551-560.

74 Szabo, B. A., Basu, P. R., Rossow, M. P., "Adaptive Finite Element Analysis Based on P-Convergence," Research in Computerized Structural Analysis and Synthesis, NASA Conference Publication 2059, 1978, pp. 43-50.

75 Tang, J. W., Turcke, D. J., "Characteristics of Optimal Grids," Computer Methods in Applied Mechanics and Engineering, Vol. 11, 1977, pp. 31-37.

76 Taylor, R. L., and Iding, R., "Application of Extended Variational Principles to Finite Element Analysis," Conference on Variational Methods in Engineering, Southampton University, England, September 1972.

77 Turcke, D. J., "Optimum Mesh Configuration in the Finite Element Method," Ph.D. Thesis, Dept. Civil Engineering, University of Waterloo, Canada, July 1974.

78 Turcke, D. J., "Why Optimized Grids in the Finite Element Method, " 14th Midwestern Mechanics Conference, University of Oklahoma, Oklahoma, March 24-26, 1975.

79 Turcke, D. J., "Further Developments in Grid Selection Procedures in the Finite Element Method," Fifth Canadian Conference of Applied Mechanics, University of New Brunswick, Canada, May 26, 1975.

80 Turcke, D. J., "On Optimum Finite Element Grid Configurations," AIAA Journal, Vol. 14, No. 2, 1976, pp. 264-265.

81 Turcke, D. J., "Optimal Piecewise Approximations in Numerical Analysis," Symposium on Innovative Numerical Analysis in Applied Engineering Science, Versailles, France, May 1977.

82 Turcke, D. J., "A Discretization Procedure for Finite Element Grids in Plate Analysis," AIAA/ASME 19th Structures, Structural Dynamics, and Materials Conference, Bethesda, Maryland, April 1978.

83 Turcke, D. J., "An Interactive Structural Modeling Technique," SAP Users Conference on Computer Methods in Engineering, Los Angeles, California, June 1978.

84 Turcke, D. J., "Equalizing Energy Levels in Optimum Finite Element Mesh Configurations," Eighth U.S. National Congress of Applied Mechanics, Los Angeles, California, June 1978.

85 Turcke, D. J., "Optimal Piecewise Approximations of Functions in Civil Engineering," International Congress on the Application of Mathematics, Weimar DDR, East Germany, July 1978.

86 Turcke, D. J., "A Preprocessing Technique for Improved Mesh Generation," Second World Congress on Finite Element Methods, Bournemouth, Dorset, England, October 1978.

87 Turcke, D. J., "Finite Element Mesh Configurations Using Isoenergetics and Equalized Energy Levels," Symposium on Future Trends in Computerized Structural Analysis and Synthesis, Washington, D. C., November 1978.

88 Turcke, D. J., "Characteristics of Piecewise Approximations in Numerical Analysis," in Finite Element Grid Optimization, edited by Shephard, M., and Gallagher, R., ASME Publication PVP-38, New York, 1979.

89 Turcke, D. J., Hoerz, D., "Techniques for Adaptive Mesh Modifications with Conformity," AIAA/ASME/ASCE/AHS 20th Structures, Structural Dynamics and Materials Conference, St. Louis, Missouri, April 1979.

90 Turcke, D. J., and Hoerz, D., "Constraint Techniques for Adaptive Mesh Modifications," Nonlinear Finite Element Analysis and Adina Conference, M.I.T., Cambridge, Mass., August 1979.

91 Turcke, D. J., and Hoerz, D., "Efficient Grid Layouts Using a Constraint Technique," Sixteenth Midwestern Mechanics Conference, Manhattan, Kansas, September 1979.

92 Turcke, D. J., McNeice, G. M., "A Variational Approach to Grid Optimization in the Finite Element Method," Proceedings Conference on Variational Mechanics in Engineering, Southampton University, England, September 1972.

93 Turcke, D. J., and McNeice, G. M., "Procedures for Selecting Near Optimum Finite Element Grids," Second International Conference on Pressure Vessel and Piping Technology, San Antonio, Texas, October 1973.

94 Turcke, D. J., McNeice, G. M., "Guidelines for Selecting Finite Element Grids Based on an Optimization Study," Computers and Structures, Vol. 4, 1974, pp. 499-519.

95 Turcke, D. J., McNeice, G. M., "Applications of Grid Selection Procedures for Improved Finite Element Stress Analysis," Proceedings International Conference on Vehicle Structural Mechanics, SAE, Detroit, 1974, pp. 203-216.

96 Turcke, D. J., and Sui, D., "Optimum Grids in Nonlinear Finite Element Analysis," Symposium on Mathematical Modeling in Structural Engineering, NASA Langley Research Center, Hampton, VA, October 1979.

97 Viviani, A., "Grid and Metric Optimization in Finite Difference and Finite Element Methods in Magnetic Problems," IEEE Transactions in Magnetics, Vol. MAG-14, No. S., September 1978, pp. 461-463.

98 White, A. B., "On Selection of Equidistributing Meshes for Two Point Boundary-Value Problems," Center for Numerical Analysis CNA-112, University of Texas at Austin, July 1976.

99 Zare, P., Rheinboldt, W. C., "Design of an Adaptive Finite Element System," Computer Science Report Transaction 593, University of Maryland, November 1977.

CHAPTER FOUR

HIGHER-ORDER, SPECIAL AND SINGULAR FINITE ELEMENTS

S. N. Atluri
Regents' Professor of Mechanics
Center for the Advancement of Computational Mechanics
School of Civil Engineering
Georgia Institute of Technology
Atlanta, Georgia

ABSTRACT

This chapter deals with the topics of (i) interpolation such that function continuity is maintained at the interelement boundaries; (ii) certain important properties of these interpolation functions; (iii) sub- or iso- or superparametric geometric transformations for elements with curved boundaries, and properties of such transformations; (iv) a discussion of problems with singularities for derivatives of the field variable; and (v) special and singular finite elements to treat problems of this kind.

SCOPE OF THE CHAPTER

In Section I we treat the topic of Lagrange interpolation on a line in one dimension, in triangles and quadrilaterals in two dimensions, and in tetrahedra, hexahedra, and prisms in three dimensions. Only interpolation functions that maintain function continuity at interelement boundaries are discussed with a view toward their application in deriving "singular" elements, which are discussed in later sections. Basis functions that maintain derivative continuity, in addition to function continuity, are discussed in the chapter by Wachpress. In Section II we consider certain elements with boundary nodes only and discuss briefly a method of elimination of internal parameters to derive the basis functions for such elements. In Section III we present sub- or iso- or superparametric geometric transformations, and their fundamental properties, to represent one, two, and three dimensional elements with curved geometries. These geometric transformations, in general, only yield approximations to the original curves and surfaces. The topic of finding "exact" basis functions for curved elements has been treated in the chapter by Wachpress. A general discussion of problems, in two and three dimensions, with singularities for the derivatives of the field variable is presented in Section IV. The relevant problems of fracture mechanics are briefly noted. Section V is devoted to the concepts underlying the development of special and singular finite elements to deal with problems with nonremovable singularities. Three types of such singular elements are considered, viz., (i) those involving singular geometric transformations which can be either introduced directly or through distorting the placement of cartesian nodes in a sub- or isoparametric geometric transformation, (ii) those whose shape functions have been modified to reflect the known singular behavior in the function derivatives, and (iii) those elements within which the known analytical asymptotic solutions for the field behavior near the singularity are included in addition, in some cases, to the usual polynomial shape functions.

Some of the material in this chapter has been presented here for the first time.

In keeping with the aims of this book, the material is presented in such a fashion, that it should be accessible to an engineer with a standard baccalaureate background.

I. Lagrange Interpolation

I.1 One-Dimensional Domain

Consider, without loss of generality, a straight line along the x-axis in a cartesian reference frame, such that $x_o \leq x \leq x_M$. Consider the nondimensional coordinate $\xi = (x-x_o)/(x_M-x_o)$ such that $0 \leq \xi \leq 1$. A complete mth order polynomial $F^{(m)}(\xi)$, (where m is assumed to be an integer), can be represented by interpolating the discrete values of the function at (m+1) equidistant points $\xi_i[i=0,\ldots m;\ \xi_i = (i/m)]$ using the Lagrange interpolation functions, $L_i^{(m)}(\xi)$, as

$$F^{(m)}(\xi) = \sum_{i=o}^{m} F_i\, L_i^{(m)}(\xi) \tag{1}$$

where $$L_i^{(m)}(\xi) = \frac{(\xi-\xi_o)(\xi-\xi_1)\ldots(\xi-\xi_{i-1})(\xi-\xi_{i+1})\ldots(\xi-\xi_m)}{(\xi_i-\xi_o)(\xi_i-\xi_1)\ldots(\xi_i-\xi_{i-1})(\xi_i-\xi_{i+1})\ldots(\xi_i-\xi_m)}$$

Henceforth, we use the notation:

$$\prod_{j=o}^{m} (a-a_j) = (a-a_o)(a-a_1)(a-a_2)\ldots(a-a_{j-1})(a-a_j)(a-a_{j+1})\ldots(a-a_m) \tag{2}$$

Thus, $$L_i^{(m)}(\xi) = \prod_{j=o,j\neq i}^{m} \left(\frac{\xi-\xi_j}{\xi_i-\xi_j}\right) \tag{3}$$

It is seen that the functions in Eq. (3) have the property, that

$$L_i^{(m)}(\xi_k) = \delta_{ik} \tag{4}$$

where $\delta_{ik} = 0(i\neq k)$ and $\delta_{ik} = 1\ (i=k)$. It is also seen that the polynomials $L_i^{(m)}$, for the given positioning of the points ξ_i, are linearly independent and that each of them is of mth order. Thus, any other polynomial $G^{(r)}(\xi)$, $r \leq m$, can be represented as:

$$G^{(r)}(\xi) = \sum_{i=o}^{m} A_i\, L_i^{(m)}(\xi) \tag{5}$$

where A_i are constants. In view of Eq. (4), it is seen that

$$G_j \equiv G^{(r)}(\xi_j) = \sum_{i=o}^{m} A_i\, \delta_{ij} = A_j \tag{6}$$

Thus, $$G^{(r)}(\xi) = \sum_{j=o}^{m} G_j\, L_j^{(m)}(\xi) \tag{7}$$

However, when m is an integer, r must be an integer and $r \leq m$, so that the representation in Eq. (7) is exact. By letting $r = o$ and $\overline{G}^{(o)}(\xi) = 1$, we obtain the useful result;

$$\sum_{i=o}^{m} L_i^{(m)}(\xi) \equiv 1 \tag{8}$$

Finally we note that since x and ξ are related linearly to each other in the present case, the function F(x) is also an mth order polynomial.

I.2 Two-Dimensional Domains

a. Triangle ($o \leq \xi, \eta, \zeta \leq 1$). Consider, without loss of generality, a triangular domain whose vertices $P_i (i=1,2,3)$ are located at coordinates (x_i, y_i) $(i=1,2,3)$ in the plane $z = o$ in a cartesian coordinate system (x,y,z). We introduce nondimensional coordinates ξ, η, ζ such that $o \leq \xi, \eta, \zeta \leq 1$. If P is an arbitrary point in the triangle whose area is represented by Δ_{123}, the parametric coordinates are such that $\xi = (\Delta_{P23})/(\Delta_{123})$, $\eta = (\Delta_{P31}/\Delta_{123})$ and $\zeta = (\Delta_{P12}/\Delta_{123})$ respectively. The relations between the (x,y) and the (ξ,η,ζ) coordinates can be seen to be:

$$x = x_1\xi + x_2\eta + x_3\zeta$$

$$y = y_1\xi + y_2\eta + y_3\zeta \tag{9}$$

The vertices of the triangle in the ξ, η, ζ system are: $P_1 = (1,0,0)$; $P_2 = (0,1,0)$; and $P_3 = (0,0,1)$. However, the three coordinates ξ, η, ζ are constrained such that

$$\xi + \eta + \zeta = 1 \tag{10}$$

we consider (m+1) equidistant points along each of the sides $\xi = 0$, $\eta = 0$, and $\zeta = 0$ respectively, such that $\xi_i = (i/m)$, $\eta_j = (j/m)$, and $\zeta_k = (k/m)(i,j,k = 0,\ldots m)$. We locate a point P_{ijk} such that it is at the intersection of the three lines, $\xi = \xi_i$; $\eta = \eta_j$, $\zeta = \zeta_k$. Thus, there are a total of (m+1)(m+2)/2 points in the domain. Because of Eq. (10), it is seen that $(i+j+k) \equiv m$. A complete mth order homogeneous polynomial $F^{(m)}(\xi,\eta,\zeta)$ can be represented exactly by interpolating the values of the function F_{ijk} at points P_{ijk} by using Lagrange interpolation, as:

$$F^{(m)}(\xi,\eta,\zeta) = \sum_{(ijk)} F_{ijk} L_{ijk}^{(m)}(\xi,\eta,\zeta) \tag{11}$$

$$\text{where, } L_{ijk}^{(m)} = \left[\prod_{r=o}^{i-1}\left(\frac{\xi-\xi_r}{\xi_i-\xi_r}\right)\right]\left[\prod_{s=o}^{j-1}\left(\frac{\eta-\eta_s}{\eta_j-\eta_s}\right)\right]\left[\prod_{t=o}^{k-1}\left(\frac{\zeta-\zeta_t}{\zeta_k-\zeta_t}\right)\right] \tag{12}$$

Alternative representations for $L_{ijk}^{(m)}$ were given in (1) and pictorial descriptions of these functions can be found in (2,3,4). The functions in Eq. (12) have the properties,

$$L_{ijk}^{(m)}(\xi_p,\eta_n,\zeta_\ell) = \delta_{ip}\,\delta_{jn}\,\delta_{k\ell}; \quad \sum_{ijk} L_{ijk}^{(m)} \equiv 1 \tag{13}$$

b. Triangle ($o \leq \eta, \zeta \leq 1$). The representation of a two-dimensional domain in terms of three parameters ξ, η, ζ, constrained by Eq. (10), is often inconvenient. It is convenient to introduce a standard non-dimensional triangle ($o \leq \eta, \zeta \leq 1$) as shown in Fig. 1. As can be seen from Eq. (9) the triangle $P_1P_2P_3$ with cartesian coordinates $(x_i, y_i)(i=1,2,3)$ is then mapped into the standard triangle, shown in Fig. 1b, through the relations:

$$(x-x_1) = (x_2-x_1)\eta + (x_3-x_1)\zeta$$

$$(y-y_1) = (y_2-y_1)\eta + (y_3-y_1)\zeta \tag{14}$$

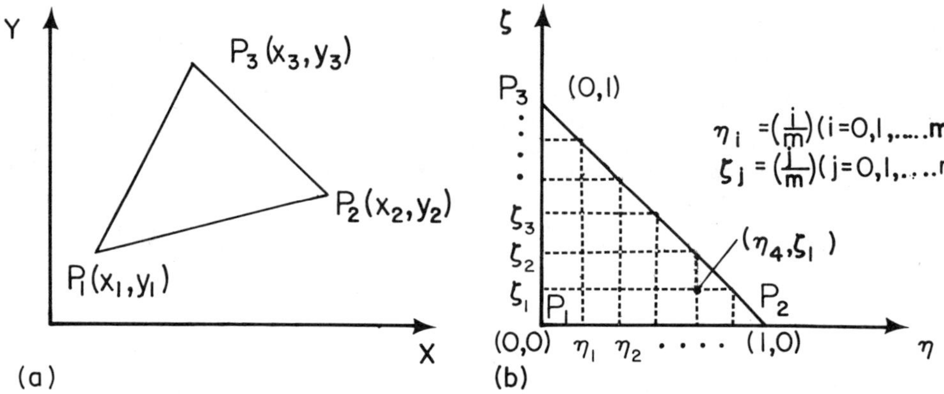

Fig. 1

Consider (m+1) equidistant points along the lines $\eta = o$ and $\zeta = o$, respectively, such that $\eta_i = (i/m)$ and $\zeta_j = (j/m)(i,j=0,1\ldots m)$. A complete mth order polynomial (m being an integer), $F^{(m)}(\eta,\zeta)$, can be exactly represented by interpolating the values of the function at the $(m+1)(m+2)/2$ symmetrically located points P_{ij} (with coordinates η_i, ζ_j) in the standard triangle, as:

$$F^{(m)}(\eta,\zeta) = \sum_{i=o}^{m} \sum_{j=o}^{m-i} F_{ij}\, L_{ij}^{(m)}(\eta,\zeta) \tag{15}$$

$$\text{where, } L_{ij}^{(m)} = \left[\prod_{r=o}^{i-1}\left(\frac{\eta-\eta_r}{\eta_i-\eta_r}\right)\right] \left[\prod_{s=o}^{j-1}\left(\frac{\zeta-\zeta_s}{\zeta_j-\zeta_s}\right)\right] \left[\prod_{t=o}^{m-(i+j+1)}\left\{\frac{<1-(\eta+\zeta) - (t/m)>}{<1-(\eta_i+\zeta_j) - (t/m)>}\right\}\right] \tag{16}$$

Referring to Fig. 1b, a simple geometric interpretation for the function in Eq. (16) is that it is an appropriately normalized product of the equations for (i) the vertical lines passing through the points $\eta_r[r=o,\ldots(i-1)]$; (ii) the horizontal lines passing through the points $\zeta_s[s=o,\ldots(j-1)]$; and (iii) the inclined lines through the points $\eta_t[t=(i+j+1),\ldots m]$. Examples of linear, quadratic, and cubic polynomials, $L_{ij}^{(1)}$, $L_{ij}^{(2)}$, and $L_{ij}^{(3)}$, respectively, are illustrated in detail in (5). Note that $L_{ij}^{(1)}$ and $L_{ij}^{(2)}$ do not need interpolation points inside the standard triangle, while $L_{ij}^{(3)}$ depends on a tenth point ($\zeta = \eta = 1/3$) inside the triangle, in addition to the nine boundary points which divide each of the three edges into the three equal segments. The normalization of the interpolation in Eq. (16) is such that

$$L_{ij}^{(m)}(\eta_k,\zeta_\ell) = \delta_{ik}\,\delta_{j\ell} \tag{17}$$

Further, the functions $L_{ij}^{(m)}$ are, for the positioning of the points (η_i, ζ_j) as in the present case, linearly independent, and each of them is an mth order polynomial (m is an integer) in η, ζ. Thus, any other polynomial $H^{(r)}(\eta,\zeta)$ [r an integer, $r \leq m$] can be expressed as a linear combination of the function in Eq. (16), as:

$$H^{(r)}(\eta,\zeta) = \sum_{i=o}^{m} \sum_{j=o}^{m-i} A_{ij} \, L_{ij}^{(m)}(\eta,\zeta) \tag{18}$$

In view of Eq. (17), it is seen that

$$H^{(r)}(\eta_k,\zeta_\ell) \equiv A_{k\ell}; \; H^{(r)}(\eta,\zeta) = \sum_k \sum_\ell H^{(r)}(\eta_k,\zeta_\ell) \, L_{k\ell}^{(m)}(\eta,\zeta) \tag{19}$$

$$\text{Thus,} \quad \sum_{k=o}^{m} \sum_{\ell-o}^{m-k} L_{k\ell}^{(m)} = 1 \tag{20}$$

We also note that due to the linearity of the relations in Eq. (14), the function $F^{(m)}$ of Eq. (15) is also an mth order polynomial in (x,y).

For purposes to be evident later, we now consider certain interesting features of the linear geometric transformation in Eq. (14). Ignoring for the moment the special cases when the lines P_1P_2 and/or P_1P_3 in Fig. (1a) may be parallel to the cartesian axes, without loss of generality, consider a straight line passing through the point P_1 (x_1,y_1) and given by the equation,

$$(x-x_1)/(y-y_1) = \beta; \; [(x_3-x_1)/(y_3-y_1)] \leq \beta \leq [(x_2-x_1)/(y_2-y_1)] \tag{21}$$

Using Eq. (21) in Eq. (14) and rearranging terms, it is seen that

$$[(x_2-x_1)+(y_1-y_2)\beta]\eta = [(x_1-x_3) + \beta(y_3-y_1)]\zeta \tag{22}$$

Thus, a straight line passing through P_1 in the (x,y) plane is mapped into a straight line passing through the origin in the (η,ζ) plane. From Eq. (22), it can be derived that,

$$(\eta+\zeta) = \left[\frac{(x_2-x_3)+\beta(y_3-y_2)}{(x_2-x_1)+\beta(y_1-y_2)}\right]\zeta \equiv \left[\frac{(x_2-x_3)+\beta(y_3-y_2)}{(x_1-x_3)+\beta(y_3-y_1)}\right]\eta \tag{23}$$

The radial length, R, measured from the point P_1 in the (x,y) plane is given by:

$$R^2 = (x-x_1)^2 + (y-y_1)^2 \equiv (1+\beta^2)[(y_2-y_1)\eta + (y_3-y_1)\zeta]^2 \tag{24}$$

wherein, use is made of Eqs. (21) and (14b). Substituting for η and ζ from Eq. (23) in Eq. (24), we also obtain

$$R^2 = \frac{(1+\beta^2)J_o}{[(x_2-x_3)+\beta(y_3-y_2)]^2} (\eta+\zeta)^2 \tag{25}$$

where $J_o = 2(\text{Area } P_1P_2P_3) = \det \begin{bmatrix} 1 & x_1 & y_1 \\ 1 & x_2 & y_2 \\ 1 & x_3 & y_3 \end{bmatrix}$

Thus it is seen from Eqs. (23 to 25) that, in the parametric system (η,ζ), the radial length, R, from P_1 in the cartesian (x,y) system is proportional to η or ζ or $(\eta+\zeta)$, and in general a linear function of η, ζ, and $(\eta+\zeta)$. It can be seen from Eq. (16) that the polynomial $L_{ij}^{(m)}$, especially L_{oo}^{m} corresponding to the point $P_1(\eta=\zeta=0)$, contains terms such as $(\eta+\zeta)^p$ (p, an integer and $p \leq m$). The polynomial $F^m(x,y)$ corresponding to Eq. (15) contains terms of the type R^p(p, an integer) when the linear transformation between the (x,y) and (η,ζ) systems, as in Eq. (14), is used.

c. Triangle (Polar Co-ordinates $0 \leq \sigma, \rho \leq 1$). Since $(\eta+\zeta)$ has been shown in the above to be proportional to the radius R measured from P_1, it is convenient to introduce $(\eta+\zeta) = \sigma$ as a new parameter in describing an arbitrary triangle in the (x,y) system by polar coordinates, σ and ρ, as follows. We rewrite Eqs. (9) or (14) as:

$$\begin{aligned} x &= x_1[1-(\eta+\zeta)] + x_2\eta + x_3\zeta \\ &= x_1[1-(\eta+\zeta)] + x_2(\eta+\zeta)\left[1 - \frac{\zeta}{\eta+\zeta}\right] + x_3(\eta+\zeta)\frac{\zeta}{\eta+\zeta} \\ &= x_1(1-\sigma) + x_2\sigma(1-\rho) + x_3\sigma\rho \end{aligned} \tag{26}$$

with similar equations for y. In the above, the parameters (σ,ρ), where,

$$\sigma \equiv (\eta+\zeta); \quad \rho \equiv \frac{\zeta}{\eta+\zeta}$$

or

$$\eta \equiv \sigma(1-\rho) \text{ and } \zeta \equiv \sigma\rho \tag{27}$$

are polar coordinates such that $0 \leq \sigma, \rho \leq 1$, as shown in Fig. 2.

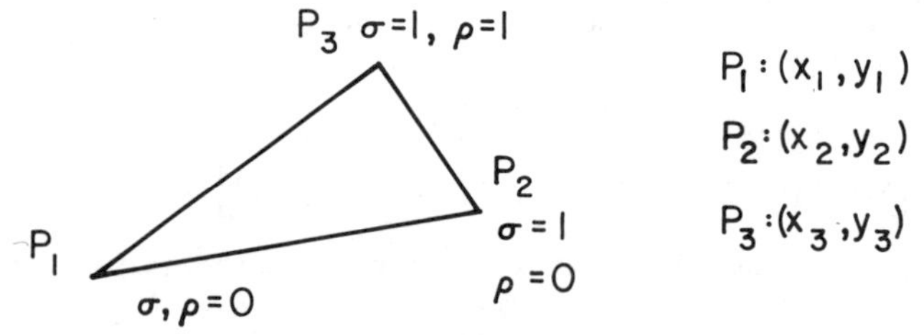

Fig. 2

By substituting for η and ζ in terms of σ and ρ from Eq. (27), the Lagrange polynomials of Eq. (16) can be written in terms of σ and ρ. It is noted that now the polynomials $L_{ij,p}^{(m)}$ especially $L_{oo}^{(m)}$ and hence $F^{(m)}$ of Eq. (15), would contain terms of the type σ, and are thus of type R^p ($p \leq m$, p an integer).

For convenience, we write Eq. (26) as:

$$(x-x_1) = [(x_2-x_1)(1-\rho) + (x_3-x_1)\rho]\sigma$$

similarly

$$(y-y_1) = [(y_2-y_1)(1-\rho) + (y_3-y_1)\rho]\sigma \tag{28}$$

Consider, without loss of generality, a straight line, $(x-x_1)/(y-y_1) = \beta$, passing through the point (x_1,y_1) in the (x,y) plane. From Eq. (18), rearranging terms, it is seen that this straight line maps into

$$\rho = [(x_2-x_1) + \beta(y_1-y_2)]/[(x_2-x_3) + \beta(y_3-y_2)] \tag{29}$$

which is a straight line in the (σ,ρ) plane. Likewise, the radial length, R, from (x,y) can be derived to be:

$$R^2 = (x-x_1)^2 + (y-y_1)^2 = \left(\frac{(1+\beta^2)J_o}{[(x_2-x_3)^2+\beta(y_3-y_2)]^2}\right)\sigma^2 \tag{30}$$

where J_o is twice the area of the triangle $P_1P_2P_3$. Thus, when a geometric transformation of the type of Eq. (28) is employed, R varies proportional to σ.

The above polar-coordinates were used in certain applications in (6,7,8,9).

d. Quadrilateral ($0 \leq \eta, \zeta \leq 1$). Consider a general quadrilateral $P_1P_2P_3P_4$, with straight-line boundaries, in the (x,y) plane with coordinates (x_i,y_i) $(i=1,\ldots 4)$. This can be mapped into a unit square ($0 \leq \eta, \zeta \leq 1$) by the bilinear transformation:

$$x = x_1(1-\eta)(1-\zeta) + x_2(1-\zeta)\eta + x_3\zeta\eta + x_4\zeta(1-\eta)$$

or

$$x-x_1 = (x_2-x_1)\eta(1-\zeta) + (x_4-x_1)\zeta(1-\eta) + (x_3-x_1)\eta\zeta \tag{31a}$$

and similarly,

$$y-y_1 = (y_2-y_1)\eta(1-\zeta) + (y_4-y_1)\zeta(1-\eta) + y_3-y_1)\eta\zeta \tag{31b}$$

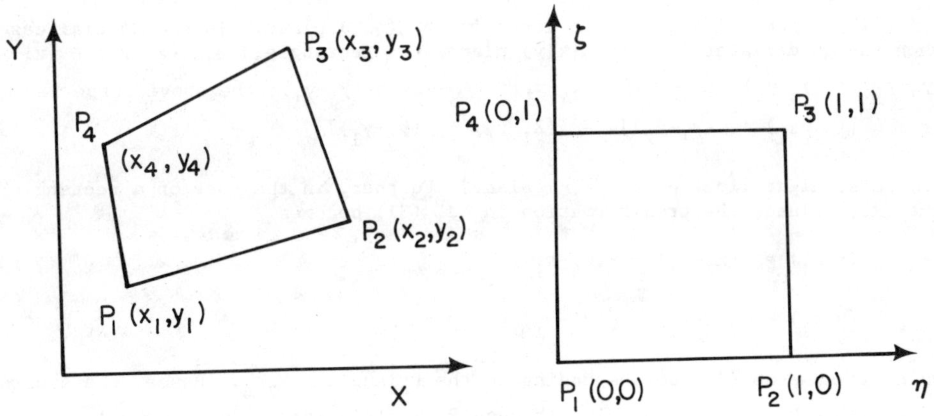

Fig. 3

As shown in Fig 3, the points P_1, P_2, P_3, and P_4 are respectively mapped into (0,0), (1,0), (1,1) and (0,1) in the (η,ζ) plane. By considering (m+1) equidistant points along the lines $\zeta = 0$ and $\eta = 0$, respectively, such that $\eta_i = (i/m)$, $\zeta_j = (j/m)$ $(i,j=0,1,\ldots m)$, we can write an interpolating function, which is of mth order in each of the ζ, η coordinates (such as bi-linear, bi-quadratic, etc.) as:

$$F_{ij}^{(m,m)}(\eta,\zeta) = \sum_{i=0}^{m} \sum_{j=0}^{m} F_{ij} L_{ij}^{(m,m)}(\eta,\zeta) \tag{32}$$

$$\text{where } L_{ij}^{(m,m)}(\eta,\zeta) = \left[\prod_{\substack{r=o\\r\neq i}}^{m} \left(\frac{\eta-\eta_r}{\eta_i-\eta_r}\right)\right] \left[\prod_{\substack{s=o\\s\neq j}}^{m} \left(\frac{\zeta-\zeta_s}{\zeta_j-\zeta_s}\right)\right] \tag{33a}$$

Once again, $L_{ij}^{(m,m)}(\eta_k,\zeta_\ell) = \delta_{ik}\,\delta_{j\ell}$. It should be noted that the above interpolation functions are not complete polynomilas of order 2m in (η,ζ) (However, at the boundaries of the domain, ie., ζ = const. or η = const., the polynomial is complete and of degree 'm' in the respective variable). Nevertheless, in view of Eq. (8), it can be seen that the above functions also possess the property that,

$$\sum_{i=o}^{m} \sum_{j=o}^{m} L_{ij}^{(m,m)}(\zeta,\eta) = 1 \tag{33b}$$

and also the property analogous to that in Eq. (19), except that they can only represent functions of the type

$$G^{(r,s)}(\eta,\zeta) = \left[G^{(r)}(\eta)\, G^{(s)}(\zeta)\right], \quad r,s \leq m$$

We consider, again without loss of generality, a straight-line, with the equation $[(x-x_1)/(y-y_1)] = \beta$, passing through P_1 in the (x,y) plane. By using Eq. (31), it is seen that the map of this straight line in the (η,ζ) plane is given by:

$$[(x_2-x_1) + \beta(y_1-y_2)]\eta(1-\zeta) + [(x_4-x_1) + \beta(y_1-y_4)]\zeta(1-\eta)$$

$$+ [(x_3-x_1) + \beta(y_1-y_3)]\eta\zeta = 0 \tag{34}$$

which is in general a quadratic curve in the (η,ζ) plane. In the special case when the quadrilateral in the (x,y) plane is a rectangle, i.e., $(x_2-x_1) \equiv (x_3-x_4)$; $(y_2-y_1) = (y_3-y_4)$; $(x_3-x_2) \doteq (x_4-x_1)$; $(y_3-y_2) = (y_4-y_1)$; the above curve becomes,

$$[(x_2-x_1) + \beta(y_1-y_2)]\eta = [(X_1-x_4) + \beta(y_4-y_1)]\zeta \tag{35}$$

i.e., a straight line in the (η,ζ) plane. Further, in the case of a rectangle in the (x,y) plane, the transformation in Eq. (31) becomes

$$(x-x_1) = \eta(x_2-x_1) + \zeta(x_4-x_1) \tag{36}$$

$$(y-y_1) = \eta(y_2-y_1) + \zeta(y_4-y_1)$$

which is same as (14) corresponding to the triangle $P_1P_2P_4$. Hence, the square of length P_1P of a line passing through P_1 in (x,y) plane is given by:

$$R^2 = (x-x_1)^2 + (y-y_1)^2 = (1+\beta^2)\{\eta(y_2-y_1) + \zeta(y_4-y_1)\}^2$$

$$= (\eta+\zeta)^2 \frac{(1+\beta^2)}{[(x_2-x_4)+\beta(y_4-y_2)]^2} \{(y_2-y_1)[(x_1-x_4)+(y_4-y_1)]$$

$$+ (y_4-y_1)[(x_2-x_1) + \beta(y_1-y_2)]\}^2 \quad (37)$$

Thus, $R \sim (\eta+\zeta)$. However, in the interpolation function of Eq. (33), terms of the type $(\eta+\zeta)^p$ ($p \leq m$, p an integer) do not occur. Thus, the function $F^m(x,y)$ of Eq. (32) does not, in general, contain terms of the type R^p.

Another comment of interest concerning the quadrilateral element can be made: suppose that points P_1 and P_4 coincide. Then, Eq. (31) reduces to:

$$x-x_1 = (x_2-x_1)\eta(1-\zeta) + (x_3-x_1)\eta\zeta$$

$$y-y_1 = (y_2-y_1)\eta(1-\zeta) + (y_3-y_1)\eta\zeta \quad (38)$$

which are equations analogous to the transformation equations for the triangle, namely Eq. (28), when η (for the quadrilateral) $\equiv \sigma$ (for the triangle) and likewise $\zeta \equiv \rho$. Likewise, if a linear interpolation function is considered in the quadrilateral and triangle respectively, and the case $F_{00} \equiv F_{01}$ is considered for the quadrilateral, it can be seen from Eqs. (33) and (27b, and 16) that $F^{(1,1)}(\eta,\zeta)$ for the quadrilateral is identical to $F^{(1)}(\sigma,\rho)$ for the triangle. This has also been noted in (10). However, the same equality cannot be expected for $F^{(r,r)}(\eta,\zeta)$ (for the degenerate quadrilateral when $F_{oj} \equiv F_{oo}$, $j=1,2,3\ldots$) and $F^{(r)}(\sigma,\rho)$ for the triangle, for any $r > 1$.

I.3 Three-Dimensional Domain

a. Tetrahedron: (ξ, η, ζ, ψ). Consider a tetrahedron $P_1P_2P_3P_4$, with plane faces, in the (x,y,z) space. This can be mapped into a unit tetrahedron with vertices (1,0,0,0), (0,1,0,0), (0,0,1,0) and (0,0,0,1) in the (ξ,η,ζ,ψ) space by the transformation:

$$x = x_1\xi + x_2\eta + x_3\zeta + x_4\psi$$

$$y = y_1\xi + y_2\eta + y_3\zeta + y_4\psi$$

$$z = z_1\xi + z_2\eta + z_3\zeta + z_4\psi$$

$$1 = \xi + \eta + \zeta + \psi \quad (39)$$

For any generic point P(x,y,z) in the tetrahedron, the coordinates ξ, η, ζ, and ψ have the interpretations that ξ = (Volume $PP_2P_3P_4$)/(Volume $P_1P_2P_3P_4$) etc. Only three of the coordinates, say, η, ζ, ψ are independent, while the fourth, say ξ, is given by Eq. (39d). A complete mth order polynomial in (η, ζ, ψ) can be represented by interpolating at 1/6 (m+1)(m+2)(m+3) symmetrically located points in the unit tetrahedron, as:

$$F^{(m)}(\eta, \zeta, \psi) = \sum_{i+j+k=0}^{m} F_{ijk}\, L_{ijk}^{(m)}(\eta,\zeta,\psi) \quad (40)$$

Further details of $L_{ijk}^{(m)}$ along with their geometric interpretations can be found in (3,4,5). Once again, the interpolates $L_{ijk}^{(m)}$ have the properties analogous to those discussed in connection with Eqs. (18-20).

b. Unit Cube: $(0 \leq \xi, \eta, \zeta \leq 1)$. Consider a general hexahedron $(P_1P_2\ldots P_8)$

identified by coordinates $(x_i,y_i)(i=1,...8)$ in the (x-y-z) cartesian space. This can be mapped into a unit cube $0 \leq \xi, \eta, \zeta \leq 1$ by using transformations entirely analogous to Eq. (31) (see for instance (3,4,5)). By considering (m+1) equidistant points along each of the axes ξ, η, and ζ respectively such that $\xi_j = (j/m)$; $\eta_k = (k/m)$; and $\zeta_l = (\ell/m)$ $(j,k,\ell=o,...m)$, we write a Lagrange interpolation function as:

$$F^{(m,m,m)}_{(\xi,\eta,\zeta)} = \sum_{i=o}^{m} \sum_{j=o}^{m} \sum_{k=o}^{m} F_{ijk}\, L_{ijk}^{(m,m,m)}(\xi,\eta,\zeta)$$

$$\text{where } L_{ijk}^{(m,m,m)} = \left[\prod_{\substack{r=o\\ r\neq i}}^{m} \left(\frac{\xi-\xi_r}{\xi_i-\xi_r}\right)\right] \left[\prod_{\substack{s=o\\ s\neq j}}^{m} \left(\frac{\eta-\eta_s}{\eta_j-\eta_s}\right)\right] \left[\prod_{\substack{t=o\\ t\neq k}}^{m} \left(\frac{\eta-\eta_t}{\eta_k-\eta_t}\right)\right] \quad (41)$$

Again, these functions possess the property analogous to that in Eq. (33b) and that in Eq. (19) except that they can represent only function of the type

$$F^{(r,s,t)}(\xi,\eta,\zeta)\left[= F^{(r)}(\xi)\, F^{(s)}(\eta)\, F^{(t)}(\zeta)\right],\ r,s,t \leq m$$

Triangular Prism Elements. These elements can be generated by multiplying the Lagrange polynomials of Eq. (16) [in the triangle coordinates η, ζ of Eq. (14) or of σ and ρ from Eq. (27)] with one dimensional Lagrange polynomials in the meridional coordinate ξ of the prism. Illustrations of such interpolants can be found in (2,3,4).

I.4 Comments on Lagrange Interpolation

The common properties of all the above interpolation functions are such that: (i) along any boundary-segment of the domain, the interpolation function is uniquely determined by the values of the function at the nodes on the particular segment only, (ii) the interpolant corresponding to the interior nodes (points) in the domain vanishes all along the boundary of the domain; (iii) because of (i) and (ii), the interpolation function is continuous at inter-domain boundaries if identical types of interpolation are used in adjoining domains (elements). (iv) all functions satisfy the condition that the sum over all the points in the domain of the individual interpolant for each point is equal to unity (see Eqs.(8, 20 and 33b, for instance).

One of the draw backs of the above interpolation functions, henceforth called Lagrange shape functions, is the occurence of nodes within the domain (henceforth called an element). These internal nodes can sometimes be eliminated by the well-known static-condensation procedures from the stiffness matrix of the element once such a matrix is generated (3), or alternatively the internal nodes can be eliminated a priori by other means (5, 11) which are labeled in (5) as methods of elimination of internal parameters.

However, in certain cases of two- and three-dimensional elements, shape functions for elements with only boundary nodes have been found by chance in (2,3,12,13). Accordingly, these elements were dubbed as "serendipity" elements for reasons of history and myth explained in (2). We now discuss these elements and their relation to the above mentioned method of elimination of internal parameters.

II. "Serendipity" Elements and a Method of Elimination of Internal Modes

Such elements need to be considered in only two- and three dimensional cases. The concepts can most simply be explained by considering a quadrilateral first.

II.1 Two-Dimensional Cases

a. Quadrilateral ($0 \leq \eta, \zeta \leq 1$). In a bilinear approximation, i.e., the case of (m,m) = (1,1) in Eq. (32), no internal nodes are present. However in a bi-quadratic, i.e., (m,m) = (2,2), a 9th node is located at $(\eta_1, \zeta_1) = (1/2, 1/2)$. The bi-quadratic interpolation of the type given in Eq. (32) can represent exactly, only a function of the type,

$$F^{(2,2)}(\eta,\zeta) = \alpha_1+\alpha_2\eta+\alpha_3\zeta+\alpha_4\eta^2+\alpha_5\zeta^2+\alpha_6\eta\zeta+\alpha_7\eta^2\zeta+\alpha_8\eta\zeta^2+\alpha_9\eta^2\zeta^2 \quad (42)$$

which is an incomplete polynomial in (η,ζ). In the above, the coefficients $\alpha_1 \ldots \alpha_9$ are related to the nine values F_{ij} (i,j=0,...2) at the nine nodes. Along any line η = const. or ζ = const., the function is a complete quadratic in the respective variable. This property, and hence the inter-element continuity of the functions, can still be retained even if the term $(\eta^2\zeta^2)$ is missing from the interpolation function of Eq. (42). The internal node, and hence F_{11}, will now be eliminated so that $\alpha_9 \equiv 0$. Consider the 9-noded interpolation for the present problem, as given in Eq. (32).

$$F^{(2,2)}(\eta,\zeta) = \sum_{i=o}^{2} \sum_{j=o}^{2} F_{ij} L_{ij}^{(2,2)}(\eta,\zeta) \quad (43)$$

Equation (33) can be written more conveniently as:

$$L_{ij}^{(m,m)} = [G(\eta)/G'(\eta_i)(\eta-\eta_i)] \times [H(\zeta)/H'(\zeta_j)(\zeta-\zeta_j)] \quad (44)$$

$$\text{where } G(\eta) = \prod_{r=o}^{m} (\eta-\eta_r) \text{ and } H(\zeta) = \prod_{s=o}^{m} (\zeta-\zeta_s) \quad (45)$$

In the above, ( )' denotes a derivative, and, for the present case m=2, $\eta_o = \zeta_o = 0$; $\eta_1 = \zeta_1 = 1/2$; and $\eta_2 = \zeta_2 = 1$. The coefficient of the term $\eta^2\zeta^2$ in the sum on the left hand side of Eq. (43) can be seen to be:

$$\alpha_9 = \sum_{i=o}^{2} \sum_{j=o}^{2} \frac{F_{ij}}{G'(\eta_i)H'(\zeta_j)} \quad (46)$$

where $G'(\eta_i) = \prod_{r=o, r\neq i}^{m} (\eta_i-\eta_r)$ etc. By setting $\alpha_9 = 0$, we obtain from Eq. (46) that:

$$F_{11} = -G'(\eta_1)H'(\zeta_1) \sum\sum_{\substack{i,j=o \\ i=j\neq 1}}^{2} \left[\frac{F_{ij}}{G'(\eta_i)H'(\zeta_j)}\right] \quad (47)$$

Noting that $G'(\eta_o) = H'(\zeta_o) = 1/2$; $G'(\eta_1) = H'(\zeta_1) = -1/4$; and $G'(\eta_2) = H'(\zeta_2) = 1/2$; we obtain for the case when $\alpha_9 = 0$ in Eq. 42 that,

$$F_{11} = 1/2(F_{10}+F_{12}+F_{01}+F_{21}) - 1/4(F_{00}+F_{02}+F_{20}+F_{22}) \quad (48)$$

When this constraint is used in Eq. 43 we obtain the modified shape functions of the 8-noded element as:

$$F(\xi,\eta) = \sum_{\substack{i=o \\ i=j\neq 1}}^{2} \sum_{j=o}^{2} F_{ij} \left[L_{ij} - \frac{G'(\eta_1)H'(\zeta_1)L_{11}}{G'(\eta_i)H'(\zeta_j)}\right] \quad (49)$$

It can be verified that the above modified shape functions are identical to those reported originally for an 8-noded "serendipity" element in (2,3,12). It is however noted that the functions given in (2,3,12), and in the form most frequently used in engineering literature, are in the nondimensional coordinates ($-1\leq\eta^*$, $\zeta^*\leq 1$) which are related to η, ζ employed here as: $\zeta^* = 2\eta - 1$; $\zeta^* = 2\zeta - 1$.

It is of interest to note (as can be verified easily) that in the 8-noded quadrilateral described above, if one introduces the additional constraint that ($F_{00} = F_{01} = F_{02}$), the thus reduced shape functions at the six nodes in the parametric coordinates ξ, η, will not be the same as the quadratic interpolation function for a 6-noded triangle, in the parameters σ, ρ, derivable from Eq. (16). These differences arise only in the interpolation functions for the nodes on σ=1 in Fig. 1c. We also note that the 6 noded triangle derivable from Eq. (16) has all the nodes at the boundary only.

Likewise, a bi-cubic interpolation in the η, ζ coordinates of the quadrilateral would involve 16 nodes, 12 on the boundary and four in the interior. Using procedures described above, the terms $\eta^2\zeta^2$, $\eta^3\zeta^2$, $\eta^2\zeta^3$, and $\eta^3\zeta^3$ can be eliminated from the bi-cubic polynomial in η, ζ and still obtain an interpolation function which is a complete cubic along each of the edges, $\zeta = 0$, $\eta = 0$, etc. When this is done, the four internal nodes can be eliminated, we obtain a 12 boundary-node element, as given in (2,3,12). It is noted that in deriving this 12 noded element, the nodal values F_{11}, F_{12}, F_{21}, and F_{22} are expressed in terms of the remaining nodal values.

b. Triangle ($0 \leq \eta$, $\zeta \leq 1$). Interpolation functions for the case m = 1 (with three nodes) and m = 2 (with (m+1)(m+2)/2 = six nodes) involve only boundary nodes. In the case of a complete cubic polynomial, m = 3, there is a tenth node inside the triangle at $(\eta_1,\zeta_1) = (1/3,1/3)$. Using the procedures indicated in Section II.1.a, it is seen that if the value of the function at the tenth node, i.e., F_{11} in the notation of Eq. (15), is expressed in terms of the other nodal values, as:

$$F_{11} = 1/4(F_{10}+F_{20}+F_{21}+F_{12}+F_{01}+F_{02}) - 1/6(F_{00}+F_{30}+F_{03}) \tag{50}$$

then the resulting interpolation function will still interpolate cubics (11) exactly. The modified shape functions for the remaining nine nodes can be expressed as:

$$L^*_{10}(\eta,\zeta) = L_{10}(\eta,\zeta) - (1/4)L_{11}(\eta,\zeta), \text{ etc.,}$$

where $L_{ij}(\eta,\zeta)$ are as in Eq. (16) for m = 2. Using Eq. (27) these modified shape functions can be expressed more conveniently in polar coordinates, σ and ρ for the triangle.

Again, it is of interest to note that, in the 12 boundary-noded quadrilateral element discussed earlier, if the additional constraint that $F_{00} = F_{01} = F_{02} = F_{03}$ is introduced, the thus reduced shape functions (in the parameters ,) at the remaining nine nodes will not be identical to those, in parameters σ and ρ, for the above nine boundary-noded triangle. However, the dependence of these two sets of shape functions on the radial coordinate σ can be shown to be the same, but their variations in the angular coordinate θ (which is related to ρ) differ.

II.2 Three-Dimensional Cases

In the hexahedral element with trilinear interpolation, i.e., the case m = 1 in Eq. (41), there are $(m+1)^3 = 8$ nodes, ie., at the corners of the element only. A tri-quadratic element would have 27 nodes with seven "undesirable" nodes, one each at the center of the six faces and the 7th at the centroid of the element. The terms $\eta^2\xi^2$, $\xi^2\zeta^2$, $\zeta^2\eta^2$, $\eta^2\xi^2\zeta$, $\eta^2\zeta^2\xi$, $\zeta^2\xi^2\eta$, and $\xi^2\zeta^2\eta^2$ can be eliminated from the polynomial $F^{(2,2,2)}(\xi,\eta,\zeta)$ of Eq. (41), using the procedures indicated earlier. The shape functions for the thus reduced 20-noded brick element can be found in (2,3,4).

Likewise, the tricubic interpolation in ξ, η, ζ requires 64 nodes, out of which only 32 nodes are at the corners and the edge lines of the element. The remaining 32 undesirable nodes, four on each face and eight in the interior of the element, can be eliminated, by eliminating from the polynomial $F^{(3,3,3)}(\xi,\eta,\zeta)$ of Eq. (41), terms other than those involving $\xi^r\eta^s\zeta^t(r+s+t \leq 4$ with $r,s,t \leq 3)$. The thus reduced shape functions for the 32-noded hexahedron can be found in (2,3,4).

Another set of useful 3-D elements is that of triangular prisms. These can be generated in a number of ways such as: (i) multiplication of triangle Lagrange-polynomials and one-dimensional Lagrange polynomials (ii) multiplication of boundary-noded triangles with one-dimensional Lagrange polynomials, (iii) by degenerating (i.e., by merging two parrellel edges on a face) 20 and 32 boundary noded hexahedra into 15 and 24 noded triangular prisms, respectively, and (iv) etc. For examples, see (2,3).

III. Elements of Curved Geometry: Isoparametric Transformations

So far the various interpolation functions were introduced in terms of the non-dimensional coordinates ξ (for a line), ξ η ζ (or $\eta\zeta$ or $\sigma\rho$) for a triangle $\eta\zeta$ for a quadrilateral, $\xi\zeta\eta$ for a hexahedron, etc. In introducing these shape functions these nondimensional coordinates were considered to map a straight line along the x-axis, or a straight-sided triangle, or a straight sided quadrilateral etc., into the "standard" unit dimensional domains. Now we consider the cases of a general curve in space, curved sided triangles or quadrilaterals, and curved faced hexahedra etc. In these cases, it can be seen that the parameters (ξ,η,ζ) or σ and ρ or Sections I and II can be treated as curvilinear coordinates defining the geometry of the domain. The geometric relation between these curvilinear coordinates ξ, η, ζ, etc. and the cartesian coordinates x, y, z of a point in space can be assumed to be approximated by interpolation functions of precisely the kind introduced in Sections I and II. The situation is entirely analogous to concepts of differential geometry (such as the relation between the global polar coordinates R, θ and cartesian coordinates x, y as: $x = R\cos\theta$, $y = R\sin\theta$, etc.), except in the present case, ξ, η, ζ etc. are nondimensional element-local curvilinear coordinates. We briefly discuss the salient features of such geometric transformations which are generated through the use of local (element) shape functions.

III.1 Properties of Geometric Transformations

Consider a curve, parametrized by the curvilinear coordinate $\xi(0 \leq \xi \leq 1)$, in a three-dimensional space with cartesian coordinates (x,y,z). The cartesian coordinates of any point P on the curve can be represented by rth order interpolation function, analogous to Eq. (1) as:

$$\begin{Bmatrix} x^{(r)} \\ y^{(r)} \\ z^{(r)} \end{Bmatrix} = \sum_{i=o}^{r} \begin{Bmatrix} x_i \\ y_i \\ z_i \end{Bmatrix} L_i^{(r)}(\xi) \tag{51}$$

wherein (x_i,y_i,z_i) are discrete values at (r+1) equidistant points $\xi_i[(i=o...r;\ \xi_i = (i/r)]$. Of course, the values (x_i,y_i,z_i) must be specified.

Likewise in a two-dimensional case of a triangle or a quadrilateral, which we consider, without loss of generality, to be lying in the plane z = 0, we represent (x,y) by interpolation functions analogous to Eq. (15), and (32), respectively, as:

$$\begin{Bmatrix} x^{(r)} \\ y^{(r)} \end{Bmatrix} = \sum_{i=o}^{r} \sum_{j=o}^{r-i} \begin{Bmatrix} x_{ij} \\ y_{ij} \end{Bmatrix} L_{ij}^{(r)}(\eta,\zeta) \qquad \text{(triangle)} \tag{52}$$

$$\begin{Bmatrix} x^{(r,r)} \\ y^{(r,r)} \end{Bmatrix} = \sum_{i=o}^{r} \sum_{j=o}^{r} \begin{Bmatrix} x_{ij} \\ y_{ij} \end{Bmatrix} L_{ij}^{(r,r)}(\eta,\zeta) \quad \text{(quadrilateral)} \tag{53}$$

where $L_{ij}^{(r)}$ and $L_{ij}^{(r,r)}$ in Eqs. (52) and (53) are given in terms of parameters η, ζ of the unit triangle and unit square, respectively, in Eqs. (16) and (33). Note that the functions $L_{ij}^{(r)}$ in Eq. (52) may also be expressed in terms of polar coordinates σ and ρ, using Eq. (27). For a hexahedron with curved faces, we can likewise represent the cartesian coordinates by interplants analogous to those in Eq. (41), as:

$$\begin{Bmatrix} x^{(r,r,r)} \\ y^{(r,r,r)} \\ z^{(r,r,r)} \end{Bmatrix} = \sum_{i=o}^{r} \sum_{j=o}^{r} \sum_{k=o}^{r} \begin{Bmatrix} x_{ijk} \\ y_{ijk} \\ z_{ijk} \end{Bmatrix} L_{ijk}^{(m,m,m)}(\xi,\eta,\zeta) \tag{54}$$

In the above, in general, x_{ijk} etc. are the cartesian coordinates of the (i,j,k)th point (i.e., corresponding to ξ_i, η_j, ζ_k) in the parametric coordinates ξ, η, ζ. These discrete cartesian coordinates must, however, be specified with care (3,5) Finally, we note that instead of the interpolants in Eqs. (52-54), we may also use the interpolants with boundary-nodes only, which were discussed in Section II, to represent the cartesian coordinates of the element in terms of the parametric coordinates.

Now let us suppose that the dependent variable (or variables), such as displacement(s) or velocity(ies), of the problem is (are) represented by a mth order interpolant of the type given by Eq. (1) (in one-dimension) or Eqs. (16-37) (in two dimensions) or Eq. (41) (in three-dimensions).

From Eqs.(1,15,32,41) and Eqs. (51-54) we can immediately notice the following properties:

(a) If the geometries (ie., x, y, z coordinates) of two neighboring elements are defined in terms of the parametric coordinates (ξ,η,ζ) using identical order (say rth order) polynomials, geometrical continuity is automatically satisfied, for reasons discussed in Section I.

(b) If the dependent variable (or variables) of the problem in two neighboring elements is (are) defined in terms of ξ, η, ζ, using identical order (say mth) polynomials, the continuity of the variable, at the interfaces between elements, is automatically satisfied due to reasons discussed in Section I.

(c) In the analysis of certain problems, such as say linear solid mechanics, one of the requirements for the shape functions for the dependent variable (say displacements) is that they represent the constant term (rigid body translation) and terms linear in x, y, z (combination of small, constant, rigid rotations and strains). To examine this condition, let us consider one component of displacement, say u, in a curved triangular element in the x, y plane. The above requirement implies that the shape function must be capable of representing:

$$u^* = \alpha_1 + \alpha_2 x + \alpha_3 y \tag{55}$$

Let the geometry be represented by a rth order interplant as in Eq. (52), and u be represented by a mth order interpolant as in Eq. (15), say. Thus

$$\begin{Bmatrix} x \\ y \end{Bmatrix} = \begin{Bmatrix} x^{(r)} \\ y^{(r)} \end{Bmatrix} = \sum_{i=o}^{r} \sum_{j=o}^{r-i} \begin{Bmatrix} x_{ij} \\ y_{ij} \end{Bmatrix} L_{ij}^{(r)}(\eta,\zeta) \tag{56}$$

$$\{u\} = \left\{u^{(m)}\right\} = \sum_{k=o}^{m} \sum_{\ell=o}^{m-k} \left\{u_{k\ell}^{(m)}\right\} L_{k\ell}^{(m)}(\eta,\zeta) \tag{57}$$

The requirement that the field of Eq. (55) be represented by the interpolation functions of Eq. (57) implies the necessary condition that:

$$\{u^*\} = \lfloor \alpha_1, \alpha_2, \alpha_3 \rfloor \begin{Bmatrix} 1 \\ x^{(r)} \\ y^{(r)} \end{Bmatrix}$$

$$= \sum_{k=0}^{m} \sum_{\ell=0}^{m-k} \lfloor \alpha_1 \alpha_2 \alpha_3 \rfloor \begin{Bmatrix} 1 \\ x_{k\ell}^{(r)}(\eta_k, \zeta_\ell) \\ y_{k\ell}^{(r)}(\eta_k, \zeta_\ell) \end{Bmatrix} L_{k\ell}^{(m)}(\eta,\zeta) \tag{58}$$

Assuming that both "r" and "m" are integers, the fact that Eq. (58) is identically satisfied can be seen from Eqs. (19) and (20), provided that $r \leq m$ (as stated in Section I).

(d) By way of definition, the cases when "r" is less than, or equal to, or greater than "m" are labeled, respectively, subparametric, isoparametric, and super parametric geometric transformations between cartesian and parametric (curvilinear) coordinates. The geometric transformations introduced in Section I are thus "subparametric" and hence posses all the properties (a-c) above. However, as can be seen easily, the isoparametric transformations are more convenient to use. Even though the super-parametric elements violate condition (c) above, they have been found to be useful in certain applications to shell elements [2,3].

(e) It can be easily seen from the discussions in Sections I and II that the properties (a-c) above are also possessed by all the so-called "serendipity" elements when internal nodes are eliminated from geometric transformations as well as variable interpolation.

(f) It can also be verified from Eq. (19) [and analogous properties of the interpolants in Eqs. (32), and (41) or the boundary-node interplants of Section II] that if one considers triangles (or quadrilaterals, or hexahedra with straight boundaries)even the 'r'th order geometric transformations will become linear (bilinear or trilinear) as in Section I provided that the discrete points x_{ij}, y_{ij}, etc. (or x_{ijk}, y_{ijk}, etc.) are equidistant at the boundaries and appropriately located in interior of the element [ie, x_{ij} etc. are determined from the "linear" transformations of Section I].

III.2 Considerations of Differential Geometry

The following discussion will be presented in the context of a general three-dimensional case, the reduction to two dimensions using (ζ,η) or (σ,ρ) coordinates, or to one dimension using ξ, is apparent. Let the position vector of a point in space be $\underset{\sim}{R} = (\underset{\sim}{e}_x x + \underset{\sim}{e}_y y + \underset{\sim}{e}_z z)$, where $\underset{\sim}{e}_x$ etc., are cartesian unit vectors. The base vectors $\underset{\sim}{G}_\xi$, $\underset{\sim}{G}_\eta$, and $\underset{\sim}{G}_\zeta$ for the curvilinear coordinates (ξ,η,ζ) are defined, by using the chain-rule differentiation, as:

$$\begin{aligned} \underset{\sim}{G}_\xi &= \frac{\partial \underset{\sim}{R}}{\partial \xi} = \underset{\sim}{e}_x \frac{\partial x}{\partial \xi} + \underset{\sim}{e}_y \frac{\partial y}{\partial \xi} + \underset{\sim}{e}_z \frac{\partial z}{\partial \xi} \\ \underset{\sim}{G}_\eta &= \frac{\partial \underset{\sim}{R}}{\partial \eta} = \underset{\sim}{e}_x \frac{\partial x}{\partial \eta} + \underset{\sim}{e}_y \frac{\partial y}{\partial \eta} + \underset{\sim}{e}_z \frac{\partial z}{\partial \eta} \\ \underset{\sim}{G}_\zeta &= \frac{\partial \underset{\sim}{R}}{\partial \zeta} = \underset{\sim}{e}_x \frac{\partial x}{\partial \zeta} + \underset{\sim}{e}_y \frac{\partial y}{\partial \zeta} + \underset{\sim}{e}_z \frac{\partial z}{\partial \zeta} \end{aligned} \tag{59}$$

or more compactly

$$\begin{Bmatrix} \underset{\sim}{G}_\xi \\ \underset{\sim}{G}_\eta \\ \underset{\sim}{G}_\zeta \end{Bmatrix} = [J] \begin{Bmatrix} \underset{\sim}{e}_x \\ \underset{\sim}{e}_y \\ \underset{\sim}{e}_z \end{Bmatrix} \tag{60}$$

where the definition of [J] is apparent. In the above $\underset{\sim}{G}_\xi$ is the vector tangent to the line of constant (η,ζ) at a generic point ξ, and is, in general, a function of (ξ,η,ζ) etc. Unlike $\underset{\sim}{e}_x$, etc., $\underset{\sim}{G}_\xi$ etc., are <u>not</u> unit vectors. Also, (x,y,z) in Eq. (59) should be understood to be the rth order polynomials as in Eq. (54). The differential volume element in the cartesian coordinates is dV = dxdydz, and that in the curvilinear coordinates is given by:

$$\begin{aligned} dV &= (\underset{\sim}{G}_\xi \times \underset{\sim}{G}_\eta) \cdot (\underset{\sim}{G}_\zeta)\ d\xi d\eta d\zeta \\ &= \det\,[J]\ d\xi d\eta d\zeta \end{aligned} \tag{61}$$

wherein use is made of Eq. (59) and the well-known result from vector analysis. Let us suppose that the dependent variable(s) of the problem, say u, is represented by an mth order interpolant as for instance in Eq. (41). In analogy with Eq. (59), the partial derivatives of u with respect to ξ, η, and ζ are given by:

$$\begin{Bmatrix} (\partial u/\partial\xi) \\ (\partial u/\partial\eta) \\ \partial u/\partial\zeta \end{Bmatrix} = [J] \begin{Bmatrix} (\partial u/\partial x) \\ (\partial u/\partial y) \\ (\partial u/\partial z) \end{Bmatrix} \tag{62}$$

However, to solve the problem on hand, we need the cartesian derivatives of u, which can be found from (62) as:

$$\begin{Bmatrix} (\partial u/\partial x) \\ (\partial u/\partial y) \\ (\partial u/\partial z) \end{Bmatrix} = [J]^{-1} \begin{Bmatrix} (\partial u/\partial\xi) \\ (\partial u/\partial\eta) \\ (\partial u/\partial\zeta) \end{Bmatrix} \tag{63}$$

However, since [J] is, in general, a function of (ξ,η,ζ), the above inversion is difficult to obtain explicitly, and numerical inversion is carried out at a point (ξ_i,η_k,ζ_1) to find the discrete values of the cartesian derivatives. These discrete values are then used in a numerical integration procedure to derive the element "properties" such as the stiffness matrix, etc. (3). Since the hexahedron is now conveniently defined by the parameters $0 \leq \xi, \eta, \zeta \leq 1$, the integral of an arbitrary function $f(\xi,\eta,\zeta)$ over the volume of the element can now be written as:

$$\int_V f(x,y,x)\, dxdydz = \int_0^1\int_0^1\int_0^1 f(\xi,\eta,\zeta) \det |J|\, d\xi d\eta d\zeta \tag{64}$$

in view of Eq. (61) the above integral is most often carried out numerically.

Also, in the development of the element load vector etc., in a solid mechanics problem, certain integrals (such as the work of the surface tractions) need to be evaluated over the boundary of the element. In the parametric system (ξ,η,ζ), such a boundary surface can be represented by, say, ζ = constant. The base vectors on the surface ζ = const. are given by:

$$\bar{G}_{\xi} = (\partial\bar{R}/\partial\xi); \quad \bar{G}_{\eta} = (\partial\bar{R}/\partial\eta) \tag{65}$$

$$\text{where } \bar{R} = R|_{\zeta=\text{const.}} = e_x\, x|_{\zeta} + e_y\, y|_{\zeta} + e_z\, z|_{\zeta} \tag{66}$$

The differential area on the above surface is then given by:

$$ds = |\bar{G}_{\xi} \times \bar{G}_{\eta}|\, d\xi d\eta \tag{67}$$

where $|\ |$ implies the modulus. The unit outward (when a proper convention is employed) normal to the above surface, η (which is also often needed), is given by:

$$\eta = (\eta_x e_x + \eta_y e_y + \eta_z e_z) = (\bar{G}_{\xi} \times \bar{G}_{\eta})/|\bar{G}_{\xi} \times \bar{G}_{\eta}| \tag{68}$$

The integral of a function such as g over the surface can now be written as:

$$\int_S g(x,y,z)\, ds = \int_0^1\int_0^1 g(\xi,\eta)|\bar{G}_{\xi} \times \bar{G}_{\eta}|\, d\xi d\eta \tag{69}$$

With the background of the previous sections, we now proceed to consider the subject of special and singular elements.

IV. Problems with Singularities for Derivative of the Field Variable

There are several problems in which, at a given point in the domain, say P, the solution function, say F, would have a singularity in its derivative. If R is the radial length measured from the point P, the solution function(s) F (or F_i, i=1,2...) would behave as R^{λ} (λ may in general be complex, and the real part of λ is less than unity), so that the first derivative of F (or F_i) at P would be infinite. Such singularities may arise at reentrant corners, tips of sharp cracks etc. in two-dimensional domains, and at vertices (where three or more planes may interesect) in three-dimensional problems. The above type of singularities may be classified as point singularities. There may also be situations where there are singularities for function derivatives at each point along a curve in three-dimensional space. This class of singularities may be termed "line singularities". An example of this category is the singularity in displacement-derivatives (or strains in a linear theory) near the border of an arbitrary shaped flaw (surface of discontinuity) in a three-dimensional solid. In this problem, at every point on the flaw border, the displacement function may behave as R^{λ} ($\lambda < 1$) where R is the radial coordinate measured from the considered point in a plane locally perpendicular to the flaw border.

Most often, the value of the above mentioned λ may be determined a priori from a classical (analytical) solution of a suitably formulated eigenvalue problem (14, 15 and see the references cited in 16). However in some instances, such as the problem of a vertex in a three-dimensional solid, or the problem of a three-dimensional solid containing a crack whose plane intersects a free surface, analytical procedures are intractable to ascertain the nature of singularity (or the value of λ) at the vertex or the point where the front of the crack intersects the free surface. The problem is all the more compounded when the crack-front intersects the free surface at an angle. In such instances, the eigenvalue problem to determine λ may itself be solved numerically, such as by using finite elements or other means (17,18).

An area in which the above singularities play a dominant role, and which is of great current interest in analyzing the safety of flawed structures, is the subject of fracture mechanics. In the case of sharp cracks in two-dimensional (plane stress and plane strain) problems of homogeneous isotropic or rectilinearly anisotropic linear-elastic solids, the complete eigen-function solution for the displacement/strain/stress state near the crack-tip can be derived (16,19). These solutions indicate that the singular solution for strain ε_{ij} near the crack-tip is of the form $R^{-1/2}F_{ij}(\theta)$, where R and θ are polar coordinates centered at the crack-tip, and displacements u_i are of the form $R^{1/2}G_i(\theta)$. In the case of cracks lying at, terminating at, or intersecting bi-material interfaces, or in the general problems of cracks in nonhomogeneous, two-dimensional, linear-elastic material domains, strain singularities of the general form $R^{-\alpha}$ $(0 < \alpha < 1)$ may occur (20,24). Similar results also exist for dynamically propagating cracks in two-dimensional solids (22,23), in which case, a complete eigenfunction solution is possible, at least for constant-velocity crack propagation. In the case of arbitrarily shaped cracks embedded in three-dimensional domains of linear elastic materials, it is known (24) that the strain singularity is again of the form $R^{-1/2}F_{ij}(\theta)$ all along the crack-front, where R and θ are polar coordinates, centered at the crack front and in a plane perpendicular, locally, to the crack front. However, the general eigenfunction solution for such embedded flaws remains intractable (25), although some recent progress has been made (26). For "surface flaws" (ie., those flaws which interesect with a free surface in a 3-D solid), the nature of strain singularity near the point of intersection of the flaw border with the free surface is not yet completely clarified (18,27,28). The plate bending stress singularity near the tip of a straight-line crack, along with complete eigenfunction expansions, based on a Kirchhoff theory has been derived (29) and again the singularity is of the $R^{-1/2}$ type. The use of Kirchhoff theory in such cases is, however, inaccurate. Using higher-order theories which account for transverse shear, it is also found (30,31) that not only the bending moments but also the transverse shear resultants, would have a singularity of the type $R^{-1/2}F(\theta)$ near the crack tip, analogous to the fully three-dimensional case of a crack in a homogeneous solid.

The above paragraph deals mainly with problems of linear elastic materials. Much less literature exists on cracks in general nonlinear materials or when the finite geometry changes near the crack-tip are treated. Considering a deformation theory, wherein no unloading is treated, as a model for material plasticity (which model essentially reduces to a nonlinear elasticity theory), it has been shown in (32,33) that for cracks in two-dimensional domains the strain singularities are of the type $R^{-n/n+1}$, the stress singularities are of the type $R^{-1/n+1}$, and displacements are of the type $R^{1/n+1}$ (n is a positive real number) near the crack-tip, when the material obeys the powerlaw that ε (uniaxial strain) varies as σ^n (σ is uniaxial stress). Thus, in the limit of perfect plasticity, ie., $n \to \infty$, the strain singularity is of type R^{-1} while the stresses are non-singular. (The θ-variation of this singular behavior has not been determined analytically, as is the general eigenfunction solution beyond the asymptotic singular solution). However, the problem of cracks propagating dynamically in nonlinear materials is largely unsolved, even though some recent progress has been made (34) in understanding the nature of singularities in such problems.

From the above discussion, it may be seen that the field function (such as displacement) in such singular problems varies as R^{λ} $(0 < \lambda < 1)$ near the singular point while the derivative (or the strain in infinitesmal strain problems) varies as $R^{\lambda-1}$. Further, the problems of fracture in homogeneous materials are characterized, for the most part, by singularities of the form R^{-1} in the density of strain energy near the crack tip. The subject of error analysis of finite element methods in such problems has been studied and reviewed in (35,36, 37,38), and the need for special methods to treat the singularities has been noted.

Fortunately, some problems in the area of fracture mechanics do not require detailed, accurate, solutions for strains and stresses near the crack-tip since fracture, as a physical process, may also be studied based on considerations of global energy. Based on the theory of invariant variational principles of (39), several conservation laws which have a bearing on the energy release rate due to an advancing crack-tip, have been derived (40). One such conservation law is characterized by the so-called J-integral (41,42), which is related to the energy-release rate under self-similar crack growth as well as to the intensity of the stress-singularity. Using nonsingular elements, attempts have been made to calculate the intensity of the singular field through the J-integral (43 to 46). Direct use of the energy release rate concept, which necessitates the solution of two problems with slightly different crack lengths was made earlier in (44,47,48,49,50). A more efficient use of this approach, through the concept of stiffness derivative (or virtual crack extensions), was made in (51-53). Calculations of stress-intensities through certain integrals on contours remote from the crack-tip (and hence do not depend accutely on the solution accuracy near the crack-tip) were also demonstrated in (54 to 58).

Extensive surveys of numerical methods in fracture have already appeared (59,60,61,62,63,64,65,66,67,68,69). Rather than duplicating these reviews, the remainder of this chapter will attempt to analyze the fundamental ideas in the generation of special and singular elements with singularities for function-derivatives, and to point out certain generalizations which are new.

V. Special and Singular Elements

V.1 Some General Comments

The problem on hand is to devise special and/or singular elements within which the field variable would vary as R^λ $(0 < \lambda < 1)$ where R is the radial distance from the point where the derivative of the function would have a singularity of the type $R^{\lambda-1}$. Without loss of generality, let (x_1) (x_1,y_1), and (x_1,y_1,z_1) be the desired points of singularity in one-, two-, and three-dimensional problems, respectively, such that, R is equal to $(x-x_1)$, $[(x-x_1)^2 + (y-y_1)^2]^{1/2}$, $[(x-x_1)^2 + (z-z_1)^2]^{1/2}$, respectively.

From Eq. (63) it is immediately noticed that the desired form of singularity may be introduced in $(\partial u/\partial x)$, $(\partial u/\partial y)$, $(\partial u/\partial z)$ by letting (i) $[J]^{-1}$ or (ii) $(\partial u/\partial \xi)$, $(\partial u/\partial \eta)$, $(\partial u/\partial \zeta)$ or (iii) both $[J]^{-1}$ and $\partial u/\partial \xi$, etc. to be singular at the desired point. The first of these three cases implies a singularity in the geometric transformation between (x,y,z) and (ξ,η,ζ) systems, while the second case corresponds to the introduction of shape functions for u in (ξ,η,ζ) parameters that have singular derivatives w.r.t. (ξ,η,ζ).

However, it should be remembered that the element shape functions derived under any of the above three cases must satisfy the properties (a), (b), and (c) discussed under Section III, namely, geometric compatibility, function continuity, and representation of rigid body and constant strain modes.

We now discuss the cases (i), (ii), and (iii) described above.

V.2 Singular Geometric Transformations

V.2.1 One-Dimensional Cases

Consider, without loss of generality, a straight line along the x-axis, $x_o \leq x \leq x_M$. Let the geometry of this line be described by an rth order polynomial as in Eq. (51) i.e.,

$$x = x^{(r)} = \sum_{i=o}^{r} x_i \, L_i^{(r)}(\xi) \tag{70}$$

where $x_i = x(\xi_i)$, and $\xi_i = (i/r)$ $(i = 0,1\ldots r)$ are $(r+1)$ equidistant points in the parametric domain $0 \leq \xi \leq 1$. (x_i, themselves may not necessarily be equidistant). Also, let the dependent variable, say u, be represented by an mth order polynomial.

$$u(\xi) = \sum_{j=m}^{m} u_j L_j^{(m)}(\xi) \tag{71}$$

where $u_j = u(\xi_j)$, but now $\xi_j = (j/m)(j=o,\dots m)$ are (m+1) equidistant points in $0 \leq \xi \leq 1$.

Suppose that in (70) the points x_i are themselves equidistant, i.e., $x_i = x_o + (x_M-x_o)(i/r) = x_o + (x_M-x_o)\xi_i$ or $(x_i-x_o) = (x_M-x_o)\xi_i$. For these values of x_i, the transformation in Eq. (70) reduces to

$$(x-x_o) = (x_M-x_o)\xi \tag{72}$$

in view of Eq. (6) and (7). Thus, because of Eq. (72), the polynomial u(x) will also be an mth (integer) order polynomial in x and hence $(\partial u/\partial x)$ will not have any singularities. If on the other hand, the geometric transformation Eq. (72) is replaced by:

$$(x-x_o) = (x_M-x_o)\xi^t \tag{73}$$

where t is a positive integer greater than unity, the function u(x) corresponding to $u(\xi)$ of Eq. (71) would be an mth order polynomial in the variable $(x-x_o)^{1/t}$ or $R^{1/t}$, and hence the derivative $(\partial u/\partial x)$ has a term which varies as $R^{(1-t)/t}$ and, for $t > 1$, would have a singularity at $x = x_o$. Again, from Eqs. (6) and (7) it is evident that the special case of Eq. (73) follows from the general rth order transformation of Eq. (70) provided that the points x_i are spaced such that

$$(x_i-x_o) = (x_M-x_o)(\xi_i)^t \equiv (x_M-x_o)(\frac{i}{r})^t \tag{74}$$

provided $t \leq r$, for reasons discussed in Section I.1. Thus, for instance when r=2, the positioning of nodes at $x = x_o$, $x = x_o + (x_M-x_o)/2$, and at $x = x_M$ would lead to the linear transformation $x \sim \xi$; on the other hand, it the nodes are placed at $x = x_o$; $x = x_o + (x_M-x_o)(1/2)^2 = x_o\ (x_M-x_o)(1/4)$, and $x = x_M$ (i.e., t=2) it would lead to $x \sim \xi^2$ and hence $\partial u/\partial x$ would have a singularity of the type $R^{-1/2}$. Since t is restricted to $t \leq r$, no other type of singularities are possible for r = 2. When r = 3, the positioning of the nodes x_i equidistant from each other will lead to a linear relation $x \sim \xi$; when x_i are chosen such that $x_i = x + (x_M-x_o)(i/3)^2(i=0,1,2,3)$, x varies as ξ^2 and thus $(\partial u/\partial x)$ varies as $R^{-1/2}$; on the other hand, if x_i are chosen such that $x_i = x_o + (x_M-x_o)(i/3)^3(i=0,1,2,3)$, x varies as ξ^3 and $(\partial u/\partial x)$ varies as $R^{-2/3}$. Thus, in general, singularities in $\partial u/\partial x$ of the type $R^{(1-t)/t}$, $t \leq r$ (t and r are integers), can be created (by geometric transformations of the type $x \sim \xi^t$) by suitably choosing the values x_i in an rth order geometric transformation of the type Eq. (70).

As discussed earlier, the property (c) of Section III.1 would be satisfied for a general representation of the type of Eqs. (70) and (71) if $r \leq m$. However, when Eq. (70) reduces to Eq. (73) due to the choice of x_i as in Eq. (74) property (c) of Section III.1 would be satisfied, if $t \leq m$. Thus for subparametric transformations, $r < m$, and $t \leq r$; while for isoparametric transformations, $r = m$, $t \leq m$.

It can be shown that choosing the values of $x(\xi_i)$ using Eq. (74) for either sub- or isoparametric transformations, results in singularities in $(\partial u/\partial x)$ of only the type $R^{(1-t)/t}$ [$t \leq r$; or $t \leq m$] where t is an integer. This is primarily due to the fact geometric transformation of the type in Eq. (73) can be affected, by polynomial sub- or isoparametric transformation of the type of Eq. (70) only if t is an integer.

If, on the other hand, one abandons the concepts of isoparametric (or subparametric) geometric transformations, one may directly assume a geometric transformation of the type:

$$(x-x_o) = (x_M-x_o)\xi^\beta \tag{75}$$

where β is a real number. However, if the finite domain (x_M-x_o) is to be mapped into the domain $0 < \xi < 1$, β cannot be negative. With the transformation of Eq. (75) it is seen that the function u(x) in Eq. (71) will be an mth (m being an integer) order polynomial in $R^{1/\beta}$, and $(\partial u/\partial x)$ will have a singularity of the type $R^{(1-\beta)/\beta}$ ($\beta > 0$, but not an integer).

However, for $(x-x_o)$ of the type of (75) with arbitrary β, the property (c) of Section III.1 cannot be satisfied when $u(\xi)$ is taken to be of the form of (71), since, in that case, ξ^β cannot be represented exactly by Eq. (72) which represents an mth order polynomial in ξ.

V.2.2 Two-Dimensional Case

(a) Triangle. Consider a straight-sided triangle P_1, P_2, P_3 (see Fig. 1a) which is mapped into a standard triangle, $0 \leq \eta, \zeta \leq 1$, through an rth order transformation of the type of Eq. (52), i.e.,

$$\begin{Bmatrix} x^{(r)} \\ y^{(r)} \end{Bmatrix} = \sum_{i=0}^{r} \sum_{j=0}^{r-i} \begin{Bmatrix} x_{ij} \\ y_{ij} \end{Bmatrix} L_{ij}^{(r)}(\eta,\zeta) \tag{76}$$

while the dependent variables, say u and v, are represented by an mth order interpolant analogous to Eq. (76) except that (x,y) are replaced by (u,v) and "r" is replaced by "m". In Eq. (76), x_{ij} $[=x(\eta_i,\zeta_j)]$ and y_{ij} are the cartesian coordinates of the point (η_i,ζ_j) $[i,j = 0,1,\ldots r$; and $\eta_i = (i/r)$ etc.). For any $r \geq 1$, it can be seen from Eq. (19) that if the x_{ij}, y_{ij} coordinates in Eq. (76) are so chosen that

$$\begin{Bmatrix} x_{ij} \\ y_{ij} \end{Bmatrix} = \begin{Bmatrix} x^{(1)}(\eta_i,\zeta_j) \\ y^{(1)}(\eta_i,\zeta_j) \end{Bmatrix} = \sum_{i=0}^{1} \sum_{j=0}^{1-i} x_{ij} L_{ij}^{(1)}(\eta_i,\zeta_j)$$

$$= \begin{Bmatrix} x_{00} + (x_{10}-x_{00})\eta_i + (x_{01}-x_{00})\zeta_j \\ y_{00} + (y_{10}-y_{00})\eta_i + (y_{01}-y_{00})\zeta_j \end{Bmatrix} \tag{77}$$

then the representation in Eq. (76) reduces to the linear transformation given in Eq. (14); hence a polynomial of mth order in (η,ζ) would represent a polynomial of the same degree in (x,y). A feature of the linear transformation of Eq. (14), which is shown through (25) is that $R \sim (\eta+\zeta)$. Thus, as mentioned in Section I, a polynomial in $(\eta+\zeta)$ would give a polynomial in R. In order to represent a function of the type R^λ, we seek to affect a nonlinear geometric relation between R and $(\eta+\zeta)$ [say of the type $R \sim (\eta+\zeta)^{1/\lambda}$] so that a polynomial in $(\eta+\zeta)$ would represent a polynomial in R^λ. The way to affect such a nonlinear transformation between R and $(\eta+\zeta)$ is clear from a close examination of Eqs. (14, 21 to 25) and the condition that the edge $(\eta+\zeta) = 1$ should map onto the edge P_2P_3.

Thus, if one modifies the geometric transformation of Eq. (14) to be of the type:

$$x^{(t)} = (x-x_{00}) = \{ (x_{10}-x_{00})\eta + (x_{01}-x_{00})\zeta\} \{ \eta+\zeta\}^{t-1}$$

$$y^{(t)} = (y-y_{00}) = \{ (y_{10}-y_{00})\eta + (y_{01}-y_{00})\zeta\} (\eta+\zeta)^{t-1} \qquad (78)$$

it is seen that Eqs.(21-23) remain unchanged, while Eqs. (24) and (25) become, respectively,

$$R^2 = (x-x_{00})^2 + (y-y_{00})^2 \equiv (1+\beta)^2 [(y_{10}-y_{00})\eta + (y_{01}-y_{00})\zeta]^2 (\eta+\zeta)^{2t-2}$$

and $$R^2 = \frac{(1+\beta^2)J_o}{[(x_{10}-x_{01}) + \beta(y_{10}-y_{01})]^2} \cdot (\eta+\zeta)^{2t} \qquad (80)$$

In the above, to keep the double-index notation in (76) consistent, we used the convention: $x_1 = x_{00}$; $x_2 = x_{10}$; $x_3 = x_{01}$ etc. Thus, it is seen that the geometric transformation of Eq. (78) leads to the result that $R \sim (\eta+\zeta)^t$. Thus, any polynomial in $(\eta+\zeta)$ would represent a polynomial in $R^{1/t}$.

Now, the transformation of Eq. (78) contains terms of order t in the parameters (η,ζ). Again, in view of the property given in Eq. (19), the functions $x^{(t)}(\eta,\zeta)$ and $y^{(t)}(\eta,\zeta)$ of Eq. (78) can be represented by an rth order transformation of the type Eq. (76) if and only if $t \leq r$ when one substitutes $x^{(t)}(\eta_j,\zeta_j)$ and $y^{(t)}(\eta_i,\zeta_j)$, respectively, for x_{ij} and y_{ij} in Eq. (76). Let the polynomial representation for the dependent variables be of order 'm'. It is seen from Eq. (16) that this polynomial contains terms of the type $(\eta+\zeta)^p$, $1\leq p\leq m$. If the geometric transformation is subparametric, $r < m$; and hence $t \leq r < m$. If, on the other hand, the geometric transformation is isoparametric, $r = m$; and $t \leq r = m$. Thus, through nonlinear geometric transformations of the type of (78), dependent function representations only of the type $R^{1/t}$ (and its integer powers), where t is an integer and $t \leq m$, are possible.

Once again, from Eq. (19) and Eq. (78) it is seen that the dependent-function representation as an mth order polynomial can exactly account for rigid body and constant strain motion provided that t is an integer and $t \leq m$.

The geometrically nonlinear transformation of the type of Eq. (78) is achieved, by taking

$$\begin{Bmatrix} x_{ij} \\ y_{ij} \end{Bmatrix} = \begin{Bmatrix} x^{(t)}(\eta_i,\zeta_j) \\ y^{(t)}(\eta_i,\zeta_j) \end{Bmatrix} = \begin{Bmatrix} (x_{10}-x_{00})\eta_i + (x_{01}-x_{00})\zeta_j \\ (y_{10}-y_{00})\eta_i + (y_{01}-y_{00})\zeta_j \end{Bmatrix} (\eta_i+\zeta_j)^{t-1} \qquad (81)$$

for (x_{ij} and y_{ij}) in the expressions for $x^{(r)}$ and $y^{(r)}$ respectively in Eq. (76). Thus Eq. (81) indicates as to how the cartesian coordinates x_{ij} and y_{ij} must be chosen to create, in general, a relation of the type in Eq. (78) from (76). For conceptual clarity, let us write (78) in terms of (σ,ρ) using Eq. (27), as:

$$(x-x_1) = [(x_2-x_1)(1-\rho) + (x_3-x_1)\rho]\sigma^t$$

$$(y-y_1) = [(y_2-y_1)(1-\rho) + (y_3-y_1)\rho]\sigma^t \qquad (82)$$

wherein, x_{00}, x_{10}, etc. of Eq. (78) are replaced by x_1, x_2, etc., since the indices for the orthogonal coordinates (ξ,η) and the polar-coordinates (σ,ρ) do not coincide. It can be seen from Fig. 4, that a point with coordinates (η_i,ζ_j) (with indices i, j) in the (η,ζ) system would correspond to the point $(\sigma_{i'},\rho_{j'})$ with indices i', j') in the (σ,ρ) system, such that $i' = (i+j)$; $j' = j$. For an rth order interpolant, $\sigma_{i'} = (i'/r)$ $(i' = o,\ldots r)$, and $\rho_{j'} = (j'/i')$ $(j' = 0,1,\ldots i')$; thus Eq. (82) can be written as:

$$(x_{i'j'}-x_1) = [(x_2-x_1)(1-\frac{j'}{i'}) + (x_3-x_1)\frac{j'}{i'}]\,(i'/r)^t$$

$$(y_{i'j'}-y_1) = [(y_2-y_1)(1-\frac{j'}{i'}) + (y_3-y_1)\frac{j'}{i'}]\,(i'/r)^t \tag{83}$$

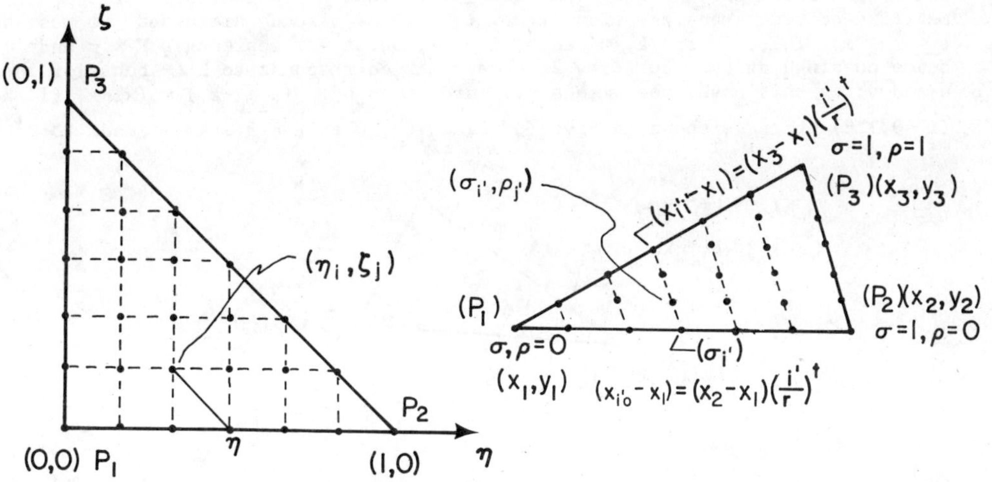

Fig. 4

The physical interpretation of Eq. (83) can be seen to be: (a) divide the lines P_2P_1 and P_3P_1 into unequal lengths according to the equations, $(x_{i'0}-x_1) = (x_2-x_1)(i'/r)^t$, and $(x_{i'i'}-x_1) = (x_3-x_1)(i'/r)^t$ ($i' = 0,1,\ldots r$), respectively, and similar equations for $(y_{i'0}-y_1)$ and $(y_{i'i'}-y_1)$ and (b) divide the line joining the points $(x_{i'0}, y_{i'0})$ and $(x_{i'i'}, y_{i'i'})$ into i' equal parts, as shown in Fig. 4.

The Jacobian of the transformation in Eq. (82) can be written as

$$\det J = \det \begin{vmatrix} (\partial x/\partial\sigma); & (\partial y/\partial\sigma) \\ (\partial x/\partial\rho); & (\partial y/\partial\rho) \end{vmatrix} = 2At\sigma^{2t-1}$$

so that:

$$(\partial\sigma/\partial x) = [(y_3-y_2)/(2tA)]\sigma^{1-t}; \quad (\partial\rho/\partial x) = -[(y_2-y_1) + (y_3-y_2)\rho](\sigma^{-t}/2A)$$

$$(\partial\sigma/\partial y) = -(x_3-x_2)\,\sigma^{(1-t)}/2tA; \quad (\partial\rho/\partial y) = [(x_2-x_1) + (x_3-x_2)\rho](\sigma^{-t}/2A) \tag{85}$$

It is clear from Eq. (85), and remembering that in the present case $\sigma \sim R^{1/t}$, that for $t > 1$, the inverse of the Jacobian matrix is singular at $\sigma = R = 0$, i.e., at point (x_1,y_1) of the triangle. Further, the cartesian derivatives which are given by:

$$\frac{\partial u}{\partial x} = \frac{\partial u}{\partial\sigma}\frac{\partial\sigma}{\partial x} + \frac{\partial u}{\partial\rho}\frac{\partial\rho}{\partial x}; \quad \frac{\partial u}{\partial y} = \frac{\partial u}{\partial\sigma}\frac{\partial\sigma}{\partial y} + \frac{\partial u}{\partial\rho}\frac{\partial\rho}{\partial y}$$

$$\frac{\partial v}{\partial x} = \frac{\partial v}{\partial \sigma}\frac{\partial \sigma}{\partial x} + \frac{\partial v}{\partial \rho}\frac{\partial \rho}{\partial x};\ \frac{\partial v}{\partial y} = \frac{\partial v}{\partial \sigma}\frac{\partial \sigma}{\partial y} + \frac{\partial v}{\partial \rho}\frac{\partial \rho}{\partial y} \tag{86}$$

would become singular at $\sigma = 0$.

Now, we consider a few examples of singular geometric transformations that can be generated through Eqs. (82) and (83). Consider either sub- or isoparametric geometric transformation, i.e., $r \leq m$. As already discussed, we must have $t \leq r \leq m$. Thus, if $r = 2$, t can be 1 or 2, but $t = 1$ represents $R \sim \sigma$ and hence no singularity. But, $t = 2$, when $r = 2$ corresponds to $R^{1/2}$ behavior in u and v; in this case, the values $x_{i'0}$ are given by: $(x_{i'0}-x_1) = (x_2-x_1)(i'/2)^2$ $(i'=0,1,2)$ etc., as shown in Fig. 5. Likewise, when $r = 3$, $t = 2$ leads to $R^{1/2}$

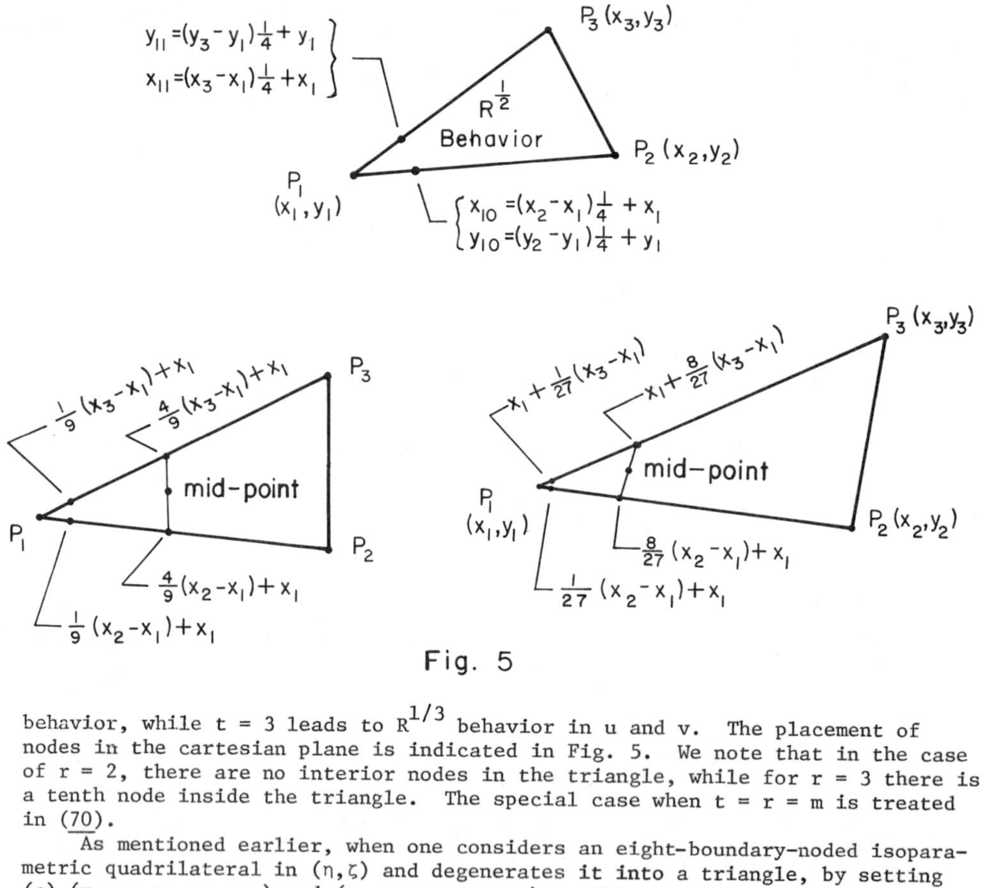

Fig. 5

behavior, while $t = 3$ leads to $R^{1/3}$ behavior in u and v. The placement of nodes in the cartesian plane is indicated in Fig. 5. We note that in the case of $r = 2$, there are no interior nodes in the triangle, while for $r = 3$ there is a tenth node inside the triangle. The special case when $t = r = m$ is treated in (70).

As mentioned earlier, when one considers an eight-boundary-noded isoparametric quadrilateral in (η,ζ) and degenerates it into a triangle, by setting (a) $(x_{00} = x_{01} = x_{02})$ and $(y_{00} = y_{01} = y_{02})$ in the geometric transformation, and (b) $U_{00} = U_{01} = U_{02}$ etc. in the function representation, it can be shown easily that the resulting expressions for x, y and u in terms of (η,ζ) of the quadrilateral, would not be the same as for a triangle in terms of the polar coordinates (σ and ρ). However, it can be shown that dependence of these two sets of functions on (η) and (σ), respectively, are the same. Since η for the degenerate quadrilateral has the same geometric meaning as σ for the triangle, it can be seen that the placement of the cartesian nodes in the degenerate quadrilateral as in the case of the triangle discussed above, would result in a singularity in the geometric transformation identical to that in the triangle as discussed above. The case of a degenerate 8-noded isoparametric quadrilateral, with the cartesian coordinates of the side nodes, on radial lines from the point of singularity, being displaced to (1/4) the length of the side from the point of singularity, (analogous to the above discussed case of $t = 2 = r = m$) was treated in (71, 72). Likewise, the case of a degenerate 12-noded isoparametric quadrilateral [analogous to the presently discussed case of $t = 2$, $r = m = 3$] was discussed in (73). Thus in both (71, 73) a derivative singularity of $R^{-1/2}$ is realized. However, an interesting feature of the degenerate quadrilaterals is that when the constraint $U_{00} = U_{01} = \ldots U_{0i}$ [i = 2 in the quadratic, and i = 3 in the cubic]is removed, and each of these nodal-function-values is allowed to be independent, a singularity of the type R^{-1} (which is the physical singularity near the crack-tip in a perfectly plastic material) in the first derivative of the function, is realized. Also, since $t \leq m$ (and t is an integer) is satisfied in both the cases of (71, 73), it is seen that the property (c) of the Section III.1 is satisfied.

Now, if one doesn't insist on using sub- or isoparametric transformations (and then distort the placement of nodes in cartesian space to acheive a singularity in geometric transformation), one can directly write, instead of (78) and (82), that

$$(x-x_1) = [(x_2-x_1)\eta + (x_3-x_1)\zeta]\,(\eta+\zeta)^{\beta-1}$$

or $$(x-x_1) = [(x_2-x_1)(1-\rho) + (x_3-x_1)\rho]\sigma^{\beta} \tag{87}$$

with similar equation for $(y-y_1)$. Now β can be any positive real number. However, if the function u is an mth order polynomial in (η,ζ) [or (σ,ρ)], it is seen that the function will now vary as $R^{1/\beta}$ near $(x_1;y_1)$. However, the property (c) of the section III.1 can no longer be satisfied for arbitrary β.

Now, consider the quadrilateral of Section I.1.b which was defined there in terms of (η,ζ). We will now change these parameters to $\bar{\eta}$, $\bar{\zeta}$, $(0 \leq \bar{\eta}, \bar{\zeta} \leq 1)$ so as to avoid confusion with the triangle parameters (η,ζ) considered in this section. From Eqs. (31b) it is clear that when $x_4 = x_1$ and $y_4 = y_1$, i.e., the quadrilateral is geometrically degenerated to a triangle.We note that, by comparison with Eq. (28), $\bar{\eta} \equiv \sigma$ and $\bar{\zeta} = \rho$, such that $0 \leq (\bar{\eta},\bar{\zeta}), (\sigma,\rho) \leq 1$. Thus the geometrical transformation for the degenerate quadrilateral, viz.,

$$(x-x_1) = [(x_2-x_1)(1-\bar{\zeta}) + (x_3-x_1)\bar{\zeta}]\bar{\eta} \tag{88}$$

and a similar relation for $(y-y_1)$ is bi-linear in $(\bar{\eta},\bar{\zeta})$. To introduce a non-linear geometric transformation, and hence possibly a singularity, at $x = x_1$, in the inverse of the Jacobian, we may introduce new parameters $\bar{\eta}^*$, $\bar{\zeta}^*$ such that; $(\bar{\eta}^*)^{\alpha} = \bar{\eta} = \sigma$; and $\bar{\zeta}^* = \bar{\zeta} = \rho$. When this is done, Eq. (88) becomes:

$$\begin{Bmatrix}(x-x_1)\\(y-y_1)\end{Bmatrix} = \left[\begin{Bmatrix}(x_2-x_1)\\(y_2-y_1)\end{Bmatrix}(1-\bar{\zeta}) + \begin{Bmatrix}(x_3-x_1)\\(y_3-y_1)\end{Bmatrix}\bar{\zeta}\right](\bar{\eta}^*)^{\alpha} \tag{89}$$

Where, $0 \leq \bar{\eta}^* \leq 1$. Now the Jacobian of the matix:

$$\begin{bmatrix}(\partial x/\partial\bar{\eta}^*) & (\partial x/\partial\bar{\zeta})\\(\partial y/\partial\bar{\eta}^*) & (\partial y/\partial\bar{\zeta})\end{bmatrix} \tag{90}$$

is equal to $2A\alpha(\bar{\eta}^*)^{2\alpha-1} = 2A\alpha\sigma^{(2\alpha-1)/\alpha}$, and hence,

$$(\partial\bar{\eta}^*/\partial x) = (\bar{\eta}^*)^{1-\alpha}(y_3-y_2)/2A\alpha = (\sigma)^{\frac{1-\alpha}{\alpha}}(y_3-y_2)/2A\alpha$$

$$(\partial\bar{\zeta}/\partial x) = -[(y_2-y_1)+(y_3-y_2)\bar{\zeta}][(\bar{\eta}^*)^{-\alpha}/2A] = -(\sigma^{-1}/2A)[(y_2-y_1)+(y_3-y_2)\bar{\zeta}]$$

$$(\partial\bar{\eta}^*/\partial y) = -(x_3-x_2)(\bar{\eta}^*)^{1-\alpha}/2A\alpha = -\sigma^{\frac{1-\alpha}{\alpha}}(x_3-x_2)/2A\alpha$$

$$\partial\bar{\zeta}/\partial y = [(x_2-x_1) + (x_3-x_2)\bar{\zeta}](\bar{\eta}^*)^{-\alpha}/2A$$

$$= [(x_2-x_1) + (x_3-x_2)\bar{\zeta}](\sigma^{-1}/2A) \tag{91}$$

However, the shape functions for the dependent variables, say, u and v, may also be assumed in the parametric variables $0 \leq (\bar{\eta}^*, \bar{\zeta}) \leq 1$, in the same form as in the first Section, (I.1.d) i.e., (η,ζ) in that section are replaced by $(\bar{\eta}^*,\bar{\zeta})$, respectively, in the degenerate quadrilateral. Thus, for instance, for a bilinear interpolation in $\bar{\eta}^*$, $\bar{\zeta}$, of a dependent varialbe, u, we have from Eq. (32)

$$u = u_1(1-\bar{\eta}^*)(1-\bar{\zeta}) + u_2(1-\bar{\zeta})\bar{\eta}^* + u_3\, \bar{\zeta}\, \bar{\eta}^* + u_4\, \bar{\zeta}(1-\bar{\eta}^*) \tag{92}$$

Thus, unlike in the previous case of the triangle wherein the function-interpolation was not altered along with the modified geometric transformation, here the function interpolation has itself been altered in addition to a singular geometric transformation. From Eq. (91) and (92) it can be seen that the derivative,

$$\frac{\partial u}{\partial x} = \frac{\partial u}{\partial \bar{\eta}^*}\frac{\partial \bar{\eta}^*}{\partial x} + \frac{\partial u}{\partial \bar{\zeta}}\frac{\partial \bar{\zeta}}{\partial x} \tag{93}$$

will have a singularity of the type $\sigma^{(1-\alpha)/\alpha}$ and σ^{-1} when $u_1 \neq u_4$, but only of the type $\sigma^{(1-\alpha)/\alpha}$ when $u_1 = u_4$.

It is interesting to observe that in Eqs. (89)-(93) the dependence of σ on R (i.e., $\sigma \sim R$) is not altered, while the new parametric coordinate $\bar{\eta}^*$ varies as $(\sigma)^{1/\alpha}$ or $(R)^{1/\alpha}$; whereas, in the case of Eq. (78) and (82) σ, and hence $\bar{\eta}$ of the degenerate quadrilateral, both vary as $(R)^{1/t}$.

The developments in Eqs. (89) - (93) appear to have been also given in (10), although the motivations behind the introduction of the nonlinear geometric transformations and the function representations as in (89) or (92) are somewhat unclear and confusing in (10), perhaps, due, in part, to the notations employed therein.

If the function representation in $\bar{\eta}^*$, $\bar{\zeta}$ (as for instance in Eq. 92) is, in general, of mth order it is clear that the condition of rigid rotation and constant strain motions will not be satisfied unless "α" in Eq. (20) is an integer and $\alpha \leq m$. This can be verified from (10) also.

V.2.2.b Quadrilateral

Eight-noded quadrilateral singular elements, wherein the placement of nodes in the cartesian space is analogous to the case of the triangle discussed above, were first proposed in (74, 75). However, it was contended in (71, 76) that the appropriate first-derivative singularity is created only along the two boundary lines emanating from the point of singularity of the quadrilateral, but not throughout the entire interior of the quadrilateral. Moreover, it was also contended (77) that the "strain-energy" of the singular quadrilateral, in linear problems, is unbounded. However, the above contentions of (71, 76, and 77) were shown (78) to be erroneous, i.e., the proper singularity exists through the quadrilateral and the strain energy is in fact bounded.

However, since the angular variation of the singular field, near the point of singularity, can be better approximated by triangular elements than by quadrilateral elements, triangular singular elements are in general preferable.

V.2.3. Three-Dimensional Case

In the tetrahedron, by appropriately placing the nodes on the faces of the tetrahedron in the cartesian space [analogous to Eq. (83)], singularities of the type $R^{\frac{1-t}{t}}$ (t an integer, $t \leq m$) can be created. Further details can be found in (79,80). These elements would be useful in representing point singularities.

In the case of line singularities, we can consider singular triangular prism elements. The base of the prism, i.e., the triangle, is treated analogous to that in subsection V.2.2.a. The meridion of the prism is represented in the usual fashion, such as by one-dimensional Lagrange polynomials [71].

V.3 Shape Functions with Singular Derivatives

In the previous subsection we discussed the possibility of introducing a singularity in $(\partial u/\partial x)$ etc., through making $[J]^{-1}$ singular. We now consider the possibility of introducing $R^{\lambda-1}$ type singularities in $(\partial u/\partial x)$ etc., through making $(\partial u/\partial \eta)$ etc., appropriately singular, while retaining the linearity of geometric transformation between (x,y,z) and (ξ,η,ζ).

We consider the two dimensional example, while the extensions to other dimensions are left to the reader. Consider a straight sided triangle whose cartesian coordinates are mapped into parametric coordinates (η,ζ) or (σ,η) as per Eq. (14) or (28). (Even if higher order sub- or isoparametric geometric transformations are employed, we assume that the cartesian coordinates of the nodes are so selected, that the actual transformation is given by Eq. (14) or (28)). Since σ is shown to be proportional to R^{λ}in Eq. (30), a function that varies as R can be directly assumed, by replacing σ by σ^{λ} or $(\eta+\zeta)$ by $(\eta+\zeta)^{\lambda}$ in the mth order interpolation functions of Eq. (15). However, if constant strain terms are to be represented in such functions, it is seen that $t\lambda$ must be equal to 1, for a t which is an integer, and $t \leq m$.

Thus, consider 1st order interpolations in the triangle, for the dependent variable, say u, when σ is replaced by σ^{λ} (See Eq. 26), i.e.,

$$u = u_1(1-\sigma^{\lambda}) + u_2\,\sigma^{\lambda}(1-\rho) + u_3\,\sigma^{\lambda}\rho \tag{94}$$

while the geometric transformation is given by:

$$x = x_1(1-\sigma) + x_2\sigma(1-\rho) + x_3\sigma\rho \tag{95}$$

and a similar expression for y. Thus it is seen that while rigid body translation can be represented by (94), constant strain (and rigid rotation) terms cannot be represented. Interpolations of the type of (94) were introduced in [6, 7, 81]. Nonincorporation of constant strain motions makes these elements undesirable in certain analyses, such as problems of thermal stresses.

Quadratic interpolation corresponding to Eq. (16), written in terms of σ and ρ and when σ is replaced by σ^{λ}, yield the following appropriately normalized [so that $L_{i'j'}(\sigma_{k'},\rho_{\ell'}) = \delta_{i'k'}\delta_{j'\ell'}$], shape functions:

$$L_{00} = (1-\sigma^{\lambda})(1-2\sigma^{\lambda}) \;;\; L_{10} = [2^{2\lambda}/(2^{\lambda}-1)]\sigma^{\lambda}(1-\rho)(1-\sigma^{\lambda})$$

$$L_{20} = \sigma^{\lambda}(1-\rho)[2\sigma^{\lambda}(1-\rho)-1] \;;\; L_{21} = 4\sigma^{2\lambda}\rho(1-\rho)$$

$$L_{22} = \sigma^{\lambda}\rho(2\sigma^{\lambda}\rho-1) \;;\; L_{11} = [2^{2\lambda}/(2^{\lambda}-1)]\,\sigma^{\lambda}\rho\,(1-\sigma^{\lambda}) \tag{96}$$

where in, $\sigma_{i'} = (i'/2)(i'=0,2)$; $\rho_{j'} = (j'/i')(j'=0,i')$. For the special case of $\lambda = 1/2$, the functions in (96) were also given in (10, Table I) except that they were not properly normalized in (10) [note that (σ and ρ) correspond to ρ and $(1+\eta)/2$, respectively in (10)]. In general, for arbitrary λ, constant strain motions cannot be represented by (96). However, for the special case of $\lambda = 1/2$, a function of the type (95), and hence constant strain motions, can be represented by (96).

For the special case of $\lambda = 1/2$, certain shape functions were proposed in (82) later modified slightly in (8). The functions in (8) are:

$$L_{00} = 1+\sqrt{2}\sigma - (1+\sqrt{2})\sigma^{1/2} \;;\; L_{10} = -2(1+\sqrt{2})(1-\rho)(\sigma-\sigma^{1/2}) \;;$$

$$L_{20} = (1-\rho)[(2+\sqrt{2})\sigma - (1+\sqrt{2} + 2\rho)\sigma^{1/2}] \;;\; L_{21} = 4\rho(1-\rho)\sigma^{1/2} \;;$$

$$L_{22} = \rho[(2+\sqrt{2})\sigma - (3+\sqrt{2} - 2\rho)\sigma^{1/2}] \;;\; L_{11} = -2(1+\sqrt{2})\rho\,(\sigma-\sigma^{1/2}) \tag{97}$$

It is seen that only the functions L_{00}, L_{20}, and L_{22} (i.e., the ones corresponding to corner nodes) in (97) differ from the corresponding ones in Eq. (96) when $\lambda = 1/2$ in Eq. (96). While the σ dependence of the functions in Eq. (96), and Eq. (97) is the same, it is the ρ (and hence the angular coordinate) dependence that is slightly different in the two cases.

Another procedure whereby shape functions for standard triangular and quadrilateral elements can be converted to singularity functions has been devised in (83). Suppose that an mth order interpolation in the standard triangle, $0 \leq \eta, \zeta \leq 1$, is considered and the node $\eta = \zeta = 0$ is the required point of singularity for the function derivative. In the procedure of (83), one defines modified shape functions:

$$L^*_{ij} = [1-(1-(1/R)]\ \delta_{io}\ \delta_{jo} + L_{ij}/S \tag{98}$$

where

$$S = [1-L_{00}]^{\beta}$$

The modified functions in Eq. (98) can represent singularities of the type $R^{-\beta}$ in the cartesian derivatives of the functions. The functions L^*_{ij} satisfy the constraint $\sum_{i=0}^{m} \sum_{j=0}^{m-i} L^*_{ij} = 1$; but cannot represent constant strain terms. Moreover, for the case of the triangle, it can be seen that Eq. (98) is, in principle, analogous to that in (7, 8, 82); while for a quadrilateral it has not been verified that the function has a $R^{1-\beta}$ variation along all the radial lines passing through the point of singularity.

If one recognizes the basic concept that the parametric coordinate σ in the unit triangle ($0 \leq \sigma, \rho \leq 1$) varies as the radial length R, shape functions for the dependent variable u that have terms such as σ^{λ}, and at the same time can represent linear terms in x, and y, (when the linear geometric transformation of Eq. (95) is used), can easily be derived. Thus, if geometrical transformations of the type Eq. (95) are used, in order to represent a function of type R^{λ}, and at the same time account for constant strain motions, one may start out by writing:

$$U(\sigma,\rho) = \alpha_1 + \alpha_2 x + \alpha_3 y + \sigma^{\lambda} F(\rho) \tag{99}$$

where α_1, α_2, α_3 are constants. Rewriting x, and y as:

$$x = x_1 + \{(x_2-x_1)(1-\rho) + (x_3-x_1)\rho\}\sigma \tag{100}$$

and a similar expression for y, it is seen that we may write,

$$u(\sigma,\rho) = \mu_1 + \sigma\{\mu_2(1-\rho) + \mu_3\rho\} + \sigma^{\lambda} F(\rho) \tag{101}$$

Interpolation functions of the above type for triangular elements with three nodes on each of the two radial boundary lines from the point of singularity, and k nodes on the third boundary line (thus involving a total of 5 + k nodes) have been derived in (9). Some additional elements with similar properties have been discussed in (80). It is noted that along any radial line (ρ = const), say $\rho = 0$, the function is of the form: $U(\sigma) = \mu_1 + \mu_2\sigma + \mu_4\sigma^{\lambda}$ where μ_4 is another undetermined parameter in $F(\rho)$ of Eq. (101).

V.4 Concluding Comments on Singular Geometric Transformations and Modified Shape Functions

Even though a singular behavior in the cartesian gradient of the function can be induced by either (i) a singular geometric transformation or (ii) directly altering the shape functions while retaining the linearity of geometric transformation attention must be paid to: (a) integration of singular integrands (such as the strain-energy density of R^{-1} type in fracture mechanics) and (b) extraction of certain parameters of physical interest, such as the strength of the singularity, or the so-called stress-intensity factors. Space does not permit a full discussion of this topic, other than noting that (a) is accomplished by numerical integration (84), and (b) is accomplished by extrapolation of displacement or stress data to the point $R \to 0$. The numerical accuracies of both (a) and (b) have not yet been satisfactorily established. Finally we note that certain transition elements that can be used in conjunction with the above discussed singularity elements have been presented in (85).

VI. Special Elements Employing Analytical Asymptotic Solutions

For the most part, the singular elements described above are used to model singularities of the type $R^{\lambda-1}$ $(0 < \lambda < 1)$ in the function derivatives, wherein λ is known a priori, through an eigenvalue or other asymptotic analyses. As mentioned before the value of λ may also be determined from a numerical analysis. In an important subclass of problems, such as linear and nonlinear fracture, the singular solution $R^{\lambda-1}F(\theta)$ can be determined analytically, along with higher-order eigenfunctions in some cases. An exception to this is the problem of the nature of singularity near the point where the crack front intersects a free surface in a three-dimensional problem.

VI.1 Enriched Isoparametric Elements

In this approach presented in (86), the function representation in a two-dimensional element, with one of its nodes as the desired point of singularity, consists of the usual polynomial interpolations of the type discussed in Section I, which are augmented by the known asymptotic solution, in the form:

$$u = \Sigma\,\Sigma\,\alpha_{ij}\,L_{ij}(\zeta,\eta) + \beta_1 R^{\lambda}(F(\theta) \tag{102}$$

where $R^{\lambda}F(\theta)$ is the known asymptotic solution (R,θ are polar coordinates centered at the point of singularity). In Eq. (102) α_{ij} are undetermined parameters for each element, while β_1 is treated as a global variable. Thus α_{ij} are expressed in terms of the nodal displacements u_{ij} (which are thus global variables) as well as β_1, from the equation:

$$u_{k\ell} = \sum_{i,j} \alpha_{ij}\,L_{ij}(\xi_k,\eta_\ell)+\beta_1 R^{\lambda}(\xi_k,\eta_\ell)\;F[\theta(\zeta_k,\eta_\ell)] \tag{103}$$

Thus,

$$u = \sum_{i,j} u_{ij}\,L_{ij}(\zeta,\eta) + \beta_1[R^{\lambda}F(\theta) - \sum_{k\ell} L_{k\ell}\;R^{\lambda}(\zeta_k,\eta_\ell)F(\theta_{k\ell})] \tag{104}$$

where $\theta_{k\ell} = \theta(\zeta_k,\eta_\ell)$. Thus, the element field is expressed in terms of global parameters u_{ij} as well as β_1 (or several β's in a problem such as mixed-mode fracture (16). It is apparent that the function of Eq. (104) in the singular element would not be compatible at its boundary with surrounding elements in which the function is represented through L_{ij}'s only. This can be remedied by defining the interpolations in the elements immediately surrounding the singular elements to be:

$$u = \sum_{ij} u_{ij}\,L_{ij} + G\beta_1[R^{\lambda}F(\theta) - \sum_{k\ell} L_{k\ell}\;(R^{\lambda}F(\theta))_{k\ell}] \tag{105}$$

wherein G is a function that is unity at the boundaries of singular elements and vanishes at the boundaries of the above "surrounding" elements, which are away from the singular elements. Thus this concept can be classified as a "global-local" approach, further details of which are discussed in Chapter 15 of this book. Details of the application of the above approach to two-dimensional fracture were given in (86). An extension to 3-D fracture, without satisfying the interelement compatibility as through Eq. (105), was given in (87).

VI.2 Hybrid Finite Element Methods for Singularity Problems

Hybrid finite elements in elasticity are based on variational formulations wherein relevant field variables in the element need not, a priori, satisfy the requirements of interelement displacement compatibility and/or interelement traction reciprocity. The constraint conditions are, however, enforced through the technique of Lagrange multipliers, which are, thus, the additional variables introduced at the element boundary in the formulation. Depending on the nature of the formulation, these Lagrange multipliers have the physical meaning of inter-element boundary displacements and/or tractions. The theoretical basis of some or all of the hybrid finite elements is discussed in several places (88, 89, 90, 91) as well as in Chapter 5 of this book and will not be repeated here.

Since the assumed displacements and/or stresses in an element in the hybrid formulation can be arbitrary, it is seen that the known asymptotic solutions for stresses and/or displacements can be incorporated in the element without worrying about the interelement conditions a priori. An added, but a very important benefit of such formulations is the ability of the methods to directly yield the solution for the strengths of the singularity (such as the stress-intensity factors); thus eliminating the need for "extrapolation techniques" as in the case of singular elements discussed in Section V. Further, since the known asymptotic solution satisfies the relevant field equations, the integration of singular strain energy densities, etc., can be performed with ease by converting such domain integrals to boundary integrals through the use of the divergence theorem.

The application of the general hybrid methods in fracture mechanics is discussed in detail in (92, 93). Here, we briefly mention these methods, with primary emphasis only on listing appropriate references for the various problem categories.

VI.2.1 Hybrid Elements Through a Boundary Variational Principle

In this case, a single element surrounds the point of singularity, but the formulation is limited to two-dimensional linear elastic fracture problems of homogeneous isotropic or anisotropic materials. In such problems, a complete series solution is known for stresses and displacements near the crack-tip. These solutions satisfy both the equations of equilibrium and compatibility. Thus the variational formulation for the crack-element must only match the elements' boundary displacements with those of the surrounding elements. This boundary variational principle can be stated as the stationary condition:

$$\pi_b = \sum_n [\int_{\partial V_n} (\frac{1}{2} \underset{\sim}{T}^T \underset{\sim}{U} - \underset{\sim}{T}^T \underset{\sim}{\tilde{u}})ds + \int_{S_{\sigma_n}} \underset{\sim}{\bar{T}}^T \underset{\sim}{\tilde{u}}\, ds \tag{106}$$

Where $\underset{\sim}{T}$ and $\underset{\sim}{U}$ are vectors of tractions and displacement, respectively, at the boundary of the element; ∂V_n, and $\underset{\sim}{T}$ are associated with the assumed stresses $\underset{\sim}{\sigma}$ (or displacements $\underset{\sim}{U}$) inside the element; and $\tilde{u}$ are independently prescribed displacements at ∂V_n, so that they match the displacements of the surrounding elements. Further, S_{σ_n} is the surface where tractions are prescribed. It is seen that the assumed series solution for $\underset{\sim}{\sigma}$ in the crack-element satisfies the crack-face traction conditions also apriori. Thus the integrals in Eq.(106) are free from singularities. The finite element method based on Eq.(106) leads to a direct evaluation of the stress-intensity factors.

The application the above method to two-dimensional linear elastic fracture can be found in (94,to97). The use of analytical series solutions without satisfying interelement continuity, however, was suggested earlier in (98,99).

VI.2.2 Stress-Hybrid Singular Elements

The variational principle for the formulation of a hybrid stress finite element model (88, 89, 90) is based on the stationary condition of the functional:

$$\pi_{mc} = \sum_n [\int_{V_n} \frac{1}{2} \underset{\sim}{\sigma}^T \underset{\approx}{S} \underset{\sim}{\sigma}\, dV - \int_{\partial V_n} \underset{\sim}{T}^T \underset{\sim}{\tilde{u}} ds + \int_{S_{\sigma_n}} \underset{\sim}{T}^T \underset{\sim}{\tilde{u}} ds] \tag{107}$$

where $\underset{\sim}{\sigma}$ represents an arbitrary equilibrated stress within an element; $\underset{\approx}{S}$ is the compliance matrix of the material; $\underset{\sim}{T}$ are tractions corresponding to the assumed $\underset{\sim}{\sigma}$; and $\underset{\sim}{\tilde{u}}$ are the independently assumed element boundary displacements which are inherently compatible at the interelement boundary. Since the assumed equilibrated stress field is arbitrary, one can assume from the singular element, $\underset{\sim}{\sigma} = \underset{\sim}{\sigma}^S + \underset{\sim}{\sigma}^R$ where $\underset{\sim}{\sigma}^S$ is the known analytical asymptotic singular solution, and $\underset{\sim}{\sigma}^R$ is any polynomial solution derivable from stress-functions. Note that $\underset{\sim}{\sigma}^S$, by its very nature, satisfies not only equilibrium, but also corresponds to compatible strains. Using this property, the complementary energy corresponding to $\underset{\sim}{\sigma}^S$ can be evaluated through a boundary-integral only. This method also leads to a direct computation of stress-intensity factors.

The method has been used in 2-D linear elastic fracture problems (100); problems of cracked plates under bending (101, 102), and 3-D linear elastic fracture (103).

V.2.3. Displacement-Hybrid Singular Element

The variational principle for the formulation of the displacement-hybrid model is based on the stationarity of the functional (90, 104).

$$\pi_{mp} = \sum_n \left[\int_{V_n} \left(\frac{1}{2} \underset{\sim}{\varepsilon}^T \underset{\approx}{c} \underset{\sim}{\varepsilon} - \bar{\underset{\sim}{F}}^T \underset{\sim}{u}\right) dV - \int_{\partial V_n} \underset{\sim}{T}^T (\underset{\sim}{u} - \tilde{\underset{\sim}{u}}) ds - \int_{S_{\sigma_n}} \bar{\underset{\sim}{T}}^T \tilde{\underset{\sim}{u}} \, ds \right. \tag{108}$$

where $\underset{\sim}{\varepsilon}$ are the assumed compatible strains (which are derived from an assumed arbitrary $\underset{\sim}{u}$) within the element, $\tilde{\underset{\sim}{u}}$ are independently assumed boundary displacements, $\underset{\sim}{T}$ are independently assumed boundary tractions, and $\underset{\approx}{c}$ is the matrix of elastic coefficients. Since the $\underset{\sim}{u}$ assumed within the element is arbitrary, one can take $\underset{\sim}{u} = \underset{\sim}{u}^R + \underset{\sim}{u}^S$, where $\underset{\sim}{u}^R$ is any polynomial field with $\underset{\sim}{\alpha}$ as undetermined parametrs, while $\underset{\sim}{u}^S$ corresponds to the known asymptotic singular solution, which has the stress-intensity factors as the undetermined parameters. Note again, that, by definition, $\underset{\sim}{u}^S$ is not only a compatible field but also leads to equilibrated stresses. Because of this, the strain energy corresponding to u^S can be evaluated through boundary-integrals only. This method also leads to a direct computation of the stress-intensity factors.

This method has been applied to problems of 2-D linear elastic fracture (105, 108), problems of 3-D fracture of homogeneous and bimaterial linear elastic solids (109 - 115), problems of 2-D elastic-plastic fracture under large-scale yielding (116 to 119), problems of elastic-plastic subcritical crack growth (120 - 122), and to problems of dynamic crack propagation in linear materials (123 to 128).

Acknowledgements

The work leading to this article was supported in part by the U.S. AFOSR under contract F49620-78-C-0085 with Dr. J.D. Morgan, III, as the program manager. The author gratefully acknowledges this support from AFOSR over the years. The author thanks K. Vijayakumar and R.B. Stonesifer for helpful discussions during the course of this writing. Critical comments received from R.H. Gallagher and P. Tong on a first draft of this article are gratefully acknowledged. The author's appreciation goes to Ms. Margarete Eiteman for her expert typing of this manuscript.

References

1. Sylvester, P., "Higher-Order Polynomial Triangular Finite Elements for Potential Problems" International Journal of Engineering Science, Vol. 7, 1969, pp. 849-861.

2. Zienkiewicz, O.C., Irons, B.M., Ergatoudis, J., Ahmad, S. and Scott, F.C., "Isoparametric and Associated Element Families for Two- and Three-Dimensional Analysis" in Finite Element Methods in Stress Analysis (I. Holland and K. Bell, Eds.) Tapir Press, Trondheim, Norway, 1969, pp. 383-432.

3. Zienkiewicz, O.C., The Finite Element Method in Engineering Science, 3rd Edition, McGraw Hill, 1977.

4. Huebner, K.H., The Finite Element Method for Engineers, John Wiley and Sons, 1975.

5. Mitchell, A.R. and Wait, R., The Finite Element Method in Partial Differential Equations, John Wiley and Sons, 1977.

6. Tracey, D.M., "Finite Element for Determination of Crack Tip Elastic Stress Intensity Factors" Engineering Fracture Mechanics, Vol. 3, pp. 255-266, 1971.

7. Tracey, D.M. and Cook, T.S., "Analysis of Power Type Singularities Using Finite Elements", International Journal for Numerical Methods in Engineering, Vol. 11, pp. 1225-1233, 1977.

8. Stern, M. and Becker, E., "A Conforming Crack Tip Element with Quadratic Variation in the Singular Fields", International Journal of Numerical Methods in Engineering, Vol. 12, pp 279-288, 1978.

9. Stern, M., "Families of Consistent Conforming Elements with Singular Bevariate Fields", International Journal for Numerical Methods in Engineering, Vol. 14, pp. 409-421, 1979.

10. Yamada, Y., Ezawa, Y. and Nishiquchi, "Reconsiderations on Singularity or Crack Tip Elements", International Journal for Numerical Methods in Engineering, Vol. 14, pp. 1525-1544, 1979.

11. Ciarlet, P.G. and Raviart, P.A., "General Lagrange and Hermite Interpolation in R^n with Applications to Finite Element Methods", Archive for Rational Mechanics and Analysis, Vol. 46, pp 177-199, 1972.

12. Ergatoudis, J.G., Irons, B.M. and Zienkiewicz, O.C., "Curved Isoparametric Quadrilateral Elements for Finite Element Analysis", International Journal of Solids and Structures, Vol. 4, pp 31-42, 1968.

13. Scott, F., "A Quartic Two-Dimensinoal Iso-parametric Element", Undergraduate Project Report, University of Wales, Swansea, 1968.

14. Lehman, R.S., "Development at an Analytic Corner of Solutions of Elliptic Partial Differential Equations", Journal of Mathematical Mechanics, Vol. 8, pp. 727-760, 1959.

15. Williams, M.L., "On the Stress Distribution at the Base of a Stationary Crack", Journal of Applied Mechanics, Vol. 24, pp. 109-114, 1957.

16. Sih, G.C. and Liebowitz, H., "Mathematical Theories of Brittle Fracture" in Fracture, Vol. 2 (Edited by H. Liebowitz), Academic Press, pp. 68-191, 1969.

17. Swedlow, J.L., "Singularity Computations", International Journal for Numerical Methods in Engineering, Vol. 12, pp. 1779-1798, 1978.

18. Bazant, Z.P., "General Numerical Method for Three-Dimensional Singularities in Cracked or Notched Solids", Fracture 1977, Vol. 1, (Proceedings of ICF4), University of Waterloo Press, pp. 371-385, 1977.

19. Rice, J.R., "Mathematical Analysis in the Mechanics of Fracture" in Fracture Vol. 2 (Edited by H. Liebowitz) Academic Press, pp. 192-314, 1968.

20. Erdogan, F., "Fracture of Nonhomogeneous Solids" in The Mechanics of Fracture, (Edited F. Erdogan) ASME-AMD Vol. 19, ASME, New York, pp. 155-170, 1976.

21. Comninou, M., "The Interface Crack", in Journal of Applied Mechanics, Vol. 44, pp. 631-636, 1977.

22. Achenbach, J.D., "Dynamic Effects in Brittle Fracture" in Mechanics Today, Vol. 1 (S. Nemat-Nasser, Ed.) Pergamon, pp. 1-57, 1972.

23. Freund, L. B., "Dynamic Crack Propagation", in The Mechanics of Fracture (F. Erdogan, Ed.) ASME-AMD Vol. 19, ASME, New York, pp. 105-134, 1976.

24. Kassir, M. D. and Sih, G. C., Three-Dimensional Crack Problems, Noordhoff, 1975.

25. Shah, R. C. and Kobayashi, A. S., "Stress Intensity Factor for an Elliptical Crack Under Arbitrary Normal Loading," Engineering Fracture Mechanics, Vol. 3, pp. 71-96, 1971.

26. Vijayakumar, K. and Atluri, S. N., "An Embedded Elliptical Crack, in an Infinite Solid, Subject to Arbitrary Crack-Face Tractions", Journal of Applied Mechanics, Vol. 48, No. 1, pp. 88-96, March 1981.

27. Folias, E. S., "On the Three-Dimensional Theory of Cracked Plates", Journal of Applied Mechanics, Vol. 42, pp. 663-674, 1975.

28. Benthem, J. P., "Three-Dimensional State of Stress at the Vertex of Quarter-Infinite Crack in a Half-Space", Report 563, Lab. of Engineering Mechanics, Delft University of Technology, 1975.

29. Williams, M. L., "The Bending Stress Distribution at the Base of a Stationary Crack", Journal of Applied Mechanics, Vol. 28, pp. 78-82, 1961.

30. Wang, N. M., "Twisting of an Elastic Plate Containing Crack", International Journal of Fracture Mechanics, Vol. 6, pp. 367-378, 1970.

31. Hartranft, R. J. and Sih, G. C., "The Use of Eigenfunction Expansions in the General Solution of Three-Dimensional Crack Problems", Journal of Mathematics and Mechanics, Vol. 19, pp. 123-138, 1969.

32. Hutchinson, J. W., "Singular Behavior at the End of a Tensile Crack in a Hardening Material", Journal of Mechanical Physics and Solids, Vol. 16, pp. 13-31, 1968.

33. Rice, J. R. and Rosengren, G. F., "Plane Strain Deformation Near a Crack Tip in a Power Law Hardening Material", Journal of Mechanical Physics and Solids, Vol. 16, pp. 1-12, 1968.

34. Achenback, J. D., Burgers, P. and Dunayevsky, V., "Near-Tip Plastic Deformations in Dynamic Fracture Problems", in Nonlinear and Dynamic Fracture Mechanics, ASME-AMD Vol. 35, (N. Perrone and S. N. Atluri, Eds.) ASME, pp. 105-124, 1979.

35. Tong, P. and Pian, T. H. H., "On the Convergence of the Finite Element Method for Problems with Singularity", International Journal of Solids and Structures, Vol. 9, pp. 313-321, 1972.

36. Barnhill, R. E. and Whiteman, J. R., "Error Analysis of Galerkin Methods for Dirichlet Problems Containing Boundary Singularities", Journal of Inst. Math. Applics., Vol. 15, pp. 121-125, 1975.

37. Schatz, A. and Wahlbin, L., "Maximum Norm Estimates in the Finite Element Method on Plane Polygonal Domains, Part I", Math. Comput., Vol. 32, pp. 73-109, 1978.

38. Whiteman, J. R. and Akin, J. E., "Finite Elements, Singularities and Fracture", in The Mathematics of Finite Elements and Applications III, MAFELAP 1978, (Ed. by J. R. Whiteman), Academic Press, London, pp. 35-54, 1979.

39. Noether, E., "Invariante Variations Problems", Gottinger Nachrichben Methematisch - Physikalische Klasse 2, p. 235, 1918.

40. Knowles, J.K. and Sternber, E., "On a Class of Conservation Laws in Linearized and Finite Elasto-Statics", Arch. Rat. Mech. and Analysis, pp. 187-211, 1972.

41. Rice, J.R., "A Path-Independent Integral and the Approximate Analysis of Strain Concentration by Notches and Cracks", Trans. ASME, Journal of Applied Mechanics, Vol. 35, pp. 379-386, 1968.

42. Eshelby, J.D., "The Continuum Theory of Lattice Defects", Solid State Physics, Vol. III, Academic Press, New York, pp. 79-144, 1956.

43. Chan, S.K., Tuba, I.S. and Wilson, W.K., "On the Finite Element Method in Linear Fracture Mechanics", Engineering Fracture Mechanics, Vol. 2, pp. 1-17, 1970.

44. Anderson, G.P., Ruggles, V.L. and Stibor, G.S., "Use of Finite Element Computer Programs in Fracture Mechanics", International Journal of Fracture Mechanics, Vol. 7, pp. 63-76, 1971.

45. Neale, B.K., "Finite Element Crack Tip Modeling When Evaluating the J-Integral", International Journal of Fracture, Vol. 11, No. 1, pp. 177-178, 1975.

46. Kobayashi, A., Chiu, S. and Beeuwkes, R., "A Numerical and Experimental Investigation of the Use of the J-Integral", Engineering Fracture Mechanics, Vol. 5, pp. 293-305, 1973.

47. Watwood, V.B., "Finite Element Method for Prediction of Crack Behavior", Nuclear Engineering and Design, Vol. 11, No. 2, pp. 323-332, March 1970.

48. Dixon, J.R. and Pook, L.P., "Stress Intensity Factors Calculated Generally by the Finite Element Techniques", Nature, Vol. 224, p. 166, 1969.

49. Dixon, J.R. and Strannigan, J.S., "Determination of Energy Release Rates and Stress-Intensity Factors by the Finite Element Method", Journal of Strain Analysis, Vol. 7, No. 2, pp. 125-131, 1972.

50. Mowbray, D.F., "A Note on the Finite Element Method in Linear Fracture Mechanics", Engineering Fracture Mechanics, Vol. 2, pp. 173-176, 1970.

51. Parks, D.M., "A Stiffness Derivative Finite Element Technique for Determination of Crack-Tip Stress Intensity Factors", International Journal of Fracture, Vol. 10, pp. 487-502, 1974.

52. Parks, D.M., "Virtual Crack Extension: A General Finite Element Technique for J-Integral Evaluation", in Numerical Methods in Fracture Mechanics (Luxmore and Owen, Eds.), Swansea, United Kingdom, pp. 464-478, 1978.

53. Hellen, T.K., "On the Method of Virtual Crack Extensions", International Journal for Numerical Methods in Engineering, Vol. 9, pp. 187-207, 1975.

54. Rybicki, E.F. and Kanninen, M., "A Finite Element Calculation of Stress Intensity Factors by a Modified Crack Closure Integral", Engineering Fracture Mechanics, Vol. 9, pp. 931-938, 1977.

55. Stern, M., Becker, E. and Dunham, R.S., "A Contour Integral Computation of Mixed Mode Stress Intensity Factors", International Journal of Fracture, Vol. 12, pp. 359-368, 1976.

56. Stern, M. and Soni, M., "The Calculation of Stress Intensity Factors in Anisotropic Materials by a Contour Integral Method", in Computational Fracture Mechanics (E. Rybicki and S. Benzley, Eds.), ASME Special Publication, pp. 161-172, 1975.

57. Hong, C.C. and Stern, M., "The Computation of Stress-Intensity Factors in Dissimilar Materials", Journal of Elasticity, Vol. 8, pp. 21-34, 1978.

58. Stern, M. and Soni, M.L., "On the Computation of Stress Intensities at Fixed-Free Corners", International Journal of Solids and Structures, Vol. 12, pp. 331-337, 1976.

59. Gallagher, R.H., "Survey and Evaluation of the Finite Element Method in Fracture Mechanics Analysis", Proceedings First International Conference on Structural Mechanics in Reactor Technology, Berlin, Vol. 6, Part L, pp. 637-653, September 1972.

60. Gallagher, R.H., "A Review of Finite Element Techniques in Fracture Mechanics", in Numerical Methods in Fracture Mechanics (A.R. Luxmore and D.R.J. Owen, Eds.), University College of Swansea, United Kingdom, pp. 1-25, 1978.

61. Rice, J.R. and Tracey, D.M., "Computational Fracture Mechanics", Numerical and Computer Methods in Structural Mechanics, Edited by S. Fenves et al., Academic Press, pp. 585-623, 1973.

62. Pian, T.H.H., "Crack Elements", Proceedings of World Congress on Finite Element Methods in Structural Mechanics, Bournemouth, England, Vol. 1, pp. F.1-F.39, 1975.

63. Apostal, M., Jordan, S. and Marcal, P.V., "Finite Element Techniques for Postulated Flaws in Shell Structures", EPRI Special Report 22, Electric Power Research Institute, Palo Alto, California, August 1975.

64. Rybicki, E., and Benzley, A. (Eds.), Computational Fracture Mechanics, ASME Special Publication, New York, 1975.

65. Oglesby, J. and Lomacky, O., "An evaluation of the Finite Element Method in Fracture Mechanics Analysis", Trans. ASME, Journal of Engineering for Industry, Vol. 95, No. 1, pp. 177-185, February 1973.

66. Broekhoven, M., "Computation of Stress Intensity Factors for Nozzle Corner Cracks by Various Finite Element Procedures", Third SMiRT Conference, London, Paper G4/6, Vol. III, G-H, Comm. of European Com., Brussels, 1975.

67. Hellen, T.K., "On Special Isoparametric Elements for Linear Elastic Fracture Mechanics", International Journal for Numerical Methods in Engineering, Vol. 11, No. 1, pp. 200-203, 1977.

68. Prij, J., "Two- and Three-Dimensional Finite Element Analysis of a Central-Cracked Crackgrowth", Trans. Fourth SMiRT Conference, Vol. 6, Paper G4/2, Comm. of European Com., Brussels, 1977.

69. Benzley, S. and Parks, D.M., "Fracture Mechanics", in Structural Mechanics Computer Programs, W. Pilkey, K. Saczalski and H. Schaeffer, Eds., University of Virginia Press, pp. 81-102, 1977.

70. Wait, R., "Singular Isoparametric Finite Elements", Journal of Inst. Maths. Applics., Vol. 20, pp. 133-141, 1977.

71. Barsoum, R.S., "Triangular Quarter Point Elements as Elastic and Perfectly-Plastic Crack Tip Elements", International Journal for Numerical Methods in Engineering, Vol. 11, No. 1, pp. 85-98, 1977.

72. Barsoum, R.S., "A Degenerate Solid Element for Linear Fracture Analysis of Plate Bending and General Shells", International Journal for Numerical Methods in Engineering, Vol. 10, No. 3, pp. 551-564, 1976.

73. Pu, S.L., Hussian, M.A. and Lorensen, W.E., "The Collapsed Cubic Isoparametric Element as a Singular Element for Crack Problems", International Journal for Numerical Methods in Engineering, Vol. 12, pp. 1727-1742, 1978.

74. Henshell, R.D. and Shaw, K.G., "Crack Tip Elements are Unnecessary", International Journal for Numerical Methods in Engineering, Vol. 9, pp. 495-509, 1975.

75. Barsoum, R.S., "On the Use of Isoparametric Finite Elements in Linear Fracture Mechanics", International Journal for Numerical Methods in Engineering, Vol. 10, No. 1, pp. 25-37, 1976.

76. Wait, R., "Finite Element Methods for Elliptic Problems with Singularity", Computational Methods for Applied Mechanics in Engineering, Vol. 13, pp. 141-150, 1975.

77. Hibbitt, H.D., "Some Properties of Singular Isoparametric Elements", International Journal for Numerical Methods in Engineering, Vol. 11, No. 1, pp. 180-184, 1977.

78. Ying, L.A., "A Note on the Singularity and the Strain Energy of Singular Elements", International Journal for Numerical Methods in Engineering, Vol. 18, No. 1, pp. 31-39, 1982.

79. Atluri, S.N. and Kumar, K.V., "$(\frac{i}{r})^t$ Point Elements, Singular Transformations, and Special Finite Elements", Center for the Advancement of Computational Mechanics, Georgia Institute of Technology, Report, 1981.

80. Ying, L.A., "Some 'Special' Interpolation Formulae for Triangular and Quadrilateral Elements", International Journal for Numerical Methods in Engineering, Vol. 18, pp. 959-966, 1982.

81. Tracey, D.M., "Finite Elements for Three-Dimensional Elastic Crack Analysis", Nuclear Engineering and Design, Vol. 16, pp. 282-290, 1977.

82. Blackburn, W.W., "Calculations of Stress Intensity Factors at Crack Tips Using Special Finite Elements", The Mathematics of Finite Elements and Applications, (Edited by J.R. Whiteman), Academic Press, London, pp. 327-336, 1973.

83. Akin, J.E., "The Generation of Elements with Singularities", International Journal for Numerical Methods in Engineering, Vol. 10, No. 6, pp. 1249-1260, 1976.

84. Dunham, R., "A Quadrature Rule for Conforming Crack Tip Elements", International Journal for Numerical Methods in Engineering, Vol. 14, pp. 287-289, 1979.

85. Lynn, P.P. and Ingraffe, A.R., "Transition Elements to be Used with Quarter-Point Crack-Tip Elements", International Journal for Numerical Methods in Engineering, Vol. 12, pp. 1030-1036, 1978.

86. Benzley, S.E., "Representation of Singularities with Isoparametric Finite Elements", International Journal for Numerical Methods in Engineering, Vol. 8, No. 3, pp. 537-545, 1974.

87. Hilton, P.D., Kiefer, B.V. and Sih, G.C., "Specialized Finite Element Procedures for Three Dimensional Crack Problems", in Numerical Methods in Fracture Mechanics, (A.R. Luxmore and D.R.J. Owen, Eds.), University College, Swansea, pp. 411-421, 1978.

88. Pian, T.H.H. and Tong, P., "The Basis of Finite Element Method for Solid Continua", International Journal for Numerical Methods in Engineering, Vol. 1, pp. 3-28, 1969.

89. Washizu, K., Variational Methods in Elasticity and Plasticity, Second Edition, Pergamon, 1975.

90. Atluri, S.N., "On Hybrid Finite Element Models in Solid Mechanics", (Linear Theory) in Advances in Computer Methods for Partial Differential Equations (R. Vishnevetsky, Ed.) AICA, Rutgers University, pp. 346-356, 1975.

91. Atluri, S.N. and Murakawa, H., "On Hybrid Finite Element Models in Nonlinear Solid Mechanics", in Finite Elements in Nonlinear Mechanics, Vol. 1, (Edited by P.G. Bergan, et al), Tapir Press, Trondheim, Norway, pp. 2-41, 1977.

92. Tong, P. and Atluri, S.N., "On Hybrid Finite Element Techniques in Crack Analysis", in Proceedings International Conference on Fracture Mechanics in Engineering and Technology (G.C. Sih, Ed.), Noordhoff Press, pp. 56-81, 1977.

93. Tong, P., Pian, T.H.H. and Orringer, O., "Fracture Mechanics Analysis with Hybrid 'Crack' Finite Elements", in Case Studies in Fracture Mechanics, AMMRC MS 77-5, Army Materials and Mechanics Research Center, pp. 2.4.-1 2.4.16, 1977.

94. Tong, P., Pian, T.H.H. and Lasry, S.J., "A Hybrid-Element Approach to Crack Problems in Plane Elasticity", International Journal for Numerical Methods in Engineering, Vol. 7, pp. 297-308, 1973.

95. Tong, P., "A Hybrid Crack Element for Rectilinear Anisotropic Material", International Journal for Numerical Methods in Engineering, Vol. 11, pp. 377-383, 1977.

96. Lin, K.Y. and Mar, J.W., "Finite Element Analysis of Stress Intensity Factors for Crack at a Bi-Material Interface", International Journal of Fracture, Vol. 12, pp. 521-531, 1976.

97. Orringer, O., "Fracture Mechanics Analysis of an Attachment Lug", ASRL TR-177-1, M.I.T.; Also, AFFDL-TR-75-51, 1976.

98. Byskov, I., "The Calculation of Stress Intensity Factors Using the Finite Element Method with Cracked Elements", International Journal of Fracture Mechanics, Vol. 6, pp. 159-167, 1970.

99. Morgan, J.D., III, "Dynamics of Cracked Structures Using Finite Elements", Ph.D. Thesis, Georgia Institute of Technology, 1974.

100. Pian, T.H.H., Tong, P. and Luk, C.H., "Elastic Crack Analysis by a Finite Element Hybrid Method", Proceedings of Third Conference on Matrix Methods in Structural Analysis, Wright Patterson Air Force Base, AFFDL-TR-71-160, pp. 661-682, Dec. 1973.

101. Rhee, H.C., Atluri, S.N., Moriya, K. and Pian, T.H.H., "Hybrid Finite Element Procedures for Analyzing Through Flaws in Plates in Bending", Trans. of Fourth SMiRT Conference, Paper M2/4, Vol. M, Comm. of European Comm., Brussels, 1977.

102. Rhee, H.C., "On the Accuracy of Finite Element Solutions of Problems of Bending of Plates with Traction Boundary Conditions", Ph.D. Thesis, Georgia Institute of Technology, 1976.

103. Pian, T.H.H. and Moriya, K., "Three-Dimensional Fracture Analysis by Assumed Stress Hybrid Elements", in Numerical Methods in Fracture Mechanics, (A.R. Luxmore and D.R.J. Owen, Eds.), University College, Swansea, pp. 363-373, 1978.

104. Tong, P., "New Displacement Hybrid Model for Solid Continua", International Journal for Numerical Methods in Engineering, Vol. 2, pp. 78-83, 1970.

105. Atluri, S.N., Kobayashi, A.S. and Nakagaki, M., "Application of an Assumed Displacement Hybrid Finite Element Procedure to Two-Dimensional Problems in Fracture Mechanics", AIAA Paper No. 74-390, Proceedings of AIAA/ASME/SAE 15th SDM Conference, Las Vegas, April 1974.

106. Atluri, S.N., Kobayashi, A.S. and Nakagaki, M., "An Assumed Displacement Hybrid Finite Element Model for Linear Fracture Mechanics", International Journal of Fracture, Vol. 11, pp. 257-271, 1975.

107. Atluri, S.N. Kobayashi, A.S. and Nakagaki, M., "A Finite Element Program for Fracture Mechanics Analysis Composite Materials", in Fracture Mechanics of Composites, ASTM STP 593 American Society for Testing and Materials, pp. 86-98, 1975.

108. Atluri, S.N., Kobayashi, A.S. and Nakagaki, M., "Fracture Mechanics Application of a Displacement Hybrid Finite Element Method", AIAA Journal, Vol. 13, pp. 734-739, 1975.

109. Atluri, S.N. and Kobayashi, A.S., "Three-Dimensional Linear Fracture Mechanics Analysis by a Displacement Hybrid Finite Element Model", Paper No. L-7/3, Third SMiRT Conference, London, Comm. of European Communities, Brussels, 1975.

110. Atluri, S.N. and Kobayashi, K., "On a 3-D Singularity Element for Computation of Combined Mode Intensity Factors", in Advances in Engineering Science, Vol. 1, NASA CP-2001, pp. 267-276, 1976.

111. Atluri, S.N., Kathiresan, K. and Nakagaki, M., "Inner Surface Cracks in an Internally Pressurized Cylinder Analysed by Displacement Hybrid Finite Element Method", in Pressure Vessel Technology, Part II, Materials and Fabrication, ASME, New York, 1977, pp. 579-593.

112. Atluri, S.N. and Kathiresan, K., "Stress Analysis of Typical Flaws in Aerospace Structural Components", in Proceedings of 19th AIAA/ASME/SAE SDM Conference, Bethesda, Maryland, pp. 340-351, 1978.

113. Atluri, S.N. and Kathiresan, K., "3-D Analysis of Surface Flaws in Thick-Walled Reactor Pressure-Vessels Using Displacement Hybrid Finite Elements", Nuclear Engineering and Design, Vol. 51, pp. 163-176, 1979.

114. Atluri, S.N. and Kathiresan, K., "Influence of Flaw Shapes on Stress Intensity Factors for Pressure Vessel Surface Flaws and Nozzle Corner Cracks", ASME Preprint 79-PVP-65; also Journal of Pressure Vessel Technology, ASME, Vol. 102, pp. 278-286, 1980.

115. Atluri, S.N., Nakagaki, M., Kathiresan, K., Rhee, H.C. and Chen, W.H., "Hybrid Finite Element Models for Linear and Nonlinear Fracture Analyses", in Numerical Methods in Fracture Mechanics, (A.R. Luxmore and D.R.J. Owens, Eds.) University College, Swansea, United Kingdom, pp. 52-66, 1978.

116. Atluri, S.N. and Nakagaki, M., "Post-Yield Analysis of a Three-Point Bend Fracture Specimen: An Embedded Singularity Finite Element Incremental Method", in Developments in Theoretical and Applied Mechanics, Vol. 8, VPI & SU, pp. 206-224, 1976.

117. Atluri, S.N. and Nakagaki, M., "J-Integral Estimates for Strain Hardening Materials in Ductile Fracture Problems", AIAA Journal, Vol. 15, pp. 842-851, 1977.

118. Atluri, S.N. and Nakagaki, M., "Fracture Analysis Under Large-Scale Yielding: A Finite Deformation, Embedded Singularity Elasto-Plastic Finite Element Solution", in Flaw Growth and Fracture, ASTM STP-631, American Society for Testing and Materials, pp. 43-61, 1977.

119. Atluri, S.N. and Nakagaki, M., "Stress Anlaysis of Cracks in the Elasto-Plastic Range", Fracture, 1977, Vol. 3 (D.M.R. Tapling, Ed.), Pergamon Press, pp. 457-463, 1977.

120. Nakagaki, M., Chen, W.H. and Atluri, S.N., "A Finite Element Analysis of Stable Crack Growth in Elastic-Plastic Fracture", ASTM STP-668 (Landes, Begley, and Clarke, Eds.) American Society for Testing and Materials, pp. 195-214, 1979.

121. Nakagaki, M. and Atluri, S.N., "Fatigue Crack Closure and Delay Effects Under Mode I Spectrum Loading: An Efficient Elastic-Plastic Analysis Procedure", Fatigue of Engineering Materials and Structures, Vol. 1, pp. 421-429, 1979.

122. Nakagaki, M. and Atluri, S.N., "An Elastic-Plastic Analysis of Fatigue Crack Closure in Modes I and II", AIAA Journal, Vol. 18, No. 9, pp. 1110-1117, 1980.

123. Atluri, S.N., Nishioka, T. and Nakagaki, M., "Numerical Modeling of Dynamic and Nonlinear Crack Propagation in Finite Bodies, by Moving Singular Elements" in Nonlinear and Dynamic Fracture Mechanics (N. Perrone and S.N. Atluri, Eds.) ASME AMD Vol. 35, pp. 37-67, ASME 1979.

124. Nishioka, T. and Atluri, S.N., "Numerical Modeling of Dynamic Crack Propagation in Finite Bodies, by Moving Singular Elements. Part I: Formulation", Journal of Applied Mechanics, Vol. 47, No. 3, pp. 570-577, 1980.

125. Nishioka, T. and Atluri, S.N., "Numerical Modeling of Dynamic Crack Propagation in Finite Bodies, by Moving Singular Elements. Part II: Results", Journal of Applied Mechanics, Vol. 47, No. 3, pp. 577-583, 1980.

126. Atluri, S.N. and Nishioka, T., "Dynamic Fracture Analysis: A Translating-Singularity Finite Element Procedure", in Advances in Fracture Research, Vol. 5, 1981.

127. Nishioka, T., Stonesifer, R.B. and Atluri, S.N., "An Evaluation of Several Moving Singularity Finite Element Models for Fast Fracture Analysis", Engineering Fracture Mechanics, Vol. 15, No. 1-2, pp. 205-218, 1981.

128. Nishioka, T. and Atluri, S.N., "Efficient Computational Techniques for Analysis of Some Problems of Fracture in Pressure Vessels and Piping", ASME Preprint 80-C2/PVP-110, June 1980, 12 pp.

CHAPTER FIVE

MULTIFIELD (MIXED AND HYBRID) FINITE ELEMENT MODELS

A. K. Noor
George Washington University Center
at NASA Langley Research Center
Hampton, Virginia

ABSTRACT

Status and some of the recent developments of multifield (mixed and hybrid) finite element models and their application to the solution of structural and nonstructural problems are summarized. Discussion focuses on a number of aspects of multifield models including: definitions and classification of multifield models; multifield variational principles; equivalence between multifield models and other single-field models; assets and liabilities of multifield models; and future directions for research. Also, an extensive list of references on the subject is included.

1. INTRODUCTION

Finite element practice continues to be based primarily on single-field formulations (sometimes referred to as *primal or primitive* formulations) of element properties. In structural and solid mechanics the primal formulations include the assumed displacement, potential energy formulation and the assumed stress, complementary energy formulation, with the former being the most-commonly used one. The single-field (primal) finite element models provided the simplest approaches to the element formulation and to the assembly of the element equations into a global system of equations in the early years of development of finite element technology. As the understanding of the finite element method deepened it became possible to broaden the practice to base element formulation on other than single field and to use schemes which differ somewhat from the concepts used in forming the global system of equations for single-field models.

The development of multifield models was largely motivated by attempts to overcome the shortcomings of conventional, single-field element models. Among these shortcomings are:

1. *Difficulty to construct compatible shape functions for* C^1 *elements* (e.g., plate and shell elements based on Kirchhoff-Love theory).
2. *Poor performance of single-field models in constrained media problems* (e.g., incompressible and nearly incompressible materials; inextensional and nearly inextensional deformations of curved beams and shells; and negligible transverse shear deformation in slender beams and in thin plates and shells).
3. *Loss of accuracy in calculating secondary fields* (e.g., stress calculations using single-field displacement models).

4. *Slow convergence for problems with high gradients* (or singularities) in the secondary field (e.g., crack propagation problems using displacement models).

The multifield element models considered in the present chapter belong to the classes of *mixed and hybrid element models*. These models were applied to several static stress analysis, eigenvalue and nonlinear structural problems. Also, their application to nonstructural problems are multiplying rapidly. In a large class of problems they were found to possess a number of distinct advantages over single-field models. The extensive literature now available on mixed and hybrid models makes a state-of-the-art summary highly desirable for engineers and researchers working on the subject.

The present chapter attempts to summarize the status and some of the recent developments of mixed and hybrid finite element models. Since the subject is very broad discussion is focused on a number of aspects which are of interest to the author and which have not been grouped together in one publication before. These aspects include:

1. Definitions and classification of multifield models
2. Multifield variational principles and variational principles based on relaxed continuity requirements
3. Equivalence between multifield models and other single-field models
4. Assets and liabilities of multifield models
5. Future directions for research.

Also, an extensive list of references is included at the end of the chapter. The references are grouped into nine sections. References in the first section deal with general topics and with topics related to mixed and hybrid models. References in subsequent sections deal with the aspects and applications of the mixed and hybrid models identified by the section headings. The references in each section are arranged alphabetically. Most of the discussion pertains to structural and solid mechanics problems. However, some consideration is given to nonstructural problems. The use of mixed formulations and mixed method in conjunction with other numerical discretization procedures is discussed in Ref. 1.13.

2. DEFINITIONS

A number of definitions have been proposed for hybrid and mixed element models (see, for example, Refs. 1.2, 1.6, 1.20 and 1.32). Most of these definitions are based on the character of the variational principle and the constraints used in the element development, as well as on the method of implementation and the nature of the resulting discrete algebraic equations. An examination of the cited references reveals that there is no universal agreement on the definitions. However, the following definitions seem to be accepted by the majority of the researchers in the field and are, therefore, adopted herein.

2.1 Hybrid Finite Element Models

Hybrid models are ones for which the formulation is based on a modified variational principle with relaxed interelement requirements. In the modified principle some or all of the interelement requirements are treated as constraints and are enforced in an *average (variational)* sense by means of Lagrange multipliers, which will be continuous functions of the boundary coordinates. Therefore, the formulation involves independent approximation of the field variable(s) within the elements and of the Lagrange multiplier(s) along the element boundaries. This definition goes well beyond the original definition of hybrid finite element models given by Pian (Refs. 1.21, 1.23 and 1.25).

Usually, all but one of the fields are described in terms of generalized parameters; that field is given in terms of physical (nodal) degrees of freedom. The appropriate variational functional is first formed in terms of both classes of parameters and then the stationary condition is applied to the generalized parameter set. This yields a system of equations relating the generalized parameters to the physical degrees of freedom. The equations are used to eliminate the generalized parameters from the expression of the variational functional. Thus, although the development of element properties starts by approximating more than one field, the final element equations are usually expressed in terms of a single field.

In structural and solid mechanics problems, hybrid finite element models are obtained by relaxing the condition of displacement continuity or traction reciprocity along the interelement boundaries. This is accomplished by using several modified variational principles which can be derived from the classical minimum potential energy and minimum complementary energy principles.

2.2 Mixed Finite Element Models

In mixed models the element parameters belong to more than one field, and *in contradistinction to hybrid models all the field variables are described within the element as well as on its boundary.* In structural and solid mechanics problems the element parameters include force (or stress) and kinematic variables (e.g., displacement and/or strains).

Two types of mixed models may be distinguished:

a. *Mixed models with continuous fields across element boundaries.* If the continuity of all field variables is enforced across element boundaries, then the size of the system analysis is expanded well beyond that which would be employed in a conventional single-field solution.

b. *Mixed models with discontinuous fields across element boundaries.* Here the continuity of a single-field only is enforced across element boundaries. The parameters used in approximating the other fields can be eliminated on the element level and the size of the system analysis is the same as that which would be employed in a single-field solution.

2.3 Hybrid-Mixed Models

A finite element model is called hybrid-mixed if it involves more than one field within the element and also contains independent variables along the interelement boundaries. Such elements are based on modified multifield variational principles with relaxed interelement requirements. In structural and solid mechanics problems, hybrid-mixed models can be obtained by relaxing some or all of the interelement continuity requirements in either the two-field Hellinger-Reissner principle or the three-field Hu-Washizu variational principle.

2.4 Comments on the Definitions of Hybrid and Mixed Models

The following comments regarding the foregoing definitions of mixed and hybrid models seem to be in order:

1. The modified variational principles used in the development of hybrid models have two major characteristics: a) they are stationary principles; and b) they are dependent on the chosen finite element grid. The latter property can be used to distinguish hybrid models from other models.

2. The condensation process used for the mixed models with discontinuous fields across the element boundaries (i.e., the elimination of the parameters used in approximating the discontinuous fields), is similar to that used for hybrid models. However, the *mixed models differ from hybrid models in the fact that all the fields are described within the element.*

3. Hybrid models and mixed models with discontinuous fields across interelement boundaries lead to elemental equations that can be incorporated into existing single-field programs. Therefore, these models can be viewed by a user of a finite element program as single-field models and can be easily combined with other single-field elements to model a physical problem.

4. The multifield (mixed and hybrid) models as defined herein are to be distinguished from mixed methods of analysis wherein mixing of the variables occurs on the system level rather than the element level (i.e., the global equations of the system contain more than one field). An example of this situation from the structural mechanics field is the analysis of a large structure by using substructuring technique, with some of the substructures analyzed by the displacement method and others by the force method. The system of equations thus obtained contain both forces and displacements as unknowns. Structures in which certain elements or substructures are considerably stiffer than others are

best suited for this mixed method. The stiff structure segments are analyzed by the displacement method and the flexible substructures are analyzed by the force method (see Refs. 1.33 and 1.34).

As an illustration, the details of the development of a variety of mixed and hybrid models for the two-dimensional heat conduction problem are given in Appendix A.

3. MULTIFIELD VARIATIONAL PRINCIPLES

Variational principles have been used extensively in the mathematical formulation of finite element models. Conversely, the remarkable success of finite element methods has given great stimulus to the development of new variational principles. In this section, a brief review is given of the various variational principles used in the development of mixed and hybrid finite element models.

3.1 Classical Multifield Principles

Multifield variational principles were first introduced in the area of solid mechanics. Hellinger presented in 1914 (Ref. 2.7) a multifield variational principle for finite elasticity problems in which stresses and displacements are varied independently. Hellinger's variational principle does not account for boundary conditions. For linear elasticity problems, Prange (Ref. 2.28) modified Hellinger's principle by including the boundary conditions. Reissner, apparently unaware of Hellinger's work, presented in 1950 (Ref. 2.31) a variational theorem for linear elasticity with independent displacement and stress fields, which includes the boundary conditions. Extension of this theorem to finite elasticity was presented in 1953 (Ref. 2.32). Hu presented in 1954 a three-field mixed variational theorem which includes independent displacement, stress and strain fields (Ref. 2.11). Similar theorem was presented independently by Washizu (Ref. 1.32). Historical accounts of multifield (mixed) variational principles in solid mechanics are given in Refs. 2.18 and 2.34 and a generalized version of Hellinger's principle in more modern notation is given in Ref. 1.31.

For elasticity problems the interrelationships among mixed and other variational principles (e.g., minimum potential energy and minimum complementary energy) are discussed in Ref. 1.32. A more elegant approach of establishing the three-field, Hu-Washizu principle, and the two-field, Hellinger-Reissner principle, is to start with the potential energy functional and successively relax conditions on the applicability of the minimum potential energy principle and effect satisfaction on certain other conditions. This approach is discussed in Ref. 1.32. A review of a number of variational principles for linear elastostatic problems is given by Tonti (Ref. 2.39).

Several extensions and applications of mixed variational principles in solid mechanics have been reported in the literature. Among these mention may be made of the applications to shells (Refs. 2.4, 2.17 and 2.33); plates (Ref. 2.36); finite elasticity problems (Ref. 2.16); continuum mechanics (Ref. 2.35); and initial value and dynamic problems (Refs. 2.1 and 2.30).

Mixed variational principles proved to be useful for the analysis of incompressible (and nearly incompressible) solids (Refs. 2.8, 2.13 and 2.38). The incompressibility of the material implies the vanishing of the mean (or volumetric) strain. The use of analysis techniques based on the single-field principle of minimum potential energy for such materials encounters computational difficulties and yields inaccurate solutions (see Refs. 1.8 and 1.22).

3.2 Multifield Variational Principles with Relaxed Continuity Requirements

The continuity requirements in classical (single-field) finite element models may in some cases lead to considerable difficulties (viz. C^1 problems). In an effort to simplify the development of finite elements in these situations, generalized variational principles with discontinuous fields at interelement boundaries in a finite element assembly were proposed. The continuity requirements along the interelement boundaries are treated as conditions of constraint and are introduced into the variational principle by means of Lagrange multipliers.

These Lagrange multipliers are recognized as the complementary boundary variables. Independent approximations are used for the field variable(s) in the interior of an element, and for the Lagrange multipliers on the boundary of that element.

The possibility of relaxing the interelement continuity requirements for the classical variational principles is one of the most versatile features of the finite element method. As mentioned previously, finite element formulations derived from such modified variational principles are called hybrid models. The first general and systematic derivation of variational principles with discontinuous fields was given by Prager (Refs. 2.26 and 2.27). These concepts were further developed by Pian (Refs. 2.22, 2.23, 2.24 and 7.60) who demonstrated the versatility of the associated hybrid finite element models. In solid mechanics problems the generalized principles allow the *a priori* relaxation of the constraints on interelement displacement continuity and/or traction reciprocity in a finite element assembly. Bufler (Ref. 2.2) and Nemat-Nasser and Lee (Refs. 2.20 and 2.21) have presented variational formulations which allow discontinuous field functions. A new interpretation of hybrid models has been provided by Fraeijs de Veubeke (Ref. 2.3) and Sander and Beckers (Ref. 1.28) in connection with the patch test for convergence of the finite element approximation. A comprehensive treatment of various modifications of Hellinger-Reissner's variational principle has been given by Knothe (Ref. 2.15).

3.3 Incremental Variational Principles

In solving highly nonlinear and path-dependent problems and problems with combined geometric and material nonlinearities, it is convenient to use incremental methods. Examples of these situations in the solid mechanics area are provided by large-rotation and large-strain problems. Several multifield variational principles of the incremental type have been developed in recent years, particularly in the solid mechanics area. These include the incremental forms of the two-field Hellinger-Reissner functional (Refs. 2.40 and 2.41) and the three-field Hu-Washizu functional given in Refs. 2.16 and 2.19. In Ref. 2.25, the effects of equilibrium imbalance and compatibility mismatch at the beginning of each loading increment are included in the variational principle. A family of incremental variational principles for hybrid formulations have been presented in Ref. 7.5. A complete review of incremental variational principles including ones suitable for mixed and hybrid formulations are given in Refs. 2.9 and 2.10.

Note that in solid mechanics problems involving nonconservative loading, the use of an incremental variational principle in conjunction with an updated Lagrangian formulation allows the nonconservative loads to be treated as piecewise conservative loads whose directions are continuously updated. The resulting stiffness matrix is, therefore, symmetric. On the other hand, if a total Lagrangian description is used, the stiffness matrix for the nonconservative loading case will be nonsymmetric.

3.4 Time-Dependent Variational Principles

Although the multifield variational principles for steady-state problems have been established, the corresponding variational principles for several transient problems (e.g., transient heat conduction) have not been derived until recently. These transient problems are, in general, not self-adjoint. Gurtin (Ref. 1.9) used the convolution method to reduce the initial value problem to an equivalent boundary-value problem, and then derived a variational principle for the reduced problem. The resulting Euler equations of the variational principle are integro-differential equations which contain the initial conditions implicitly. For linear initial-value problems of the parabolic and hyperbolic types, multifield variational principles were given in Ref. 2.30.

In elasto-dynamic problems, several multifield variational principles have been proposed. Most of these variational principles are extensions of the multifield principles used in time-independent (static) problems. One approach for deriving multifield principles in elasto-dynamics is to start with the functional of Hamilton's principle (the Lagrangian or action integral for conservative systems) and successively relax continuity in space and time using Lagrange multipliers, and restore the meaning of some of the multipliers using appropriate variational derivatives (see Ref. 2.6). Among the resulting variational principles mention may be made of the three-field mixed canonical principle in which the primary fields subject to variation are the displacement, velocity and stress fields; the two-field mixed principles of displacements and stresses; displacements and velocities (Refs. 2.5, 2.12 and 2.14); and the two-field hybrid variational principles (see Refs. 2.6, 2.29 and 2.37).

3.5 Comments on Multifield Variational Principles

The following comments concerning multifield variational principles seem to be in order:

1. The major advantage of multifield variational principles over single-field principles is the flexibility they provide in generating a finite element model. On the other hand, the multifield variational principles have the drawback of increasing the number of unknown fields; and consequently, the number of degrees of freedom in the finite element model.
2. Multifield variational principles are stationary principles, and unlike single-field principles, they do not provide bounds on the global system properties.
3. In a multifield variational principle not all the unknown fields are necessarily taken to be continuous at interelement boundaries. For example, some of the Lagrange multiplier fields can be discontinuous at interelement boundaries (see Appendix A).

4. FORMULATION OF THE DISCRETE ELEMENT EQUATIONS FOR MIXED MODELS

In general, there are three approaches for formulating the discrete element equations for mixed finite element models, namely:

1. *The Direct Method* in which the fundamental equations in their natural or primitive form are combined directly for each element. In structural and solid mechanics problems the fundamental equations include equations of motion (or equilibrium), constitutive relations, and strain-displacement relations.
2. *The Weighted Residual Approach* in which the approximations for the different fields are substituted directly into the mixed governing differential equations of the problem and an attempt is made to minimize a weighted integral of the residuals over the region of the finite element according to some criterion. The resulting formulation is referred to as a weak formulation.
3. *The Variational Approach* based on the use of mixed variational principles.

The first approach is useful for simple elements such as truss and beam elements in structural mechanics (especially in the presence of geometric and material nonlinearities). However, it becomes difficult to apply to more complex elements (e.g., shells). Some of the early applications of mixed finite elements in structural mechanics used the direct method (see Refs. 3.1 to 3.6). More recently, the direct method was applied to nonlinear static and dynamic analysis of pin-jointed space trusses (Refs. 3.7 and 3.8).

The weighted residual approach has broader scope than either of the direct or variational approaches. It does not require the existence of a variational principle. The weighting functions may be chosen in a variety of ways, and each choice corresponds to a different criterion in the method of weighted residuals (see Ref. 1.7). Most of the reported applications have used either Galerkin or least-square weighted-residual criterion (see, for example, Refs. 4.1 to 4.7). For linear self-adjoint problems the Galerkin criterion of the method of weighted residuals yields results which are identical with those obtained by variational approaches. It may be mentioned that the least-square weighted residual criterion involves more computational effort than the other criteria. However, it has the advantage that the resulting algebraic equations are always symmetric and positive definite. Therefore, iterative methods may be successfully used for their solution.

5. COMPUTATIONAL ASPECTS OF MULTIFIELD ELEMENTS

Efficiency of multifield models and their effectiveness in solving practical problems depend, among other things, on:

1. The algorithm used for generating the element characteristic arrays; and,
2. The technique used for the assembly and solution of the resulting equations.

Some of the approaches used for reducing the computational effort involved in generating the elemental arrays and solving the resulting equations, for different multifield models, are listed subsequently.

5.1 Mixed Models with Continuous Fields Across Element Boundaries

If the number of fundamental unknowns in the formulation and the number of element degrees of freedom is large (e.g., shear-flexible shell element with thirteen degrees of freedom at each node), the element characteristic arrays need not be formed in full. Rather, the submatrices representing nodal contributions are formed and stored on disk files. Only a few of these submatrices need to reside in the central memory at any one time during the assembly process. For the convenience of the assembly process, each of the submatrices is stored as a separate record in the disk files. Large-size problems can be handled by using the hypermatrix (or block matrix) storage scheme (Ref. 6.53). This procedure is suitable for computers with a random-access backing store such as a disk or drum.

The global (system) matrices are obtained by assembling the nodal contributions from different elements. This is accomplished by submatrix additions. An address (or pointer) matrix is used to identify the location of nonzero submatrices in the global matrix (hypermatrix). A zero entry in the address matrix denotes a zero submatrix which is neither generated nor stored.

The hypermatrix storage scheme combines the following advantages for handling the large system of equations of the mixed model:

1. Independence of the central memory requirements on the problem type and size.
2. A controllable ratio between central processing unit (CPU) time and data transfer (I/O) time.
3. High modularity of both program and data.

The difficulties associated with the nondefinite character of the resulting algebraic equations are overcome by assembling the discontinuous fields first (e.g., stress resultant field for shell elements), followed by the continuous field parameters (nodal displacements for shell elements). Gaussian elimination technique is then used for the solution of the equations, and no reordering or pivoting will be needed. However, the number of arithmetic operations and the storage requirements in the solution process can be significantly larger than those resulting from assembling the parameters of the different fields at each node. To remedy this drawback a nested dissection scheme is used. The nested dissection scheme is an ordering strategy for the node numbers which is closely related to multilevel substructuring (see Ref. 6.55).

The questions of numerical accuracy, stability, and conditioning of the indefinite equations of the mixed method with continuous fields have not been adequately studied. In particular, the effect of the nested dissection ordering strategy on the numerical accuracy of the solutions requires more investigation. Reference 6.54 shows that for the case of curved beams, appropriate nondimensionalization of the fundamental unknowns can lead to considerable reduction in the condition number of the resulting algebraic equations.

5.2 Mixed Models with Discontinuous Fields Across Element Boundaries

Because the parameters associated with the discontinuous fields are local to the individual elements, they are usually eliminated from the governing equations, on the element level. The computational effort involved in the elimination of these parameters can be reduced if the interpolation functions for the discontinuous fields are chosen to be orthogonal polynomials, thereby reducing the array that needs to be inverted into a block diagonal matrix.

The same simplification can be made for hybrid-mixed models, based on modified multifield variational principles with relaxed continuity requirements (see Ref. 1.26).

6. MATHEMATICAL ASPECTS OF MULTIFIELD ELEMENT MODELS

The mathematical aspects of mixed and hybrid finite element models have recently attracted the attention of many investigators. The condition for the stability of mixed models has been given by Ladyszhenskaya (1.12), Babuska (5.2), and Brezzi (5.6). This condition is referred to in the literature as the LBB stability condition, and its importance has first been presented in the engineering literature by Oden, Kikuchi and Song (Ref. 5.27). If the LBB condition is satisfied, no stability problems are encountered in the solution. On the other hand, if the LBB condition is not satisfied there are always problems (with admissible input data) in which instability will be encountered with the finite element model used. However, these instabilities do not necessarily occur in every problem. The class of problems for which instability is not encountered have been called in Ref. 5.1 the *class of perfect solutions*. For simple problems it is possible to identify the class of perfect solutions. However, for more complicated situations perfect solutions cannot be identified *a priori*. Therefore, it is desirable to have LBB condition satisfied. Examples of perfect solutions using mixed elements which violate the LBB condition are given in Refs. 5.4 and 5.28. Convergence properties and *a priori* error estimates have also been developed for a number of variational-based and weighted-residual mixed elements (see Refs. 5.5, 5.7, 5.8, 5.9, 5.10, 5.11, 5.12, 5.14 to 5.26, and 5.29 to 5.34). However, most of the aforementioned mathematical studies go through the extra step of decomposing the higher-order differential operators (e.g., Laplace or biharmonic operators) into lower-order ones, instead of using, from the start, the *natural* lower-order operators associated with the fundamental equations of mechanics.

The mathematical theory of hybrid models is more involved than that of mixed models. Convergence properties of hybrid models and of hybrid-mixed models are discussed in Refs. 5.3 and 5.13.

7. APPLICATIONS OF MIXED AND HYBRID FINITE ELEMENT MODELS

Multifield finite element models have been applied to a large number of linear and nonlinear problems. Most of the applications, however, have been in the structures and solid mechanics field. In this section a review is made of some of the reported applications of mixed and hybrid element models. Detailed accounts of the applications of mixed models to structural mechanics problems are given in Ref. 1.13. Several examples of the application of hybrid models to a variety of solid mechanics and fracture mechanics problems are given in Refs. 7.2, 7.5, 7.6, 7.9, 7.10, 7.15, 7.16, 7.21, 7.22, 7.23, 7.29, 7.60, 7.63, 7.81 and 7.82.

7.1 Applications of Mixed Finite Element Models

The variational approach to formulating the mixed finite element equations is by far the most commonly used to-date among the three approaches outlined in Section 4. Almost all the reported applications of the variational approach in the structures and solid mechanics field are based on the two-field Hellinger-Reissner mixed variational principle or modifications thereof. The first application of a variational principle to develop mixed finite elements is due to Herrmann (6.34 and 6.35), who developed two triangular elements for the linear static bending analysis of thin plates. The first element is based on a linear variation for the transverse displacement w and constant distributions for the three stress couples $M_{\alpha\beta}$ (α, $\beta = 1, 2$). The second element is based on linear variation for each of w and $M_{\alpha\beta}$. Since the publication of Ref. 6.34, several mixed finite elements have been developed for the analysis of plates and shells. Among the various applications of these models, mention may be made of static free vibration and stability analysis of plates (6.2 to 6.4, 6.14, 6.18, 6.19, 6.22, 6.42, 6.43, 6.51, 6.59, 6.63 and 6.75), linear static analysis and free vibrations of cylindrical and shallow shells (6.1, 6.5, 6.6, 6.7, 6.20, 6.21, 6.24, 6.36, 6.60, 6.61, 6.68, 6.71 and 6.76), and analysis of shells of revolution (6.10, 6.16, 6.25, 6.31 and 6.32). In Ref. (6.53), mixed shear-flexible finite elements were applied to the stress and free vibration analysis of laminated composite plates and shells. Other linear problems analyzed by mixed finite elements include plane stress (Refs. 6.23 and 6.48), curved beams (Ref. 6.29), Saint-Venant torsion (Ref. 6.52), plane problems with sharp cracks (Ref. 6.57), incompressible and nearly incompressible solids (Ref. 6.11), rubber-like materials (Ref. 6.64), contact problems (Refs. 6.58, 6.74 and 9.5), and waves in elastic composites (Ref. 6.50).

Mixed finite elements have also been applied to a number of nonlinear problems including inelastic plane frames (Ref. 6.67), elasto-plastic analysis with hardening (Ref. 6.41), elastoplastic analysis of plates (Refs. 6.8, 6.9 and 6.66), large deflection static analysis and large amplitude free vibrations of plates (Refs. 6.28, 6.33, 6.47 and 6.62), geometrically nonlinear analysis of shells of revolution (Refs. 6.17 and 6.73), geometrically nonlinear analysis of cylindrical and shallow shells (Refs. 6.28, 6.55, 6.60, 6.69 and 6.70), limit analysis of plates (Ref. 6.15), and geometrically nonlinear analysis of curved beams (Ref. 6.54).

Applications of mixed finite elements to transient response problems are given in Ref. 6.13 for three-dimensional solids, in Ref. 6.17 for shells of revolution, and in Ref. 6.56 for curved beams. In the first reference both geometric and material nonlinearities are included.

The superiority of mixed models with discontinuous stress fields at interelement boundaries, over those with continuous fields, has been demonstrated in Ref. 8.5 for the nonlinear analysis of curved beams, and in Refs. 8.7 and 8.6 for the free vibration and geometrically nonlinear analysis of shallow shells, respectively.

Most of the applications of mixed models to nonstructural problems have been in the fluid mechanics area and are based on the weighted residual approach (with a Galerkin or a least-square criterion). These include potential flow (Ref. 6.46), rotational flow with internal sources (Ref. 6.65), viscous incompressible flow (Refs. 4.6, 6.12, 6.30, 6.37 and 6.39), inviscid compressible flow (Ref. 6.27), transonic flow (Ref. 6.77), solution of Navier-Stokes equations (Refs. 6.38, 6.40, 6.44 and 6.72), transonic flutter analysis (Refs. 4.2, 4.3 and 6.26), hydrocapillary vibration analysis (Ref. 6.49), and steady fluid and metal flow problems (Ref. 6.78). Application of mixed models to soil-structure interaction problems is reported in Ref. 6.45.

7.2 Applications of Hybrid and Hybrid-Mixed Models

The first application of hybrid models is due to Pian (Ref. 7.57), who developed a hybrid stress model for plane elasticity problems. The element was based on a modified complementary energy principle with relaxed traction reciprocity at interelement boundaries. Further developments of plane stress elements have been reported in Refs. 7.30, 7.58, 7.59 and 7.72. Rectangular, triangular and quadrilateral hybrid models for plate bending were presented in Refs. 7.31, 7.34, 7.53, 7.68, 7.69 and 7.79. The last three references include the transverse shear deformation (which can be important for multilayered and sandwich plates). In Refs. 7.2 and 7.26 hybrid models were applied to the vibration and transient response analysis of plates. A large number of studies have been devoted to assess the performance of hybrid models in predicting the response of curved shells. These studies included linear static analysis of shells of revolution, cylindrical shells and shallow shells (Refs. 7.4, 7.7, 7.32, 7.33, 7.35, 7.36, 7.37, 7.77, 7.83 and 7.91).

Other linear problems analyzed by hybrid models include Saint-Venant torsion of elastic bars (Ref. 7.87), plane strain problems of incompressible, and nearly-incompressible materials (Refs. 7.71 and 7.78); axisymmetric solids (Refs. 7.75 and 7.76); laminated anisotropic plates (Refs. 7.49, 7.50 and 7.67); three-dimensional solids (Refs. 7.1, 7.46, 7.73 and 7.74); thick plates (Ref. 7.70); thick walled pressure vessels (Ref. 7.3); and elastic response near a fastener hole (Ref. 7.56).

Hybrid finite element models have also been applied to a number of nonlinear structural and solid mechanics problems including plane stress analysis of nonlinearly elastic and elasto-plastic materials (Refs. 7.51, 7.52 and 7.63); creep problems (Refs. 7.61 and 7.62); Saint-Venant torsion of elasto-plastic bars (Ref. 7.88); elasto-plastic analysis of plates (Ref. 7.2); geometrically nonlinear analysis of curved beams (Ref. 7.5); large deflection analysis of plates and shallow shells (Refs. 7.24, 7.25 and 7.38); elasto-plastic analysis of thick shells of revolution (Ref. 7.66).

Hybrid stress models are particularly useful for use in fracture mechanics applications. It is possible to include special terms which account for the correct stress singularity near the crack tip. Among the linear fracture mechanics applications of hybrid stress and displacement models are uniaxial tension of a plate with an edge or central crack (Refs. 7.8 and 7.80), cracks in composite plates (Refs. 7.14 and 7.54); three-dimensional cracks (Refs. 7.11, 7.12, 7.17, and 7.19); and through-flaws in plates subjected to bending (Ref. 7.64). Hybrid models were also applied to study the ductile fracture for strain-hardening materials (Ref. 7.20), and the post-yield response of a three-point bend fracture test specimen with a single edge crack (Ref. 7.18).

Nonstructural applications of hybrid models include indentation of a monkey brain (Ref. 7.13); soil-structure interaction problems (Ref. 7.65); potential flow problems (Ref. 7.55); Stokes flow (Refs. 7.27, 7.28 and 7.90); solution of Navier-Stokes equations (Ref. 7.89).

In a number of solid mechanics applications, the use of hybrid-mixed models were shown to overcome three major drawbacks of the hybrid stress model (Ref. 1.26); namely, a) difficulty of choosing the assumed stress terms; b) requirement of inverting the flexibility matrix in the process of constructing the element stiffness matrix; and c) difficulty of choosing equilibrating stresses in the case of complex structures such as shells. The formulation of hybrid-mixed models is based on the modified Hellinger-Reissner and Hu-Washizu variational principles with relaxed continuity requirements. The stress equilibrium conditions are not introduced initially but are brought in through the use of additional internal displacement parameters.

7.3 Simplified Hybrid Models

Since the initial development of hybrid models, a number of attempts have been made to generalize and improve the efficiency of these models (see, for example, Refs. 7.42, 7.47, 7.84, 7.85 and 7.86). One of the popular modified models is the simplified hybrid model which is based on the use of generalized variational principles with relaxed interelement continuity requirements and the *a priori* replacement of the Lagrange multipliers by their expressions in terms of the primary field variable. The result of using this approach is to add to the single-field element equations corrective terms which represent the counterbalancing effect, in the global model, to using nonconforming element shape functions. Several applications have been reported using the simplified hybrid models (see Refs. 7.39, 7.40, 7.41, 7.43, 7.44 and 7.45). However, careful examination has shown that the simplified hybrid models may become unstable. Furthermore, the models are, in general, incapable of restoring interelement compatibility in an integral sense (see Ref. 7.48) and, consequently, they must be used with caution.

8. ASSETS AND LIABILITIES OF MULTIFIELD MODELS

The studies made with multifield models have identified the following major advantages over single-field models:

1. *Simplicity of Element Formulation*

a. Because the Euler equations of the mixed functionals are the more basic equations of mechanics (or physics) with lower-order derivatives, the interelement continuity requirements on the assumed fields are of lower order than for the conventional single-field variational principles. Examples of these situations are provided by thin plates and shells where only C^0 continuity is required for the shape functions of the multifield models.

b. The development of the characteristic arrays for multifield models involves fewer arithmetic operations than that of their equivalent single-field models. This is particularly true if: i) the interpolation functions for the fields that are local to the element are selected to be orthogonal polynomials, and ii) the theory of group representation is used to take advantage of the similarities in algebraic form of the various integrals appearing in the characteristic arrays of the multifield models (see Refs. 6.52 and 6.53).

c. For some nonlinear problems, multifield models lead to algebraic equations of a lower order than those obtained by a single field model. An example of this situation is provided by moderate rotation, geometrically nonlinear solid mechanics problems. The resulting finite element equations of the mixed formulation contain bilinear and quadratic terms in the force and kinematic variables. By contrast, the finite element equations of the single-field (displacement) models are cubic in the nodal displacements (see Ref. 8.6).

2. *Uniform Accuracy for the Different Fields.*

a. For both the mixed models with discontinuous fields and the hybrid models, the approximations for the discontinuous fields within the individual elements can be arbitrary. Therefore, the local known information can be exploited in the construction of element characteristics. For example, in crack propagation problems the singular behavior of stresses near the crack tip, obtained from the theory of elasticity, can be used to construct special elemental matrices around the crack tip, while polynomials are used to construct elemental matrices for other elements in regions where stress gradients are not high.

b. In some applications, multifield models can directly yield quantities of practical interest, thus eliminating the need to use further approximations or extrapolation techniques. Examples of these situations are provided by the stress computations in solid mechanics and the evaluation of stress intensity factors in fracture mechanics.

3. *Versatility.* Multifield models of the hybrid and mixed-hybrid types provide a convenient way to:

a. Match approximate solutions for different regions which make them eminently suited for analyzing nonhomogeneous media with discontinuous properties.

b. Satisfy, to any desired degree of accuracy, the natural boundary conditions along arbitrarily curved boundaries (see Refs. 1.1 and 1.35).

4. *Insensitivity of the Performance of the Model to Variations in the Geometric and Physical Characteristics of the Problem.* Three examples can be cited from the solid mechanics field where the performance of multifield models was shown to be considerably less sensitive to variations in the geometric and material characteristics of the structure than that of the single field (displacement) models (see Ref. 1.24). The first is the case of nearly incompressible materials, where the mean (or volumetric) strain is close to zero. The second example is the application of shear-flexible plate (or shell) elements to analyze thin plates (or shells) with negligible shear deformation. The third problem is the use of shell elements, which do not include the rigid body modes explicitly, to analyze very thin shells with negligible extensional energy. For all three problems the single-field displacement models encounter computational difficulties.

While there are a number of advantages in using multifield finite element models, four difficulties arise:

1. The first difficulty is due to the nondefiniteness of the matrix of the resulting algebraic equations. Since these equations are not positive definite, some efficient algorithms used with the single-field models cannot be applied.

2. The second difficulty results from the use of multifield variational principles. Since these principles are stationary and not extremum principles, a bound on the numerical solution cannot be obtained.

3. The third difficulty is associated with mixed models with continuous fields at interelement boundaries. The increase in the number of degrees of freedom results in a substantial increase in the size of the elemental matrices, and in the number of simultaneous equations, as compared with the single-field models.

4. The fourth difficulty is that some of the hybrid models and the mixed models with discontinuous fields at interelement boundaries contain spurious mechanisms (associated with zero eigenvalues) which, if excited, result in a poor performance of the element.

The first and third difficulties can be greatly alleviated (or possibly nullified) by using the computational procedure described in the section on computational aspects of multifield finite elements. The second difficulty is not a practical one although bounds on the solution can be a nice feature to have in a numerical procedure. The fourth difficulty, the zero-energy spurious modes, can be suppressed by using the techniques presented in Refs. 1.3, 1.11, 1.18, 1.19, 1.27 and 1.29.

9. USE OF REDUCTION METHODS IN CONJUNCTION WITH MULTIFIELD MODELS FOR NONLINEAR ANALYSIS

In recent years considerable work has been devoted to the development of techniques for reducing the total number of degrees of freedom of the discretized system without sacrificing the accuracy. Such techniques are called *reduction methods*. A possible approach for applying reduction methods in conjunction with multifield formulation is to use multifield finite element models for the initial discretization of the system, resulting in a large system of nonlinear equations with the unknowns belonging to more than one field. The vector of unknown parameters within each element is expressed as a linear combination of a small number of global approximation (or basis) vectors. A Bubnov-Galerkin (or Rayleigh-Ritz) technique is then used to approximate the finite element equations of the initial discretization by a reduced system of nonlinear equations.

The success of reduction methods depends to a great extent on the proper choice of global approximation vectors. For nonlinear steady-state problems an effective choice for the global approximation vectors was found to consist of a nonlinear solution and its various order path derivatives (derivatives with respect to a load, displacement or path parameter). The advantages of these vectors and their effectiveness in solving nonlinear structural mechanics and thermal problems are demonstrated in Refs. 1.14 to 1.17.

For some nonlinear transient problems, a good choice of global approximation vectors was found to be a combination of two sets of eigenvectors; namely, the eigenvectors of the linear system, and the eigenvectors of the steady-state nonlinear system (see Ref. 1.15).

10. EQUIVALENCE BETWEEN MULTIFIELD MODELS AND SOME CLASSES OF SINGLE-FIELD MODELS

In recent years a number of studies have been devoted to the establishment of the equivalence between multifield models and some classes of single-field models. These studies have enhanced the understanding of a number of special classes of single-field models such as reduced/selective integration models, penalty-finite element models, and nonconforming single-field models. In this section, a definition of equivalent finite element models is given and then two of the classes of single-field models which are equivalent to some mixed models are discussed.

10.1 Definition

Two finite element models are said to be *equivalent* if their governing finite element equations, when expressed in terms of a common set of nodal variables and/or parameters are *identical*. The other nodal variables and/or parameters not contained in the common set must be local to the individual elements and do not affect the assembly process. The two models are said to be *nearly equivalent* if their finite element equations expressed in terms of a common set of variables, are *almost identical* (e.g., if the corresponding numerical coefficients in both sets of equations differ by a small percentage).

Two classes of single-field models which are equivalent to some mixed models, are described subsequently. The two classes are: reduced/selective integration models, and penalty finite element models.

10.2 Reduced/Selective Integration Single-Field Models

Reduced integration technique refers to using a lower-order quadrature formula than the *normal* one in evaluating the characteristic arrays of a single-field model. This *underintegration* of the element characteristic arrays was shown to result in a significant improvement in the performance of single-field models for constrained media applications (e.g., incompressible solids and fluids; and shear-flexible beams, plates and shells). The procedure was first suggested by Zienkiewicz, Taylor and Too (Ref. 1.36), and was later applied to a number of constrained media problems. However, the use of such low-order quadrature formula was shown to diminish the rank of the elemental matrices and may occasionally lead to undesirable zero energy spurious modes or mechanisms (see Refs. 1.10 and 8.2).

To remedy this, the reduced/selective integration concept was introduced in which the variational functional is decomposed into components. A low-order quadrature formula is used in evaluating the constrained components, and the "normal" quadrature formula is used in evaluating the remaining components.

In a number of applications, selective integration was shown to maintain the attributes of reduced integration while mitigating rank-deficiency problems. Also, a generalization of the selective integration procedure has been given in Ref. 8.3 for the cases where the segregation of the constrained components of the functional is not possible.

Mixed models with discontinuous fields which are equivalent to single-field models based on either normal or reduced/selective integration have been identified in Refs. 8.1, 8.2, 8.4, 8.5, 8.6 and 8.7 for a variety of structural and fluid mechanics applications. The conditions for the equivalence of these models are given in Refs. 8.6 and 8.7. It was shown in Refs. 8.5 and 8.6 that choosing polynomial interpolation functions for the discontinuous fields, which are local to the individual element, of the same degree (or higher than) those used for the continuous field, can result in degrading the performance of the mixed model.

10.3 Penalty Finite Element Models

Penalty finite element models refer to finite elements based on a variational formulation with penalty, in which the functional being minimized is appended by a term containing the product of a penalty number and the equality constraint. Despite its wide use in mathematical programming and optimization, the penalty function method was not regarded, until recently, as a powerful basis for finite element computations. This is because in practical applications, the penalty terms misbehave without the proper selection of the approximate functions and/or integration formulas. The use of reduced integration to evaluate the penalty terms (coefficients of the penalty parameters) circumvented this difficulty, and resulted in a wide acceptance of the method. Penalty finite element models have been successfully applied to a broad class of constrained media problems including shear-flexible beams, plates and shells (Refs. 9.2, 9.7 and 1.37); plastic flow of metals (Ref. 9.9); and nonlinear incompressible solids and fluids (Refs. 9.3, 9.4 and 9.6). A detailed historical account of the penalty method and a list of applications of the method is presented in Ref. 9.8.

The understanding of the penalty finite element models was considerably enhanced by the establishment of the equivalence between these models and a class of mixed models based on "perturbed Lagrangian" formulations (see Ref. 9.1).

10.4 Comments on the Equivalence Between Multifield Models and Single-Field Models

In spite of the equivalence discussed in the preceding subsections, multifield models possess a number of advantages over their equivalent single-field models. Some of these advantages are listed subsequently:

1. The development of mixed models with discontinuous fields is simpler and more straightforward than the development of reduced/selective integration single-field models. This is particularly true for: a) cases where the decomposition of the functional into constrained and unconstrained components cannot be easily made; and b) cases where the functional of the mixed variational

principle is simpler than that of the single-field principle (e.g., geometrically nonlinear shell problems).

2. The evaluation of the element characteristic arrays for mixed models with discontinuous fields involve fewer arithmetic operations than the formulation of the corresponding arrays in the single-field models. This was demonstrated in Ref. 8.6 for the case of geometrically nonlinear shell elements.

3. When reduction methods are used in conjunction with multifield models, the following two advantages can be identified (see Refs. 1.14 and 8.6).

a) *Simplicity of generation of global approximation (or basis) vectors*, in the sense of fewer arithmetic operations required for the generation of these vectors than those required in the corresponding single-field models.

b) *Better approximation properties.* Numerical studies have demonstrated the higher accuracy of the solutions obtained by reduction method-mixed models than those obtained by the corresponding single-field models.

11. FUTURE DIRECTIONS FOR RESEARCH

Among the different aspects of multifield models which appear to have high potential for research are the following:

1. *Development of simple and accurate multifield models with no spurious modes.* This includes the rational selection of shape functions for the different fields, and an investigation of whether it is necessary to have the individual elements free of spurious modes, or it is sufficient to remove the spurious modes from the total finite element model through the application of some constraints (such as the use of a few normally-integrated elements near the boundary). An attempt to rationalize the selection of shape functions for single-field models, in order to eliminate the spurious modes and maintain high accuracy for constrained problems, has been made in Ref. 1.30.

2. *Adaptive refinement strategy for use with multifield models.* This includes an investigation of the merits of using the h and the p versions (and possibly their combination) with multifield models.

3. *Application of reduction methods in conjunction with multifield models.* Although results to-date demonstrate the high potential of applying reduction methods in conjunction with multifield models for solution of nonlinear problems, further improvements in the computational algorithms are needed to realize the full potential of these methods. This is particularly true for transient (time-dependent) problems and inelastic solid mechanics problems.

4. *Application of multifield models to complex practical problems.* The opportunities provided by mixed and hybrid models have not been fully explored, particularly in areas where multifield models appear to be eminently suited, such as reanalysis techniques required in the automated optimum design of complex engineering systems; contact-impact problems; study of frictional sliding between two or more bodies; and solution of various nonlinear coupled problems.

CONCLUDING REMARKS

The status and some of the recent developments of multifield (mixed and hybrid) finite element models and their application to the solution of structural and nonstructural problems have been summarized. A number of aspects of the multifield models are considered herein including: definitions and classification of multifield models; multifield variational principles; equivalence between multifield models and other single-field models; and computational aspects. The major advantages and drawbacks of multifield models are outlined and a number of aspects of multifield models which have high potential for research are identified.

REFERENCES

General

1.1 Atluri, S. N. and Rhee, H. E., "Traction Boundary Conditions in Hybrid Stress Finite Element Model," AIAA Journal, Vol. 16, No. 5, May 1978, pp. 529-531.

1.2 Atluri, S. N., Gallagher, R. H., and Zienkiewicz, O. C., eds., Hybrid and Mixed Finite Element Models, John Wiley, 1983.

1.3 Belytschko, T., Liu, W. K., and Kennedy, J. M., "Hour-Glass Control in Linear and Nonlinear Problems," in Computer Methods for Nonlinear Solids and Structural Mechanics, ed. by S. N. Atluri and N. Perrone, AMD Vol. 54, American Society of Mechanical Engineers, 1983, pp. 37-63.

1.4 Biot, M. A., Variational Principles in Heat Transfer, Oxford at the Clarendon Press, 1970.

1.5 Carslaw, H. S. and Jaeger, J. C., Conduction of Heat in Solids, second edition, Oxford University Press, 1959.

1.6 Carey, G. F. and Oden, J. T., Finite Elements: A Second Course, Vol. II, Prentice-Hall, 1982.

1.7 Finlayson, B. A., The Method of Weighted Residuals and Variational Principles, Academic Press, 1972.

1.8 Fried, I., "Finite Element Analysis of Incompressible Material by Residual Energy Balancing," International Journal of Solids and Structures, Vol. 10, 1974, pp. 993-1002.

1.9 Gurtin, M. E., "Variational Principles for Linear Initial-Value Problems," Quarterly of Applied Mathematics, Vol. 22, No. 3, 1964, pp. 252-256.

1.10 Hughes, T. J. R. and Cohen, M., "The 'Heterosis' Finite Element for Plate Bending," Computers and Structures, Vol. 9, 1978, pp. 445-450.

1.11 Kosloff, D. and Frazier, G. A., "Treatment of Hour-Glass Patterns in Low-Order Finite Element Codes," International Journal for Numerical Analysis Methods in Geomechanics, Vol. 2, 1978, pp. 57-72.

1.12 Ladyszhenskaya, O. A., The Mathematical Theory of Viscous Incompressible Flows, Gordon Breach, New York, 1969.

1.13 Noor, A. K., "Mixed Method of Analysis," Structural Mechanics Software Series, The University Press of Virginia, Vol. 3, 1980, pp. 263-305.

1.14 Noor, A. K. and Peters, J. M., "Nonlinear Analysis Via Global-Local Mixed Finite Element Approach," International Journal for Numerical Methods in Engineering, Vol. 15, 1980, pp. 1363-1380.

1.15 Noor, A. K., "Recent Advances in Reduction Methods for Nonlinear Problems," Computers and Structures, Vol. 13, Nos. 1/2, 1981, pp. 31-44.

1.16 Noor, A. K., "On Making Large Nonlinear Problems Small," Computer Methods in Applied Mechanics and Engineering, 1982, Vol. 34, pp. 955-985.

1.17 Noor, A. K., Balch, C. D., and Shibut, M. A., "Reduction Methods for Nonlinear Steady-State Thermal Analysis," NASA TP-2098, March 1983. Also to be published in International Journal for Numerical Methods in Engineering.

1.18 Onate, E., Hinton, E., and Glover, N., "Techniques for Improving the Performance of Ahmad Shell Elements," Report C/R/313/78, Department of Civil Engineering, University of Wales, Swansea.

1.19 Parisch, H., "A Critical Survey of the Nine-Node Degenerated Shell Element with Special Emphasis on Thin Shell Application and Reduced Integration," Computer Methods in Applied Mechanics and Engineering, Vol. 20, 1979, pp. 323-350.

1.20 Pian, T. H. H. and Tong, P., "Basis of Finite Element Methods for Solid Continua," International Journal for Numerical Methods in Engineering, Vol. 1, 1969, pp. 3-28.

1.21 Pian, T. H. H., "How Did I Think of the Assumed Stress Hybrid Method," (in English), Outline of Variational Principles in Elasticity (in Japanese), by K. Washizu, Series in Computer Oriented Structural Engineering, Vol. II-3-A, Baifukan Publishing Company, Tokyo, 1972, pp. 100-103.

1.22 Pian, T. H. H. and Lee, S. W., "Notes on Finite Elements for Nearly Incompressible Materials," AIAA Journal, Vol. 14, No. 6, June 1976, pp. 824-826.

1.23 Pian, T. H. H., "A Historical Note About 'Hybrid Element'," International Journal for Numerical Methods in Engineering, Vol. 12, No. 5, 1978, pp. 891-892.

1.24 Pian, T. H. H. and Tong, P., "Reissner's Principle in Finite Element Formulations," Mechanics Today, Vol. 5, 1980, pp. 377-395.

1.25 Pian, T. H. H., "Reflections and Remarks on Hybrid and Mixed Finite Element Methods," in Hybrid and Mixed Finite Element Methods, ed. by S. N. Atluri, R. H. Gallagher and O. C. Zienkiewicz, John Wiley and Sons, 1983, pp. 565-576.

1.26 Pian, T. H. H., Chen, D. P., and Kang, D., "A New Formulation of Hybrid/Mixed Finite Element," Computers and Structures, Vol. 16, 1983, pp. 81-87.

1.27 Rubinstein, R., Punch, E. F., and Atluri, S. N., "An Analysis of, and Remedies for, Kinematic Modes in Hybrid-Stress Finite Elements: Selection of Stable, Invariant Stress Fields," Computer Methods in Applied Mechanics and Engineering, Vol. 38, 1983, pp. 63-92.

1.28 Sander, G. and Beckers, P., "Delinquent Finite Elements for Shell Idealization," Proceedings of the World Congress on Finite Element Methods in Structural Mechanics, Bournemouth, Dorset, England, Vol. II, Oct. 1975, pp. 2.1 to 2.31.

1.29 Sani, R. L., Gresho, P. M., Lee, R. L., and Griffiths, D. F., "The Cause and Cure (?) of the Spurious Pressures Generated by Certain Finite Element Solutions of the Incompressible Navier-Stokes Equations," International Journal for Numerical Methods in Fluids, Vol. 1, 1981, Part 1, pp. 17-43; Part 2, pp. 171-204.

1.30 Tessler, A. and Hughes, T. J. R., "Auxiliary Convergence Criteria for Mindlin Plate Elements and Their Application to the Four-Node Quadrilateral," Proceedings of the AIAA/ASME/ASCE/AHS 24th Structures, Structural Dynamics and Materials Conference, May 2-4, 1983, Lake Tahoe, Nevada, Part 1, pp. 154-160.

1.31 Truesdell, C. and Toupin, R., The Classical Field Theories, Encyclopedia of Physics, ed. by S. Flugge, Vol. 3/1, Springer, Berlin, 1960.

1.32 Washizu, K., Variational Methods in Elasticity and Plasticity, third edition, Pergamon Press, 1982.

1.33 Wiberg, N. E., Diacoptics and Codiacoptics - Two Dual Mixed Methods for Analyzing Elastic Structures, Report 67:8, Chalmers University of Technology, Goteborg, 1967.

1.34 Wiberg, N. E., "Matrix Structural Analysis with Mixed Variables," International Journal for Numerical Methods in Engineering, Vol. 8, 1974, pp. 167-194.

1.35 Wolf, J. P., "Systematic Enforcement of Stress Boundary Conditions in the Assumed Stress Hybrid Model Based on the Deformation Method," Proceedings of the First International Conference on Structural Mechanics in Reactor Technology, Berlin, Vol. 6, Part M, 1971, pp. 464-484.

1.36 Zienkiewicz, O. C., Taylor, R. L., and Too, J. M., "Reduced Integration Technique in General Analysis of Plates and Shells," International Journal for Numerical Methods in Engineering, Vol. 3, 1971, pp. 275-290.

1.37 Zienkiewicz, O. C., The Finite Element Method, third edition, McGraw-Hill Book Company, New York, 1977.

Multifield Variational Principles

2.1 Barr, A. D. S., "An Extension of the Hu-Washizu Variational Principle in Linear Elasticity for Dynamic Problems," Journal of Applied Mechanics, Vol. 33, No. 2, June 1966, p. 465.

2.2 Bufler, H., "Generalized Variational Principles with Relaxed Continuity Requirements for Certain Nonlinear Problems, With an Application to Nonlinear Elasticity," Computer Methods in Applied Mechanics and Engineering, Vol. 19, 1979, pp. 235-255.

2.3 de Veubeke, B. Fraeijs, "Variational Principles and the Patch Test," International Journal for Numerical Methods in Engineering, Vol. 8, No. 4, 1974, pp. 783-801.

2.4 Elias, Z. M., "Mixed Variational Principles for Shells," International Conference on Variational Methods in Engineering, Southampton, Sept. 1972, in Variational Methods in Engineering, ed. by C. A. Brebbia and H. Tottenham, Southampton University Press, 1973, pp. 3/33-3/45.

2.5 Geradin, M., Sander, G., and Nyssen, C., "Mixed Variational Formulations in Linear and Nonlinear Structural Dynamics," Proceedings of the Symposium of Applications of Computer Methods in Engineering, Los Angeles, CA, Aug. 23-26, 1977.

2.6 Geradin, M., "Variational Methods of Structural Dynamics and Their Finite Element Implementation," in Advanced Structural Dynamics, ed. by J. Donea, Applied Science Publishers, Ltd., London, 1980, pp. 1-41.

2.7 Hellinger, E., "Der Allgemeine Ansatz der Mechanik der Kontinua," Encyclopadie der Mathematischen Wissenschaften, Vol. 4, Part 4, 1914, pp. 602-694.

2.8 Herrmann, L. R., "Elasticity Equations for Incompressible and Nearly Incompressible Materials by a Variational Theorem," AIAA Journal, Vol. 3, 1965, pp. 1896-1900.

2.9 Horrigmoe, G., "Nonlinear Finite Element Models in Solid Mechanics," Report No. 76-2, Division of Structural Mechanics, The Norwegian Institute of Technology, The University of Trondheim, Norway, Aug. 1976.

2.10 Horrigmoe, G. and Bergan, P. G., "Incremental Variational Principles and Finite Element Models for Nonlinear Problems," Computer Methods in Applied Mechanics and Engineering, Vol. 7, No. 2, 1976, pp. 201-217.

2.11 Hu, H. C., "On Some Variational Principles in the Theory of Elasticity and the Theory of Plasticity," Scientia Sinica, Vol. 4, 1955, pp. 33-45.

2.12 Karnopp, B. H., "Reissner's Variational Principle and Elasto-Dynamics," Acta Mechanica, Vol. 6, 1968, pp. 158-164.

2.13 Key, S. W., "A Variational Principle for Incompressible and Nearly Incompressible Anisotropic Elasticity," International Journal of Solids and Structures, Vol. 5, 1969, pp. 824-826.

2.14 Hughes, T. J. R., "A Reduction Scheme for Problems of Structural Dynamics," International Journal of Solids and Structures, Vol. 12, 1976, pp. 744-767.

2.15 Knothe, K., "Variationsprinzipien der Elastostatik mit gelockerten Stetigkeitsforderungen und ihre Verwandbarkeit im Rahmen der Methode der finiten Elemente," Institut fur Luft-und Raumfahrt, Technische Universitat Berlin, Report No. ILP-13, 1974.

2.16 Lee, K. N. and Nemat-Nasser, S., "Mixed Variational Principles, Finite Elements and Finite Elasticity," in Computational Methods in Nonlinear Mechanics, ed. by J. T. Oden, et al., The Texas Institute for Computational Mechanics, Austin, 1974, pp. 637-649.

2.17 Naghdi, P. M., "On a Variational Theory in Elasticity and Its Application to Shell Theory," Journal of Applied Mechanics, Vol. 31, 1964, pp. 647-653.

2.18 Nemat-Nasser, S., "General Variational Principles in Nonlinear and Linear Elasticity with Applications," Mechanics Today, Vol. 1, 1972, pp. 214-261.

2.19 Nemat-Nasser, S., "On Variational Methods in Finite and Incremental Elastic Deformation Problems with Discontinuous Fields," Quarterly of Applied Mathematics, July 1972, pp. 143-156.

2.20 Nemat-Nasser, S. and Lee, K. N., "Finite Element Formulations for Elastic Plates by General Variational Statements with Discontinuous Fields," Developments in Mechanics, Vol. 7, Proceedings of the Thirteenth Midwestern Mechanics Conference, 1973, pp. 979-995.

2.21 Nemat-Nasser, S. and Lee, K. N., "Application of General Variational Methods with Discontinuous Fields to Bending, Buckling and Vibration of Beams," Computer Methods in Applied Mechanics and Engineering, Vol. 2, No. 1, 1973, pp. 33-41.

2.22 Pian, T. H. H., "Variational Formulations of Numerical Methods in Solid Continua," Computer Aided Engineering, Proceedings of the Symposium, University of Waterloo, Waterloo, Ontario, Canada, May 11-13, 1971, pp. 421-448.

2.23 Pian, T. H. H., "Finite Element Formulation by Variational Principles with Relaxed Continuity Requirements," in The Mathematical Foundations of the Finite Element Method with Applications to Partial Differential Equations, ed. by K. A. Aziz, Academic Press, 1972, pp. 671-687.

2.24 Pian, T. H. H., "Finite Element Methods by Variational Principles with Relaxed Continuity Requirements," in Variational Methods in Engineering, ed. by C. A. Brebbia and H. Tottenham, Southampton University Press, 1973, pp. 3/1-3/24.

2.25 Pian, T. H. H., "Variational Principles for Incremental Finite Element Methods," Journal of the Franklin Institute, Vol. 302, Nos. 5 and 6, Nov./Dec. 1976, pp. 473-488.

2.26 Prager, William, "Variational Principles of Linear Elastostatics for Discontinuous Displacements, Strains and Stresses," in Recent Progress in Applied Mechanics, The Folke-Odqvist Volume, B. Broberg, J. Hult and F. Niordson, Sweden, 1967, pp. 463-474.

2.27 Prager, William, "Variational Principles for Elastic Plates with Relaxed Continuity Requirements," International Journal of Solids and Structures, Vol. 4, No. 9, 1968, pp. 837-844.

2.28 Prange, G., "Das Extremum der Formanderungsarbeit," Habilitation Thesis, Hannover, 1916.

2.29 Raasch, I., "A Variational Principle for Nonlinear Elastodynamics and Its Application to the Hybrid Stress Model," International Journal of Nonlinear Mechanics, Vol. 10, No. 5, 1975, pp. 215-222.

2.30 Reddy, J. N., "A Note on Mixed Variational Principles for Initial-Value Problems," Quarterly Journal of Mechanics and Applied Mathematics, Vol. 28, Part 1, 1975, pp. 123-132.

2.31 Reissner, E., "On a Variational Theorem in Elasticity," Journal of Mathematics and Physics, Vol. 29, 1950, pp. 90-95.

2.32 Reissner, E., "On a Variational Theorem for Finite Elastic Deformations," Journal of Mathematics and Physics, Vol. 32, 1953, pp. 129-135.

2.33 Reissner, E., "On the Form of Variationally Derived Shell Equations," Journal of Applied Mechanics, ASME, Vol. 31, June 1964, pp. 233-238.

2.34 Reissner, E., "Variational Methods and Boundary Conditions in Shell Theory," Studies in Optimization, Proceedings of the Symposium on Optimization, Vol. 1, Society of Industrial and Applied Mathematics, 1970, pp. 78-94.

2.35 Sandhu, R. S. and Pister, K. S., "Variational Principles for Boundary Value and Initial-Boundary Value Problems in Continuum Mechanics," International Journal of Solids and Structures, Vol. 7, 1971, pp. 639-654.

2.36 Sandhu, R. S. and Pister, K. S., "Variational Principles for Plate Bending - A Unified Approach," in Variational Methods in Engineering, ed. by C. A. Brebbia and H. Tottenham, Southampton University Press, 1973, pp. 2/68-2/80.

2.37 Tabarrok, B., "A Variational Principle for the Dynamic Analysis of Continua by the Hybrid Finite Element Method," International Journal of Solids and Structures, Vol. 7, No. 3, 1971, pp. 251-268.

2.38 Taylor, R. L., Pister, K. S., and Herrmann, L. R., "On a Variational Theorem for Incompressible and Nearly-Incompressible Orthotropic Elasticity," International Journal of Solids and Structures, Vol. 4, 1968, pp. 875-883.

2.39 Tonti, E., "Variational Principles in Elastostatics," Meccanica, Vol. 2, Dec. 1967, pp. 201-208.

2.40 Wempner, G. A., "Discrete Approximations Related to Nonlinear Theories of Solids," International Journal of Solids and Structures, Vol. 7, No. 11, 1971, pp. 1581-1599.

2.41 Wempner, G. A., "Discrete Approximations of Elastic-Plastic Bodies by Variational Methods," in Variational Methods in Engineering, ed. by C. A. Brebbia and H. Tottenham, Southampton University Press, 1973, pp. 7/1-7/35.

Analysis of Pin-Jointed Trusses and Framed and Skin Type Structures

3.1 Klein, B., "A Simple Method of Matric Structural Analysis," Journal of the Aeronautical Sciences, Vol. 24, No. 1, Jan. 1957, pp. 39-46.

3.2 Klein, B., "A Simple Method of Matric Structural Analysis: Part II - Effects of Taper and a Consideration of Curvature," Journal of the Aeronautical Sciences, Vol. 24, No. 11, Nov. 1957, pp. 813-820.

3.3 Klein, B., "A Simple Method of Matric Structural Analysis: Part III - Analysis of Flexible Frames and Stiffened Cylindrical Shells," Journal of the Aeronautical Sciences, June 1958, Vol. 25, No. 6, pp. 385-394.

3.4 Klein, B., "A Simple Method of Matric Structural Analysis: Part V - Structures Containing Plate Elements of Arbitrary Shape and Thickness," Journal of the Aerospace Sciences, Vol. 27, No. 11, Nov. 1960, pp. 859-866.

3.5 Klein, B. and Chirico, M., "New Methods in Matric Structural Analysis," Proceedings of the Second Conference on Electronic Computation, ASCE, Structural Division, 1960, pp. 213-223.

3.6 Klein, B., "Application of a New Matrix Method to Vibration Analysis of Structures," Journal of the Aerospace Sciences, Vol. 29, March 1962, pp. 350-351.

3.7 Noor, A. K., "Nonlinear Analysis of Space Trusses," Journal of the Structural Division, ASCE, Vol. 100, No. ST3, March 1974, pp. 533-546.

3.8 Noor, A. K. and Peters, J. M., "Nonlinear Dynamic Analysis of Space Trusses," Computer Methods in Applied Mechanics and Engineering, Vol. 21, 1980, pp. 131-151.

Weighted Residual Approach

4.1 Chatterjee, A. and Setlur, A. V., "A Mixed Finite Element Formulation for Plate Problems," International Journal for Numerical Methods in Engineering, Vol. 4, No. 1, 1972, pp. 67-84.

4.2 Fix, G. J. and Gunzburger, M. D., "On Least Squares Approximations to Indefinite Problems of the Mixed Type," International Journal for Numerical Methods in Engineering, Vol. 12, 1978, pp. 453-469.

4.3 Fix, G. J., Gunzburger, M. D. and Nicolaides, R. A., "On Mixed Finite Element Methods II. The Least Squares Method," Computers and Mathematics with Applications, Vol. 5, 1979, pp. 87-98.

4.4 Rossow, M. P., "The Least-Square Variational Principle for Finite Element Applications," Journal of Applied Mechanics, Dec. 1975, pp. 900-901.

4.5 Salaam, U. and Sandhu, R. S., "A Finite Element Galerkin Formulation and Its Numerical Performance," International Journal for Numerical Methods in Engineering, Vol. 10, 1976, pp. 1077-1095.

4.6 Zienkiewicz, O. C. and Taylor, C., "Weighted Residual Processes in Finite Element Method with Particular Reference to Some Transient and Coupled Problems," Lectures on Finite Element Methods in Continuum Mechanics, ed. by J. T. Oden and E. R. A. Oliveira, University of Alabama Press, Huntsville, Alabama, 1973, pp. 415-458.

4.7 Zienkiewicz, O. C., Owen, D. R. J., and Lee, K. N., "Least-Square Finite Element for Elasto-Static Problems - Use of 'Reduced' Integration," International Journal for Numerical Methods in Engineering, Vol. 8, 1974, pp. 341-358.

Mathematical Aspects

5.1 Arnold, D. N., Babuska, I., and Osborn, J., "Finite Element Methods: Principles for Their Selection," Technical Note BN-997, Laboratory for Numerical Analysis, Institute for Physical Science and Technology, University of Maryland, Feb. 1983.

5.2 Babuska, I., "The Finite Element Method with Lagrangian Multipliers," Numerische Mathematik, Vol. 20, 1973, pp. 179-192.

5.3 Babuska, I., Oden, J. T., and Lee, J. K., "Mixed-Hybrid Finite Element Approximations of Second-Order Elliptic Boundary-Value Problems," Computer Methods in Applied Mechanics and Engineering, Vol. 11, 1977, pp. 175-206.

5.4 Bercouvier, M., "Perturbation of Mixed Variational Problems," R.A.I.R.O., Vol. 12, No. 3, 1978, pp. 211-236.

5.5 Bhandari, D. R. and Oden, J. T., "General Mixed Finite Element Methods of Nonlinear Continua," Zeitschrift fur Angewandte Mathematik und Mechanik, Vol. 53, 1973, pp. 441-451.

5.6 Brezzi, F., "On the Existence, Uniqueness and Approximation of Saddle-Point Problems Arising From Lagrangian Multipliers," R.A.I.R.O., R-2, 1974, pp. 129-151.

5.7 Brezzi, F., Johnson, C., and Mercier, B., "Analysis of a Mixed Finite Element Method for Elasto-Plastic Plates," Mathematics of Computations, Vol. 31, No. 140, 1977, pp. 809-817.

5.8 Brezzi, F. and Raviart, P. A., "Mixed Finite Element Methods for Fourth-Order Elliptic Equations," Topics in Numerical Analysis III, edited by J. J. H. Miller, Academic Press, London, 1977, pp. 33-56.

5.9 Ciarlet, P. G. and Raviart, P. A., "A Mixed Finite Element Method for the Biharmonic Equation," Mathematical Aspects of Finite Elements in Partial Differential Equations, ed. by C. de Boor, Academic Press, New York, 1974, pp. 125-145.

5.10 Fortin, M., "An Analysis of the Convergence of Mixed Finite Element Methods," R.A.I.R.O., Vol. 11, R-3, 1977, pp. 341-354.

5.11 Johnson, C., "On the Convergence of a Mixed Finite Element Method for Plate Bending Problems," Numerische Mathematik, Vol. 21, 1973, pp. 43-62.

5.12 Johnson, C. and Pitkäranta, J., "Analysis of Some Mixed Finite Element Methods Related to Reduced Integration," Mathematics of Computation, Vol. 38, No. 158, 1982, pp. 375-400.

5.13 Kikuchi, F., "Some Considerations of the Convergence of Hybrid Stress Method," 1973 Tokyo Seminar on Finite Element Analysis, Tokyo, Nov. 1973, in Theory and Practice in Finite Element Structural Analysis, ed. by Y. Yamada and R. H. Gallagher, University of Tokyo Press, 1973, pp. 25-42.

5.14 Kikuchi, F. and Ando, Y., "On the Convergence of a Mixed Finite Element Scheme for Plate Bending," Nuclear Engineering Design, Vol. 24, No. 3, 1973, pp. 357-373.

5.15 Mercier, B., "Numerical Solution of the Biharmonic Problem by Mixed Finite Element of Class C^o," Report Laboratorio di Analisi Numerical Del C.N.R., Pavia, 1973.

5.16 Mirza, F. A., "Convergence of Mixed Methods in Continuum Mechanics and Finite Element Analysis," Ph.D. Thesis, University of British Columbia, Canada, 1977.

5.17 Mignot, A. L. and Surry, C., "A Mixed Finite Element Family in Plane Elasticity," Applied Mathematical Modeling, Vol. 5, No. 4, 1982, pp. 259-262.

5.18 Miyoshi, I., "Finite Element Method of Mixed Type and Its Convergence in Linear Shell Problems," Kumamoto Journal of Science (Mathematics), Vol. 10, 1973, pp. 35-38.

5.19 Oden, J. T., "Generalized Conjugate Functions for Mixed Finite Element Approximations of Boundary-Value Problems," in The Mathematical Foundations of the Finite Element Method with Applications to Partial Differential Equations, ed. by A. K. Aziz, Academic Press, New York, 1972, pp. 629-669.

5.20 Oden, J. T. and Reddy, J. N., "Mixed Conjugate Finite Element Approximations of Linear Operators," Journal of Structural Mechanics, Vol. 1, No. 1, 1972, pp. 113-131.

5.21 Oden, J. T., "A Theory of Mixed Finite Element Approximations of Non-Self-Adjoint Boundary-Value Problems," Proceedings of the Seventh U.S. National Congress of Applied Mechanics, Boulder, Colorado, June 1974, pp. 19-51.

5.22 Oden, J. T., "Some Contributions to the Mathematical Theory of Mixed Finite Element Approximations," Theory and Practice in Finite Element Structural Analysis, ed. by Y. Yamada and R. H. Gallagher, Proceedings of the 1973 Tokyo Seminar on Finite Element Analysis, The University of Tokyo Press, 1974, pp. 3-23.

5.23 Oden, J. T., Goos, G., and Harminas, J., "Formulation and Application of Certain Primal and Mixed Finite Element Models of Finite Deformations of Elastic Bodies," Lecture Notes in Computer Science, Vol. 10, Computer Methods in Applied Science and Engineering, Part 1, Springer-Verlag, Berlin-Heidelberg, 1974, pp. 334-365.

5.24 Oden, J. T. and Reddy, J. N., "Some Observations on Properties of Certain Mixed Finite Element Approximations," International Journal for Numerical Methods in Engineering, Vol. 9, No. 4, 1975, pp. 933-938.

5.25 Oden, J. T. and Lee, J. K., "Theory of Mixed and Hybrid Finite Element Approximations in Linear Elasticity," Lecture Notes in Mathematics, Proceedings of the IUTAM/IUM Symposium on Applications of Methods of Functional Analysis to Problems of Mechanics, Marseille, France, Sept. 1975, Springer-Verlag, Berlin, Vol. 603, 1976, pp. 90-109.

5.26 Oden, J. T. and Reddy, J. N., "On Mixed Finite Element Approximations," SIAM Journal of Numerical Analysis, Vol. 13, No. 3, June 1976, pp. 393-404.

5.27 Oden, J. T., Kikuchi, N. and Song, Y. J., "Reduced Integration and Exterior Penalty Method for Finite Element Approximations of Contact Problems in Incompressible Elasticity," TICOM Report 80-2, Texas Institute for Computational Mechanics, The University of Texas, Austin, 1980.

5.28 Oden, J. T., Kikuchi, N., and Song, Y. J., "Penalty Finite Element Methods for the Analysis of Stokesian Flows," Computer Methods in Applied Mechanics and Engineering, Vol. 31, No. 3, Aug. 1982, pp. 297-329.

5.29 Reddy, J. N., "A Mathematical Theory of Complementary-Dual Variational Principles and Mixed Finite Element Approximations of Linear Boundary Value Problems in Continuum Mechanics," Ph.D. Dissertation, University of Alabama, Huntsville, 1973.

5.30 Reddy, J. N. and Oden, J. T., "Convergence of Mixed Finite Element Approximations of a Class of Linear Boundary-Value Problems," Journal of Structural Mechanics, Vol. 2, No. 2, 1973, pp. 83-108.

5.31 Reddy, J. N., "Some Mathematical Properties of Certain Mixed Galerkin Approximations in Nonlinear Elasticity," Proceedings of the International Conference on Computational Methods in Nonlinear Mechanics, University of Texas, Austin, Sept. 23-25, 1974, pp. 627-635.

5.32 Reddy, J. N. and Oden, J. T., "Mixed Finite Element Approximations of Linear Boundary Value Problems," Quarterly of Applied Mathematics, Vol. 33, No. 3, 1975, pp. 255-280.

5.33 Sheu, M. G., "On Theories and Applications of Mixed Finite Element Methods for Linear Boundary-Value Problems," Computers and Mathematics with Applications, Vol. 4, No. 4, 1978, pp. 333-347.

5.34 Talaslidis, D., "On the Convergence of a Mixed Finite Element Approximation for Cylindrical Shells," ZAMM, Vol. 59, 1979, pp. 431-436.

Applications of Mixed Models

6.1 Abbas, S. and Will, G. T., "A Mixed Finite Element Formulation for Shells Through a Reduced Reissner's Principle in Elastodynamics," Acta Mechanica, Vol. 37, 1980, pp. 75-85.

6.2 Akay, H. U., "An Investigation of First and Second-Order Mixed Plate Bending Elements," International Journal for Numerical Methods in Engineering, Vol. 15, 1980, pp. 351-360.

6.3 Allman, D. J., "Finite Element Analysis of Plate Buckling Using a Mixed Variational Principle," Proceedings of the Third Conference on Matrix Methods in Structural Mechanics, Wright Patterson Air Force Base, Ohio, October 1971, AFFDL-TR-71-160, pp. 683-702.

6.4 Altman, W. and Venancio-Filho, F., "Stability Analysis of Plates Using a Mixed Finite Element Formulation," Computers and Structures, Vol. 4, 1974, pp. 437-443.

6.5 Altman, W. and Iguti, F., "A Thin Cylindrical Shell Finite Element Based on a Mixed Formulation," Computers and Structures, Vol. 6, 1976, pp. 149-155.

6.6 Altman, W. and Bismarck-Nasr, M. N., "Vibration of Thin Cylindrical Shells Based on a Mixed Finite Element Formulation," Computers and Structures, Vol. 8, 1978, pp. 217-221.

6.7 Ando, Y., Yagawa, G., Kikuchi, F., Iida, K., and Kawai, T., "On the Application of Mixed Finite Element Methods to the Stress Concentration Problems of Cylindrical Shells with a Circular Cutout or a Crack," Bulletin of the Japan Society of Mechanical Engineers, Vol. 15, 1972, pp. 647-656.

6.8 Backlund, J., "Mixed Finite Element Analysis of Plates in Bending," Department of Structural Mechanics, Chalmers Institute of Technology, Goteborg, Publication 71:4, 1971.

6.9 Backlund, J., "Mixed Finite Element Analysis of Elasto-Plastic Plates in Bending," Archives of Mechanics, Vol. 24, No. 3, 1972, pp. 319-335.

6.10 Barony, S. Y. and Tottenham, H., "The Analysis of Rotational Shells Using a Curved Ring Element and the Mixed Variational Formulation," International Journal for Numerical Methods in Engineering, Vol. 10, 1976, pp. 861-872.

6.11 Bercovier, M., "Finite Elements for Incompressible or Nearly-Incompressible Materials," Proceedings of the ADINA Conference, Massachusetts Institute of Technology, Cambridge, MA, Aug. 1977, pp. 384-400.

6.12 Bercovier, M. and Engleman, M., "A Finite Element for the Numerical Solution of Viscous Incompressible Flows," Journal of Computational Physics, Vol. 30, Feb. 1979, pp. 181-201.

6.13 Biffle, J. H. and Key, S. W., "Finite Element Formulations for Transient Dynamic Problems in Solids Using Explicit Time Integration," Computer Methods in Applied Mechanics and Engineering, Vol. 12, Dec. 1977, pp. 323-336.

6.14 Bron, J. and Gurbachan, D., "Mixed Quadrilateral Elements for Bending," AIAA Journal, Vol. 10, No. 10, Oct. 1972, pp. 1359-1361.

6.15 Casciaro, R. and DiCarlo, A., "Mixed Finite Element Models in Limit Analysis," International Conference on Computational Methods in Nonlinear Mechanics, Austin, Texas, Sept. 1974, in Computational Methods in Nonlinear Mechanics, ed. by J. T. Oden, et al., The Texas Institute for Computational Mechanics, Austin, 1974, pp. 171-181.

6.16 Chan, A. S. L. and Trbojevic, V. M., "Thin Shell Finite Element by the Mixed Method Formulation - Part 1," Computer Methods in Applied Mechanics, Vol. 9, 1976, pp. 337-367.

6.17 Chan, A. S. L. and Trbojevic, V. M., "Thin Shell Finite Element by the Mixed Method Formulation - Parts 2 and 3," Computer Methods in Applied Mechanics and Engineering, Vol. 10, 1977, pp. 75-103.

6.18 Ciarlet, P. G. and Raviart, P. A., "A Mixed Finite Element Method for the Biharmonic Equation," Mathematical Aspects of Finite Elements in Partial Differential Equations, ed. by C. de Boor, Academic Press, New York, 1974, pp. 125-145.

6.19 Connor, J., "Mixed Models for Plates," in Finite Element Techniques in Structural Mechanics, ed. by H. Tottenham and C. Brebbia, Stress Analysis Publishers, Southampton, 1971, pp. 125-151.

6.20 Connor, J., "Mixed Models for Shells," in Finite Element Techniques in Structural Mechanics, ed. by H. Tottenham and C. Brebbia, Stress Analysis Publishers, Southampton, 1971, pp. 181-207.

6.21 Connor, J. J. and Will, G. T., "A Mixed Finite Element Shallow Shell Formulation," in Recent Advances in Matrix Methods of Structural Analysis and Design, ed. by R. H. Gallagher, Y. Yamada and J. T. Oden, University of Alabama Press, Huntsville, 1971, pp. 105-137.

6.22 Cook, R. D., "Eigenvalue Problems with a 'Mixed' Plate Element," AIAA Journal, Vol. 7, No. 5, May 1969, pp. 982-983.

6.23 Dunham, R. S. and Pister, K. S., "A Finite Element Application of the Hellinger-Reissner Variational Theorem," Proceedings of the Second Conference on Matrix Methods in Structural Mechanics, Wright Patterson Air Force Base, Ohio, Oct. 1968, AFFDL-TR-68-150, pp. 471-487.

6.24 Eatock-Taylor, W. R., "Discrete Element Analysis of Shells," Ph.D. Thesis, Stanford University, California, August 1968.

6.25 Elias, Z. M., "Mixed Finite Element Method for Axisymmetric Shells," International Journal for Numerical Methods in Engineering, Vol. 4, No. 2, 1972, pp. 261-278.

6.26 Fix, G. J., Gunzburger, M. D., and Nicolaides, R. A., "On Mixed Finite Element Methods for First-Order Elliptic Systems," Numerische Mathematik, Vol. 37, 1981, pp. 29-48.

6.27 Fletcher, C. A. J., "A Primitive Variable Finite Element Formulation for Inviscid Compressible Flow," Journal of Computational Physics, Vol. 33, 1979, pp. 301-312.

6.28 Gass, N. and Tabarrok, B., "Large Deformation Analysis of Plates and Cylindrical Shells by a Mixed Finite Element Method," International Journal for Numerical Methods in Engineering, Vol. 10, 1976, pp. 731-746.

6.29 Gellert, M. and Laursen, M. E., "Formulation and Convergence of a Mixed Finite Element Method Applied to Elastic Arches of Arbitrary Geometry and Loading," Computer Methods in Applied Mechanics and Engineering, Vol. 7, 1976, pp. 285-302.

6.30 Glowinski, R. and Pironneau, O., "On a Mixed Finite Element Approximation of the Stokes Problem (I)," Numerische Mathematik, Vol. 33, 1979, pp. 397-424.

6.31 Gould, P. L. and Sen, S. K., "Refined Mixed Method Finite Elements for Shells of Revolution," Proceedings of the Third Conference on Matrix Methods in Structural Mechanics, Wright Patterson Air Force Base, Ohio, Oct. 1971, AFFDL-TR-71-160, pp. 397-421.

6.32 Gould, P. L., "Condensation for Mixed Dynamic Finite Element Analysis of Rotational Shells," Computers and Structures, Vol. 10, 1979, pp. 251-253.

6.33 Harbord, R., Kröplin, and Schröder, R., "Schalenelemente in gemischer Darstellung: Theorie-Kritik-Beispiele," Ingenieur-Archiv, Vol. 47, 1978, pp. 207-222.

6.34 Herrmann, L. R., "A Bending Analysis of Plates," Proceedings of the Conference on Matrix Methods in Structural Mechanics, AFFDL-TR-66-80, 1966, pp. 577-604.

6.35 Herrmann, L. R., "Finite Element Bending Analysis for Plates," Journal of the Engineering Mechanics Division, ASCE, Vol. 93, No. EM5, Oct. 1967, pp. 13-26.

6.36 Herrmann, L. R. and Mason, W. E., "Mixed Formulations for Finite Element Shell Analysis," Conference on Computer-Oriented Analysis of Shell Structures, Report No. AFFDL-TR-71-79, June 1971, pp. 290-336.

6.37 Hutton, S. G., Exeter, M. K., Fussey, D. E., Webster, J. J., and Rigon, C., "Primitive Variable Finite Element Formulations for Steady Viscous Flows," International Journal for Numerical Methods in Engineering, Vol. 15, 1980, pp. 209-223.

6.38 Huyakorn, P. A., Taylor, C., Lee, R. L., and Gresho, P. M., "A Comparison of Various Mixed Interpolation Finite Elements in the Velocity-Pressure Formulation of the Navier-Stokes Equations," Computers and Fluids, Vol. 6, 1978, pp. 25-35.

6.39 Jackson, C. P. and Cliffe, K. A., "Mixed Interpolation in Primitive Variable Finite Element Formulations for Incompressible Flow," International Journal for Numerical Methods in Engineering, Vol. 17, 1981, pp. 1659-1688.

6.40 Johnson, C., "A Mixed Finite Element Method for Navier-Stokes Equations," Research Report 77-IAR, Department of Computer Science, Chalmers Institute of Technology, 1977.

6.41 Johnson, C., "A Mixed Finite Element Method for Plasticity with Hardening," SIAM Journal for Numerical Analysis, Vol. 14, 1977, pp. 575-584.

6.42 Kikuchi, F. and Ando, Y., "Rectangular Finite Element for Plate Bending Analysis Based on Hellinger-Reissner's Variational Principle," Journal of Nuclear Science and Technology, Vol. 9, No. 1, 1972, pp. 28-35.

6.43 Lee, S. W. and Pian, T. H. H., "Improvement of Plate and Shell Finite Element by Mixed Formulations," AIAA Journal, Vol. 16, No. 1, 1978, pp. 29-34.

6.44 LeTallec, P., "A Mixed Finite Element Approximation of the Navier-Stokes Equations," Numerische Mathematik, Vol. 35, 1980, pp. 381-404.

6.45 Lightner, J. G., "A Mixed Finite Element Procedure for Soil-Structure Interaction Including Construction Sequences," Ph.D. Dissertation, Virginia Polytechnic Institute and State University, Blacksburg, 1981.

6.46 Meissner, U., "A Mixed Finite Element Model for Use in Potential Flow Problems," International Journal for Numerical Methods in Engineering, Vol. 6, No. 4, 1973, pp. 467-473.

6.47 Miyoshi, T., "A Mixed Finite Element Method for the Solution of the von Karman Equations," Numerische Mathematik, Vol. 26, 1976, pp. 255-269.

6.48 Mirza, F. A. and Olsen, M. D., "The Mixed Finite Element Method in Plane Elasticity," International Journal for Numerical Methods in Engineering, Vol. 15, 1980, pp. 273-289.

6.49 Morand, H. and Ohayon, R., "Variational Formulations of the Hydrocapillary Vibration Problems," in Colloque International sur la Stabilisation des Vehicules Spatiaux et les Problemes, Technologiques et Dynamiques Poses par les Liquides, European Space Agency and Centre National d'Etudes Spatiales, Toulouse, France, Oct. 10-12, 1977, pp. 105-119 (French).

6.50 Nemat-Nasser, S., "General Variational Methods for Waves in Elastic Composites," Journal of Elasticity, Vol. 2, No. 2, June 1972, pp. 73-90.

6.51 Newsom, C. D., "Finite Element Formulation of Mixed and Stress Variational Principles for Structural Dynamic Analysis," Ph.D. Thesis, The University of Texas at Austin, 1972.

6.52 Noor, A. K. and Andersen, C. M., "Mixed Isoparametric Elements for Saint-Venant Torsion," Computer Methods in Applied Mechanics and Engineering, Vol. 6, No. 2, 1975, pp. 195-218.

6.53 Noor, A. K. and Andersen, C. M., "Mixed Isoparametric Finite Element Models of Laminated Composite Shells," Computer Methods in Applied Mechanics and Engineering, Vol. 11, 1977, pp. 255-280.

6.54 Noor, A. K., Greene, W. H., and Hartley, S. J., "Nonlinear Finite Element Analysis of Curved Beams," Computer Methods in Applied Mechanics and Engineering, Vol. 12, 1977, pp. 289-307.

6.55 Noor, A. K. and Hartley, S. J., "Nonlinear Shell Analysis Via Mixed Isoparametric Elements," Computers and Structures, Vol. 7, 1977, pp. 615-626.

6.56 Noor, A. K. and Knight, N. F., Jr., "Nonlinear Dynamic Analysis of Curved Beams," Computer Methods in Applied Mechanics and Engineering, Vol. 23, 1980, pp. 225-251.

6.57 Olson, M. D. and Mirza, F. A., "A Mixed Finite Element Method for Calculation of Stress Intensity Factors," Numerical Methods in Fracture Mechanics, ed. by A. R. Luxmore and D. R. J. Owen, University College of Swansea, 1978, pp. 798-803.

6.58 Olson, M. D., "The Mixed Finite Element Method in Elasticity and Elastic Contact Problems," Hybrid and Mixed Finite Element Methods, ed. by S. N. Atluri, R. H. Gallagher and O. C. Zienkiewicz, John Wiley and Sons, 1983, pp. 19-49.

6.59 Poceski, A., "A Mixed Finite Element Method for Bending of Plates," International Journal for Numerical Methods in Engineering, Vol. 9, No. 1, 1975, pp. 3-15.

6.60 Prato, C. A., "A Mixed Finite Element for Thin Shell Analysis," Sc.D. Dissertation, Massachusetts Institute of Technology, Cambridge, MA, 1968.

6.61 Prato, C. A., "Shell Finite Element Method Via Reissner's Principle," International Journal of Solids and Structures, Vol. 5, No. 10, 1969, pp. 1119-1133.

6.62 Reddy, J. N. and Stricklin, J. D., "Large Deflection and Large Amplitude Free Vibrations of Thin Rectangular Plates Using Mixed Isoparametric Elements," Proceedings of the Symposium on Applications of Computer Methods in Engineering, Los Angeles, CA, Aug. 23-26, 1977, Vol. 2, University of Southern California, Los Angeles, 1978, pp. 1323-1335.

6.63 Sander, G. and Carnoy, E., "Equilibrium and Mixed Formulations in Stability Analysis Plate Bending Finite Element Derivation Using Variational Principle," Proceedings of the International Conference on Finite Elements in Nonlinear Solid and Structural Mechanics, Aug. 29-Sept. 1, 1977, Geilo, Norway, Vol. 1, pp. 87-108.

6.64 Scharnhorst, T. and Pian, T. H. H., "Finite Element Analysis of Rubber-Like Materials by a Mixed Model," International Journal for Numerical Methods in Engineering, Vol. 12, 1978, pp. 665-676.

6.65 Schmid, G., "Finite Element Approximation to Rotational Flow with Internal Sources," Proceedings of the Conference on Numerical Methods in Fluid Mechanics, Koln, Germany, Oct. 8-10, 1975, pp. 189-196.

6.66 Simo, J. C., Taylor, R. L., and Slater, J. H., "Mixed Finite Element Approximations for Nonlinear Plates," Computer Methods for Nonlinear Solids and Structural Mechanics, ed. by S. N. Atluri and N. Perrone, AMD Vol. 54, American Society of Mechanical Engineers, 1983, pp. 227-237.

6.67 Slater, J. M. and Taylor, R. L., "Mixed Model Finite Element Analysis of Inelastic Plane Frames," Report CE299, Department of Civil Engineering, University of California, Berkeley, 1980.

6.68 Sodhi, D. S., "Mixed Finite Element Method for Vibration Analysis of Shallow Shells," Proceedings of the Fourth Canadian Congress of Applied Mechanics, Montreal, May 28-June 1, 1973, pp. 527-528.

6.69 Tahiani, C., "Analysis of Geometrically Nonlinear Thin Shells by Mixed Elements," D.Sc. Thesis, Laval University, Quebec, Canada, Aug. 1971 (in French).

6.70 Tahiani, C. and Lachance, L., "Linear and Nonlinear Analysis of Thin Shallow Shells by Mixed Finite Elements," Computers and Structures, Vol. 5, 1975, pp. 167-177.

6.71 Talaslidis, D. and Wunderlich, W., "Static and Dynamic Analysis of Kirchhoff Shells Based on Mixed Finite Element Formulation," Computers and Structures, Vol. 10, No. 1/2, 1979, pp. 239-249.

6.72 Taylor, C. and Hood, P., "A Numerical Solution of the Navier-Stokes Equations Using the Finite Element Technique," Computers and Fluids, Vol. 1, No. 1, 1973, pp. 73-100.

6.73 Tottenham, H., Barony, S. Y., "Mixed Finite Element Formulation for Geometrically Nonlinear Analysis of Shells of Revolution," International Journal for Numerical Methods in Engineering, Vol. 12, 1978, pp. 195-201.

6.74 Tseng, J. and Olson, M. D., "The Mixed Finite Element Method Applied to Two-Dimensional Elastic Contact Problems," International Journal for Numerical Methods in Engineering, Vol. 17, No. 7, July 1981, pp. 991-1014.

6.75 Visser, W., "A Refined Mixed-Type Plate Bending Element," AIAA Journal, Vol. 7, No. 9, Sept. 1969, pp. 1801-1803.

6.76 Visser, W., "The Application of a Curved Mixed-Type Shell Element," IUTAM Symposium, Liege, Belgium, Aug. 1970, in High Speed Computing of Elastic Structures, ed. by Fraeijs B. de Veubeke, University of Liege, 1971, pp. 321-356.

6.77 Wellford, I. C., Jr. and Hafez, M. M., "Mixed Finite Element Models and Dual Iterative Methods for Transonic Flow," Second International Symposium on Finite Element Methods in Flow Problems, Santa Margherita Ligure, Italy, June 14-18, 1976.

6.78 Yamada, Y., Ito, K., Yokouchi, Y., Tamano, T., and Ohtsubo, T., "Finite Element Analysis of Steady Fluid and Metal Flow," Finite Elements in Fluids, ed. by R. H. Gallagher, J. T. Oden, C. Taylor, and O. C. Zienkiewicz, Vol. 1, John Wiley and Sons, 1975, pp. 73-94.

Application of Hybrid and Hybrid-Mixed Models

7.1 Ahmad, S. and Irons, B. M., "An Assumed Stress Approach to Refined Isoparametric Finite Elements in Three Dimensions," Proceedings of the 1974 International Conference on Finite Element Methods in Engineering, University of New South Wales, Australia, Aug. 28-30, 1974, pp. 85-100.

7.2 Ali, R., Gopalacharyulu, S., and Sharman, P. W., "The Development of a Series of Hybrid Stress Finite Elements," World Congress on Finite Element Methods in Structural Mechanics, Vol. 2, ed. by J. Robinson, Robinson and Associates, Verwood, Dorset, England, 1975, pp. 13.1-13.27.

7.3 Appa Rao, T. V. S. R., "An Assumed Stress Hybrid Finite Element Model for the Analysis of An Axisymmetric Thick Walled Pressure Vessel," Proceedings of the First International Conference on Structural Mechanics in Reactor Technology, Vol. 6, Part M, Berlin, 1971, pp. 315-335.

7.4 Atluri, S. N. and Pian, T. H. H., "Theoretical Formulation of Finite Element Methods in Linear Elastic Analysis of General Shells," Journal of Structural Mechanics, Vol. 1, No. 1, 1972, pp. 1-41.

7.5 Atluri, S. N., "On the Hybrid Stress Finite Element Model for Incremental Analysis of Large Deflection Problems," International Journal of Solids and Structures, Vol. 9, No. 10, 1973, pp. 1177-1191.

7.6 Atluri, S. N., "On the Hybrid Stress Finite Element Model in Linear Elastodynamic Analysis," AIAA Journal, Vol. 11, 1973, pp. 1028-1031.

7.7 Atluri, S. N. and Pian, T. H. H., "Finite Element Analysis of Shells of Revolution by Two Doubly-Curved Quadrilateral Elements," Journal of Structural Mechanics, Vol. 1, No. 3, 1973, pp. 393-416.

7.8 Atluri, S. N., Kobayashi, A. S., and Nakagaki, M., "Application of an Assumed Displacement Hybrid Finite Element Procedure to Two-Dimensional Problems in Fracture Mechanics," AIAA/ASME/SAE Fifteenth Structures, Structural Dynamics and Materials Conference, April 17-19, 1974, Las Vegas, Nevada, AIAA Paper No. 74-390.

7.9 Atluri, S. N., "Hybrid Finite Element Models in Solid Mechanics - Linear Theory," Advances in Computer Methods for Partial Differential Equations, ed. by R. Visnevetsky, AICA, Rutgers University Press, 1975, pp. 351-362.

7.10 Atluri, S. N., "On Hybrid Finite Element Models in Solid Mechanics," Advances in Computer Methods for Partial Differential Equations, ed. by R. Visnevetsky, AICA, Rutgers University Press, 1975, pp. 346-356.

7.11 Atluri, S. N. and Kathiresan, K., "An Assumed Displacement Hybrid Finite Element Model for Three-Dimensional Linear-Fracture Mechanics Analysis," Proceedings of the Twelfth Annual Meeting of the Society of Engineering Science, Austin, Texas, Oct. 1975, pp. 391-403.

7.12 Atluri, S. N., Kathiresan, K., and Kobayashi, A. S., "Three-Dimensional Linear Fracture Mechanics Analysis by a Displacement-Hybrid Finite Element Model," Transactions of the Third International Conference on Structural Mechanics in Reactor Technology, London, Sept. 1-5, 1975, Paper L 7/3.

7.13 Atluri, S. N., Kobayashi, A. S., and Cheng, J. S., "Brain Tissue Fragility - A Finite Strain Analysis by a Hybrid Finite Element Method," Journal of Applied Mechanics, ASME, Vol. 42, No. 2, 1975, pp. 269-273.

7.14 Atluri, S. N., Kobayashi, A. S., and Nakagaki, M., "A Finite Element Program for Fracture Mechanics Analysis of Composite Material," Fracture Mechanics of Composites, ASTM STP-593, American Society for Testing and Materials, 1975, pp. 86-98.

7.15 Atluri, S. N., Kobayashi, A. S., and Nakagaki, M., "An Assumed Displacement Hybrid Finite Element Model for Linear Fracture Mechanics," International Journal of Fracture, Vol. 11, No. 2, 1975, pp. 257-271.

7.16 Atluri, S. N., Kobayashi, A. S., and Nakagaki, M., "Fracture Mechanics Application of An Assumed Displacement Hybrid Finite Element Procedure," AIAA Journal, Vol. 13, No. 6, 1975, pp. 734-739.

7.17 Atluri, S. N. and Kathiresan, K., "On A Three-Dimensional Singularity Element for Computation of Combined Mode Stress Intensities," Advances in Engineering Science, Vol. 1, NASA CP-2001, Nov. 1976, pp. 267-275.

7.18 Atluri, S. N. and Nakagaki, M., "Post-Yield Analysis of a Three-Point Bend Fracture Test Specimen: An Embedded Singularity Finite Element Incremental Method," Proceedings of the Eighth Southeastern Conference on Theoretical and Applied Mechanics, April 29-30, 1976, Virginia Polytechnic Institute and State University, Blacksburg, Virginia.

7.19 Atluri, S. N., Kathiresan, K., Kobayashi, A. S., and Nakagaki, M., "Inner Surface Cracks in an Internally Pressurized Cylinder Analyzed by a Three-Dimensional Displacement Hybrid Finite Element Method," Pressure Vessel Technology, Part II, Materials and Fabrication (Third International Conference, Tokyo, Japan), American Society of Mechanical Engineers, New York, April 1977, pp. 527-533.

7.20 Atluri, S. N. and Nakagaki, M., "J-Integral Estimates for Strain-Hardening Materials in Ductile Fracture Problems," AIAA Journal, Vol. 15, No. 7, July 1977, pp. 923-931.

7.21 Atluri, S. N. and Murakawa, H., "On Hybrid Finite Element Models in Nonlinear Solid Mechanics," Finite Elements in Nonlinear Mechanics, ed. by P. G. Bergan, et al., Vol. 1, TAPIR, Trondheim, Norway, 1978, pp. 3-41.

7.22 Atluri, S. N., Nakagaki, M., Kathiresan, K., Rhee, H. C., and Chen, W. H., "Hybrid Finite Element Models for Linear and Nonlinear Fracture Analysis," Numerical Methods in Fracture Mechanics, ed. by A. R. Luxmoore, et al., Swansea, Wales, 1978, pp. 52-67.

7.23 Atluri, S. N., Nakagaki, M., and Kathiresan, K., "Hybrid Finite Element Analysis of Some Nonlinear and Three-Dimensional Problems of Engineering Fracture Mechanics," Computers and Structures, Vol. 12, 1980, pp. 511-520.

7.24 Boland, P. L., "Large Deflection Analysis of Thin Elastic Structures by the Assumed Stress Hybrid Finite Element Method," Department of Aeronautics and Astronautics, Massachusetts Institute of Technology, Ph.D. Thesis, October 1975.

7.25 Boland, P. L. and Pian, T. H. H., "Large Deflection Analysis of Thin Elastic Structures by the Assumed Stress Hybrid Finite Element Method," Computers and Structures, Vol. 7, Feb. 1977, pp. 1-12.

7.26 Brandt, K., "Calculation of Vibration Frequencies by a Hybrid Element Method Based on a Generalized Complementary Energy Principle," International Journal for Numerical Methods in Engineering, Vol. 11, 1977, pp. 231-246.

7.27 Bratiana, C. and Atluri, S. N., "A Stress-Hybrid Finite Element Method for Stokes' Flows," Letters in Heat and Mass Transfer, Vol. 7, 1980, pp. 227-233.

7.28 Bratiana, C. and Atluri, S. N., "A Hybrid Finite Element Method for Stokes Flows: Part I - Formulation and Numerical Studies," Computer Methods in Applied Mechanics and Engineering, Vol. 36, 1983, pp. 23-37.

7.29 Cheng, J. S., Atluri, S. N., and Kobayashi, A. S., "Assumed Displacement Hybrid Finite Element Method for Nonlinear Elastic and Elastic-Plastic Analyses," Eighteenth Structures, Structural Dynamics and Materials Conference, March 21-23, 1977; and Aircraft Composites: The Emerging Methodology for Structural Assurance, San Diego, California, March 24-25, 1977, Technical Papers, Vol. A, AIAA, pp. 279-289.

7.30 Cook, R. D. and Al-Abdulla, J. K., "Some Plane Quadrilateral Hybrid Finite Elements," AIAA Journal, Vol. 7, 1969, pp. 2184-2185.

7.31 Cook, R. D., "Two Hybrid Elements for the Analysis of Thick, Thin and Sandwich Plates," International Journal for Numerical Methods in Engineering, Vol. 5, No. 2, 1972, pp. 277-288.

7.32 Deak, A. L. and Atluri, S. N., "Nonlinear Hybrid Stress Finite Element Analysis of Laminated Shells," Computational Methods in Nonlinear Mechanics, ed. by J. T. Oden, et al., The Texas Institute for Computational Mechanics, Austin, 1974, pp. 79-88.

7.33 Edwards, G. and Webster, J. J., "Hybrid Cylindrical Shell Finite Elements," Finite Elements for Thin Shells and Curved Members, ed. by D. Ashwell and R. Gallagher, Wiley Interscience, 1976, pp. 171-195.

7.34 Harvey, J. W. and Kelsey, "Triangular Plate Bending Elements with Enforced Compatibility," AIAA Journal, Vol. 9, No. 6, June 1971, pp. 1023-1026.

7.35 Henshell, R. D., Neale, B. K., and Warburton, G. B., "A New Hybrid Cylindrical Shell Finite Element," Journal of Sound and Vibration, Vol. 16, No. 4, 1971, pp. 519-531.

7.36 Henshell, R. D., Neale, B. K., and Warburton, G. B., "On Hybrid Cylindrical Shell Elements," Journal of Sound and Vibration, Vol. 21, No. 3, 1972, pp. 373-378.

7.37 Henshell, R. D., "A Theoretical Basis for Hybrid Finite Elements in Dynamic Problems," Journal of Sound and Vibration, Vol. 39, No. 4, 1975, pp. 520-522.

7.38 Horrigmoe, G., "Large Displacement Analysis of Shells by a Hybrid Stress Finite Element Method," IASS World Congress on Space Enclosures, Montreal, July 1976.

7.39 Kikuchi, F. and Ando, Y., "Finite Element Analysis of Vibration of Thin Elastic Plates by Simplified Hybrid Displacement Method," Journal of Nuclear Science and Technology, Vol. 9, No. 3, 1972, pp. 189-190.

7.40 Kikuchi, F. and Ando, Y., "Simplified Hybrid Displacement Method Applied to Plate Buckling Problems," Journal of Nuclear Science and Technology, Vol. 9, No. 8, 1972, pp. 497-499.

7.41 Kikuchi, F. and Ando, Y., "Some Finite Element Solutions for Plate Bending Problems by Simplified Hybrid Displacement Method," Nuclear Engineering and Design, Vol. 23, 1972, pp. 155-178.

7.42 Kikuchi, F. and Ando, Y., "A New Variational Functional for the Finite Element Method and Its Application to Plate and Shell Problems," Nuclear Engineering and Design, Vol. 21, 1972, pp. 95-113.

7.43 Kikuchi, F. and Ando, Y., "Application of Simplified Hybrid Displacement Method to Large Deflection Analysis of Elastic-Plastic Plates and Shells," Journal of the Faculty of Engineering, University of Tokyo (B), Vol. 32, No. 1, 1973, pp. 117-135.

7.44 Kikuchi, F. and Ando, Y., "Application of Simplified Hybrid Displacement Method to Plate and Shell Problems," International Conference on Structural Mechanics in Reactor Technology, Berlin, Sept. 1973, Paper No. M5/5.

7.45 Kikuchi, F. and Ando, Y., "Simplified Hybrid Displacement Method for Linear Finite Element Analysis of General Shells," International Journal for Pressure Vessels and Piping, Vol. 2, No. 2, 1974, pp. 155-164.

7.46 Lee, S. W., "An Assumed Stress Hybrid Finite Element for Three-Dimensional Elastic Structural Analysis," Massachusetts Institute of Technology, ASRL-TR-170-3 (AFOSR-TR-75-0087), May 1974.

7.47 Mang, H. A., "Derivation of General Algebraic Constraint Conditions for 'Weak' C^1 Continuity for Thin Shells," International Journal for Numerical Methods in Engineering, Vol. 11, 1977, pp. 1593-1604.

7.48 Mang, H. A. and Gallagher, R. H., "A Critical Assessment of the Simplified Hybrid Displacement Method," International Journal for Numerical Methods in Engineering, Vol. 11, No. 2, 1977, pp. 145-167.

7.49 Mau, S. T. and Witmer, E. A., "Static Vibration and Thermal Stress Analysis of Laminated Plates and Shells by the Hybrid Stress Finite Element Method with Transverse Shear Deformation Effects Included," Massachusetts Institute of Technology, ASRL-TR-169-2, Oct. 1972.

7.50 Mau, S. T., Pian, T. H. H., and Tong, P., "Vibration Analysis of Laminated Plates and Shells By a Hybrid Stress Element," AIAA Journal, Vol. 11, No. 10, 1973, pp. 1450-1452.

7.51 Murakawa, H. and Atluri, S. N., "Finite Elasticity Solutions Using Hybrid Finite Elements Based on a Complementary Energy Principle," Journal of Applied Mechanics, ASME, Vol. 45, No. 3, 1978, pp. 539-547.

7.52 Murakawa, H. and Atluri, S. N., "Finite Elasticity Solutions Using Hybrid Finite Elements Based on a Complementary Energy Principle, Part 2: Incompressible Materials," Journal of Applied Mechanics, ASME, Vol. 46, March 1979, pp. 71-77.

7.53 Neale, B. K., Henshell, R. D., and Edwards, G., "Hybrid Plate Bending Elements," Journal of Sound and Vibration, Vol. 23, No. 1, 1972, pp. 101-112.

7.54 Nishioka, T. and Atluri, S. N., "An Efficient 'Assumed-Stress' Finite Element Procedure for the Analysis of Multilayer Anisotropic Laminates," Fifteenth Society of Engineering Science Meeting, University of Florida, Dec. 4-6, 1978.

7.55 Oden, J. T. and Lee, J. K., "Mixed-Hybrid Methods for the Analysis of Potential Flow," Second International Symposium on Finite Element Methods in Flow Problems, Santa Margherita Ligure, Italy, June 14-18, 1976.

7.56 Orringer, O. and Stalk, G., "A Hybrid Finite Element for Stress Analysis of Fastener Details," Journal of Engineering Fracture Mechanics, Vol. 523, 1976, pp. 1-11.

7.57 Pian, T. H. H., "Derivation of Element Stiffness Matrices by Assumed Stress Distributions," AIAA Journal, Vol. 2, 1964, pp. 1333-1336.

7.58 Pian, T. H. H., "Element Stiffness Matrices for Boundary Compatibility and for Prescribed Boundary Stresses," Proceedings of the Conference on Matrix Methods in Structural Mechanics, AFFDL-TR-66-80, 1965, pp. 457-477.

7.59 Pian, T. H. H. and Tong, P., "Rationalization in Deriving Element Stiffness Matrix by Assumed Stress Approach," Proceedings of the Second Conference on Matrix Methods in Structural Mechanics, AFFDL-TR-68-150, 1968, pp. 441-469.

7.60 Pian, T. H. H., "Hybrid Models," Numerical and Computer Methods in Structural Mechanics, ed. by S. J. Fenves, et al., Academic Press, 1973, pp. 59-78.

7.61 Pian, T. H. H., "Nonlinear Creep Analysis by Assumed Stress Finite Element Methods," AIAA Journal, Vol. 12, 1974, pp. 1756-1758.

7.62 Pian, T. H. H., Spilker, R. L., and Lee, S. W., "Elastic-Plastic and Creep Analysis by Assumed Stress Finite Elements," Transactions of the Third International Conference on Structural Mechanics in Reactor Technology, London, Vol. 5, Part M, Paper M 2/1, Sept. 1-5, 1974.

7.63 Pian, T. H. H., Tong, P., Luk, C. H., and Spilker, R. L., "Elasto-Plastic Analysis by Assumed Stress Hybrid Model," Proceedings of the 1974 International Conference on Finite Element Methods in Engineering, University of New South Wales, Australia, Aug. 28-30, 1974, pp. 419-434.

7.64 Rhee, H. C., Atluri, S. N., Moriya, K., and Pian, T. H. H., "Hybrid Finite Element Procedure for Analyzing Through Flaws in Plates in Bending," Fourth International Conference on Structural Mechanics in Reactor Technology, San Francisco, 1977.

7.65 Sagrand, S. M., "A Hybrid Finite Element Procedure for Soil-Structure Interaction Including Construction Sequences," Ph.D. Dissertation, Virginia Polytechnic Institute and State University, Blacksburg, 1981.

7.66 Spilker, R. L., "A Study of Elastic-Plastic Analysis by the Assumed Stress Hybrid Finite Element Model with Application to Thick Shell of Revolution," Massachusetts Institute of Technology, ASRL-TR-175-1. Also, Sc.D. Thesis, Department of Aeronautics and Astronautics, Dec. 1974.

7.67 Spilker, R. L., Chou, S. C., and Orringer, O., "Alternate Hybrid-Stress Elements for Analysis of Multilayer Composite Plates," Journal of Composite Materials, Vol. 11, 1977, pp. 51-70.

7.68 Spilker, R. L. and Munir, N. I., "A Serendipity Cubic Displacement Hybrid Stress Element for Thin and Moderately Thick Plates," International Journal for Numerical Methods in Engineering, Vol. 15, 1980, pp. 1261-1278.

7.69 Spilker, R. L., "Invariant Hybrid-Stress Elements for Thin and Moderately-Thick Plates," New Concepts in Finite Element Methods, ASME AMD Vol. 44, 1981, pp. 225-246.

7.70 Spilker, R. L., "High-Order Three-Dimensional Hybrid Stress Elements for Thick-Plate Analysis," International Journal for Numerical Methods in Engineering, Vol. 17, 1981, pp. 53-69.

7.71 Spilker, R. L., "Improved Hybrid-Stress Axisymmetric Elements Including Behavior for Nearly-Incompressible Materials," International Journal for Numerical Methods in Engineering, Vol. 17, 1981, pp. 483-501.

7.72 Spilker, R. L., Maskeri, S. M., and Kania, E., "Plane Isoparametric Hybrid-Stress Elements: Invariance and Optimal Sampling," International Journal for Numerical Methods in Engineering, Vol. 17, No. 10, Oct. 1981, pp. 1469-1496.

7.73 Spilker, R. L. and Singh, S. P., "Three-Dimensional Hybrid-Stress Isoparametric Quadratic Displacement Elements," International Journal for Numerical Methods in Engineering, Vol. 18, No. 3, March 1982, pp. 445-465.

7.74 Sung, W. L., "An Assumed Stress Hybrid Finite Element for Three-Dimensional Elastic Structural Analysis," Report No. ASRL-TR-170-3, Department of Aeronautics and Astronautics, Massachusetts Institute of Technology, Cambridge, MA, 1974.

7.75 Spilker, R. L. and Pian, T. H. H., "A Study of Axisymmetric Solid of Revolution Elements Based on Assumed-Stress Hybrid Model," Computers and Structures, Vol. 9, 1978, pp. 273-279.

7.76 Spilker, R. L. and Daugirda, D. M., "Analysis of Axisymmetric Structures Under Arbitrary Loading Using the Hybrid Stress Model," International Journal for Numerical Methods in Engineering, Vol. 17, 1981, pp. 801-828.

7.77 Tabarrok, B. and Hoa, V. S., "Thermal Stress Analysis of Plates and Shallow Shells by Hybrid Finite Element Method," Journal of Strain Analysis, Vol. 9, No. 3, 1974, pp. 152-158.

7.78 Tong, P., "An Assumed Stress Hybrid Finite Element Method for an Incompressible and Nearly-Incompressible Material," International Journal of Solids and Structures, Vol. 5, No. 5, 1969, pp. 455-461.

7.79 Tong, P., "New Displacement Hybrid Finite Element Models for Solid Continua," International Journal for Numerical Methods in Engineering, Vol. 2, No. 1, 1970, pp. 73-83.

7.80 Tong, P., Pian, T. H. H., and Lasry, S. J., "A Hybrid Element Approach to Crack Problems in Plane Elasticity," International Journal for Numerical Methods in Engineering, Vol. 7, No. 3, 1973, pp. 297-308.

7.81 Tong, P., Pian, T. H. H., and Orringer, O., "Fracture Mechanics Analysis with Hybrid 'Crack' Finite Elements," Case Studies in Fracture Mechanics, AMMRC MS77-5, Army Materials and Mechanics Research Center, 1977, pp. 2.4.1-2.4.16.

7.82 Tong, P. and Atluri, S. N., "On Hybrid Finite Element Technique for Crack Analysis," Proceedings of the International Conference on Fracture Mechanics and Technology, Hong Kong, March 21-25, 1977, Vol. 2, Alphen aan den Rijn, Netherlands, Sigthoff and Nordhoff International Publishers, 1977, pp. 1445-1466.

7.83 Weißgerber, V., "Hybride Schalenelemente mit einer Anwendung auf Wendelschalen," Ingenieur-Archiv, Vol. 44, No. 2, 1975, pp. 103-112.

7.84 Wolf, J. P., "Structural Averaging of Stresses in the Hybrid Stress Model," AIAA Journal, Vol. 10, No. 6, 1972, pp. 843-845.

7.85 Wolf, J. P., "Generalized Hybrid Stress Finite Element Models," AIAA Journal, Vol. 11, No. 3, 1973, pp. 386-388.

7.86 Wolf, J. P., "Alternate Hybrid Stress Finite Element Models," International Journal for Numerical Methods in Engineering, Vol. 9, No. 3, 1975, pp. 601-615.

7.87 Yamada, Y., Nakagiri, S., and Takatsuka, K., "Analysis of Saint-Venant Torsion Problem by a Hybrid Stress Model," Monthly Journal of the Institute of Industrial Science, University of Tokyo, Vol. 21, No. 11, 1969.

7.88 Yamada, Y., Nakagiri, S., and Takatsuka, K., "Elastic Plastic Analysis of Saint-Venant Torsion Problem by a Hybrid Stress Model," International Journal for Numerical Methods in Engineering, Vol. 5, No. 2, 1972, pp. 193-207.

7.89 Yang, C. T., Rubinstein, R., and Atluri, S. N., "On Some Fundamental Studies into the Stability of Hybrid-Mixed Finite Element Methods for Navier-Stokes Equations in Solid/Fluid Mechanics," Proceedings of the Sixth Invitational Symposium on the Unification of Finite Elements - Finite Differences and Calculus of Variations, ed. by H. Kardestuncer, University of Connecticut, May 1982, pp. 24-76.

7.90 Ying, L. A. and Atluri, S. N., "A Hybrid Finite Element Method for Stokes Flow: Part II - Stability and Convergence Studies," Computer Methods in Applied Mechanics and Engineering, Vol. 36, 1983, pp. 39-60.

7.91 Yoshida, Y., "A Hybrid Stress Element for Thin Shell Analysis," Finite Element Methods in Engineering, ed. by V. Pulmano and A. Kabaila, University of New South Wales, Australia, 1974, pp. 271-284.

Equivalence Between Multifield Models and Single-Field Models

8.1 Hughes, T. J. R., "Equivalence of Finite Elements for Nearly Incompressible Elasticity," Journal of Applied Mechanics, ASME, March 1977, pp. 181-183.

8.2 Hughes, T. J. R., Cohen, M., and Haroun, M., "Reduced and Selective Integration Techniques in the Finite Element Analysis of Plates," Nuclear Engineering and Design, Vol. 46, No. 1, 1978, pp. 203-222.

8.3 Hughes, T. J. R., "Generalization of Selective Integration Procedures to Anisotropic and Nonlinear Media," International Journal for Numerical Methods in Engineering, Vol. 15, Sept. 1980, pp. 1413-1418.

8.4 Malkus, D. S. and Hughes, T. J. R., "Mixed Finite Element Methods - Reduced and Selective Integration Techniques: A Unification of Concepts," Computer Methods in Applied Mechanics and Engineering, Vol. 15, No. 1, July 1978, pp. 63-81.

8.5 Noor, A. K. and Peters, J. M., "Mixed Models and Reduced/Selective Integration Displacement Models for Nonlinear Analysis of Curved Beams," International Journal for Numerical Methods in Engineering, Vol. 17, 1981, pp. 615-631.

8.6 Noor, A. K. and Andersen, C. M., "Mixed Models and Reduced/Selective Integration Displacement Models for Nonlinear Shell Analysis," International Journal for Numerical Methods in Engineering, Vol. 18, 1982, pp. 1429-1454.

8.7 Noor, A. K. and Peters, J. M., "Mixed Models and Reduced/Selective Integration Displacement Models for Vibration Analysis of Shells," Hybrid and Mixed Finite Element Methods, ed. by S. N. Atluri, R. H. Gallagher and O. C. Zienkiewicz, John Wiley, 1983, pp. 537-564.

Penalty Finite Element Models

9.1 Bercouvier, M., "Perturbation of Mixed Variational Problems," R.A.I.R.O., Vol. 12, No. 3, 1978, pp. 211-236.

9.2 Brockman, R. A., "A Penalty Function Approach for the Nonlinear Finite Element Analysis of Thin Shells," Ph.D. Dissertation, University of Dayton, Ohio, 1979.

9.3 Hughes, T. J. R., Liu, W. K., and Brooks, A., "Finite Element Analysis of Incompressible Viscous Flows by the Penalty Function Formulation," Journal of Computational Physics, Vol. 30, 1979, pp. 1-60.

9.4 Malkus, D. S., "Finite Elements with Penalties in Nonlinear Elasticity," International Journal for Numerical Methods in Engineering, Vol. 16, 1980, pp. 121-136.

9.5 Oden, J. T., "Mixed Finite Element Approximations Via Interior and Exterior Penalties for Contact Problems in Elasticity," Hybrid and Mixed Finite Element Methods, ed. by S. N. Atluri, R. H. Gallagher and O. C. Zienkiewicz, John Wiley, 1983, pp. 467-486.

9.6 Reddy, J. N., "On the Finite Element Model with Penalty for Incompressible Fluid Flow Problems," The Mathematics of Finite Elements and Applications III, ed. by J. R. Whiteman, Academic Press, 1979, pp. 227-235.

9.7 Reddy, J. N., "A Penalty Plate-Bending Element for the Analysis of Laminated Anisotropic Composite Plates," International Journal for Numerical Methods in Engineering, Vol. 15, 1980, pp. 1187-1206.

9.8 Reddy, J. N. (ed.), Penalty-Finite Element Methods in Mechanics, AMD Vol. 51, American Society of Mechanical Engineers, 1982.

9.9 Zienkiewicz, O. C. and Godbole, P. N., "Penalty Function Approach to Problems of Plastic Flow of Metals with Large Surface Deformations," Journal of Strain Analysis, Vol. 10, 1975, pp. 180-183.

APPENDIX A - MULTIFIELD MODELS FOR TWO-DIMENSIONAL STEADY-STATE HEAT CONDUCTION

The fundamental equations and the basic characteristics of a number of multifield (mixed and hybrid) finite element models for the two-dimensional steady-state heat conduction problem are given in this appendix.

A.1 Fundamental Equations

The two fundamental equations are (see Ref. 1.5):

Conservation of thermal energy: $$-\partial_\alpha q_\alpha + Q = 0 \quad (1)$$

and, Fourier's law of conduction: $$q_\alpha = -k_{\alpha\beta}\,\partial_\beta T \quad (2)$$

or $$\partial_\alpha T = -f_{\alpha\beta}\,q_\beta \quad (3)$$

where T is the temperature field; q_α are the components of the flux field; $k_{\alpha\beta}$ ($=k_{\beta\alpha}$) are thermal conductivity coefficients of the material; $f_{\alpha\beta}$ are thermal resistivities (inverses of thermal conductivities); Q is the rate of heat generation per unit area; and $\partial_\alpha \equiv \partial/\partial x_\alpha$. The range of the Greek subscripts α, β is 1 to 2 and a repeated subscript in the same term denotes summation over the full range. In general, both the $k_{\alpha\beta}$ and $f_{\alpha\beta}$ are functions of the temperature T.

Equations 1 and 2 can be combined to give the following single differential equation in terms of the temperature field:

$$\partial_\alpha(k_{\alpha\beta}\,\partial_\beta T) + Q = 0 \quad (4)$$

The boundary conditions can include:

specified temperature: $$T = \tilde{T} \quad (5)$$

and/or specified flux: $$q_\alpha\,n_\alpha = \tilde{q} \quad (6)$$

where n_α are the components of the outward normal to the boundary; and the prescribed quantities are denoted with a tilde.

Equations 4 to 6 are the Euler equations of the following single-field variational principle. (For a detailed discussion of variational principles in heat transfer see Ref. 1.4.)

$$\delta\pi(T) = \int_S [k_{\alpha\beta}\,\partial_\beta T\,\delta(\partial_\alpha T) - Q\,\delta T]\,dS + \int_{C_q} \tilde{q}\,\delta T\,dC = 0 \quad (7)$$

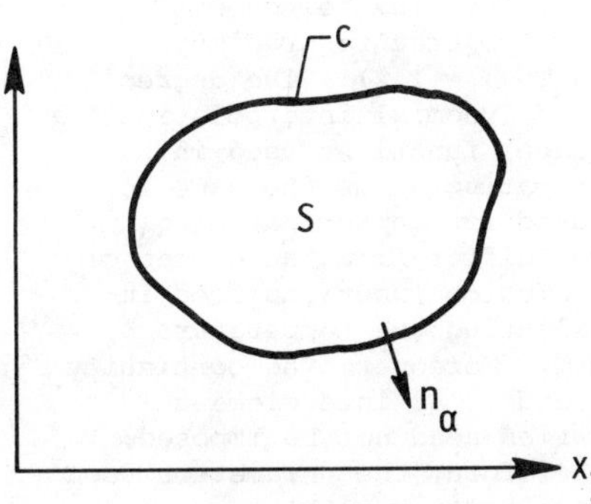

where S is the solution domain and C_q is the portion of the boundary where the flux components are prescribed.

A.2 Single-Field Finite Element Model

The governing equations of the single-field model are obtained by dividing the domain S into finite elements $S^{(e)}$ and using the following approximation for the temperature field T in each element

$$T = N_i\,T_i \quad (8)$$

where N_i are interpolation (or shape) functions and T_i are nodal temperatures, and the range of the subscript i is 1 to m (number of nodes in the element).

The finite element equations for each individual element can be cast in the following form:

$$K_{ij}\, T_j = Q_i \tag{9}$$

where K_{ij} are the conductivity coefficients of the element and Q_i are the nodal thermal loads. In case of temperature-dependent thermal conductivities, $k_{\alpha\beta} = k_{\alpha\beta}(T)$, K_{ij} are functions of T_j and Eqs. 9 are nonlinear equations. On the other hand, if $k_{\alpha\beta}$ are independent of T, Eqs. 9 are linear.

A.3 Mixed Finite Element Models

Two classes of mixed models are considered herein. The first class is based on a three-field variational principle and the second is based on a two-field variational principle. Henceforth, the two classes of models will be referred to as three-field and two-field mixed models, respectively.

Three-Field Mixed Models

The variational principle for this model is given by:

$$\delta\pi(T,q_\alpha,\phi_\alpha) = \sum_{\text{elements}} \int_{S^{(e)}} [(k_{\alpha\beta}\,\phi_\beta + q_\alpha)\,\delta\phi_\alpha + (\phi_\alpha - \partial_\alpha T)\,\delta q_\alpha - q_\alpha\,\delta(\partial_\alpha T) - Q\,\delta T]\, dS = 0 \tag{10}$$

where $S^{(e)}$ is the element domain, and the boundary integrals have been dropped, for convenience.

The fundamental unknowns used in the development of these models consist of: the temperature field T; the flux components q_α; and the temperature gradients $\phi_\alpha = \partial_\alpha T$ ($\alpha = 1,2$). The degree of the polynomial interpolation (or shape) functions used in approximating ϕ_α is the same as that used for approximating q_α and can differ from the degree of interpolation functions used in approximating the temperature field T. Moreover, the continuity of q_α and ϕ_α at interelement boundaries need not be imposed, and therefore, the parameters used in approximating both q_α and ϕ_α can be eliminated on the element level.

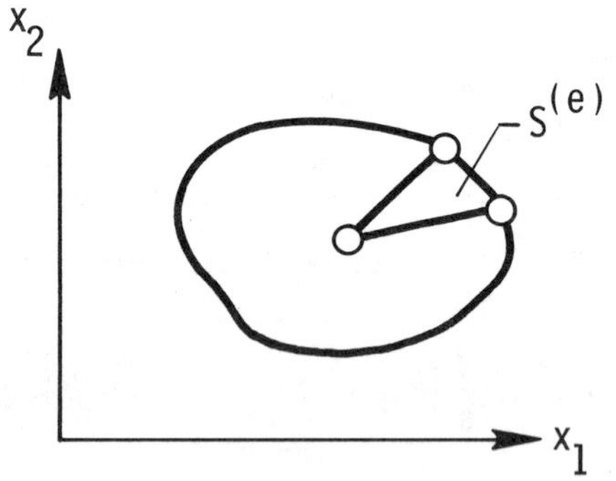

The finite element equations for the individual elements can be cast in the following form:

$$\mathcal{K}_{IJ}\,\phi_J + \mathcal{S}_{IJ}\,q_J = 0 \tag{11}$$

$$(\mathcal{S}^t)_{IJ}\,\phi_J - \mathcal{B}_{Ij}\,T_j = 0 \tag{12}$$

$$-(\mathcal{B}^t)_{iJ}\,q_J = Q_i \tag{13}$$

where ϕ_J, q_J and T_j are the parameters used in approximating ϕ_α, q_α and T, respectively; the $\mathbb{K}$, $\mathcal{S}$ and $\mathcal{B}$ are "generalized" heat transfer coefficients, and the superscript t denotes transposition. The range of the uppercase Latin subscripts is 1 to 2n, where n is the number of parameters used in approximating each of the flux (or the temperature gradient) components; and the range of the lowercase Latin indices is 1 to m (where m is the number of temperature nodes). A repeated subscript in the same term denotes summation over the full range of that subscript.

For nonlinear problems with temperature-dependent thermal conductivities, $\mathbb{K}_{IJ}$ are functions of the nodal temperatures T_j. On the other hand, for linear problems $\mathbb{K}_{IJ}$ are independent of T_j.

If the flux and temperature-gradient parameters are eliminated from Eqs. 11, 12 and 13, one obtains the following equations in the nodal temperatures T_i:

$$K_{ij}\, T_j = Q_i \tag{14}$$

where K_{ij} are the linear conductivity coefficients defined as follows:

$$K_{ij} = (\mathcal{B}^t)_{iJ}\, (\mathcal{S}^{-1})_{JI}\, \mathbb{K}_{IL}\, (\mathcal{S}^{-t})_{LK}\, \mathcal{B}_{Kj} \tag{15}$$

$(\mathcal{S}^{-1})_{IJ}$ and $(\mathcal{S}^{-t})_{IJ}$ denote the inverse and transpose inverse of the $\mathcal{S}_{IJ}$.

Two-Field Mixed Models

These are similar to the three-field mixed models except that the fundamental unknowns consist of the temperature field and the flux components only. The two-field variational principle used in the development of this model is given by:

$$\delta\pi(T,q_\alpha) = \sum_{\text{elements}} \int_{S^{(e)}} [(f_{\alpha\beta}\, q_\beta + \partial_\alpha T)\, \delta q_\alpha + q_\alpha\, \delta(\partial_\alpha T) + Q\, \delta T]\, dS = 0 \tag{16}$$

Again, the boundary integrals have been dropped, for convenience.

The finite element equations for the individual elements can be cast in the following form:

$$\mathcal{F}_{IJ}\, q_J + \mathcal{B}_{Ij}\, T_j = 0 \tag{17}$$

$$(\mathcal{B}^t)_{iJ}\, q_J = -Q_i \tag{18}$$

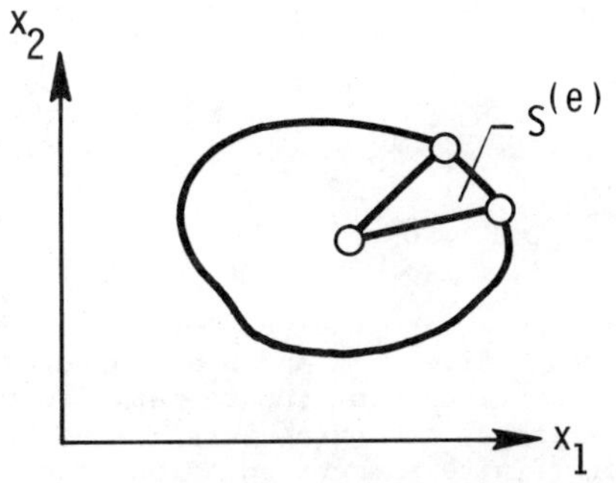

where the $\mathcal{F}$ terms are the thermal resistivity coefficients. The other terms were defined previously in connection with Eqs. 11 to 13.

For linear problems, the flux parameters can be eliminated from Eqs. 17 and 18 on the element level, and the resulting equations have the same form as Eqs. 11, with the linear conductivity coefficients K_{ij} defined as follows:

$$K_{ij} = (\mathcal{B}^t)_{iI}\, (\mathcal{F}^{-1})_{IJ}\, \mathcal{B}_{Jj} \tag{19}$$

where $(\mathcal{F}^{-1})_{IJ}$ denotes the inverse of the array $\mathcal{F}_{IJ}$.

A.4 Hybrid Finite Element Models

A number of different hybrid models can be developed each based on a modified variational principle with relaxed continuity requirements. Herein three hybrid models are developed for the *linear* two-dimensional heat conduction problem.

The models are analogous to the three models presented in Ref. 1.32 for linear elasticity problems. The models differ in the manner the temperature constraint is imposed at interelement boundaries.

Hybrid Model I. This model is based on the modified variational principle with the following functional:

$$\pi(T,\lambda) = \sum_{\text{elements}} \int_{S^{(e)}} \left(\frac{1}{2} k_{\alpha\beta}\, \partial_\alpha T\, \partial_\beta T - QT\right) dS + \sum \int_{C^{(ab)}} \lambda \left(T^{(a)} - T^{(b)}\right) dC \tag{20}$$

where λ is a Lagrange multiplier; $T^{(a)}$ and $T^{(b)}$ represent the approximations of the temperature field in the adjacent elements (a) and (b) joining on the interface $C^{(ab)}$; and a repeated subscript in the same term denotes summation over its full range. Note that the second summation sign in Eq. 20 is carried over all interelement boundaries.

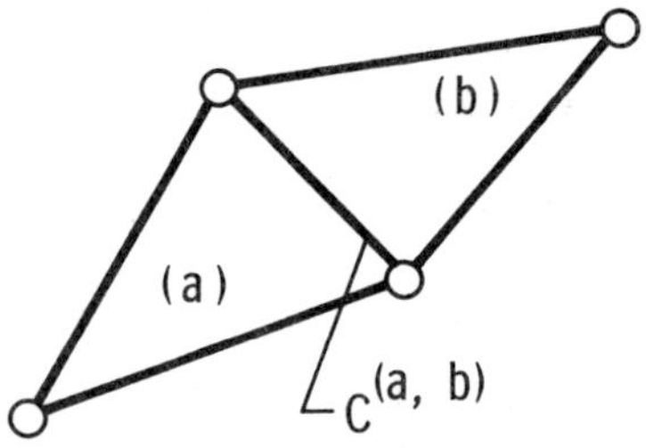

The fundamental unknowns used in the development of this hybrid model consist of the temperature field T, and the Lagrange multiplier field λ. The temperature field is approximated inside the element and the Lagrange multiplier is approximated on the common interface with adjacent elements. The model has been called *the hybrid model with single-layer interface* in Ref. 1.37.

The finite element equations for the individual elements can be written in the following form:

$$\bar{K}_{ij}\, T_j + \bar{\mathcal{S}}_{iJ}\, \lambda_J = Q_i \tag{21}$$

$$(\bar{\mathcal{S}}^t)_{Ij}\, T_j = 0 \tag{22}$$

where T_j and λ_J are the parameters and nodal variables used in approximating T and λ, respectively; $\bar{K}$ and $\bar{\mathcal{S}}$ are generalized heat transfer coefficients. Note that the continuity of the temperature T is not imposed at interelement boundaries and, therefore, the parameters T_j can be eliminated on the element level. The resulting finite element equations can be cast in the following form:

$$(\bar{\mathcal{S}}^t)_{Ii}\, (\bar{K}^{-1})_{ij}\, \bar{\mathcal{S}}_{jJ}\, \lambda_J = (\bar{\mathcal{S}}^t)_{Ii}\, (\bar{K}^{-1})_{ij}\, Q_j \tag{23}$$

where $(\bar{K}^{-1})_{ij}$ denotes the inverse of the array $\bar{K}_{ij}$.

Hybrid Model II. This model differs from hybrid model I in that different Lagrange multipliers are introduced in elements (a) and (b) such that:

$$\lambda^{(a)} + \lambda^{(b)} = 0 \tag{24}$$

The functional of the modified principle can be expressed as follows:

$$\bar{\pi}(T,\lambda,\mu) = \sum_{\text{elements}} \int_{S^{(e)}} (\tfrac{1}{2}\, k_{\alpha\beta}\, \partial_\alpha T \;\; \partial_\beta T - QT)\, dS$$

$$+ \sum \int_{C^{(ab)}} [\lambda^{(a)} T^{(a)} + \lambda^{(b)} T^{(b)} - \mu(\lambda^{(a)} + \lambda^{(b)})]\, dC \tag{25}$$

where μ is a Lagrange multiplier defined on the common interface.

The finite element equations for the individual elements can be written in the following form:

$$\bar{K}_{ij}\, T_j + \bar{\mathcal{S}}_{iJ}\, \lambda_J = Q_i \tag{26}$$

$$(\bar{\mathcal{S}}^t)_{Ij}\, T_j + \bar{B}_{IJ}\, \mu_J = 0 \tag{27}$$

and $$(\bar{B}^t)_{IJ}\, \lambda_J = 0 \tag{28}$$

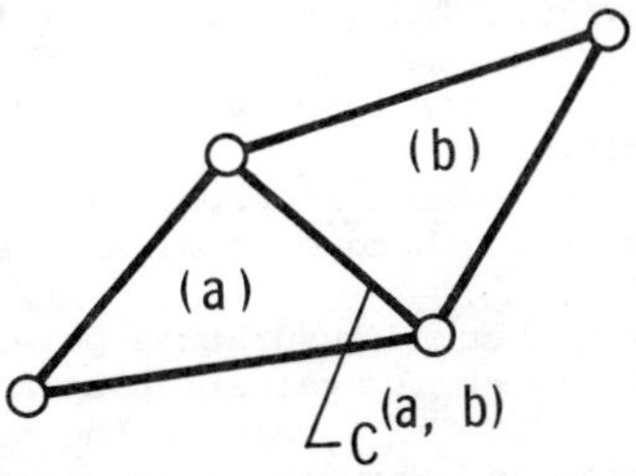

where T_j and λ_J are the parameters used in approximating T within the element and λ on the interfaces of each element, respectively; and μ_J are the nodal variables used in approximating μ on the common interface. Note that both T_j and λ_J can be eliminated on the element level. The resulting finite element model has been called the *hybrid model with double-layer interface* in Ref. 1.37.

Hybrid Model III. The modified variational principle of this model is obtained from that of the preceding model by using the stationary conditions on $C^{(ab)}$ to eliminate $\lambda^{(a)}$ and $\lambda^{(b)}$. The stationary conditions can be written in the following form:

$$\lambda^{(a)} = -k_{\alpha\beta}\, \partial_\alpha T^{(a)}\, n_\beta = q_\beta^{(a)}\, n_\beta \tag{29}$$

and

$$\lambda^{(b)} = -k_{\alpha\beta}\, \partial_\alpha T^{(b)}\, n_\beta = q_\beta^{(b)}\, n_\beta \tag{30}$$

The functional of the modififed variational principle can be expressed as follows:

$$\bar{\bar{\pi}}(T,\mu) = \sum_{\text{elements}} \int_{S^{(e)}} (\tfrac{1}{2}\, k_{\alpha\beta}\, \partial_\alpha T \;\; \partial_\beta T - QT)\, dS$$

$$+ \sum \Big[\int_{\overset{*}{C}{}^{(ab)}} q_\beta^{(a)}\, n_\beta\, (T^{(a)} - \mu)\, dC \tag{31}$$

$$+ \int_{\overset{*}{C}{}^{(ba)}} q_\beta^{(b)}\, n_\beta\, (T^{(b)} - \mu)\, dC \Big]$$

The independent fields subject to variation are T and μ. The temperature $T^{(a)}$ in element a may be chosen independently of the temperature $T^{(b)}$ in element b, while μ should be common to $\overset{*}{C}^{(ab)}$ and $\overset{*}{C}^{(ba)}$. The final elemental equations can be expressed in terms of the nodal parameters μ_J.

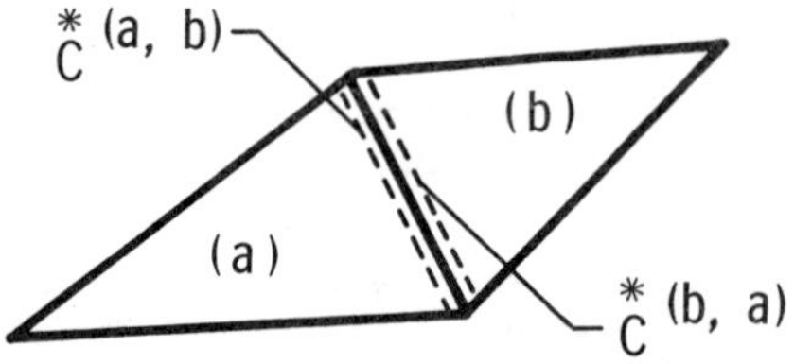

A.5 Equivalence Between Mixed Models and Single-Field Models

The three-field and the two-field mixed models are said to be equivalent to the single-field model if Eqs. 11 for the mixed models are identical with Eqs. 9 of the single-field model, where K_{ij} in the three-field and the two-field mixed models are defined by Eqs. 15 and 19, respectively. The conditions for the equivalence are:

1. The same number of nodes and Lagrangian interpolation functions are used for approximating the temperature T in both the single-field and mixed finite element models.

2. The polynomial interpolation functions for the fields q_α and ϕ_α are of the same degree as those of the temperature, and are discontinuous at interelement boundaries.

3. The number of quadrature points in the Gauss-Legendre quadrature formula used for the numerical evaluation of all terms of the mixed and single-field models is equal to the square of the number of temperature nodes.

The following comments on the equivalence seem to be in order:

1. The aforementioned equivalences hold for the case of temperature-dependent thermal conductivities provided the same approximation is used for the thermal conductivities in both the mixed and their equivalent single-field models.

2. The finite element equations for the individual elements, Eqs. 11, 12, 13, 17 and 18 remain unchanged when the degree of the approximating polynomials for each of q_α and ϕ_α is increased by one provided the numbers of quadrature points are not changed.

3. The aforementioned equivalent mixed and single-field models become nearly-equivalent when: a) the number of quadrature points is increased (for example, in the case of curved-sided elements); and/or b) different approximations are made for the thermal conductivities in mixed and single-field models (for example, thermal resistivities are approximated in the mixed models while thermal conductivities are approximated in single-field models).

CHAPTER SIX

SOLUTION OF LINEAR FINITE ELEMENT EQUATIONS

J. K. Reid
Computer Science and Systems Division
AERE Harwell
Oxfordshire, England

ABSTRACT

The principle direct methods for solving finite element sets of linear equations are described and compared. All are variants of Gaussian elimination so the relevant properties of this are first introduced, including its numerical stability and the effect of errors. Two iterative methods that have come to prominence recently are described and, finally, some brief comments on solving very large problems are made.

INTRODUCTION

In this chapter we consider the solution of sets of n linear equations

$$[A]\{x\} = \{b\} \tag{1}$$

that have arisen from finite element applications. The $n \times n$ matrix [A] is usually symmetric ($[A]^T = [A]$), and positive definite ($\{z\}^T[A]\{z\} > 0$ unless $\{z\} = \{0\}$) because an energy minimizing principle underlies the mathematical model. These properties are very helpful for both direct and iterative methods and for most of this chapter we assume that they hold, but we do not neglect the general case. The matrix [A] and vector {b} always originate as sums

$$[A] = \sum_k [B^{(k)}], \quad \{b\} = \sum_k \{c^{(k)}\} \tag{2}$$

of contributions from the finite elements. Each element k is associated with only a few variables and the matrix $[B^{(k)}]$ and the vector $\{c^{(k)}\}$ have nonzeros only in those rows and columns that correspond to these few variables. Therefore, $[B^{(k)}]$ and $\{c^{(k)}\}$ may be stored in the computer in packed form in arrays with dimensions equal to the number of variables in element k, provided there is an associated index list specifying which variables are involved (i.e., to which row of the overall matrix each row of the packed form corresponds). The resulting overall matrix is sparse and may be treated by any sparse matrix technique, for example, as a band matrix if the variables are suitably ordered. However, we may go further and exploit the explicit form (2). In the frontal method this form is exploited to the extent that the matrix [A] is never formed explicitly, but instead its triangular factors are formed, probably to be held away from main storage.

This chapter concentrates on direct methods because these are almost always used in practice, but does describe two iterative methods that have become prominent lately: preconditioned conjugate gradients and multigrid iteration. Direct methods are widely used, and because they are based on Gaussian elimination we begin by describing its properties, particularly in connection with roundoff and other errors. In the following sections we describe the principle variants in a self-contained manner. We end with a short discussion of input-output operations and the use of parallel and vector hardware. For a comprehensive bibliography of references for structural engineers see Meyer (1,2).

GAUSSIAN ELIMINATION

All direct methods for solving sets (1) of linear equations are based on variants of Gaussian elimination. It is essential to pay careful attention to the sparsity of the matrix [A], perhaps by exploiting its special form (2), if large problems are to be solved, and much of this chapter is devoted to this. However, it is very worthwhile first to review the properties of the basic method as applied to full matrices. In particular, the error analysis of Wilkinson (3, 4) tells us when we can rely on the computed results and is essentially simple though not widely understood by nonspecialists.

If no changes are in use, then the steps performed at the kth major step of the elimination are

$$a_{ij}^{(k+1)} = a_{ij}^{(k)} - a_{ik}^{(k)} (a_{kk}^{(k)})^{-1} a_{kj}^{(k)} \qquad (i,j > k) \qquad (3)$$

$$b_{i}^{(k+1)} = b_{i}^{(k)} - a_{ik}^{(k)} (a_{kk}^{(k)})^{-1} b_{k}^{(k)} \qquad (i > k) \qquad (4)$$

commencing with $[A^{(1)}] = [A]$, $\{b^{(1)}\} = \{b\}$. After (n-1) such steps we have a system of linear equations whose matrix is upper-triangular and which can be solved by the back substitution

$$x_k = (a_{kk}^{(k)})^{-1} (b_k^{(k)} - \sum_{j=k+1}^{n} a_{kj}^{(k)} x_j), \quad k = n, n-1, \ldots, 1. \qquad (5)$$

The operations (3) are numerically stable in the presence of roundoff provided that the numbers do not grow drastically in size. That growth may cause loss of accuracy and may be seen by considering the four-decimal example

$$1.234 + 402.1 = 403.3 \qquad (6)$$

where it is immediately apparent that the last two decimals of 1.234 have been ignored. It is often supposed that numerical stability requires that no "pivot" $a_{kk}^{(k)}$ be small and/or that no "multiplier" $a_{ik}^{(k)} (a_{kk}^{(k)})^{-1}$ be large, but actually neither condition is necessary. Instead, it is important to avoid letting the whole product $a_{ik}^{(k)} (a_{kk}^{(k)})^{-1}$ to become large; controlling the size of the pivot or of the multiplier is a possible means to this end.

If we use the notation

$$d_{kk} = a_{kk}^{(k)}; \quad \ell_{ik} = a_{ik}^{(k)} d_{kk}^{-1}, \quad i \geq k \; ; \quad u_{kj} = d_{kk}^{-1} a_{kj}^{(k)}, \quad j \leq k \qquad (7)$$

and collect all the operations (3) that are applied to a particular element a_{ij} we find the relations

$$a_{ij}^{(j)} = \ell_{ij}d_{jj} = a_{ij} - \sum_{k=1}^{j-1} \ell_{ik}\, d_{kk}\, u_{kj} \;, \quad i > j \tag{8a}$$

$$a_{ii}^{(i)} = d_{ii} = a_{ii} - \sum_{k=1}^{i-1} \ell_{ik}\, d_{kk}\, u_{ki} \tag{8b}$$

$$a_{ij}^{(i)} = d_{ii}u_{ij} = a_{ij} - \sum_{k=1}^{i-1} \ell_{ik}\, d_{kk}\, u_{kj} \;, \quad i < j \tag{8c}$$

Since (7) implies that the equalities $\ell_{kk} = u_{kk} = 1$ hold, in all three cases the left-hand side may be incorporated into the sum on the right to give

$$0 = a_{ij} - \sum_{k=1}^{\min(i,j)} \ell_{ik}\, d_{kk}\, u_{kj} \tag{9}$$

which in turn may be expressed in the matrix form

$$[A] = [L][D][U] \tag{10}$$

if [L] is the lower triangular matrix with lower triangular elements ℓ_{ij}, [D] is the diagonal matrix with diagonal elements d_{ii} and [U] is the upper triangular matrix with upper triangular elements u_{ij}.

If all the symbols refer to computed quantities, then an additonal term $\varepsilon_{ij}^{(k)}$ must be added to (3) to represent the error in that computation. As a consequence, (8) and (9) must contain the additional term

$$e_{ij} = \sum_{k=1}^{m} \varepsilon_{ij}^{(k)} \;, \quad m = \min(i,j) - 1 \tag{11}$$

and which factors exactly a perturbed matrix

$$[A] + [E] = [L][D][U] \tag{12}$$

where [E] has elements (11). Inspection of (3) shows at once that the associated error $\varepsilon_{ij}^{(k)}$ will be comparable with a round-off on the larger of $a_{ij}^{(k)}$ and $a_{ij}^{(k+1)}$. In fact, a detailed analysis (Reid, (5)) yields the bound

$$e_{ij} \leq (3.01)\, \varepsilon\, n \max_k |a_{ij}^{(k)}| \tag{13}$$

where ε (assumed less than 10^{-3}) is the relative precision. This result emphasizes the importance of avoiding growth in the size of the matrix coefficients.

If [A] is symmetric ($a_{ij} = a_{ji}$), then it is readily verified from (3) that symmetry is preserved (i.e., $a_{ij}^{(k)} = a_{ji}^{(k)}$, $i,j > k$) and, hence, that the final factorization may be written

$$[A] = [L][D][L]^T \tag{14}$$

For the case where [A] is also positive definite, Wilkinson (3) has shown that no overall growth in the size of matrix elements can occur, in the sense that the inequality

$$|a_{ij}^{(k)}| \leq \max_{i,j} |a_{ij}| \tag{15}$$

holds. This highly satisfactory result means that in this case the algorithm is unconditionally stable.

In the unsymmetric case it is usual to include row and/or column interchanges with the aim of avoiding growth. For instance, if row interchanges are introduced to make the inequalities

$$|a_{kk}^{(k)}| \geq u|a_{ik}^{(k)}|, \; i > k \tag{16}$$

hold, where u is a preset parameter in the range

$$0 < u \leq 1 \tag{17}$$

then an immediate deduction from (3) is that the inequality

$$\max_{i,j} |a_{ij}^{(k+1)}| \leq (1+u^{-1}) \max_{i,j} |a_{ij}^{(k)}| \tag{18}$$

holds. The same result holds if column interchanges are used to ensure that the inequalities

$$|a_{kk}^{(k)}| \geq u|a_{kj}^{(k)}|, \; j > k \tag{19}$$

hold. For full matrices there is no disadvantage in taking $u = 1$, that is, choosing for pivot $a_{kk}^{(k)}$ the largest element of the row or column, but for sparse matrices there are advantages in using another value for u to permit some freedom to choose pivots on sparsity grounds. Note also that for a sparse matrix there are fewer occasions for growth to occur. If there are ρ_j nonzeros in column j, then from (16) we may deduce the overall bound

$$\max_{i} |a_{ij}^{(k)}| \leq (1+u^{-1})^{\rho_j - 1} \max_{i} |a_{ij}| \tag{20}$$

The symmetric nondefinite case which occurs, for example, when performing inverse iteration for the eigenvalue problem about a shift in the middle of the spectrum, may be treated as unsymmetric. Of course, once any row interchanges are performed, the symmetry is lost, so both the work and storage requirements will be about double that needed without any interchanges. Bunch (6) solves the problem by using block 2 x 2 pivots as well as ordinary pivots. Equations (3) to (10) and (14) are valid for this more general situation if we regard the rows and columns as grouped into blocks of length 1 or 2 and labeled by the subscripts. For instance, the pivot $a_{kk}^{(k)}$ in (3) and (4) may be an ordinary pivot or it may be a 2 x 2 block pivot. Symmetric interchanges are used either to make a large diagonal element into a 1 x 1 pivot or to bring a large off-diagonal element into a 2 x 2 pivot as its off-diagonal element. For details of possible interchange strategies see Bunch (6), Bunch et al. (7), and (for the sparse case) Duff et al. (8).

The symmetric nondefinite case is also frequently treated by using ordinary pivots from the diagonal and "hoping for the best". In fact, it is perfectly straightforward to monitor the size of the intermediate numbers and, hence, provide a warning of any instability. In the case of inverse iteration, a small alteration of the eigenvalue shift will probably provide a cure. Although not often included in codes, such stability monitoring is to be advised, except in the unconditionally stable symmetric and positive definite case, because if the bound (20) is actually attained we are likely to have lost all accuracy.

Possible instability in Gaussian elimination should not be confused with possible ill-conditioning of the original equation (1). Informally, the condition number (ratio of largest eigenvalue to smallest eigenvalue in the symmetric case and ratio of singular values in the unsymmetric case) bounds the amount by which relative errors in the problem are magnified in the solution (see also Roy (9)). Symmetric positive-definite matrices for which Gaussian elimination is stable (in the sense that we explained at the beginning of this section), can be arbitrarily ill-conditioned. For a fuller discussion, see Stewart (10).

Iterative refinement can be used to mitigate these effects and estimate the error in the solution. Given an approximate solution $\{\tilde{x}\}$, a correction to it may be obtained by solving

$$[A]\{\delta\} = \{b\} - [A]\{\tilde{x}\} \tag{21}$$

Note that if the factorization (10) is preserved, then this equation is easy to solve. Note also that if $[A]$ is ill-conditioned, then the residual $\{b\} - [A]\{\tilde{x}\}$ may be small although $\{\tilde{x}\}$ has a large error. It is traditional (see Forsythe and Moler (11), for example) to use double-length arithmetic to compute the right-hand side of equation (21) with the aim of repeatedly correcting until the solution settles down, at which point it will have virtually full single-precision accuracy. However, such a procedure makes no sense unless $\{b\}$ and $[A]$ are represented exactly in single-precision or are available to more than single-precision accuracy (see the experimental results of Roy (9)). We prefer Wilkinson's suggestion (private communication) to use single precision arithmetic and regard the size of $\{\delta\}$ as an indicator of the likely error in $\tilde{x}$. Actually, one can go further (Marlow and Reid (12)) and introduce into the right-hand side of equation (21) pseudo-random perturbations at the level of the uncertainties in $[A]$ and $\{b\}$ so that $\{\delta\}$ indicates the effect of these uncertainties on the solution.

BAND MATRIX TECHNIQUES

If the variables can be so ordered that those associated with any one finite element have indices that differ by at most m, then it is apparent from (2) that $a_{ij} = 0$ if $|i-j| > m$: that is, that the matrix $[A]$ is a band matrix of bandwidth $2m+1$ and semi-bandwidth m. It is also apparent from inspection of (3) that (without interchanges) this property is preserved in the reduced matrices. Of course, it often happens that the bandwidth varies and Jennings (13) has demonstrated that it can be very worthwhile to exploit such variability. In fact, it is clear from (3) that no fill-in can ever be created ahead of the first nonzero in a row (or the first nonzero in a column), and code to work with a varying bandwidth is scarcely any more complicated than that for a fixed bandwidth. However, between the first nonzero of a row (or column) and the diagonal there is usually total fill-in. In fact, George and Liu (14) have shown that if all rows (columns) after the first have a nonzero to the left of (above) the diagonal then they all fill in totally between this nonzero and the diagonal. FORTRAN code for the symmetric positive definite case is given by Felippa (15).

Unfortunately, if interchanges are included for the sake of numerical stability, then these properties no longer hold. If only row interchanges are used then the variable (or fixed) band form is preserved in the lower triangular part but it widens in the upper-triangular part. For a fixed bandwidth matrix, the upper triangular semi-bandwidth at most doubles and many codes have been written which allocate exactly double and hold explicit zeros at the head of columns whose lengths do not increase so much. It would be possible to write code that dynamically allocated more space for the columns of a variable band matrix whenever necessary, but the author knows of no such code.

It is often natural to order the variables so that a small bandwidth results, for instance, by using a page-wise ordering for a rectangular region but, in general, an automatic renumbering system is obviously desirable. Most algorithms regard two variables as "neighbors" if an element has them both as associated variables and groups them into "level sets" S_i, the first of which contains a single starting variable. Later all variables which are neighbors of variables in S_j, but are not in any of the sets S_i, $i \leq j$, are taken to be in set S_{j+1}. Once these sets S have been constructed, then the ordering of variables from set S_1 followed by those from set S_2, etc., gives a resulting matrix [A] which is block triangular with diagonal blocks corresponding to the sets S_i. For example,

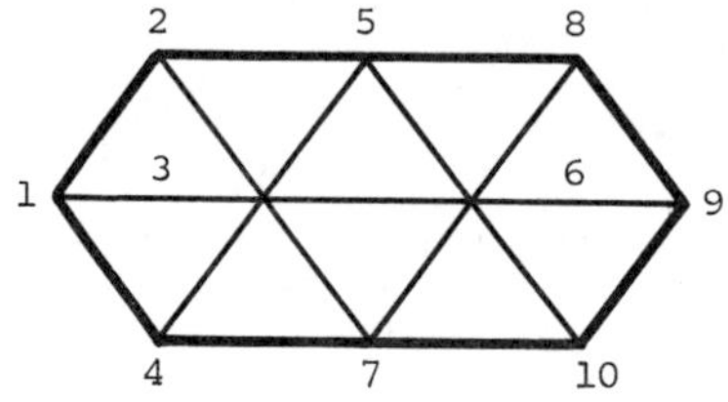

Fig. 1 A problem with six linear elements.

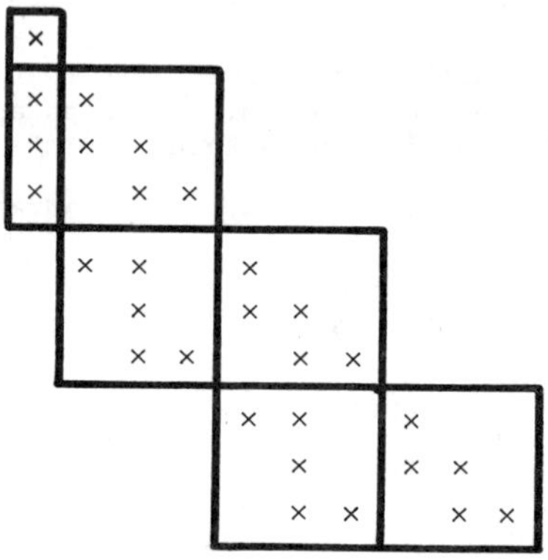

Fig. 2 The lower triangular part of the matrix corresponding to Fig. 1.

the region of Fig. 1, with three-variable triangular elements, has level sets {1}, {2, 3, 4}, {5, 6, 7}, {8, 9, 10} and the lower triangular part of the resulting matrix is shown in Fig. 2. To order within each block S_i, Cuthill and McKee (16) (see also Cuthill (17)) suggest taking first those variables that are neighbors of the first variable in S_{i-1}, then those that are neighbors of the second node in S_{i-1}, and so on; the several other orderings that have been proposed since then do not appear to offer any significant advantages. Chan and George (18) explain how this can be implemented efficiently.

Rather surprisingly, George (19) found that reversing the order obtained often yielded a worthwhile improvement. A simple proof that reversing the order cannot increase the number of nonzeros within the variable-band profile is given by Jennings (20, pp. 162-163). We illustrate with the simple example involving six-node quadratic triangular elements shown in Fig. 3. The Cuthill-McKee ordering is shown in Fig. 3 and the pattern of the lower triangular part of the resulting matrix is shown in Fig. 4a. The zeros between the first nonzero of each row and the diagonal all fill and are shown as explicit zeros in Fig. 4a. On reversing the order, the rows have the structure of the columns of Fig. 4 but now the zeros at the ends of columns 2, 6, 7 and 0 are zeros at the beginnings of corresponding rows and, therefore, no longer fill (see Fig. 4b). In fact, in this case reversing the order reduces the number of fills from 20 to 8. Notice that variables 2, 7 and 10 belong to just one element and variable 6 belongs only to adjacent elements of a level set. In general, such variables will give rise to a column with few nonzeros below the diagonal, and the reverse Cuthill-McKee order will gain from their presence. Indeed, George (19) found that the number of fills more than halved on large problems with elements having interior and/or edge nodes. Jennings' proof (20) that reversing the order can only help, is based on the observation that the Cuthill-McKee algorithm automatically gives a row-oriented profile that is not reentrant whereas the column oriented profile may be reentrant (see Figs. 4a and 4b, for example).

So far we have made no mention of the choice of starting node. It is clear that for small bandwidth we should aim for the level sets S_i to be small and numerous. For a cigar-shaped region this obviously requires starting at an end rather than the middle of a side, but a good choice is not always so apparent. Cuthill and McKee (16) suggested trying several starting variables with small numbers of neighbors. Collins (21) tries starting from every variable, but abandons each attempt immediately when he encounters a bandwidth greater than

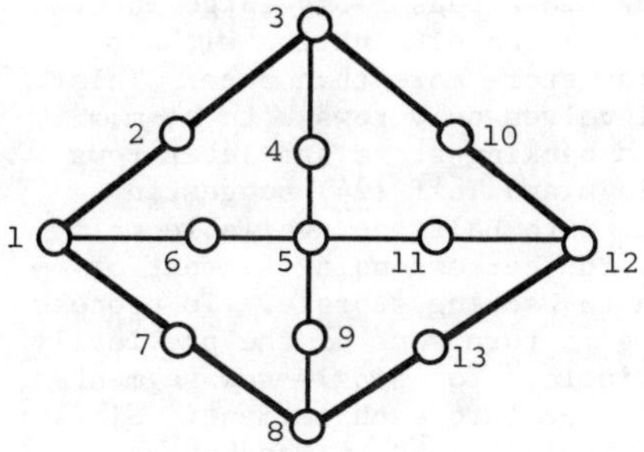

Fig. 3 A problem with four quadratic triangular elements.

	1	2	3	4	5	6	7	8	9	10	11	12	13
1	×												
2	×	×											
3	×	×	×										
4	×	×	×	×									
5	×	×	×	×	×								
6	×	×	×	×	×	×							
7	×	o	o	o	×	×	×						
8	×	o	o	o	×	×	×	×					
9	×	o	o	o	×	×	×	×	×				
10			×	×	×	o	o	o	o	×			
11			×	×	×	o	o	×	×	×	×		
12			×	×	×	o	o	×	×	×	×	×	
13					×	o	o	×	×	o	×	×	×

Fig. 4a Lower triangular part of matrix corresponding to Fig. 3.

	13	12	11	10	9	8	7	6	5	4	3	2	1
13	×												
12	×	×											
11	×	×	×										
10		×	×	×									
9	×	×	×	o	×								
8	×	×	×	o	×	×							
7					×	×	×						
6					×	×	×	×					
5	×	×	×	×	×	×	×	×	×				
4		×	×	×	o	o	o	×	×	×			
3		×	×	×	o	o	o	×	×	×	×		
2								×	×	×	×	×	
1					×	×	×	×	×	×	×	×	×

Fig. 4b Lower triangular part of matrix corresponding to Fig. 3, but with reverse ordering.

the smallest so far obtained. Gibbs, Poole and Stockmeyer (22) suggest that each variable in the final level set S_k should be tried as a starting node. If one gives more than k level sets, then it is used to replace the starting node and the new level sets are examined, continuing until no further increase in the number of level sets is obtained. Gibbs et al. reported that in all their test examples the number of level sets was actually maximized. George and Liu (23) experimented with several variants of the algorithm, including one akin to the algorithm of Collins (21) which they called "short circuiting". They chose the variant that looks at a single node of minimal degree in the last level set and published code to implement it. "Short circuiting" gave better results but was about 50% slower on average.

It frequently happens that even with a good ordering of the variables, the variable band matrix is too large to fit into main storage and, therefore, has to be held on backing store (e.g., disc). If the greatest semi-bandwidth is m and we have storage for $1/2(m+1)(m+2)$ variables and a reasonably large input-output buffer then it is straightforward to organize the elimination without writing any elements of the factors out to backing store more than once. This is possible because stage k of the elimination involves only rows k to $k+m$. The earlier rows can have already been written to backing store and later rows are not yet required. For bigger problems Jennings and Tuff (24) suggested grouping the rows into segments each of which fit into half the available main storage. Each segment in turn is overwritten by the corresponding segment of the lower triangular factor [L] and then written to backing storage. To process a particular segment in this way requires reading in turn some of the previously written segments of [L]. The method works in principle for single-row segments but will be efficient only if many rows are collected into each segment. Similar algorithms are proposed by Wilson, Bathe and Doherty (25) and by Mondkar and Powell (26) and both these papers include actual Fortran code. Mondkar and Powell also discuss how the right-hand side (load) vectors should be stored.

This assembly (2) of the individual matrices $[B^{(k)}]$ into the overall variable-band matrix [A] is reasonably straightforward. If backing storage is not in use, then we may hold the rows in sequence, with storage allocated for all the positions between the first nonzero in the row and the diagonal with pointers to the positions of the diagonal elements. The matrices $[B^{(k)}]$ may be added easily into this structure in any order. If backing storage is in use, then it is usual to read a file containing the packed $[B^{(k)}]$ several times, on each occasion accumulating as many rows of [A] as will fit into store at once. It can be very helpful to compute the largest and smallest variable number associated with each matrix $[B^{(k)}]$ for if the range of rows being assembled does not overlap the range of variables associated with $[B^{(k)}]$, then $[B^{(k)}]$ makes no contribution and need not be read.

FRONTAL TECHNIQUES

Although used in computer programs during the 1980's, the frontal method was first explained in the published literature by Irons (27) and the method is, hence, firmly linked with his name. It depends on the observation that the assembly operations (see (2))

$$\begin{aligned} a_{ij} &:= a_{ij} + b_{ij}^{(k)} \\ b_i &:= b_i + c_i^{(k)} \end{aligned} \tag{22}$$

need not be completed before elimination operations (see (3))

$$\begin{aligned} a_{ij} &:= a_{ij} - a_{ik}\, a_{kk}^{-1}\, a_{kj} \\ b_i &:= b_i - a_{ik}\, a_{kk}^{-1}\, b_k \end{aligned} \tag{23}$$

are commenced. Because addition and subtraction are associative (apart from roundoff effects) the operations (23) may be performed before all assembly operations (22) for a_{ij} have been completed, although it is necessary for a_{ik}, a_{kk}, a_{kj}, and b_k to be fully assembled or the wrong quantities will be subtracted. Irons eliminates each variable as soon as its row and column is fully summed; that is, performs all operations (23) as soon as row and column k are fully summed.

After this, row and column k play no further part in the elimination and may be written away to backing store. At a typical intermediate stage we work only with those rows and columns that have been partially summed. These correspond to those variables that are associated with one or more assembled elements and with one or more unassembled elements. These variables lie on the border between the set of assembled elements and the rest, and as the assembly and elimination progresses they form a front that moves across the region. For example, in Fig. 5, if the elements labeled a have been assembled then the front consists of variables 4, 5, 6 and 8; when the element with nodes 4, 5, 8 is assembled, variable 4 becomes fully assembled, and can be eliminated so that the front reduces to 5, 6 and 8; when the element 6, 8, 9 is assembled, variable 9 is added to the front but variable 6 can be eliminated. It is usual to hold the active rows and columns, corresponding to variables in the front, in a full matrix labeled with an index list of associated variables. In Fig. 5 the lists would successively be (4, 5, 6, 8), (5, 6, 8), (5, 6, 8, 9), (5, 8, 9). The front matrix may contain explicit zeros, so before eliminating a matrix coefficient it is worthwhile to check whether it is already zero and to skip the associated operations if it is.

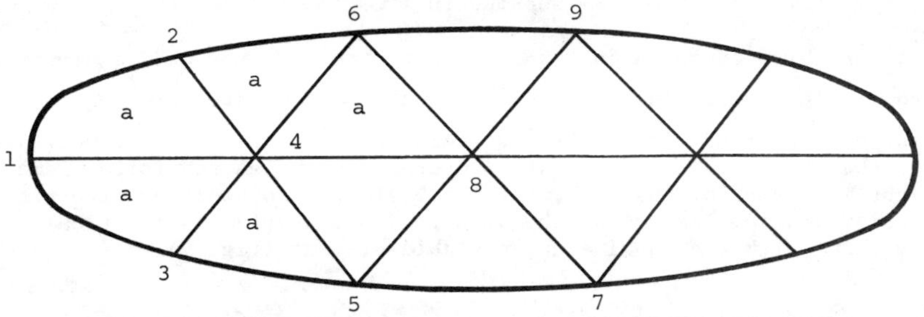

Fig. 5 A cigar-shaped problem.

Notice that the elimination order is now implied by the order of element assemblies and this order should be chosen with a view to a small front width. Working manually this is an easier and more natural task than that of ordering the more numerous variables for small bandwidth. For automatic ordering, the Cuthill-McKee algorithm (see last section) is available. The position of an element in the assembly order may be taken from the earliest position of an associated variable (or preferably) we may work with the obvious variant that uses element adjacencies in place of variable adjacencies. Again the Gibbs-Poole-Stockmeyer (22) pseudo-diameter or the variant of George and Liu (23) may be used to choose the starting variable or element.

The advantages associated with reversing the Cuthill-McKee ordering for band matrices are automatically obtained in the frontal method since each variable is eliminated immediately when it is fully summed. Thus a variable associated with a single element enters the front with the assembly of its element and immediately leaves it by elimination, and a variable associated only with a pair of elements enters the front with the first element and leaves it with the second.

The fact that variables leave the front in an order different than that in which they enter is important to the efficiency of the method, but does lead to slight programming complications. An initial pass through the index lists associated with the matrices $[B^{(k)}]$ is needed to determine when each variable appears for the last time (i.e., when it can be eliminated). There is also some complication in organizing the actual assemblies and eliminations within the (full) frontal array. Normally, the freshly entering rows and columns are placed at the end of the array and the eliminations are performed from the middle with the revised matrix closed up to fill the gaps. There is, of course, a need to maintain an index array to indicate which are the associated variables and their order.

So far we have assumed that the eliminations are numerically stable, which they certainly are in the symmetric positive definite case (see second section).

For the unsymmetric case Hood (28) suggests delaying eliminations until the front reaches a critical size then choosing as pivot the largest component in the submatrix of fully assembled rows and columns. Rather more subtle pivotal strategies based on Hood's ideas have been used by Cliffe et al. (29), and Duff's adaptation of their code is in the Harwell Subroutine Library (see Hopper (30)) and called MA32. The principle change is that any component in the submatrix of fully summed rows and columns that satisfies one of the relative pivot criteria (16) and (19) is immediately used as a pivot. This permits eliminations to be performed when the front is much smaller than its maximum permissible size and, indeed, means that the front size is usually only slightly bigger than it would have been without any pivoting. Note that because Hood's idea permits off-diagonal pivots to be chosen, separate index lists will be needed for the rows and columns (or at least for the fully assembled ones).

For the symmetric indefinite case, Hood's idea could be used in conjunction with the use of a mixture of 1×1 and 2×2 pivots (Bunch (6), see second section).

SUBSTRUCTURING

If a variable occurs in just one element, then its row and column is fully assembled within the single matrix $[B^{(k)}]$ and the associated elimination operations can be performed within $[B^{(k)}]$. This is known as "static condensation" and means that the true cost of adding internal variables to finite elements is very slight indeed. For instance, the algebraic cost of working with nine-variable biquadratic elements as shown in Fig. 6 is virtually identical with that of working with the usual eight-variable element (Fig. 7).

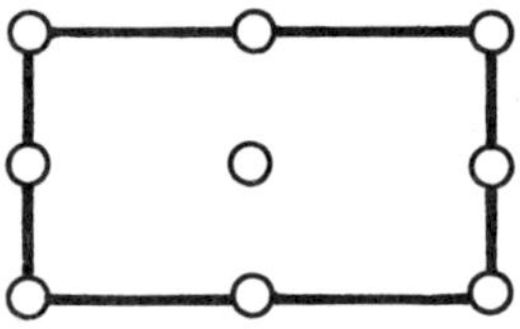

Fig. 6 Nine-node biquadratic element

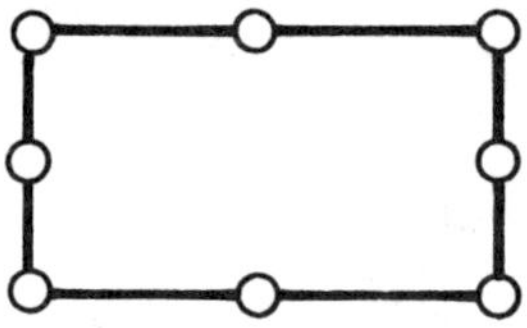

Fig. 7 Eight-node element (biquadratic less term in x^2y^2)

This idea extends naturally to groups of elements (Przemienicki, (31)). Any variables that are internal to a group may be eliminated by operations involving only those matrices $[B^{(k)}]$ that are associated with the group. There results a matrix whose rows and columns are associated with variables on the boundary of the group and which has a structure just like that of a large element parameterized by these variables. Indeed, the term "generalized element" is often used. A simple example is at an intermediate stage of frontal elimination: if ℓ elements have been assembled then the equation for the variables $\{x^{(\ell)}\}$ not so far eliminated is

$$([F^{(\ell)}] + \sum_{k > \ell} [B^{(k)}])\{\underline{x}^{(\ell)}\} = \{\underline{b}^{(\ell)}\} + \sum_{k > \ell} \{\underline{c}^{(k)}\} \tag{24}$$

where $[F^{(\ell)}]$ and $\{\underline{b}^{(\ell)}\}$ are the current frontal matrix and frontal right-hand side.

Where a problem has several natural substructures (for example, the wings, fuselage and tailplane of an aircraft) it is natural to treat each of them independently, in just this way. The overall problem then involves only the variables on the boundaries of the substructures but has the usual form (2) if the summation is interpreted as over the substructures and the matrices $[B^{(k)}]$

are those that result from elimination of internal variables from substructure k. Once the overall problem has been solved, the internal variables may be calculated by back substitution by recalling the pivotal rows stored during elimination. Very similar ideas have been used by Kron (32) for unsymmetric sets of equations arising from electrical networks.

Several advantages accrue from substructuring in this way. The calculations involved with each substructure may be performed in separate computer runs or even on separate computer systems. If any change is made in one of the substructures then the eliminations associated with it and with the overall structure must be recomputed, but not those associated with the other substructures. Really enormous problems may need several disk packs if treated as a whole, whereas data associated with each substructure and with the overall interconnection may each fit on a pack. If several substructures are identical then the elimination operations may be performed just once on a "master" copy, though the forward and backward substitution operations must be performed for each since they are likely to be different on each substructure. Finally, the total number of arithmetic operations may be reduced because the front size within the substructures is less than it would have been if the whole structure had been treated together.

The idea of substructuring may be nested, that is, each substructure may itself be substructured and to any depth. For example, seven levels of substructures were used by Araldsen (33) to analyze the structure of an oil tanker, and he made great use of identical substructures. For further comments on the advantages of this approach see the reviews of Noor et al. (34) and Dodds and Lopez (35).

A tree (see, for example, Fig. 9, representing the propeller of Fig. 8) is a suitable data structure to represent nested substructuring. Associated with each terminal node is a finite element, and associated with each node is a substructure whose members are associated with its "sons" in the tree. It is convenient to associate with each terminal node the corresponding matrix $[B^{(k)}]$ and vector $\{c^{(k)}\}$ together with the associated list of variables. Similarly, other nodes may have associated lists of boundary variables for substructures and matrices and vectors $[B^{(k)}]$, $\{c^{(k)}\}$ obtained by assembly of components and elimination of interior variables. The processing required for each node is just like the processing of the whole of a simple problem. Providing the index lists and the quantities $[B^{(k)}]$ and $\{c^{(k)}\}$ are available they can be treated as if we had ordinary elements. For example, we might use the frontal method at each node.

No node of the tree may be processed before all its sons, but there is nevertheless, considerable freedom in the ordering. Separate substructures may be handled by separate processors; for instance, the four first level substructures of Fig. 9 might be treated on four separate processors which pass their results to a fifth processor. On the other hand, if a single processor is in use there is some advantage in ordering according to a depth-first tree search. For instance, for the case shown in Fig. 9 we would process the substructures in the order 23, 24, 27, 25, 28, 26, 29. The advantage of a depth-first search is that intermediate results can be held in a stack. The stack contents for our example would be data associated with nodes (23), (23, 24), (27), (27, 25), (28), (28, 26), (29).

So far we have assumed that there is a natural way of substructuring, usually because a complicated design is assembled from simpler subassemblies. It makes sense to exploit these natural substructures, but it can also be advantageous to introduce artificial ones. For example, George (36) showed that a two-dimensional problem consisting of a regular $q \times q$ grid of square elements could be solved in $O(q^3)$ operations and $O(q^2 \log q)$ storage locations instead of $O(q^4)$ and $O(q^3)$, respectively, for band or frontal methods. He did this by dividing the elements into four groups with a "+" shaped cut, then dividing each group into four parts again with a "+" shaped cut and so on. Following a suggestion from Birkoff he called this "nested dissection" and this name has become well established. Actual gains for practical values of q, though worthwhile, are not enormous because the multiplying factors disfavor nested dissection.

George's figures (36) show, for instance, that if q = 32 the number of operations is reduced to about 38% and the number of storage locations needed excluding overheads to about 52% of the corresponding figures for band elimination using pagewise ordering.

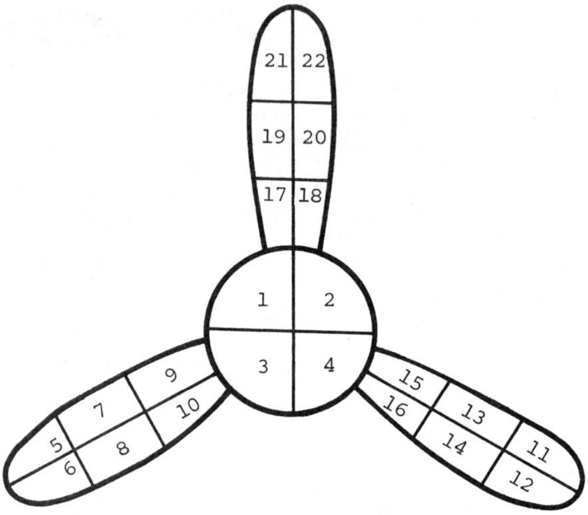

Fig. 8 A propeller

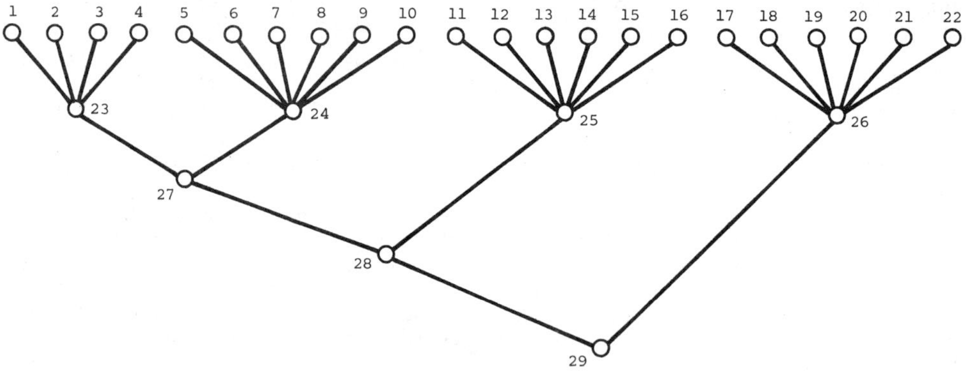

Fig. 9 Tree representing propeller

George and Liu (37) have a proposal for automating the dissection. They use the algorithm of Gibbs, Poole and Stockmeyer (22) to find a pseudo-diameter and a set of level sets and take the middle level set as a separator. They then repeat on the halves, and so on. On the regular square problem they found results were very nearly as good as with the theoretical dissection of George (36) They also make comparisons on a sequence of problems associated with using successively finer triangulations at the reentrant corner of an L-shaped region. They compared with variable band solution based on a reverse Cuthill-McKee ordering (see third section) and with treating the matrix as a general sparse matrix and using the Yale sparse matrix package (Eisenstat et al. (38). The results showed surprisingly little difference in execution time, with the band algorithm performing more operations but making up with a faster speed per operation because of its simpler data structure. Nested dissection did gain on storage utilization, even allowing for its extra overheads, for example, by about 25% over the band algorithm on the biggest problem, which had order 2233. Of course, nested dissection is asymptotically superior and none of these problems were particularly large.

To obtain some indication of the behavior on a bigger problem, the author has experimented with one kindly supplied by T. A. Manteuffel. Manteuffel himself (39) describes this problem and shows a diagram. It is a cylindrical shell with some irregularities and is built from 784 twenty-node (sixty-variable) bricks to give a total of 17928 variables. Manteuffel estimates that a band technique would involve a semi-bandwidth of 1300, storage for 23×10^6 nonzeros and 15×10^9 arithmetic operations. The SPARSPAK code of George and Liu (40, 41) is unable to handle such a big problem, but we can make estimates from its analysis of the equivalent problem with one degree of freedom per node. This indicates that the reverse Cuthill-McKee algorithm would reduce the storage required by about the factor 2 and that nested dissection would further reduce it by about the factor 2.4.

A pivotal strategy that has proved remarkably successful for any sparse symmetric matrix is that of "minimum degree". At each stage of the elimination it chooses as pivot the diagonal element of a row with least nonzeros. Traditionally, this has been implemented by holding all the nonzeros in a suitable list structure which expands with the fill-ins that result from the eliminations. Williams (42) pointed out that sparse matrix elimination without row interchanges can be expressed as nested substructuring (apart from the order of additions and subtractions) and, interestingly, minimum degree can also be represented in terms of nested substructuring. We begin by computing the numbers of nonzeros there would be in the rows of the matrix if we assembled it. For each row this is just the total number of variables in the union of the elements that contain the variable that corresponds to the row, and it may be computed directly from the lists of variables in the elements. Elimination of the variable of minimum degree may be achieved by a local assembly of all the elements in which it is involved into a substructure. The chosen variable is, of course, interior to this substructure. Following its elimination any other variables have degree one less and, therefore, must have minimum degree overall. Thus having established the substructure we should eliminate all internal variables in the usual way. The resulting substructure, with its internal variables eliminated, can now be treated just like an ordinary element. The algorithm can thus be continued to build successively larger substructures. This process of substructure generation can be made efficient since only the variable lists need be manipulated (they are merged for assemblies and then internal variables are removed) and it is possible to update the degrees of the variables (only those adjacent to or in the assembled substructure change). The algorithms of George and Liu (43, 44) use similar ideas. The author has applied an experimental code of this kind, but with a different strategy (essentially a local minimum fill-in strategy) to Manteuffel's matrix and in only two seconds of IBM 370/168 time it showed that the required storage would be for 4.8×10^6 reals and the number of operations would be 1.12×10^9. The storage gain over Manteuffel's estimate is very near to that predicted by SPARSPAK for automatic nested dissection and, indeed, SPARSPAK also tells us that on this problem minimum degree and nested dissection give similar performance. Notice that the minimum degree strategy has reduced Manteuffel's operation count by the factor 13 to make the computation a much more practicable proposition.

HYPERMATRICES

An approach that has been used with success by Argyris and his collaborators (see, for example, Schrem (45)) is to store matrices by blocks, using a full matrix of pointers to indicate actual storage positions. Any block that is zero is indicated by a pointer that has value zero so that the block itself need not be stored. A simple example is shown in Fig. 10; the zeros marked explicitly are held explicitly and the pointers indicate that A_{11} is held from location 1 of an array, A_{33} from location 7, etc.

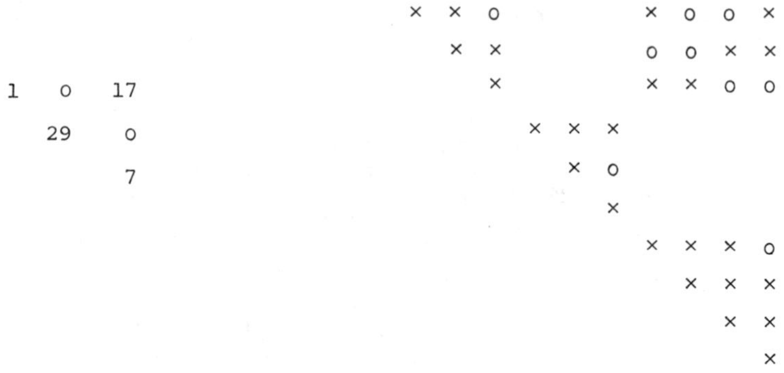

Fig. 10 An upper triangular blocked matrix and its associated matrix of pointers.

The technique can be nested with the first level pointers indicating where matrices of second level pointers are held, and so on, with only the last level pointing to real numbers. Three levels are probably as many as are ever likely to be useful.

The hypermatrix approach permits really huge problems to be handled with modest demands on main storage, but care is needed to avoid excessive input-output operations. For this reason the block sizes are usually chosen to suit hardware characteristics.

TWO ITERATIVE METHODS

Large systems of finite-difference equations have traditionally been solved by iterative methods (see, for example, Varga (46), Young (47), Wachspress (48), Walsh (49)) and, indeed, sparsity was being exploited effectively here long before it was effectively exploited for direct methods. Nevertheless, they have been little used for finite element problems. The principle reason for this is probably that the rate of convergence of the simpler methods is closely related to the condition number. For structural problems this is often very high. For instance, Manteuffel (39) estimates that his matrix (to which we referred in the section on Substructuring) has condition number 10^8. This causes no serious problems to Gaussian elimination with the long word-length normally used for major calculations on a large computer, but leads to very slow convergence of simple iterative methods. Further reasons why iterative methods have not been used are the need for estimating parameters and the general uncertainty about the likely rate of convergence. We propose here not to discuss any of the classical iterative methods (the reader may refer to the books mentioned at the beginning of this paragraph) but rather to consider two promising recent developments: preconditioned conjugate gradients and multigrid methods.

The method of conjugate gradients (Hestenes and Stiefel (50); see also Reid (51)) requires a starting iterate $\{x^{(0)}\}$ and thereafter mechanically produces iterates $\{x^{(i)}\}$ without any need for parameter estimation and requires access to $[A]$ only in that at each step it provides a vector $\{p^{(i)}\}$ and requires the product $[A]\{p^{(i)}\}$. It can be shown (see Reid (51) for example) that the residual

$$\{r^{(k)}\} = \{b\} - [A]\{x^{(k)}\} \tag{25}$$

corresponding to $\{x^{(k)}\}$ can be written

$$\{r^{(k)}\} = P_k([A])\{r^{(0)}\} \tag{26}$$

where P_k is a polynomial of degree k with constant coefficient unity. The power of the method lies in the fact that, of all such vectors, $\{r^{(k)}\}$ minimizes the error measure

$$Q(\{r\}) = \{r\}^T[A]^{-1}\{r\} \tag{27}$$

To understand the behavior, suppose that A has eigensolutions $(\lambda_i, \{e^{(i)}\})$ and expand $\{r^{(0)}\}$ as

$$\{r^{(0)}\} = \sum_i \gamma_i\{e^{(i)}\} \tag{28}$$

then $\{r^{(k)}\}$ has the expansion

$$\{r^{(k)}\} = \sum_i \gamma_i P_k(\lambda_i)\{e^{(i)}\} \tag{29}$$

If, therefore, there is a polynomial that is small on all the eigenvalues then $\{r^{(k)}\}$ will be small. Notice that there is no need for any actual eigen-analysis. Conjugate gradients automatically find a good P_k. The method works very well if the eigenvalues are clustered. The recent development is the realization that it may be possible to transform the problem to one with clustered eigenvalues by performing an approximate symmetric factorization

$$[A] \simeq [L][L]^T \tag{30}$$

and then working with the "preconditioned" equation

$$([L]^{-1}[A][L]^{-T})([L^T]\{x\}) = [L]^{-1}\{b\} \tag{31}$$

(The matrix [L] here should be compared with $[L][D]^{1/2}$ of equation (14)). If the factorization (30) is reasonably accurate, we may expect $[L]^{-1}[A][L]^{-T}$ to be near the identity matrix and, therefore, have eigenvalues clustered near unity so that conjugate gradients applied to (31) should converge rapidly. Meijerink and van der Vorst (52) proposed such a method based on ignoring fill-ins and showed that it is stable for M-matrices ($a_{ij} \leq 0$ for $i \neq j$ and $[A]^{-1} > 0$, a condition not often holding for finite element matrices). A variety of other approximate factorizations are possible. For instance, Vinsome (53) performs an approximate Gaussian elimination in which no off-diagonal elements are modified, based on the ideas of Dupont et al. (54); Gustafsson (55) worked within a fixed sparsity pattern but instead of simply dropping fill-ins, introduced more complicated modifications to ensure that $[L^{-1}][A][L]^T = O(h^{-1})$ where [A] corresponds to a discretization of an elliptic partial differential equation with mesh size h; Jennings and Malik (56) ignore elements that are small and perturb the diagonal too, in order to maintain positive definiteness; Munsgaard (57) also ignores small elements and makes additions to the diagonal, and his code (MA31 in the Harwell Library) contains a parameter which may be adjusted to control the size of dropped elements; Munksgaard's ideas have been applied by Axelsson and Munksgaard (58) to a mixed finite-element discretization of the biharmonic operator; Manteuffel (39) uses the original sparsity pattern but adds to the diagonal to maintain stability. Yet another possibility is to exploit the fact that the iteration matrix for symmetric successive over-relaxation is similar to a symmetric positive definite matrix. For a discussion of this technique, see Axelsson (59).

The second promising iterative technique that we wish to mention is applicable to equations that have arisen from finite-element discretization of partial differential equations. It is based on the property that iterative methods reduce highly oscillatory errors much more rapidly than smooth errors. Therefore, after a few iterations have been performed, the residual

$$\{r^{(i)}\} = \{b\} - [A]\{x^{(i)}\} \tag{32}$$

can be represented well on a coarser discretization. The corresponding set of equations

$$[A_1]\{\delta_1^{(i)}\} = \{r_1^{(i)}\} \tag{33}$$

is then solved on the coarse discretization for a correction $\{\delta_1^{(i)}\}$. This correction is extended by interpolation to a correction $\{\delta^{(i)}\}$ for $\{x^{(i)}\}$ on the fine discretization. Of course, the interpolation will introduce oscillatory errors but further iterations will reduce their size. After some more iterations on the fine grid a further correction is calculated by recourse to the coarse grid, and so on until convergence is obtained. In practice the idea is nested; that is, (33) is itself solved by iteration with the aid of a coarser discretization and, of course, it is not necessary to obtain a very accurate solution to (33). For fuller discussions of the technique we refer the reader to Brandt (60, 61). Nicolaides (62) shows the method in a very favorable light and it has been used with success by Bank and Sherman (63). It has been considered for the eigenvalue problem by Hackbush (64). All these authors aim to solve the equations in little more storage than is required to hold the several levels of problems and in a number of operations that is a modest multiple of the number of unknowns, n.

LARGE PROBLEMS

Computers are getting more capabilities and lower price tags, so that what ten years ago might have been regarded as a large out-of-core problem may nowadays be solved on a desktop machine. Virtual memories have become quite common too. It is important to regard a virtual memory as a very convenient way to program input-output and not as a means of providing a huge random-access memory, because truly random fashion, appalling page-thrashing can result. For example, Taylor reports (Du Croz et al. (65)) that a full linear equation solver that accesses elements by rows in FORTRAN can display quite a sharp cut-off between working satisfactorily and, for a slightly larger problem, never producing a result.

Band-matrix techniques are well-suited to efficient input-output provided the active part of the matrix can reside in main store. Frontal schemes have always been intended for efficient two-level working. Provided there is room in main storage for the frontal matrix, the method is efficient, and it handles assembly too, an awkward process out of main storage. Once the front is too big for main storage, however, the simpler frontal scheme is unsatisfactory, because each element is likely to cause the whole front to roll in and out for the sake of a small number of eliminations. Here the substructuring approach looks more attractive because the problem will not hit us until we are assembling massive structures which have many internal variables that can immediately be eliminated.

Iterative methods are far more economical in storage than direct methods and can often be expected to work entirely in main storage. Where they cannot, it is usual to keep the iterates in main storage and read [A] and {b} once per iteration.

The situation with respect to the use of our present algorithms on modern parallel and vector hardware seems to the author to be quite encouraging. The most heavily used loop in band matrix code and frontal code is essentially that of Gaussian elimination on a full matrix, which these machines handle very well.

The assembly loop, on the other hand, is essentially scalar in form but it is not executed nearly so frequently. Where complete processors working in parallel are available, the substructuring approach looks attractive, since each can be working on a separate part of the assembly tree.

ACKNOWLEDGEMENTS

The help from Professor A. Jennings, Dr. I. S. Duff and the referees who read a draft of this chapter and suggested improvements and additional references is greatly appreciated.

REFERENCES

1 Meyer, C., "Solution of Linear Equations - State-of-the-Art," Journal of the Structural Division, ASCE, Vol. 99, No. ST7, July 1973, pp. 1507-1526.

2 Meyer, C., "Special Problems Related to Linear Equation Solvers," Journal of the Structural Division, ASCE, Vol. 101, No. ST4, April 1975, pp. 869-890.

3 Wilkinson, J. H., "Error Analysis of Direct Methods of Matrix Inversion," Journal of ACM, Vol. 8, No. 3, July 1961, pp. 281-330.

4 Wilkinson, J. H., The Algebraic Eigenvalue Problem, 1965, Clarendom Press, Oxford.

5 Reid, J. K., "A Note on the Stability of Gaussian Elimination," Journal Inst. Math. Appl., Vol. 8, No. 3, December 1971, pp. 374-375.

6 Bunch, J. R., "Partial Pivoting Strategies for Symmetric Matrices," SIAM Journal on Numerical Analysis, Vol. 11, No. 3, June 1974, pp. 521-528.

7 Bunch, J. R., Kaufman, L. and Parlett, B. N., "Decomposition of a Symmetric Matrix," Num. Math., Vol. 27, No. 1, 1976, pp. 95-109.

8 Duff, I. S., Reid, J. K., Munksgaard, N. and Nielsen, H. B., "Direct Solution of Sets of Linear Equations Whose Matrix is Sparse, Symmetric and Indefinite," Journal Inst. Math. Appl., Vol. 23, No. 2, March 1979, pp. 235-250.

9 Roy, J. R., "Numerical Error in Structural Solutions," Journal of the Structural Division, ASCE, Vol. 97, No. ST4, April 1971, pp. 1039-1054.

10 Stewart, G. W., Introduction to Matrix Computations, Academic Press, New York, 1973.

11 Forsythe, G. E. and Moler, C. B., Computer Solution of Linear Algebraic Equations, Prentice-Hall, New Jersey, 1967.

12 Marlow, S. and Reid, J. K., "FORTRAN Subroutines for the Solution of Linear Equations, Inversion of Matrices and Evaluation of Determinants," Harwell Report R.6899, HMSO, 1971.

13 Jennings, A., "A Compact Storage Scheme for the Solution of Symmetric Linear Simultaneous Equations," Computer, Vol. 9, No. 3, November 1966, pp. 281-285.

14 George, A. and Liu, J. W. H., "A Note on Fill for Sparse Matrices," SIAM Journal on Numerical Analysis, Vol. 12, No. 3, June 1975, pp. 452-455.

15 Felippa, C. A., "Solution of Linear Equations with Skyline-Stored Symmetric Matrix," Computers and Structures, Vol. 5, No. 1, April 1975, pp. 13-29.

16 Cuthill, E. and McKee, J., "Reducing the Bandwidth of Sparse Symmetric Matrices," Proceedings of the 24th National Conference ACM, Brandon Systems Press, New Jersey, 1969, pp. 157-172.

17 Cuthill, E., "Several Strategies for Reducing the Bandwidth of Matrices," in Sparse Matrices and Their Applications, edited by D. J. Rose and R. A. Willoughby, Plenum Press, New York, 1972, pp. 157-166.

18 Chan, W. M. and George, A., "A Linear Time Implementation of the Reverse Cuthill-McKee Algorithm," BIT, Vol. 20, No. 1, 1980, pp. 8-14.

19 George, J. A., "Computer Implementation of the Finite Element Method," Stanford University, Computer Science Department Report STAN-CS-71-208, 1971.

20 Jennings, A., Matrix Computation for Engineers and Scientists, Wiley, New York, 1977.

21 Collins, R. J., "Bandwidth Reduction by Automatic Renumbering," International Journal for Numerical Methods in Engineering, Vol. 6, No. 3, 1973, pp. 345-356.

22 Gibbs, N. E., Poole, W. G., Jr., and Stockmeyer, P. K., "An Algorithm for Reducing the Bandwidth and Profile of a Sparse Matrix," SIAM Journal Numer. Analysis, Vol. 13, No. 2, April 1976, pp. 236-250.

23 George, A. and Liu, J. W. H., "An Implementation of a Pseudoperipheral Node Finder," ACM Trans. on Math. Software, Vol. 5, No. 3, September 1979, pp. 284-295.

24 Jennings, A. and Tuff, A. D., "A Direct Method for the Solution of Large Sparse Symmetric Simultaneous Equations," in Large Sparse Sets of Linear Equations, edited by J. K. Reid, Academic Press, London, 1971.

25 Wilson, E. L., Bathe, K. J., and Doherty, W. P., "Direct Solution of Large Systems of Linear Equations," Computers and Structures, Vol. 4, No. 2, March 1974, pp. 363-372.

26 Mondkar, D. G. and Powell, G. H., "Large Capacity Equation Solver for Structural Analysis," Computers and Structures, Vol. 4, No. 4, August 1974, pp. 699-728.

27 Irons, B. M., "A Frontal Solution Program for Finite Element Analysis," International Journal for Numerical Methods in Engineering, Vol. 2, No. 1, 1970, pp. 5-32.

28 Hood, P., "Frontal Solution Program for Unsymmetric Matrices," International Journal for Numerical Methods in Engineering, Vol. 10, No. 2, 1976, pp. 379-399.

29 Cliffe, K. A., Jackson, C. P., Rae, J., and Winters, K. H., "Finite Element Flow Modeling Using Velocity and Pressure Variables," Harwell Report R.9202, Oxford, England, 1978.

30 Hopper, M. J., "Harwell Subroutine Library, A Catalogue of Subroutines," Harwell Report R.9185, Oxford England, 1979.

31 Przemieniecki, J. S., "Matrix Structural Analysis of Substructures," AIAA Journal, Vol. 1, No. 1, January 1963, pp. 138-147.

32 Kron, G., Diakoptics, Macdonald, London, 1963.

33 Araldsen, P. O., "An Example of Large-Scale Structural Analysis. Comparison Between Finite Element Calculation and Full-Scale Measurement on Oil Tanker ESSO NORWAY, 1972," Seminar at Det norske Veritas.

34 Noor, A. K., Kamel, H. A., and Fulton, R. E., "Substructuring Techniques - Status and Projections," Computers and Structures, Vol. 8, No. 5, May 1978, pp. 621-632.

35 Dodds, R. H. and Lopez, L. A., "Substructuring in Linear and Nonlinear Analysis," International Journal for Numerical Methods in Engineering, Vol. 15, No. 4, April 1980, pp. 583-597.

36 George, A., "Nested Dissection of a Regular Finite Element Mesh," SIAM Journal Numer. Anal., Vol. 10, No. 2, April 1973, pp. 345-363.

37 George, A. and Liu, J. W. H., "An Automatic Nested Dissection Algorithm for Irregular Finite Element Problems," SIAM Journal Numer. Anal., Vol. 15, No. 5, October 1978, pp. 1053-1069.

38 Eisenstat, S. C., Gursky, M. C., Schultz, M. H., and Sherman, A. H., "The Yale Sparse Matrix Package. I: The Symmetric Codes; and II: The Non-symmetric Codes," Reports 112 and 114, Department of Computer Science, Yale University, New Haven, Connecticut, 1977.

39 Manteuffel, T. A., "An Incomplete Factorization Technique for Positive Definite Linear Systems," Mathematics of Computations, Vol. 34, No. 150, April 1980, pp. 473-497.

40 George, J. A. and Liu, J. W. H., "User Guide for SPARSPAK: Waterloo Sparse Linear Equations Package," University of Waterloo Report CS-78-30, 1978.

41 George, A. and Liu, J. W. H., "The Design of a User Interface for a Sparse Matrix Package," ACM Trans. Math. Software, Vol. 5, No. 2, June 1979, pp. 139-162.

42 Williams, F. W., "Comparison Between Sparse Stiffness Matrix and Sub-structure Methods," International Journal for Numerical Methods in Engineering, Vol. 5, No. 3, January-February 1973, pp. 383-394.

43 George, A. and Liu, J. W. H., "A Minimal Storage Implementation of the Minimum Degree Algorithm," SIAM Journal Numer. Anal., Vol. 17, No. 2, April 1980, pp. 282-299.

44 George, A. and Liu, J. W. H., "A Fast Implementation of the Minimum Degree Algorithm Using Quotient Graphs," ACM Trans. on Math. Software, Vol. 6, No. 3, September 1980, pp. 337-358.

45 Schrem, E., "Computer Implementation of the Finite-Element Procedure," in Numerical and Computer Methods in Structural Mechanics, Academic Press, New York, 1973, pp. 79-121.

46 Varga, R. S., Matrix Iterative Analysis, Prentice-Hall, New Jersey, 1962.

47 Young, D. M., Iterative Solution of Large Linear Systems, Academic Press, New York, 1971.

48 Wachspress, E. L., Iterative Solution of Elliptic Systems, Prentice-Hall, New Jersey, 1966.

49 Walsh, J. E. (Editor), Numerical Analysis - An Introduction, Academic Press, New York, 1966.

50 Hestenes, M. R. and Stiefel, E., "Methods of Conjugate Gradients for Solving Linear Systems," J. Res. Nat. Bur. Standards, Vol. 49, No. 6, December 1952, pp. 409-436.

51 Reid, J. K., "On the Method of Conjugate Gradients for the Solution of Large Sparse Systems of Equations," in Large Sparse Sets of Linear Equations, edited by J. K. Reid, Academic Press, London, 1971, pp. 231-254.

52 Meijerink, J. A. and van der Vorst, H. A., "An Iterative Solution Method for Linear Systems of Which the Coefficient Matrix is a Symmetric M-Matrix," Mathematics of Computations, Vol. 31, No. 137, January 1977, pp. 148-162.

53 Vinsome, P. K. W., "Orthomin, An Iterative Method for Solving Sparse Sets of Simultaneous Linear Equations," Soc. Pet. Eng. of A.I.M.E., 1976, SPE 5729.

54 Dupont, T., Kendall, R. P., and Rachford, H. H., Jr., "An Approximate Factorization Procedure for Solving Self-Adjoint Elliptic Difference Equations," SIAM Journal Numer. Anal., Vol. 5, No. 3, September 1968, pp. 559-573.

55 Gustafsson, I., "A Class of First Order Factorization Methods," BIT, Vol. 18, 1978, pp. 142-156.

56 Jennings, A. and Malik, G. M., "Partial Elimination," Journal Inst. Maths. Appl., Vol. 20, No. 3, November 1977, pp. 307-316.

57 Munksgaard, N., "Solving Sparse Symmetric Sets of Linear Equations by Preconditioned Conjugate Gradients," ACM Trans. Math. Software, Vol. 6, No. 2, June 1980, pp. 206-219.

58 Axelsson, O. and Munksgaard, N., "A Class of Preconditioned Conjugate Gradient Methods for the Solution of a Mixed Finite Element Discretization of the Biharmonic Operator," International Journal for Numerical Methods in Engineering, Vol. 14, No. 7, 1979, pp. 1001-1019.

59 Axelsson, A., "Solution of Linear Systems of Equations: Iterative Methods," in Sparse Matrix Techniques, edited by V. A. Barker, Springer-Verlag, Lecture Notes in Mathematics, Vol. 572, 1976, pp. 1-51.

60 Brandt, A., "Multi-Level Adaptive Techniques (MLAT) for Partial Differential Equations: Ideas and Software," in Mathematical Software III, edited by J. R. Rice, Academic Press, New York, 1977.

61 Brandt, A., "Multi-Level Adaptive Solutions to Boundary-Value Problems," Mathematics of Computations, Vol. 31, No. 138, April 1977, pp. 333-390.

62 Nicolaides, R. A., "On Some Theoretical and Practical Aspects of Multigrid Methods," Mathematics of Computations, Vol. 33, No. 147, July 1979, pp. 933-952.

63 Bank, R. E. and Sherman, A. H., "Algorithmic Aspects of the Multi-Level Solution of Finite Element Equations," in Sparse Matrix Proceedings, edited by I. S. Duff and G. W. Stewart, SIAM, Philadelphia, 1979.

64 Hackbush, W., "On the Computation of Approximate Eigenvalues and Eigenfunctions of Elliptic Operators by Means of a Multigrid Method," SIAM Journal Numer. Anal., Vol. 16, No. 2, April 1979, pp. 201-215.

65 Du Croz, J. J., Nugent, S. M., Reid, J. K., and Taylor, D. B., "Solving Large Full Sets of Linear Equations in a Paged Virtual Store," ACM Trans. Math. Software, Vol. 7, No. 4, December 1981, pp. 527-536.

CHAPTER SEVEN

SOLUTION TECHNIQUES FOR NONLINEAR FINITE ELEMENT EQUATIONS

W. C. Rheinboldt
Department of Mathematics and Statistics
University of Pittsburgh
Pittsburgh, Pennsylvania

E. Riks
National Aerospace Laboratory NLR
The Netherlands

INTRODUCTION

In recent years the nonlinear analysis of structural systems has become increasingly important in many engineering applications. Correspondingly, the literature on nonlinear solution techniques has grown rapidly, and, in the space available here, it would be impossible to give a meaningful survey of this literature. The aim of this chapter is to present an introduction to the terminology and concepts of the numerical analysis of systems of nonlinear equations and to the continuation or incremental techniques for solving the systems arising in many structural applications.

The sources of nonlinearity in structural problems may be classified naturally into four groups (see Refs. [1] and [2]).

(i) Geometric nonlinearity, due to nonlinear strain-displacement relations,

(ii) Material nonlinearity, due to nonlinear constitutive equations,

(iii) Force nonlinearity, due to nonlinear stress boundary conditions,

(iv) Kinematic constraint nonlinearity, due to nonlinear displacement boundary conditions.

The source of nonlinearity affects the form of the resulting nonlinear equations and, hence, influences the effectivity of the solution techniques. The corresponding numerical problems are as yet not completely analyzed and understood. This is particularly true for some of the nonlinearities of type (ii) and (iii), as, for instance, those generated by plasticity or creep behavior. We shall indicate some of these questions, but obviously it would be beyond the scope of this brief overview to enter into details.

In the next section some background material about the numerical analysis of systems of nonlinear equations in several variables is presented. Then some of the iterative methods are discussed which play a role in the solution of the problems arising in structural mechanics and are used for solving such systems. These systems always contain a number of intrinsic parameters representing, for example, load directions and intensities, load points, and physical or geometrical properties. This leads to a discussion of the concept of the solution set as an equilibrium surface in the combined space of behavior variables and parameters. Then the use of natural algorithms for analyzing such equilibrium surfaces, namely the continuation methods or incremental methods, as they are also called, are discussed. Finally, further results, including the computation of limit points and of bifurcation branches, the determination of critical boundaries, errors along the continuation curve, the combination of continuation methods and mesh-refinement, reduction techniques, and some of the questions relating to material nonlinearities are discussed.

NOTATION AND BASIC CONCEPTS

We denote by R^n, the real n-dimensional linear space of all column vectors, as

$$\{x\} = \begin{Bmatrix} x_1 \\ \cdot \\ \cdot \\ \cdot \\ \cdot \\ x_n \end{Bmatrix} \tag{1}$$

Let f_i, $i = 1, \ldots, n$ be n given functions which assign to each $\{x\} \in R^n$ a real number $y_i = f_i\{x\}$. In mathematical terms we say that the f_i are mappings from R^n into R^1 and write this as $f_i : R^n \to R^1$, $i = 1, \ldots, n$. Our basic problem is then to find solutions $\{x\} \in R^n$ of the system of n equations in n unknowns:

$$\begin{aligned} f_1(x_1, \ldots, x_n) &= 0 \\ &\cdot \\ &\cdot \\ &\cdot \\ f_n(x_1, \ldots, x_n) &= 0 \end{aligned} \tag{2}$$

For ease of notation, we introduce the vector function

$$\{F(x)\} = \begin{Bmatrix} f_1(x_1, \ldots, x_n) \\ \cdot \\ \cdot \\ \cdot \\ f_n(x_1, \ldots, x_n) \end{Bmatrix}, \quad \{x\} \in R^n \tag{3}$$

which associates with each vector $\{x\} \in R^n$ another vector $\{F(x)\} \in R^n$ and, hence, represents a mapping $F : R^n \to R^n$ from R^n to R^n. Our system of equations can then be written in the shorter form:

$$\{F(x)\} = \{0\} \tag{4}$$

where $\{0\}$ is the null-vector in R^n.

Simple examples of functions of one variable show that such a system need not have any solution or that it may have any number of them. In particular, in most structural problems the resulting systems (for fixed values of the intrinsic parameters) often have none or many solutions, and in the latter case it is insufficient to compute only one of these solutions. For a discussion of some of the existence results for systems of the form of Eq. (4), see Refs. [3], [4] and [5] which also have extensive references.

As usual, we measure distances in R^n in terms of some norm. The best known of these, of course, is the Euclidean norm

$$\| \{x\} \|_2 = +\sqrt{x_1^2 + x_2^2 + \ldots + x_n^2} \tag{5}$$

but for numerical calculations either one of the norms

$$\| \{x\} \|_1 = |x_1| + |x_2| + \ldots + |x_n|$$

or (6)

$$\| \{x\} \|_\infty = \max(|x_1|, |x_2|, \ldots, |x_n|)$$

is usually more convenient. We will use $\| \{x\} \|$ to denote any one of these norms. The distance between two points $\{x\}$ and $\{y\}$ of R^n is then the number

$$\| \{x\} - \{y\} \| \tag{7}$$

and we can define the open ball centered at $\{y\}$ with radius $r > 0$ as the set

$$\mathcal{B}(\{y\}, r) = \{\{x\} \in R^n; \quad \| \{x\} - \{y\} \| < r\} \tag{8}$$

For the numerical determination of any specific solution $\{x^*\} \in R^n$ of the system (4), it is important to know whether $\{x^*\}$ is an isolated solution, that is, whether there is some ball $\mathcal{B}(\{x^*\}, r)$ with a positive - although possibly small - radius $r > 0$ which contains no other solution of (4) other than $\{x^*\}$. An answer may be obtained from consideration of the derivative or Jacobian of the mapping F. This is the matrix:

$$[DF(x)] = \begin{bmatrix} \frac{\partial f_1}{\partial x_1} & \cdots & \frac{\partial f_1}{\partial x_n} \\ \cdot & & \\ \cdot & & \\ \cdot & & \\ \frac{\partial f_n}{\partial x_1} & \cdots & \frac{\partial f_n}{\partial x_n} \end{bmatrix} \tag{9}$$

formed from all partial derivatives of the component functions $f_1, \ldots, f_n$ of F. The indicated result may now be phrased as follows:

Theorem 1: Suppose that $\{x^*\}$ is a solution of (4) and that all partial derivatives entering into the Jacobian $[DF(x)]$ are continuous functions of $\{x\}$ at the point $\{x^*\}$. If the matrix $[DF(x)]$ is nonsingular, then $\{x^*\}$ is an isolated solution of (4).

This is only a sufficient condition; in other words, a solution may turn out to be isolated even though $[DF(x)]$ has no inverse. For a study of this topic see, for instance, [6]. For our purposes, the result of Theorem 1 is sufficient. In fact, the nonsingularity of the Jacobian at the solution turns out to be a very important condition for most of the subsequent discussions.

Round-off errors may affect the desired result of the numerical computation of a solution of Eq. (4) in many ways. In particular, the evaluation of the component functions $f_1, \ldots, f_n$ of F may be subject to very severe round-off errors. As an example, consider the case $n = 1$ and the polynomial

$$p(x) = x^4 - 202x^3 + 15{,}299x^2 - 514{,}898x + 6{,}497{,}400 \tag{10}$$

which turns out to have the four isolated roots $x^* = 49$, 50, 51, and 52. Yet, if we use the standard Horner algorithm for some values of x between 51.9 and 52.1, then with eight-decimal-digit, rounded arithmetic, we obtain the results shown in Fig. 1. Actually, between each point of the figure there are many further oscillations of the computed function values.

Clearly, there is an uncertainty interval $|x-52| < \delta$ around the root $x^* = 52$ of p where due to round-off we cannot obtain any meaningful values of $p(x)$. In our present case, we do not achieve even one accurate digit for $|x-52| \leq 0.1$.

Generally, a root x^* of a given function F is called ill-conditioned if near x^* we encounter difficulties of the type described here. Ill-conditioning is a qualitative property, and its effect on the computations depends on many factors.

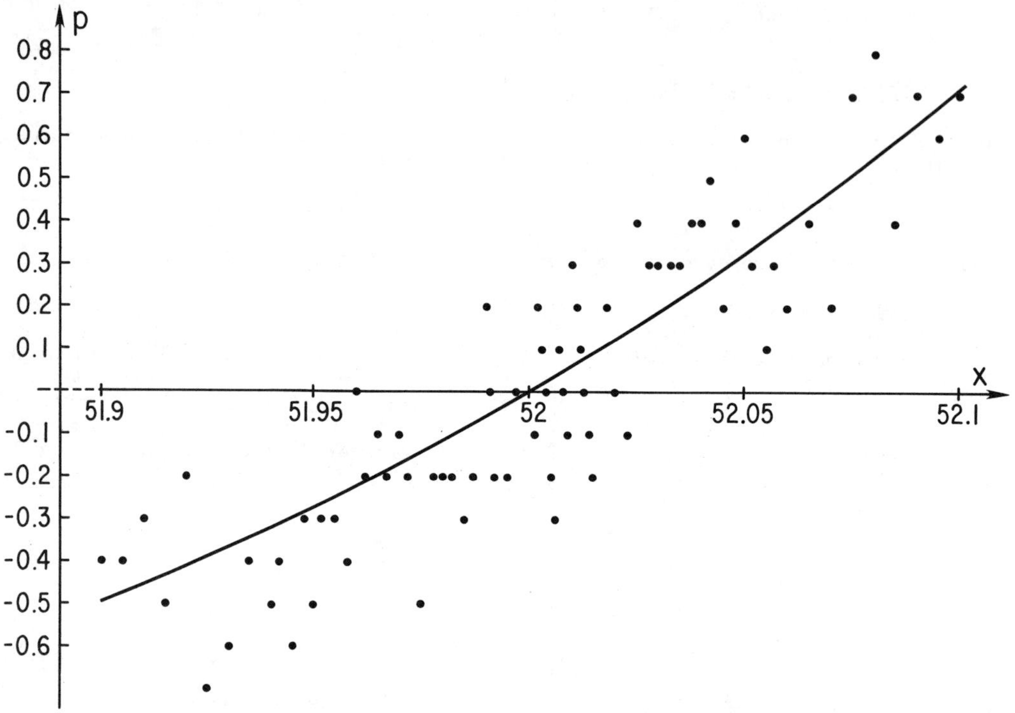

Figure 1 - The effect of ill-conditioning for (10)

One such factor is certainly the precision used in the calculation, as Table 1 shows.

Table 1 - Values of (10) computed with different precision

n decimal digit arithmetic	computed value of p(52.015)	relative error in %
8	-.200 000 00	316.2
10	.950 000 000 0 (-1)	3.789
12	.924 800 000 000 (-1)	0.1652(-1)
14	.924 956 000 000 00 (-1)	0.3237(-4)
19	.924 495 300 625 000 000 0 (-1)	0

Another factor is the algorithm used for the evaluation. For example, in our case, both the shifted form

$$p(52 + \varepsilon) = \varepsilon^4 + 6\varepsilon^3 + 11\varepsilon^2 + 6\varepsilon \tag{11}$$

and the multiplicative form

$$p(x) = (x-49)(x-50)(x-51)(x-52) \tag{12}$$

do not share the difficulties encountered with (10); but, of course, neither one is readily accessible.

Some measures of ill-conditioning of zeros of nonlinear equations have been discussed in Refs. [7] and [8]. All nonisolated roots must be considered ill-conditioned to a certain extent, but our example shows that isolated roots may have this property as well.

SOME ITERATIVE METHODS

Let us consider again the system of n equations in n variables

$$\{F(x)\} = \{0\} \tag{13}$$

with a given mapping $F: R^n \to R^n$. In special cases we may hope to find an explicit expression for a solution $\{x^*\}$. For example, for a linear F there are various elimination processes which produce $\{x^*\}$ after finitely many arithmetic operations; or for $n=1$, and quadratic or cubic polynomials F, explicit formulas for the solutions are known. But in general, the only approach for obtaining $\{x^*\}$ at least approximately is to apply some iterative process.

In principle, an iterative process is any algorithm $\mathcal{J}$ which produces a sequence $\{x^0\}$, $\{x^1\}$, $\{x^2\}$, ... of points in R^n with the property that $\lim_{k\to\infty} \{x^k\} = \{x^*\}$.

There are many different iterative processes and the choice of a specific one depends on many factors, but there exists no best method in any sense. For surveys of iterative methods for equations of the form (13) in R^n see Refs. [3], [4], [5], [9] and [10]. In this chapter we can summarize only a few of the processes that have been applied to structural problems (see also [11]).

As noted before, for linear F we know, at least in principle, how to solve Eq. (13) explicitly. Hence, it is not surprising that a large class of iterative methods for (13) are based on successive linearizations of F. Suppose that $\{x^k\}$ is some approximation of a solution $\{x^*\}$ for (13). Then the central idea of all these linearization methods is the construction of some $n \times n$ matrix $[A_k]$ and of the vector function

$$\{L_k(x)\} = [A_k](\{x\} - \{x^k\}) + \{F(x^k)\} \tag{14}$$

which agrees with F at $\{x^k\}$ and hopefully approximates F in some neighborhood of that point. If $[A_k]$ is a nonsingular matrix, then the equation

$$\{L_k(x)\} = \{0\} \tag{15}$$

has a unique solution, namely; $\{x\} = \{x^k\} - [A_k]^{-1}\{F(x^k)\}$, which we use as the next approximation $\{x^{k+1}\}$ of $\{x^*\}$. In other words, our process may be written in the explicit form

$$\{x^{k+1}\} = \{x^k\} - [A_k]^{-1}\{F(x^k)\},\ k = 0, 1, \ldots \tag{16}$$

where $\{x^0\}$ is a given starting point. For dimension $n=1$ this process is schematically shown in Fig. 2.

Even though Eq. (16) gives $\{x^0\}$, $\{x^1\}$, ... explicitly, this formula represents a poor way to proceed computationally. In fact, the explicit evaluation of an inverse matrix should be avoided wherever possible. It is not only more costly than a direct solution of a system of linear equations, but for large dimensions n and sparse matrices $[A_k]$, as they occur in structural mechanics, the inverse $[A_k]^{-1}$ is usually a full matrix with few zeros.

In a schematic language, an algorithm for a linearization process may be written about as follows:

1. Input $\{x, \varepsilon_{abs}, \varepsilon_{rel}, k_{max}\}$;

   <Initialization>

2. Evaluate $\{F(x)\}$;

3. k: = 0;

<Main loop>

4. Construct the approximating matrix [A];

5. Use elimination to decompose the matrix [A];

6. If [A] turns out to be numerically singular, then "error return (1)";

7. Use back-substitutions to solve the linear system $[A]\{y\} = \{F(x)\}$;

8. $\{x\}: = \{x\} - \{y\}$;

9. Evaluate $\{F(x)\}$;

<Test for acceptability>

10. If $(\|\{F(x)\}\| \leq \varepsilon_{abs})$ and $(\|\{y\}\| \leq \varepsilon_{abs} + \varepsilon_{rel}\|\{x\}\|)$, then "return with {x} as solution";

<Test for maximal number of iterative steps>

11. If $(k \geq k_{max})$ then "error return (2)";

12. k: = k + 1;

13. Go to 4.

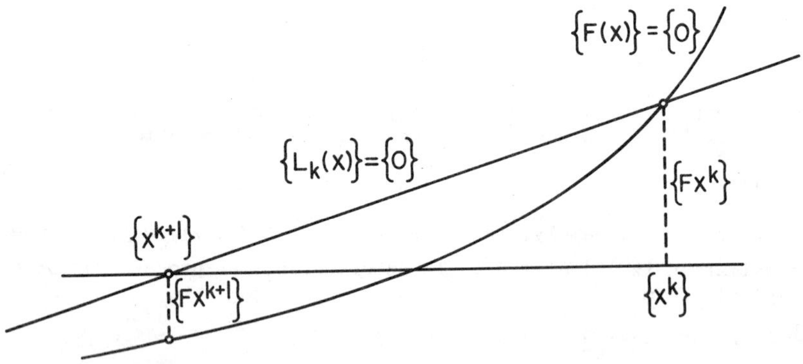

Figure 2 - Schematic step of a linearization method

The simplest choice of the approximating matrices $[A_k]$ in a linearization process such as (16) is a constant, nonsingular matrix $[A_o]$. These are the so-called parallel-chord methods, a name derived from the fact that for $n = 1$ the lines defined by the L_k will all be parallel. The use of a constant matrix has obvious advantages; in fact, in our algorithm it allows us to take the steps 4, 5 and 6 out of the main loop and then to change step 13 to, say, "Go to 7". Clearly, this may produce considerable savings, since the decomposition of a (full) $n \times n$ matrix requires of the order of n^3 arithmetic operations, while the backsubstitutions of step 7 use only of the order of n^2 operations.

A familiar parallel chord process arises when F can be written in the form

$$\{F(x)\} = [B]\{x\} - \{G(x)\} \tag{17}$$

where [B] is a nonsingular matrix and G a nonlinear mapping. In that case with the choice $[A_o] = [B]$ the linearization process reduces to

$$\{x^{k+1}\} = \{x^k\} - [B]^{-1}\{F(x)\} = [B]^{-1}\{G(x)\}, \; k = 0, 1, \ldots \tag{18}$$

A special case of this arises when [B] is the identity matrix [I], and hence, equation (13) has the form

$$\{x\} = \{G(x)\} \tag{19}$$

Then (18) becomes the process of successive approximations

$$\{x^{k+1}\} = \{G(x^k)\}, \; k = 0, 1, \ldots \;. \tag{20}$$

Clearly, the linearization L_k of F given in (14) cannot be expected to approximate F well when the $[A_k]$ are held fixed. A linearization which is better in this respect is derived from the first order Taylor approximation

$$\{F(x)\} \approx \{F(x^k)\} + [DF(x^k)](\{x\} - \{x^k\}) \tag{21}$$

involving the Jacobian matrix (9); in this case we use the matrices $[A_k] = [DF(x^k)]$ and the process (16) becomes the familiar Newton method

$$\{x^{k+1}\} = \{x^k\} - [DF(x^k)]^{-1}\{F(x^k)\}, \; k = 0, 1, \ldots \tag{22}$$

Since the evaluation of the Jacobians may be very costly, many variations of Newton's method have been proposed. The simplest is the parallel chord method with $[A_o] = [DF\{x^o\}]$, often called the modified or simplified Newton method. If $[DF\{x\}]$ is not explicitly available, then we may consider the linearization methods (16) in which $[A_k]$ is a discrete approximation of $[DF\{x^k\}]$ as, for example, the matrix $[A_k]$ with the elements

$$a_{ij}^{(k)} = \frac{1}{h_k}\left(f_i(x_1^k, \ldots, x_{j-1}^k, x_j^k + h_k, x_{j+1}^k, \ldots, x_n^k) - f_i(x_1^k, \ldots, x_n^k)\right) \tag{23}$$

$$i, j = 1, \ldots, n$$

with suitably small $h_k > 0$. Obviously, other discretizations of the n^2 partial derivatives occurring in $[DF\{x^k\}]$ may be chosen. For large sparse matrices a controlling issue here is the number of evaluations of F. Let $\{e^1\}, \ldots, \{e^n\}$ denote the natural basis vectors of R^n; that is, all components of $\{e^i\}$ are zero except for the i-th one which equals one. Then the i-th column of the matrix $[A_k]$ with the elements of Eq. (23) is the vector

$$\{F(x^k + h_k e^j)\} - \{F(x^k)\} \tag{24}$$

We require (n+1) function evaluations of F to compute $[A_k]$. For sparse matrices this can be reduced considerably, as was first observed in [12]. In brief, select a subset of columns of $[DF(x^k)]$ such that any row of the matrix has at most one nonzero element in these columns. From the remaining columns select another subset with the same properties, and continue this process until no more columns remain. For example, for a tri-diagonal matrix,

$$
\begin{bmatrix}
a_{11} & a_{12} & & & \\
a_{21} & a_{22} & a_{23} & 0 & \\
 & a_{32} & a_{33} & & \\
 & & & & a_{n-1,n} \\
 & 0 & & a_{n,n-1} & a_{nn}
\end{bmatrix} \tag{25}
$$

we may use columns 1, 4, 7, ... as the first set, columns 2, 5, 8, ... as the second, and columns 3, 6, 9, ... as the third. Generally, let the ℓ-th set contain the columns with the indices i_1, i_2, ... and introduce the vector $\{d^\ell\} = \{e^{i_1}\} + \{e^{i_2}\} + \ldots$. Then the difference

$$\{F(x^k + h_k d^\ell)\} - \{F(x^k)\}$$

defines all nonzero elements of the difference-approximation of $[DF(x^k)]$ in the columns of the ℓ-th set. Hence, if there were altogether q sets of columns, then we obtain a difference approximation of $[DF(x^k)]$ with $q+1$ function evaluations. For instance, our tridiagonal example (25) would require four function evaluations. This technique can provide considerable savings and its use may make the discretized Newton method a very attractive process. For some applications of this approach to structural problems we refer to [13].

When the basic equations (13) have a special form, as in the cases of Eqs. (17) and (19), then other linearizations are often natural. In particular, in structural applications the mapping F frequently has the so-called quasilinear form

$$\{F(x)\} = [B(x)]\{x\} - \{G(x)\} \tag{26}$$

where $[B(x)]$ is now an $n \times n$ matrix with elements that depend on $\{x\}$. In generalizing Eq. (18) we may then choose $[A_k] = [B(x^k)]$, in which case the linearization process (16) becomes

$$\{x^{k+1}\} = \{x^k\} - [B(x^k)]^{-1}\{F(x^k)\} = [B(x^k)]^{-1}\{G(x^k)\}, \; k = 0, 1, \ldots. \tag{27}$$

In finite displacement analysis we have usually

$$[B(x)] = [K] + [N(x)] \tag{28}$$

where K is the linear stiffness matrix while N incorporates the higher order (geometric) stiffness terms. Then Eq. (27) is the so-called direct iteration. Of course, with Eq. (28) we may also write F in the form of Eq. (27) with $[B] \equiv [K]$ and $\{G(x)\}$ replaced by $\{G(x)\} - [N(x)]\{x\}$. The corresponding parallel chord method (28) is sometimes termed the simplified direct iteration.

To see how these two processes for Eq. (26) compare with Newton's method for the same equation, suppose that $[B(x)]$ has the elements $b_{ij}(x_1,\ldots,x_n)$, $i,j = 1,\ldots,n$, then the Jacobian of (26) is

$$[DF(x)] = [B(x)] + [DB(x)]\{x\} \tag{29}$$

where

$$[DB(x)]\{x\} = [\sum_{\ell=1}^{n} \frac{\partial}{\partial x_j} b_{i\ell}(x_1,\ldots,x_n)x_\ell;\; i,j = 1,\ldots,n] \tag{30}$$

Hence, the direct iteration (Eq. (27)) is obtained from Newton's method (22) by dropping the term $[DB(x)]\{x\}$ in the definition of the Jacobian (Eq. (29)). In other words, we suppose here that the first order changes of the stiffness matrix with respect to $\{x\}$ are not too rapid.

Finally, a class of linearization methods in which the matrices $[A_k]$ or their inverses are updated from step to step should be mentioned. A survey of such quasi-Newton methods is given in Ref. [14]. One of the oldest of these methods is the so-called DFP-process, [15], which has the basic form of Eq. (16) with $[A_k]^{-1} = [H_k]$ where the matrices $[H_k]$ are updated by the formula

$$[H_{k+1}] = [H_k] + \frac{1}{\{s^k\}^T\{y^k\}} \{s^k\}\{s^k\}^T - \frac{1}{\{y^k\}^T[H_k]\{y^k\}} [H_k]\{y^k\}\{y^k\}^T[H_k] \quad (31)$$

with

$$\{s^k\} = \{x^{k+1}\} - \{x^k\}, \quad \{y^k\} = \{F(x^{k+1})\} - \{F(x^k)\} \quad (32)$$

In most applications this update formula has been superseded by the BFGS formula ([16], [17], [18], [19])

$$[H_{k+1}] = ([I] - \frac{\{s^k\}\{y^k\}^T}{\{y^k\}^T\{s^k\}})[H_k]([I] - \frac{\{y^k\}\{s^k\}^T}{\{y^k\}^T\{s^k\}}) + \frac{\{s^k\}^T\{s^k\}}{\{y^k\}^T\{s^k\}} \quad (33)$$

Both choices satisfy the basic secant condition

$$[H_{k+1}]\{y^k\} = \{s^k\} \quad (34)$$

which ensures that the updated matrix is consistent with the step $\{s^k\}$ and the corresponding change of F.

Evidently, if H_k is symmetric, then for both formulas the updated matrix $[H_{k+1}]$ is again symmetric. Moreover, it can be shown that when $[H_k]$ is also positive definite then both updated matrices $[H_{k+1}]$ will be positive definite (in real arithmetic) if and only if $\{y^k\}^T\{s^k\} > 0$. However, in general, neither one of the formulas preserves the sparsity of the matrices involved. For the high-dimensional problems arising in structural mechanics this is a severe handicap. Several approaches have been discussed in the literature for exploiting sparsity in the matrix updating process; we mention here only Refs. [20], [21], [22], [23], [24] and [25]. Numerical results for structural problems with some of these strategies are given in Ref. [13]. It appears that for highly non-linear, large-scale problems these approaches do not perform, as yet, very satisfactorily.

Both formulas (31) and (33) are based on additive corrections of rank two. It is also possible to use multiplicative corrections; for instance, the BFGS-update may be written in the form

$$[H_{k+1}] = ([I] + \{u^k\}\{v^k\}^T)[H_k]([I] + \{v^k\}\{u^k\}^T) \quad (35)$$

with

$$\{u^k\} = \frac{1}{\{s^k\}^T\{y^k\}} \{s^k\}$$

$$\{v^k\} = \{F(x^k)\}\left((1+\{s^k\}\left(\frac{\{F(x^k)\}^T[H_k]\{y^k\}}{\{s^k\}^T\{F(x^k)\}}\right)^{1/2}\right) - \{F(x^{k+1})\} \quad (36)$$

The advantage of this formulation is that the matrix multiplications need not be carried out. Instead, only the vectors $\{u^k\}$ and $\{v^k\}$ are stored and used in the next iteration. Except for possible multiplications involving $[H_o]$, this requires only evaluations of terms of the form

$$([I] + \{a\}\{b\}^T)\{c\} \quad (37)$$

each of which needs 2n multiplications. If the number of iteration steps is not too large, the resulting total work is rather modest. The approach appears to show considerable promise for structural applications. As discussed in

Refs. [26], [27], [28] and [29] such tests have been carried out on the ADINA system and the method has become part of that system [30] and [31].

Three principal questions arise in connection with any iterative process for solving Eq. (13); namely:

(i) Is the process well-defined, that is, can it be continued to a satisfactory end?

(ii) Do the iterates converge and, if so, is the limit a solution of (13)?

(iii) How economical is the entire operation?

In most instances, only partial answers can be given to these questions. For example, for linearization processes of the form (16), the first question asks, for instance, whether all the matrices $[A_k]$ are nonsingular. Except in special cases, it is difficult to specify the set of initial data for which this can be guaranteed. The answers to the second question are convergence theorems for the particular method under consideration. The most frequent and usually simplest of these convergence results are the local attraction theorems. Generally, an iterative process $\mathcal{J}$ is locally convergent at the point x^* if there exists a ball $\mathcal{B}(x^*,r)$ with a positive radius $r > 0$ such that when started anywhere in $\mathcal{B}(x^*,r)$, the iterates of $\mathcal{J}$ are well-defined and converge to x^*. As an example we cite a classical result of this type for Newton's method:

<u>Theorem 2</u>: Let F be continuously differentiable and x^* a solution of (13) where the Jacobian $[DF(x^*)]$ is nonsingular. Then Newton's method (22) is locally convergent at x^*.

These local theorems are very important for the theory of the particular processes but they are of little help for the applications. In general, the radius $r > 0$ of a local attraction ball $\mathcal{B}(x^*,r)$ turns out to be rather small, and hence, the theorem guarantees only that the process will converge to x^* if it is started very close to that point. At the same time, without severe restrictions on the properties of F it is rarely possible to assure convergence in a much larger domain.

The third question concerns the computational complexity of a process and is at present the least well-understood one among the three. We may distinguish several interrelated subquestions:

(i) What is the "cost" of any one step of the iterative process?

(ii) How "fast" does the sequence converge?

(iii) How "sensitive" is the process to changes of the operator or the initial data and how does it behave in spaces with different dimensions?

These questions are only meaningful once quantitative measures are specified for the terms "cost", "fast", and "sensitive". No entirely satisfactory definition has been found for the first and third of these terms. Once again, the last of the questions is the least explored one among the three, and yet, this general question of stability plays a most central role, since many of the algorithms now in use are decidedly sensitive to certain changes.

The term "fast" is usually specified only in an asymptotic sense. In other words, for any sequence of iterates $\{x^k\}$ generated by $\mathcal{J}$ and converging to $\{x^*\}$, statements are made about the behavior of the errors $\varepsilon_k = \| \{x^k\} - \{x^*\} \|$, $k = 0,1, \ldots$, when k tends to infinity. Various measures of asymptotic rates of convergence have been proposed in the literature; for a general account see Ref. [3]. Only a few typical results are given here as examples.

Let the process $\mathcal{J}$ have the general form

$$\{x^{k+1}\} = \{T(x^k)\}, \quad k = 0,1,\ldots. \tag{38}$$

This includes most of the methods mentioned before, such as the parallel chord methods (18), Newton's method (22), and the direct iteration (27). The behavior of the errors ε_k is essentially controlled here by the spectral radius of the Jacobian of T. Recall that for any $n \times n$ matrix [A] the spectral radius $\rho(A)$ is the maximum of all the eigenvalues of A in modulus.

Theorem 3: Let T: $R^n \to R^n$ be continuously differentiable in a neighborhood of the point $\{x^*\}$ where $\{x^*\} = \{T(x^*)\}$ and the spectral radius $\sigma = \rho(DT(x^*))$ satisfies $\sigma < 1$. Then the process (38) is locally convergent at $\{x^*\}$. Moreover, for any sequence $\{x^*\}$ converging to $\{x^*\}$ and any $\delta > 0$, $0 < \sigma + \delta < 1$, there exists an integer $k_o = k_o(\delta) \geq 0$ such that

$$\| \{x^k\} - \{x^*\} \| \leq (\sigma + \delta)^k, \quad k = k_o, k_o + 1, \dots \tag{39}$$

The inequality (39) asserts that the errors tend to zero at least as quickly as the numbers in the geometric sequence $\{\alpha^k\}$ with $\alpha = \sigma + \delta < 1$. This type of convergence is called linear, and for $\sigma = 0$ in (39) we speak of superlinear convergence. It turns out that, under the assumptions of Theorem 2, the iterates produced by Newton's method converge superlinearly.

The inequality (39) represents a so-called ratio-measure of the rate of convergence. Another approach is to work with inequalities between the errors ε_{k+1} and ε_k of two successive iterates. This leads to the so-called quotient measures. A typical result follows.

Theorem 4: Let T: $R^n \to R^n$ be twice continuously differentiable in a neighborhood of the point $\{x^*\}$ where $x^* = Tx^*$ and $[DT(x^*)] = 0$. Then, by Theorem 3 the process (38) is locally convergent at x^*, and in this case any sequence $\{x^*\}$ started inside the local convergence ball satisfies

$$\| \{x^{k+1}\} - \{x^*\} \| \leq \gamma \| \{x^k\} - \{x^*\} \|^2, \quad k = 0, 1, \dots \tag{40}$$

Sequences satisfying Eq. (40) are said to be (at least) quadratically convergent (under the quotient measure). Theorem 4 applies directly to Newton's method; in fact, it is not difficult to show that for it the Jacobian of the iteration function T is zero at x^*. In other words, as a direct corollary of the theorem we have the following result.

Theorem 5: Let F: $R^n \to R^n$ be twice continuously differentiable in a neighborhood of a point $x^* \in R^n$ where $[DF(x^*)]$ is nonsingular. Then Newton's method is locally convergent at x^* and any sequence $\{x^k\}$ started in the local convergence ball satisfies Eq. (40).

The quadratic convergence of Newton's method asserted in this theorem represents one of the principal reasons for its relatively widespread use. In contrast, the parallel chord methods are only linearly convergent, the quasi-Newton methods usually show only superlinear convergence, and the convergence of the discretized Newton methods can be made quadratic only for very special choices of the discretizations, although it is, in general, somewhat better than superlinear.

PARAMETRIZED SYSTEMS

In the previous sections we reviewed some basic aspects of the solution of nonlinear equations without special reference to the physical models they represent. We will now discuss the more particular problem of the solution of equations that govern the behavior of a mechanical system.

The term "behavior" is used here to mean the deformation of the structure in response to the action of external influence quantities such as loads, changes in material properties, and geometrical data, etc. This means that the equations which govern the deformation or behavior variables also depend on a set of influence parameters.

We will denote such a system of equations by

$$\{F(q,\lambda)\} = \{0\} \tag{41}$$

where the vector $\{q\} \in R^n$ represents the deformation variables, $\{\lambda\} \in R^m$ the influence parameters, and F is now a nonlinear mapping F: $R^n \times R^m \rightarrow R^n$ from R^{n+m} into R^n. The study of the response of a given mechanical system thus involves determination of the solutions $(\{q\},\{\lambda\}) \in R^n \times R^m$ of (41) under variation of $\{\lambda\}$.

In analogy to the Jacobian (9) we have to consider now the $n \times (n+m)$ derivative of F

$$[DF(q,\lambda)] = \begin{bmatrix} \frac{\partial f_1}{\partial q_1} \cdots\cdots \frac{\partial f_1}{\partial q_n} & \frac{\partial f_1}{\partial \lambda_1} \cdots\cdots \frac{\partial f_1}{\partial \lambda_m} \\ \vdots \qquad\quad \vdots & \vdots \qquad\quad \vdots \\ \frac{\partial f_n}{\partial q_1} \cdots\cdots \frac{\partial f_n}{\partial q_n} & \frac{\partial f_n}{\partial \lambda_1} \cdots\cdots \frac{\partial f_n}{\partial \lambda_m} \end{bmatrix} \tag{42}$$

For rectangular matrices such as this it makes no sense to speak of nonsingularity. Instead, we are interested in points where the rank of $[DF(q,\lambda)]$, namely, the number of linearly independent columns, is maximal. Of course, the rank can be at most equal to n and, hence, we call a solution $(\{q\},\{\lambda\}) \in R^n \times R^m$ of (41) regular if rank $[DF(q,\lambda)] = n$.

In general, there are many regular solutions of (41). In fact, if all partial derivatives occurring in Eq. (42) are continuous, then the set of all regular solutions of (41) in $R^n \times R^m$ represents a so-called m-dimensional manifold (of class C^1) in $R^n \times R^m$, which, loosely speaking, is a smooth m-dimensional surface in $n+m$ dimensional space. This solution set is now usually called the equilibrium surface of the mechanical system (see, e.g., Refs. [32], [33], [34], and [35]). Such equilibrium surfaces have been considered also - albeit implicitly - in the context of imperfection sensitivity studies (see, e.g., Refs. [36], [37], [38], [39], [40], [41], and [42]).

Naturally, the more free parameters come into play, the more involved the computation of such a surface will become. This means that in most practical situations, one tries to obtain only the most relevant parts of the solution surface. The standard approach is to restrict the variation of the parameter vector $\{\lambda\}$ to the variation of one component at a time or to a variation of all m components as prescribed functions $\lambda_i = \lambda_i(\eta)$, $i = 1,\ldots, m$, of a single variable $\eta \in R^1$. In either case, the solutions of (41) corresponding to the chosen combination of parameter values with one degree of freedom constitute a curve on the equilibrium surface of the system.

From a mathematical viewpoint the restriction to a combination of parameter values with one degree of freedom is equivalent to the reduction of our basic problem (41) to the case of one parameter. In other words, we are led to the most common case of study, equations of the form

$$\{F(q,\lambda)\} = \{0\}, \quad \{q\} \in R^n, \quad \lambda \in R^1 \tag{43}$$

where now the nonlinear function F maps $R^n \times R^1$ into R^n. In many applications the single parameter represents the intensity of a load system to which the structure under study is subjected. The load can correspond to a set of tractions, prescribed displacements, or it can be the result of a temperature distribution, etc.

As noted already, the solutions of Eq. (43) define a curve. More specifically, the regular solutions, $(\{q\},\lambda) \in R^n \times R^1$, of (43) constitute a one-dimensional manifold in $R^n \times R^1$. Such a manifold has to be a smooth, one-to-one image either of a segment of the real line or of a circle. In other words, it is either an open-ended curve segment or a closed curve, and it cannot cross itself. A simple (nonmechanical) example is given by the equation

$$4q^2 - 8q + \lambda^2 = 0, \quad q \in R^1, \quad \lambda \in R^1 \tag{44}$$

for which the solution-curve is the ellipse in Fig. 3.

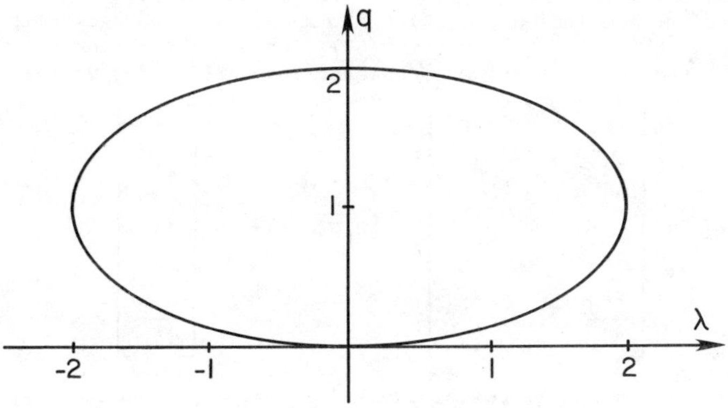

Fig. 3 - The solution curve of Eq. (44)

In order to start the computation of any such solution curve we must know at least one point on it; that is, we need to know at least one (regular) solution $(\{q^o\},\lambda_o) \in R^n \times R^1$ of (43). In practice, the equations usually are defined such that

$$[F(0,0)] = 0 \tag{45}$$

If $\{q\}$ represents a deformation vector and λ a load intensity, then this means simply that in the unloaded case the structure is undeformed. We call $(\{0\},0)$ our starting point.

In practice, we wish to compute some segment of the solution curve beginning with the starting point. In general, the segment of interest is characterized by the requirement for information about the extent to which the load can be applied before the structure will reach the limit of acceptable deformation. This limit may be determined by, for instance, bounds put on the deformations themselves, or by bounds on the induced stresses, or - and this is often the more intricate situation - by bounds that originate from stability considerations. In the latter case, the limits of deformation are very much determined by the shape of the solution curve itself (see Refs. [32], [36], [37] and [39]). We shall return to these stability concepts later.

When Eq. (45) holds, then for increasing load intensities $\lambda > 0$ the structure is expected to be loaded with a response $\{q\} \neq \{0\}$. Accordingly, it is often assumed that the desired segment of the solution-curve can be written in the form

$$\{q\} = \{q(\lambda)\}, \quad \lambda \in [0,\lambda^*] \tag{46}$$

But already the example in Fig. 3 shows that, in general, not every segment of the solution curve of Eq. (43) can be represented by Eq. (46). For instance, any segment of the ellipse which includes either one of the points $q = 1$, $\lambda = 2$ or $q = 1$, $\lambda = -2$ cannot be parametrized in terms of the parameter λ. A more general representation of the solution-curve has the form

$$\{q\} = \{q(s)\}, \quad \lambda = \lambda(s), \quad s \in [0,s^*] \tag{47}$$

where s is a suitable parameter. A possible choice for s, not restricted to any particular segment of the curve, is the arc length or chord length. But often other parameters are available and more practical. For instance, in the case of Eq. (44), we may consider the representation

$$q = 1 - \cos s, \quad \lambda = 2\sin s, \quad s \in [0,2\pi] \tag{48}$$

of the solution which is valid for the entire ellipse of Fig. 3.

By definition, a solution $(\{q\},\lambda) \in R^n \times R^1$ of (43) is regular if the $n \times (n+1)$ matrix $[DF(q,\lambda)]$, (the matrix (42) with $m=1$) has rank n. The first n columns of (42) and the last column represent the partial derivatives

$$[D_qF(q,\lambda)] = \begin{bmatrix} \frac{\partial f_1}{\partial q_1} & \cdots\cdots & \frac{\partial f_1}{\partial q_n} \\ \cdot & & \cdot \\ \cdot & & \cdot \\ \cdot & & \cdot \\ \frac{\partial f_n}{\partial q_1} & \cdots\cdots & \frac{\partial f_n}{\partial q_n} \end{bmatrix}, \quad [D_\lambda F(q,\lambda)] = \begin{bmatrix} \frac{\partial f_1}{\partial \lambda} \\ \cdot \\ \cdot \\ \cdot \\ \frac{\partial f_n}{\partial \lambda} \end{bmatrix} \tag{49}$$

of F with respect to q and λ, respectively. In structural mechanics, $[D_qF(q,\lambda)]$ corresponds to the so-called current stiffness matrix and $[D_\lambda F(q,\lambda)]$ to the current load direction.

Clearly any solution $(\{\hat{q}\},\hat{\lambda}) \in R^n \times R^1$ of (43) where $[D_qF(\hat{q},\hat{\lambda})]$ is nonsingular must be regular. Moreover, by Theorem 1 the solution $\{q\} = \{\hat{q}\}$ of the equation $[F(q,\hat{\lambda})] = [0]$ is isolated. On the other hand, a solution $(\{q\},\lambda)$ of (43) may well be regular even though $[D_qF(q,\lambda)]$ is singular. Such solutions are called limit points or turning points. They have to be distinguished from the singular points of the system, that is, the solutions $(\{q\},\lambda)$ where the $n \times (n+1)$ matrix $[DF(q,\lambda)]$ has a rank less than n.

At any of the critical points, that is, at any limit point or singular point encountered on the solution curve, the mechanical structure may suffer a loss of stability. Such a loss of stability actually corresponds to a dynamical phenomenon whereby the structure undergoes a "sudden" change of deformation. The dynamics of this phenomenon are not described by the equations (41) or (43), but it is possible to deduce from the shape of the static equilibrium solution(s) what type of "sudden" changes may be expected. We illustrate this with some typical examples.

In the example in Fig. 4 the point denoted by (1) is a limit point. Increase of the load intensity λ beyond the value λ_c results in a jump from (1) to (presumably) (2). This type of behavior is called a snap-through, snapping or collapse. An assessment of the seriousness of the situation usually requires the knowledge of the solution curve past the limit point (1) as indicated in the figure. This is a case where the parametrization (46) of the curve certainly leads to difficulties.

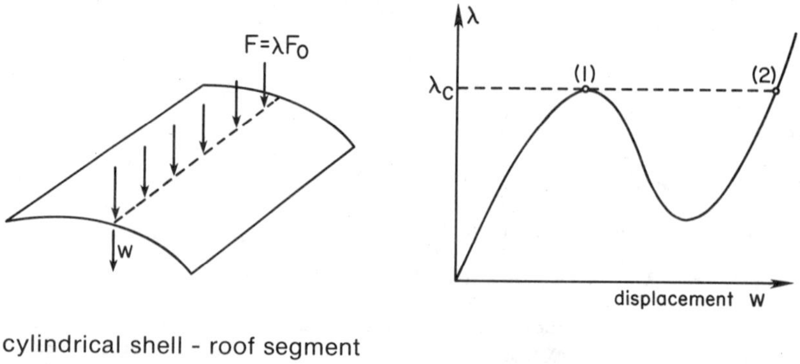

Fig. 4 - Collapse Behavior

A second example is given in Fig. 5. In this case, the solution corresponding to the point (1) is a singular solution as evidenced by the intersection of the two solution curves, which is impossible at a regular solution. In this case, the instability phenomenon is related to the bifurcation of the solutions at (1). This behavior is called buckling. It is well known that stable and unstable forms of bifurcation can be encountered. A classical example of the first type is shown in Fig. 5. Buckling in this case means a distinct change in the character of the deformation when the load intensity λ passes the bifurcation or buckling load λ_c, but it does not lead to failure of the structure at this point. On the other hand, the second type of buckling behavior, pictured in Fig. 6, is also violent. In this case we observe a dynamic departure from the bifurcation point to some other state (presumably the equilibrium state (2)).

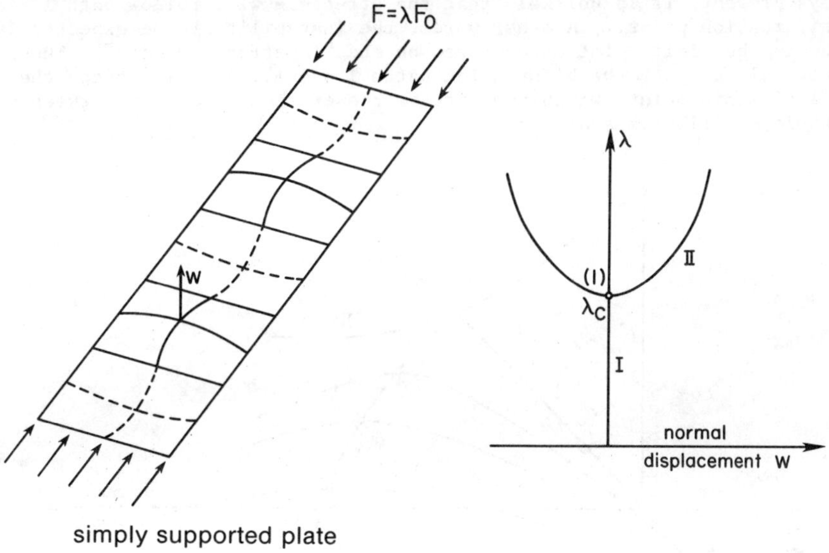

Fig. 5 - Stable Buckling

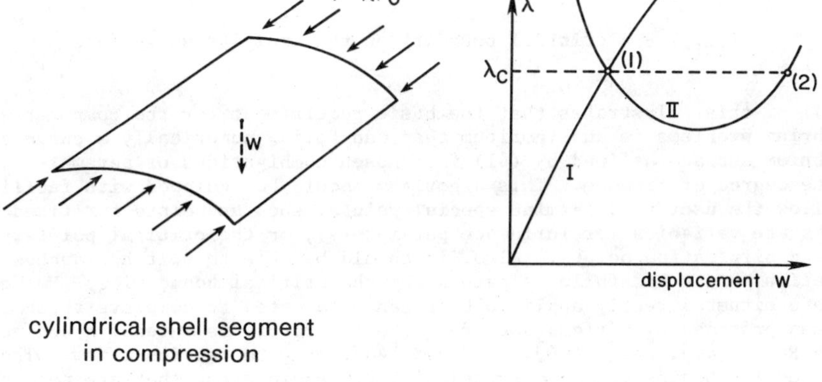

Fig. 6 - Unstable Buckling

The geometrical shape of the bifurcation branch II is the determining factor in the question of whether the bifurcation point is stable or not. Stable points do not have branches that exist simultaneously for values of λ below λ_c in some small neighborhood of the bifurcation point (see, e.g., Refs. [36], [37] and [43]).

All of these observations indicate that for a proper understanding of a given problem it is necessary to obtain a complete picture of the "solution field" of (43). At the same time we have to recall that (43) was actually obtained from (41) by introducing a combination of parameter values with one degree of freedom. In other words, for a more profound understanding of the behavior of a mechanical system we should analyze the shape of the full equilibrium surface. For instance, if the parameter μ denotes the magnitude of some deviations from the cylindrical shape of the panel of Fig. 6, then the solution curves for various fixed values $\mu_1, \mu_2, \mu_3, \ldots$ of μ have a form as shown in Fig. 7. Since small imperfections are always present, it is unlikely that the structure will follow path I leading to the bifurcation point. In other words, the instability to be expected is probably due to the limit point encountered on the "imperfection path". Thus, we should not only compute the bifurcation paths I and II, but also trace the curve III of limit points which constitutes the critical boundary between stable and unstable equilibrium states.

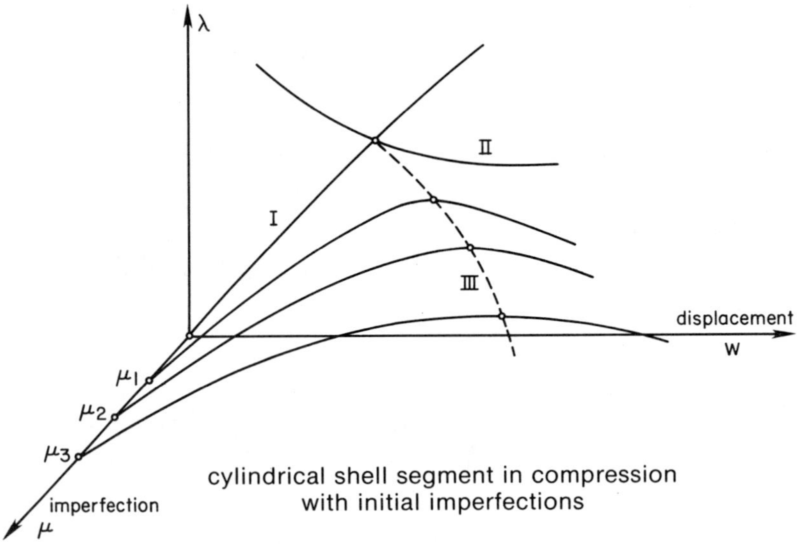

Fig. 7 - A critical boundary on the equilibrium surface

All of this illustrates that the basic requirement for the computation of equilibrium problems is an algorithm that can follow numerically a curve on the equilibrium surface defined by (41) for chosen combinations of parameter values with one degree of freedom. This algorithm should be equipped with facilities that allow the user to determine special points, such as points for fixed values of the state variables (or influence parameters), or the critical points, that is, limit and bifurcation points. Also, it should be able to switch branches at bifurcation points and follow a path along the critical boundaries. Methods which are either directly applicable or can be adopted to complete these tasks have been proposed by various authors. The literature is extensive and we refer here to Refs. [44], [45], [46], [47] and [48], only to mention a few. The following section begins with a discussion of the basic steps that are necessary for tracing a single solution curve.

represents the normal to the surface at the point $\{x\}$. If $\{x\} = \{x(s)\}$ is a point on the curve (50), and $\theta(s)$ is the angle between $\{N\}$ and the tangent $\{\dot{x}(s)\}$, then it can be shown that (54) is nonsingular exactly if

$$|\theta(s)| \neq \pi/2 \tag{56}$$

Two typical situations are sketched in Fig. 8.

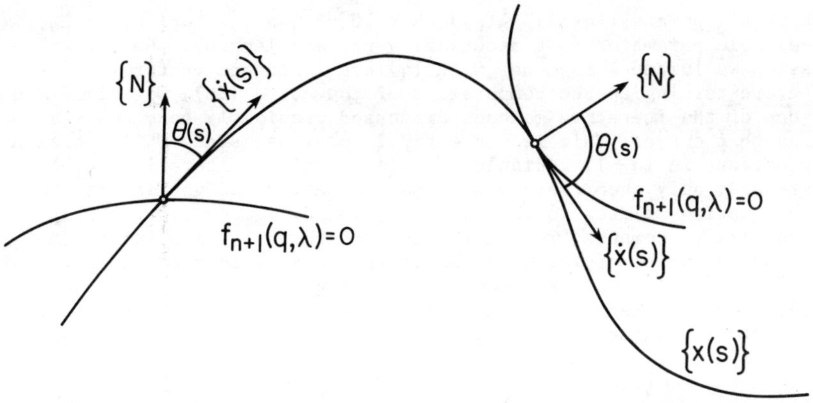

Fig. 8 - Failure of a choice of augmenting equation

Once an appropriate augmented system of equations (51) has been selected, we can apply one of the iterative methods discussed before to compute the desired solution of (51). Thus, the computation of a point on the curve consists of the following steps:

(i) Select an augmented system (51) that defines the point on the curve;

(ii) Construct a suitable approximation of the desired point from where an iterative process may be started; and,

(iii) Start from the approximate point and apply some iterative process to solve the equations.

In general, the applicable iterative processes are only locally convergent and, hence, the selection of the starting point is a critical question. As a consequence, the solution points on the curve are hardly ever obtained in any arbitrary order. Instead, we proceed sequentially along the curve and utilize information about earlier computed points to aid in the computation of the next one. More specifically, suppose that, in terms of the representation (50), we have already computed the points

$$\{x^{(i)}\} = \{x(s_i)\}, \quad i = 0,1,\ldots,k, \quad s_o = 0 < s_1 < \ldots < s_k \leq s^* \tag{57}$$

Then an approximating curve $\{\pi(\eta)\}$ can be constructed from information available at a selected number of these points. Usually, this curve is required to pass through $\{x^{(k)}\}$, and it is useful to set $\{\pi(0)\} = \{x^{(k)}\}$. We denote the parameter by η because it is rarely possible to provide for a parametrization that is equal to that of the curve (50). Now a suitable step η_{k+1} is taken to obtain a point $\{\pi(\eta_{k+1})\}$ which is to serve as the initial point for the iterative process for computing the next point $\{x^{(k+1)}\}$ further along the curve. Clearly, the step η_{k+1} must be properly chosen such that the point $\{\pi(\eta_{k+1})\}$ is within the domain of convergence of the iterative process selected to compute $\{x^{(k+1)}\}$. The

THE BASIC CONTINUATION APPROACH

As we have seen in the previous section, our interest centers on continuous paths

$$\{x\} = \{x(s)\} = \begin{Bmatrix} \{q(s)\} \\ \lambda(s) \end{Bmatrix} \in R^{n+1}, \quad s \in [0,s^*] \tag{50}$$

for which all points $(\{q(s)\}, \lambda(s))$, $s \in [0,s^*]$, are solutions of Eqs. (43) and s is a suitable parameter (not necessarily the arc length). Note that for ease of discussion we lumped λ together with $\{q\} \in R^n$ into one vector $\{x\} \in R^{n+1}$.

Before turning to the computation of the curve (50), we will discuss how to apply one of the iterative methods discussed previously to compute a specific point on that curve. This is not entirely obvious, since (43) represents a set of n equations in (n+1) variables, while all of the iterative methods discussed earlier apply only when there are as many equations as variables. Obviously, the missing equation relates to the specification of the particular point on the curve we wish to compute. A natural way of specifying a point on (50) is to define it as the point of intersection of the curve with a particular n-dimensional surface in R^{n+1}. Such a surface is usually given by a single equation $f_{n+1}(q,\lambda) = 0$ and, hence, a point of intersection of the curve with this surface must satisfy the augmented equations

$$\{\hat{F}(q,\lambda)\} \equiv \begin{Bmatrix} \{F(q,\lambda)\} \\ f_{n+1}(q,\lambda) \end{Bmatrix} = \{0\} \tag{51}$$

In most cases we use simple surfaces of intersection. For example, the equation

$$f_{n+1}(q,\lambda) \equiv \lambda - \hat{\lambda} = 0 \tag{52}$$

specifies an n-dimensional plane in R^{n+1}, orthogonal to the λ-axis. In that case it is, of course, easy to eliminate the (n+1)st equation in (51); in fact, clearly for f_{n+1} given by (53), Eqs. (51) are equivalent to the n-dimensional equation

$$\{F(q,\hat{\lambda})\} = \{0\} \tag{53}$$

in the unknown vector $\{q\} \in R^n$. This is really the case of the parametrization (46).

Clearly, the choice of the surface equation $f_{n+1}(q,\lambda) = 0$ cannot be arbitrary. In fact, we have to select f_{n+1} so as to ensure that the curve and surface actually intersect. Moreover, the part of the intersection under consideration should constitute an isolated solution of Eqs. (51); that is, in view of Theorem 1, at the point of intersection the derivative

$$[J(x)] \equiv [D\hat{F}(q,x)] = \begin{bmatrix} [D_qF(q,\lambda)] & \{D_\lambda F(q,\lambda)\} \\ D_qF_{n+1}(q,\lambda) & D_\lambda f_{n+1}(q,\lambda) \end{bmatrix}, \quad \{x\} = \begin{Bmatrix} \{q\} \\ \lambda \end{Bmatrix} \tag{54}$$

should be nonsingular. The latter condition has a simple geometric meaning. In fact, the last row of the matrix (54) or, more specifically, the column vector

$$\left\{ \{N\} = \begin{matrix} \dfrac{\partial f_{n+1}}{\partial q_1} \\ \vdots \\ \dfrac{\partial f_{n+1}}{\partial q_n} \\ \vdots \\ \dfrac{\partial f_{n+1}}{\partial \lambda} \end{matrix} \in R^{n+1} \right\} \tag{55}$$

process is then repeated to obtain $\{x^{(k+2)}\}$, and so on.

This type of procedure is basic to what is known as the continuation approach (or incremental-iterative approach) for the computation of equilibrium curves (50); that is, deformation paths in mechanics. The three steps given above may be called (i) augmentation, (ii) prediction, and (iii) correction, respectively. Once again we note that the overall method requires at least one known point on the curve from which to start. At this starting point the predictor (the extrapolation process sketched above) usually takes a simplified form.

The following simple scheme illustrates the continuation approach:

(i) Augmentation: Use the simple augmenting equation (52) in which case the system (51) can be reduced to Eq. (53).

(ii) Prediction: Select a value $\lambda_{k+1} = \lambda_k + \eta_{k+1}$, $\eta_{k+1} > 0$, and set

$$\{\pi(\eta_{k+1})\} = \{x^{(k)}\} + \eta_{k+1}\{e^{n+1}\} \tag{58}$$

that is, use the last computed point with a modified λ-component.

(iii) Corrector: Use Newton's method to solve Eq. (53) with $\hat{\lambda} = \lambda_{k+1}$, i.e., apply the process

$$\{p^{(0)}\} = \{q^{(k)}\} \tag{59}$$

$$\{p^{(j+1)}\} = \{p^{(j)}\} - [D_q F(p^{(j)}, \lambda_{k+1})]^{-1}[F(p^{(j)}, \lambda_{k+1})],$$

$$j = 0, 1, \ldots.$$

If this process is stopped with $p^{(\ell)}$ then set $\{q^{(k+1)}\} = \{p^{(\ell)}\}$.

Early applications of the continuation approach in mechanics often relied on this simple scheme (see the review articles [49], [50], [51], and [52]). It suffers, however, from a number of distinct weaknesses which restrict the usefulness of the method considerably. The objections pertain here to all three steps of the computational procedure:

(i) As we saw in the last section, the parametrization (52) is poor and breaks down in the neighborhood of any limit point.

(ii) The predictor is crude and requires more correction steps than necessary.

(iii) Newton's method is too expensive for large equations.

The undesirable property of algorithms based on the parametrization (52), that is, on load incrementation, is well known and several remedies to overcome the difficulty have been proposed in the past (see Refs. [21], [53], [54], [55], [56], [57], [58], [59], [60], [61], and [62]. Some of these proposals tried to retain the basic load-incrementation but introduced modifications near the points where it fails (see, e.g., [21], [55], [56], [58], and [64]). We shall not consider these approaches here but shall discuss only some techniques for choosing parametrizations, i.e., augmented equations (51), which do not exhibit the difficulties in the neighborhood of limit points.

In order to define the points of the desired segment of the solution curve (50) we have to use suitable families of surfaces $f_{n+1} = 0$. In line with the concept of the overall continuation approach, if $\{x^{(k)}\}$ represents the last computed point, then a new family of surfaces

$$f_{n+1}(x, x^{(k)}, \eta) = 0 \tag{60}$$

is defined which depends on $\{x^k\}$ and on a parameter η. We assume that the surface with $\eta = 0$ passes through $\{x^{(k)}\}$,

$$f_{n+1}(x^{(k)}, x^{(k)}, 0) = 0 \tag{61}$$

and that the velocity with which the surface "moves" with varying η is not zero:

$$\frac{\partial f_{n+1}}{\partial \eta}(x, x^{(k)}, \eta) \neq 0 \tag{62}$$

Moreover, we require, of course, that for each fixed η in some interval, say, $0 \leq \eta < \delta$, the corresponding surface intersects the curve (50) at a unique point $\{\bar{x}(s)\}$ where the matrix (54) is nonsingular. Hence, there is a well-defined correspondence between the surface parameter η, $0 \leq \eta < \delta$, and the parameter s of our representation of the curve.

Clearly, it would be advantageous to ensure that $\eta = s - s_k$ for all s near s_k, especially when s is the arc length of the curve. However, there are no computable functions f_{n+1} to ensure this. The approach has, therefore, been to choose f_{n+1} such that η approximates in some way the arc length.

Before defining three choices of f_{n+1} that have been discussed in the literature, we note that when $\{x^{(k)}\}$ is a regular point of F then, by definition, the $n \times (n+1)$ matrix $[DF(x^{(k)})]$ has a null-space of dimension one. Hence, the vector $\{v\} \in R^{n+1}$ satisfying

$$[DF(x^{(k)})]\{v\} = 0, \quad \{v\}^T\{v\} = 1 \tag{63}$$

is uniquely defined up to a factor ± 1. It is possible to define the sign uniquely in the entire regularity domain of F (see Ref. [65]). We denote the resulting vector $\{v\}$ by $\{\dot{x}^{(k)}\}$. Evidently, if $\{x^{(k)}\} = \{x(s_k)\}$ then we have $\{\dot{x}^{(k)}\} = \{\dot{x}(s_k)\}$.

The indicated three choices of f_{n+1} can now be written as:

$$\begin{aligned}
&(a) \quad f_{n+1} = \{\dot{x}^{(k)}\}^T(\{x\} - \{x^{(k)}\}) - \eta \\
&(b) \quad f_{n+1} = \{e^{i_k}\}^T(\{x\} - x^{(k)}\}) - \eta \\
&(c) \quad f_{n+1} = (\{x\} - \{x^{(k)}\})^T(\{x\} - \{x^{(k)}\}) - \eta^2
\end{aligned} \tag{64}$$

where in the case of (64b) the vector $\{e^{i_k}\}$ is the k-th natural basis vector of R^{n+1} corresponding to the maximum component (in modulus) of $\{\dot{x}^{(k)}\}$. A geometric interpretation of these equations for $\{x^{(k)}\} = \{x(s_k)\}$ is given in Fig. 9.

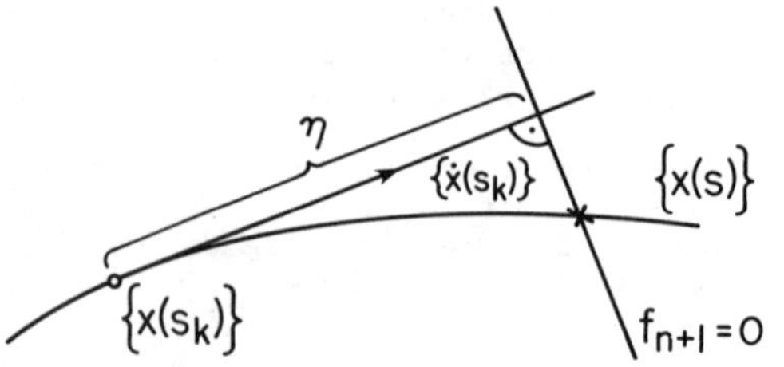

(a)

Fig. 9 - Geometry of the three parametrizations (64)

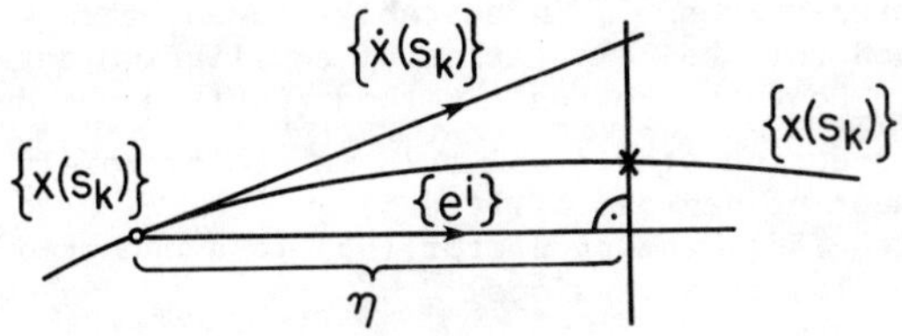

(b)

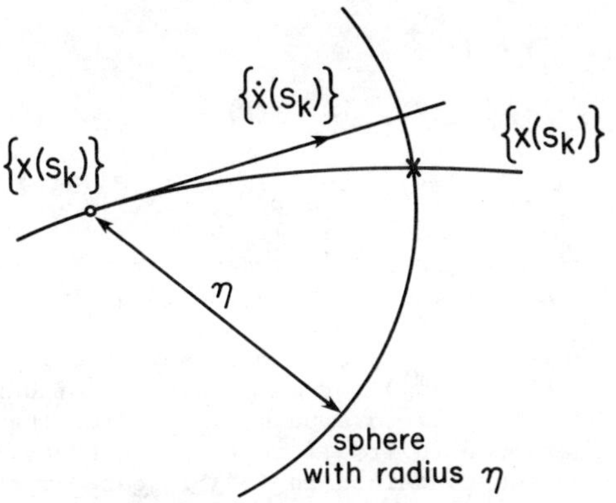

(c)

Fig. 9 - Geometry of the three parametrizations (64) - (Cont'd.)

It appears that the basic idea behind this approach was presented first in Ref. [66] but this paper went unnoticed until recently. Independent developments of procedures based on these and related choices can be found in Refs. [44], [45], [47], [59], [63], [65], [67], [68], [69], and [70]. See also some recent evaluations of this approach in [71], [72], [73], [74] and [75] or the applications in [76] and [77].

With any one of the three augmentations (64) we may now introduce the following predictor-corrector combination as a prototype of an adaptive parameter continuation approach:

Predictor: Use the so-called Euler-prediction

$$\pi(\eta) = \{x^{(k)}\} + \eta\{\dot{x}^{(k)}\} \tag{65}$$

Corrector: Apply Newton's method to the augmented equations (51) that is

$$\begin{aligned} &\{y^{(0)}\} = \{\pi(\eta_{k+1})\} \\ &\{y^{(j+1)}\} = \{y^{(j)}\} - [J(y^{(j)})]^{-1}[\hat{F}(y^{(j)})], \quad j = 0,1,\ldots,\ell \\ &\{x^{(k+1)}\} = \{y^{(\ell+1)}\} \end{aligned} \tag{66}$$

The direction vector $\{\dot{x}^{(k)}\}$ is computed after the last corrector step as

$$\{v\} = [J(y^{(\ell)})]^{-1}\{e^{n+1}\}, \quad \{\dot{x}^{(k)}\} = \pm \frac{1}{\| v \|} v \tag{67}$$

with the appropriate sign corresponding to the direction of the curve.

As long as the step-size η_{k+1} is suitably chosen, this algorithm turns out to be a reliable method for the computation of equilibrium curves ([46], [47], [65], [70] and [78]). However, Newton's method requires the decomposition of $[J(y^{(j)})]$ for each correction step j and this may be extremely costly for problems involving a large number of degrees of freedom.

In comparison with (58), the predictor (65) is a one step improvement within the class of truncated Taylor expansions

$$\{\pi(\eta)\} = \{x^{(k)}\} + \eta\{\dot{x}^{(k)}\} + \frac{1}{2}\eta^2\{\ddot{x}^{(k)}\} + \ldots \tag{68}$$

where the vectors $\{\dot{x}^{(k)}\}$, $\{\ddot{x}^{(k)}\}$, ... are determined by the equations

$$\begin{aligned} &[J(x^{(k)})]\{\dot{x}^{(k)}\} = \{r^{(1)}\} = \{e^{n+1}\} \\ &[J(x^{(k)})]\{\ddot{x}^{(k)}\} = \{r^{(2)}\} = \{r^{(2)}(x^{(k)}, \dot{x}^{(k)})\} \\ &[J(x^{(k)})]\{\dddot{x}^{(k)}\} = \{r^{(3)}\} = \{r^{(3)}(x^{(k)}, \dot{x}^{(k)}, \ddot{x}^{(k)})\} \end{aligned} \tag{69}$$

etc., which arises if we differentiate (51) repeatedly with respect to η. The solutions of (69) require the decomposition of $[J(x)]$ at the last iterate of the previous step and evaluation of the right hand side $\{r^{(m)}\}$, $m = 1,2,\ldots$. This presents no problem for $m = 1$, but it becomes more involved for increasing m caused by the circumstance that $\{r^{(m)}\}$ for $m > 1$ is built of derivatives of f_i of order higher than 1. Apart from this drawback, increasing the degree of the expansion (68) is not a guarantee in itself that the accuracy of it will be increased because all information contained in (68) is based purely on local properties of the path near $\{x^{(k)}\}$. Predictors of a degree beyond two are therefore hardly ever used. They do not, in general, save more work for the corrector than is expended in the construction of the extra terms beyond two in (68).

It should be pointed out that the Taylor expansion (68) by itself can serve as an approximate solution of $\{x(\eta)\}$ in some neighborhood of $\{x^{(k)}\}$. Such solutions are known as perturbation or asymptotic solutions in structural mechanics [79]. By their very nature and in view of what has just been said about Eq. (68), they have, in general, only a limited range of validity. Nevertheless, for the analysis of the initial postbuckling behavior of structures of the type represented by the examples in Figs. 5 and 6, the "perturbation" method as embodied by Eqs. (69) has produced some useful results, especially in the area of shell structures [80]. In this particular version of the perturbation technique, the basis of which was laid in [37], the evaluation of Eqs. (69) is carried out at the bifurcation point (where $[y(x)]$ is singular!) so that the expansion (68) serves as an approximation for the postbuckling part II branching from I. For details we refer to the literature on elastic stability theory [33], [37], [40], [42], [43], [80], [81], [82], and [83]. Descriptions of computer oriented adaptations of this approach can be found in Refs. [79], [84], [85], [86], [87], [88], [89], [90], [91], [92], [93], and [94].

The predictor of the type (68) is useful only if we have available the decomposed $[J(x^k)]$. This may not be the case, due, for example, to a choice of the corrector that does not use $[J((x)]$. An alternative to the Taylor expansion (68) is then, for instance, Lagrange interpolation. Suppose a number of points have been computed. Select from these the last ℓ and construct the polynomial

$$\pi(\eta) = \sum_{i=0}^{\ell-1} \{y^{(i)}\}\eta^i, \quad \pi(\eta_j) = \{x^{(j)}\}, \quad j = k,k-1,\ldots,k-\ell+1 \tag{70}$$

It is noted that also with this type of predictor, expansions beyond degree two rarely give better results for reasons already mentioned.

In discussing iterative methods we encountered several variations of Newton's method that have been proposed to counter the costly operations connected with this method. In principle, as long as we are not interested in aspects of stability, we can try to replace the corrector (66) by any of the variants discussed earlier. This has been done in the past with varying degrees of success ([49], [51] and [95]).

This freedom of choice is much reduced, however, when we deal with the computation of critical and post-critical equilibrium states because, in general, it is not possible to detect critical points without decomposition of $[S] = [D_q F(q,\lambda)]$ along parts of the curve where these points are anticipated. Since $[S]^{-1}$ can be constructed from elements of $[J(x)]^{-1}$, the last observation holds for $[J(x)]$. For instance, the decomposed matrix [S] provides a means to compute the determinant det [S]. A zero of this function along the path is an indication of a critical state. We, therefore, would like to monitor the value of det [S] during the computations if we are interested in the stability aspects of the solution curve.

Consequently, in the case of stability analysis we would like to have a corrector which is more efficient than Newton's method but which makes a quick return to the Jacobian [J(x)] possible. The most obvious alternative is then the modified or simplified Newton's method which we already encountered. In the continuation procedure described by (65) and (66) this type of corrector is usually applied in the form of a parallel chord method with either one of the two choices

$$\text{(a)} \quad [A_o] = [J(x^{(k)})], \qquad \text{(b)} \quad [A_o] = [J(\pi(\eta_{k+1}))] \tag{71}$$

In most cases, a decomposition of the derivative is carried out once per continuation step (although it is also possible to skip decomposition in a number of steps, see the STAGS algorithm [96] and [97]). The total amount of work is usually considerably reduced by these changes. The first approach (71a) has the advantage that we can use Eq. (65) as the predictor and will have relatively accurate values of the determinant det [S] for the detection of critical points. On the other hand, the choice of (71b) offers a somewhat better behavior as far as convergence is concerned because this variant is more "like" Newton's method than the first variant, [48].

To improve on either of the two correctors we could try to use for each corrector step updates of the type discussed in (31). Such "acceleration" techniques have been tested, for instance in Refs. [71], [72] and [98] and they seem to offer a slightly better overall performance as compared to the case where they are not used.

We need now to discuss an aspect of adaptive parametrization that concerns the structure of the Jacobian matrix [J(x)]. In many problems in structural engineering the stiffness matrix [S] is not only symmetric but it is also sparse and banded along the main diagonal. However, with any of the schemes defined by (64), this symmetry is lost in [J(x)] because the extra column and row that are added to [S] cannot be interchanged. Frontal decomposition would then not only lead to a nonsymmetric semi-inverse, but it also would destroy the band structure originally present in [S]. Consequently, decomposition of [J(x)] requires special attention to overcome this difficulty.

One particular solution to this problem is based on the decomposition of [S]. The corrector equations based on (71) are then solved in two steps involving two back substitutions [44], [54], [73] and [99]. The advantage of this approach is that existing algorithms that follow a fixed parametrization with λ can easily be adapted to the strategies (64). A disadvantage is, however, that since [S] becomes ill-conditioned in a close neighborhood of limit-points, it is not possible to compute an envelope of limit-points with this method. In [45], in connection with the parameter choice (16b), another solution of the problem has been given which is also effective, without making the method sensitive to limit-points.

Also, it seems possible to design a special decomposition method that deals with [J(x)] effectively, taking into account the sparseness of [S] and its symmetry so that altogether it does not require considerably more work and storage than the decomposition of [S] alone.

To conclude this section, we will briefly comment on the control of the stepsize η_{k+1} along the path. This aspect is important because it influences both the robustness and efficiency of the continuation process.

Ideally, we would like to have a set of measures that determines the stepsize η_{k+1} at each step $(k+1)$ such that the desired stretch of the solution curve can be obtained at a minimum of computational expense. This turns out to be impossible in general. For instance, for such a type of stepsize control we need to know, at the start of each new step, the answers to questions as, for instance:

(i) How far is the initial iterate from the expected solution?

(ii) Is it in the convergence domain of the corrector?

(iii) How many iterates are necessary to arrive at a satisfactory solution?

It turns out that this is simply beyond our reach. Of course, we could try to obtain the desired information from an evaluation of the performance of the algorithm at points already computed (see, e.g., [100]), but this turns out to be problematic as well. For instance, it is not possible to deduce the domain of convergence of the corrector at some solution point from the sequence of iterates that converged to it as has recently been shown in [101].

It is not surprising, therefore, that most steplength control algorithms are based on some heuristic arguments and often take a form determined by trial and error. One of such approaches is, for instance

$$\eta_{k+1} = \left(\frac{\ell_k}{\ell^*}\right)^{\alpha} \eta_k \tag{72}$$

where

ℓ_k = total number of corrections in the k-th step,

ℓ^* = desired number of iterations/step (prescribed by the user),

α = some power, usually, < 1,

which has been used in algorithms described in [73] and [74], and gives a reasonable performance. A more sophisticated scheme has recently been discussed in [46] and [101]. It is based on an estimate of the quality of the convergence of the corrector (at previous points) and on an estimate of the distance of the predictor to the actual solution. This step-length control strategy has shown a very satisfactory performance in many applications.

It follows from experience, however, that most convergence failures of the corrector are the result of a sudden change of the curvature $\| x(s) \|$ of the path not anticipated by the step control, so that the predictor falls outside the convergence domain of the corrector. Some assessment of curvature changes is used in [46] yet it is impossible to prevent divergence from occurring altogether. Therefore, measures have to be included to "recover" from such instances either automatically or by a stop and restart capability that allows to adjust the stepsize accordingly.

We conclude this section by showing two example problems as defined in Figs. 10 and 11. The solutions were obtained with the STAGS-A code [97] equipped with a solution procedure based on the parametrization (64a) [61] and [74]. The stepsize selector used in these cases was of the type (72). The first problem was described by 432 degrees of freedom, the second by 3076.

To complete the solution beyond the limit point, the first example requires considerably fewer solution points than the second. Although it cannot be deduced from the graphs shown, this is due to curvature changes of the solution curve which are much stronger in the second case than in the first one.

OUTLOOK ON FURTHER RESULTS

In this section we summarize some further problems and computational approaches relating to the topic here under discussion. But, for reasons of space, the presentations have to be kept rather brief, and the reader is referred to the cited literature for all details.

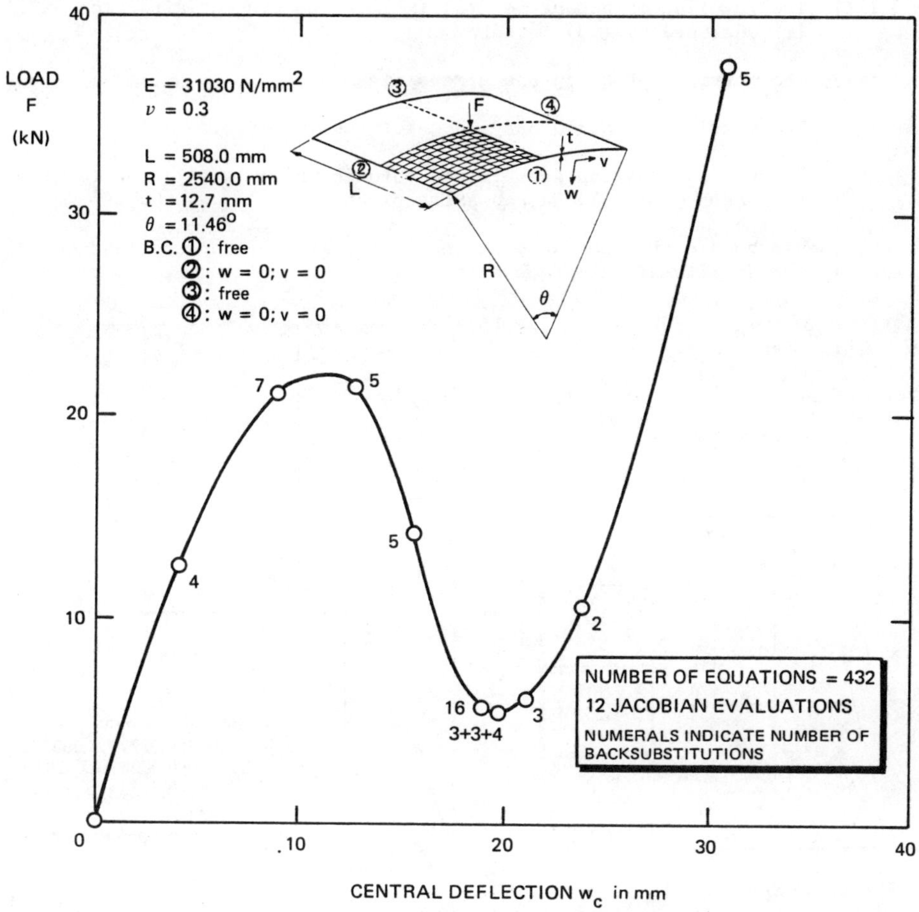

Fig. 10 - Cylindrical shell roof under central load

Computation of Limit Points

As stated previously, it is desirable to have facilities for computing the exact location of limit points where the mechanical structure under study may snap through or collapse. In view of the significance of this problem it is not surprising that a number of algorithms have been proposed for the computation of limit points. Without claim of completeness we mention here the methods described in Refs. [46], [47], [48], [70], [78], [102], [103], [104], [105], [106], [107], and [108].

There are two basic classes of methods for computing limit points; namely, (i) local iterative processes; and (ii) methods utilizing the continuation path. The members of the first class may be started anywhere in a neighborhood of the limit point $\{x^*\}$ while those in the second class require as input some point (or points) on the continuation path through $\{x^*\}$. In practice, this distinction loses much of its significance since also in the first case a continuation process is needed to reach a neighborhood of $\{x^*\}$.

The methods may be further categorized in terms of the characterization of the limit point. In essence, for a limit point $\{x^*\}$ of the problem (43) with respect to λ, five such characterizations are available.

(i) The determinant of $[D_qF(q,\lambda)]$ vanishes at $\{x^*\}$.

(ii) The (n+1)st component $\{e^{n+1}\}^T\{\dot{x}^*\}$ of the tangent-direction $\{\dot{x}^*\}$ at $\{x^*\}$ defined by (63) is zero.

(iii) The matrix $[D_qF(q,\lambda)]$ has a zero eigenvalue. (73)

(iv) The matrix $[D_qF(q,\lambda)]$ has a non-zero null vector.

(v) On the continuation path $\{x(s)\}$ through $\{x^*\} = \{x(s^*)\}$ the (n+1)st component of $\{x(s)\}$ has an extremum at $s = s^*$.

However, the methods differ not only in the choice of the characterization (73) but also in the details of the process itself.

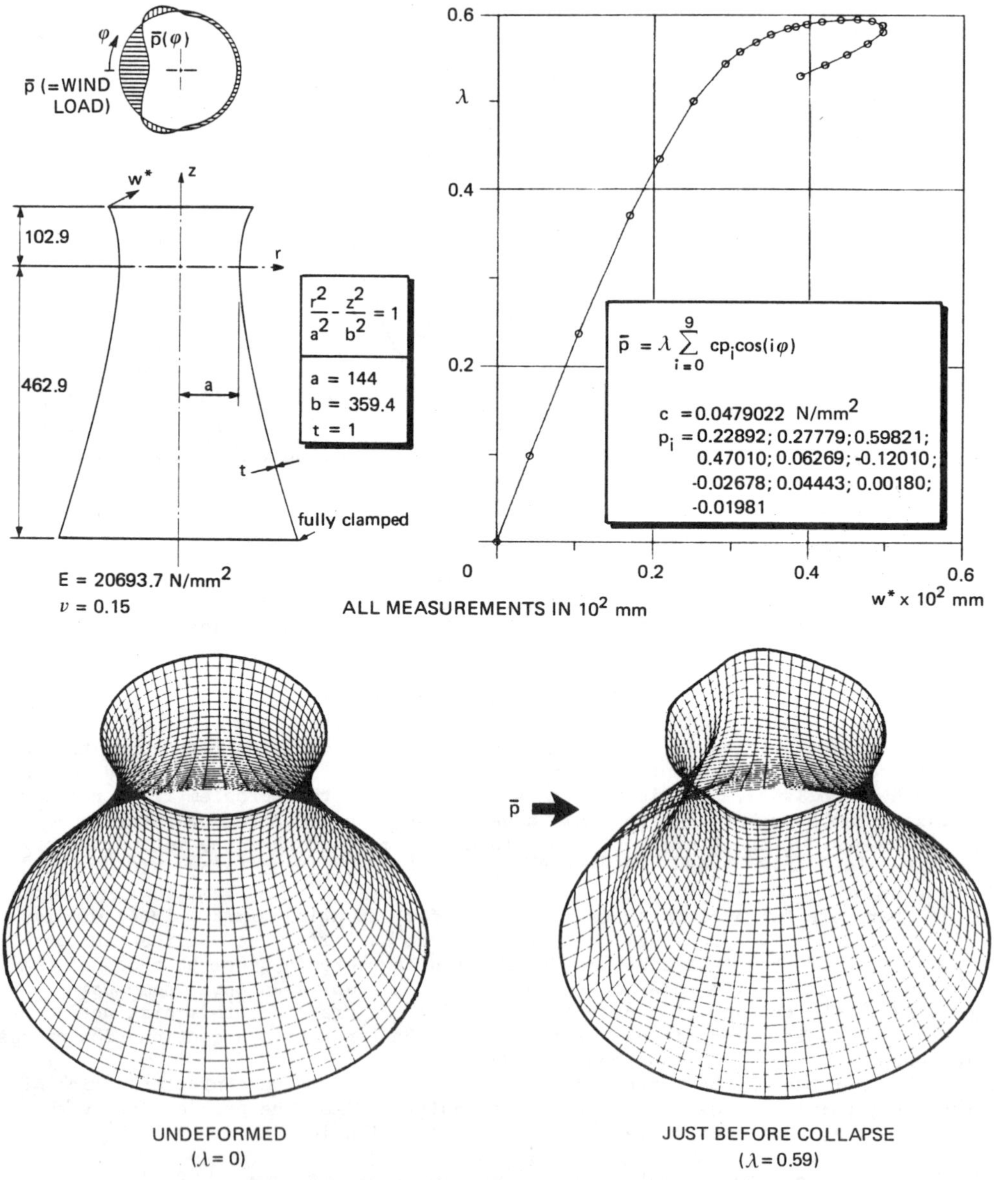

Fig. 11 - Collapse analysis of hyperboloid cooling tower

It should be noted that all methods are guaranteed to work only for the computation of simple limit points, that is, points $\{x(s^*)\}$ on the continuation curve where the real function $\tau(s) = \{e^{n+1}\}^T\{\dot{x}(s)\}$ has an isolated zero in the sense that $\dot{\tau}(s^*) \neq 0$. During the continuation process such a point is detected whenever at two succeeding points $\{x(s_k)\}$, $\{x(s_{k+1})\}$ we have

$$\text{sign}\{e^{n+1}\}^T\{\dot{x}(s_k)\} \neq \text{sign}\{e^{n+1}\}^T\{\dot{x}(s_{k+1})\} \tag{74}$$

For the specific details of the various mentioned methods we refer to the cited articles. In [109] experimental comparisons of the methods for a set of test problems were presented and some guidelines for their applicability given. It appears from this investigation that the method developed in [46] and [105], which uses the continuation path and is based on (73(ii)), shows the best overall performance in terms of reliability and speed.

Computation of Bifurcation Branches

The second type of critical point mentioned earlier is the bifurcation point where several solution branches cross and the mechanical structure may be expected to buckle. As with limit points there is considerable interest in algorithms for determining the solution structure near such bifurcation points. But the development of such algorithms is at present by far not as well-advanced as that in the case of limit points. One of the underlying reasons for this is the fact that bifurcation points are no longer regular points of the given function [F]. As a consequence the corrector iterations discussed in the previous section fail to converge there and, hence, the overall continuation process may be expected to break down if it comes too close to such a point.

These comments already indicate that there are a number of computational problems near any bifurcation point including, for example, the following ones:

(i) Detection of a bifurcation point;

(ii) Behavior of the continuation process in the neighborhood of such such a point; (75)

(iii) Switchover of the process from one branch emanating from the bifurcation point to another such branch; and,

(iv) Determination of the entire branching diagram.

These problems are interrelated and their analysis requires extensive use of results from bifurcation theory. The literature in this area is extensive and in the space available here it is not possible to enter into any details. For some reviews of bifurcation phenomena see, for instance, Refs. [110], [111], [112], or alternatively the literature on elastic stability [33], [39], [41], [42], [78], [81], [82], and [113].

The detection of a bifurcation point on some equilibrium surface depends critically on the information available, and is certainly difficult if a path is not known which leads to the point. Computationally the simplest case arises when a continuation path passes smoothly through a bifurcation point. Any regular continuation path $\{x(s)\}$ may be oriented by defining its direction to be positive or negative if the determinant

$$J(s) = \det \begin{bmatrix} [DF(x(s))] \\ \{\dot{x}(s)\}^T \end{bmatrix} \tag{76}$$

is positive or negative, respectively. If $\{\dot{x}(s)\}$ is continuous then the direction can change at best at a bifurcation point. In mechanical applications the situation shown in Fig. 10 occurs frequently; that is, two paths pass smoothly through a bifurcation point, their directions change and their angle of intersection is not too acute. In this case, most continuation processes will "jump" over $\{x^*\}$ - provided they are capable of taking sufficiently large steps. By monitoring the direction, that is, the sign of $J(s)$, we may then detect the presence of the bifurcation point.

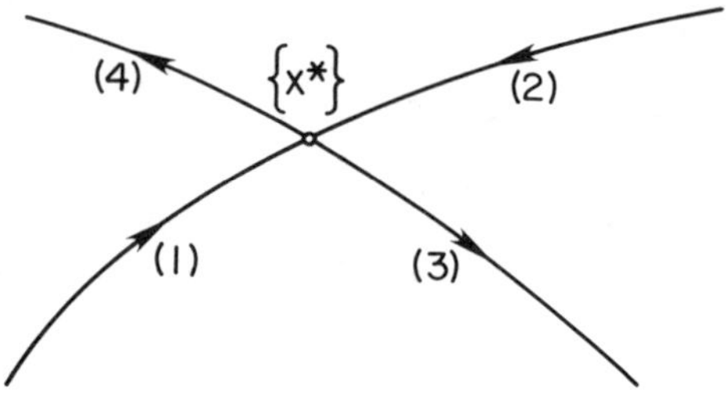

Fig. 12 - Directions at a bifurcation point

As indicated before, the continuation processes discussed in the previous section may be expected to fail near a bifurcation point. The exact nature of this failure and any remedies depend on many factors. For some discussion about this topic we refer, for example, to Refs. [114], [115], [116], [117], [118], and [119] and the references given there.

Various algorithms have been proposed for switching from one branch to another at a bifurcation point. Several of the perturbation approaches cited before may serve this purpose. In addition, we mention here the methods given in Refs. [47], [78], [115], [120], [121], [122], [123], [124], [125], and [126]. In general, these processes are guaranteed to work only in the situation of Fig. 10. While some of them are theoretically extendable to more general situations, no reliable computational algorithm appears to be available for this. The same is true for the last of our four problems (75).

Determination of Critical Boundaries

As we saw when discussing iterative methods the location of the first limit point encountered on a solution path is of considerable interest. Typically, it signifies a point where the mechanical structure may be expected to snap-through or collapse. It is then natural to raise the question of the variation of this limit point under changes of the other parameters of the system. The situation is illustrated in Fig. 7, where we are interested in the location of the path III in the critical boundary.

The standard computational approach appears to consist in the computation of a number of solution paths for different parameter combinations and in the exact determination of the first limit point on each one of these paths. Obviously, if any reasonable resolution is demanded for the desired curve in the critical boundary, then this procedure will have to be repeated many times at considerable cost. Moreover, it is usually difficult to obtain suitable starting points of the various solution curves which are guaranteed to lead to a reasonably spaced set of points on the critical curve.

In view of this it is desirable to provide for algorithms which permit a direct computation of a path in the critical boundary once a starting point on this path has been found by the above mentioned standard procedure. Several such algorithms have been presented in [105], but space does not permit us to enter into details here.

One group of methods in [105] is based on the use of a local iterative method for computing limit points as described in the beginning of this section. More specifically, one of the methods introduced in [127] or [104] is used as a corrector, and a suitable prediction-strategy is introduced to permit a trace of the desired curve in the critical boundary. The resulting process requires substantial additions to the original continuation programs and appears to be best suited for problems of moderate dimension.

Another type of process discussed in [105] does not share these restrictions. It works essentially with a basic continuation program which allows the trace of any curve on the equilibrium surface defined by a parameter-combination with one degree of freedom. This program is combined with one of the methods for computing limit points which utilize the continuation path through that point. In order to sketch the basic idea of the method for tracing a critical path, suppose that our basic equation (41) involves a two-dimensional parameter-vector $\{\lambda\} \in R^2$. Then the equilibrium surface defined by this equation is a two-dimensional surface in R^{n+2}. For the trace of a particular segment of the critical path two families of curves on the equilibrium surface are selected which, in essence, form a grid as shown in Fig. 13. The procedure then begins in tracing a curve which has approximately the direction of the critical path and then switches over to one of the intersecting curves on which then the first limit point is computed. The role of the two families of curves may change at any points as the figure shows, and there are various technical details about step-lengths, etc., which have to be taken into account. For these we refer to the cited article where also several numerical examples are given. For a further example involving the collapse behavior of a circular arch see Ref. [128].

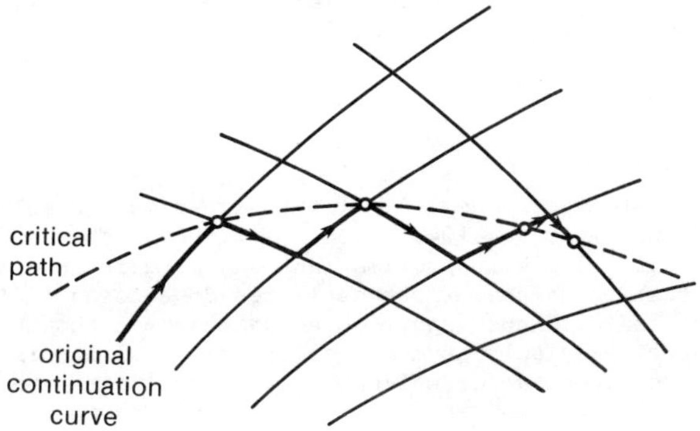

Fig. 13 - Schematic of the trace of a critical boundary

The approach indicates once again the value of considering general equilibrium surfaces and of working with continuation processes that are not limited to simple load parametrizations but permit a trace of many curves on the equilibrium surface.

Errors Along the Continuation Curve

In general, the objective of a computational solution of a physical problem is to obtain an acceptably accurate and reliable prediction of the behavior of the physical phenomena under study. For this the computation should produce not only an approximate numerical solution but also some reliable information about its accuracy. A priori error bounds, as important as they are for the theory, are rarely very realistic for practical problems. Hence, there is a need for a posteriori error estimates which utilize information obtained during the solution process.

For the finite element solution of certain linear problems in structural mechanics such a posteriori estimates were introduced and analyzed in sequence of papers [129]-[136]. Not unexpectedly, for nonlinear problems the situation is considerably more difficult and much remains to be done. In the second part of [135] and in [128], results are presented for the finite element solution of nonlinear problems in one-space dimension which show that a posteriori error estimates are also highly effective in such nonlinear cases even though the corresponding theory is as yet far from complete.

As noted before, we are interested in specific features of the equilibrium surface; as, for instance, the location of limit points. For this we require estimates of the error of the critical load as well as of the computed limit point itself. Some such a posteriori error estimates were also developed in [128] and shown to be very effective. The results show furthermore that, as predicted by the theory, the convergence of the critical loads is faster than that of the corresponding solution errors.

Nonlinear problems of the type arising in structural mechanics often have the property that the discretized equations have solutions which do not correspond to solutions of the exact problem. Such solutions have been called spurious, or numerically irrelevant. They have been observed by many authors (see [137] and [138], and the references given there).

The phenomenon is easily observed in the case of the classical Euler rod defined by the two-point boundary value problem

$$\frac{d^2u}{ds^2} = \lambda \sin u, \qquad u(0) = u(1) = 0 \tag{77}$$

For $\lambda < 0$ there exists no other solution than $u \equiv 0$. This is physically plausible since under pure tension the rod should remain straight. For the trivial mesh $s_o = 0$, $s_1 = 1/2$, $s_2 = 1$, a simple finite-difference approximation leads to the single equation

$$u_1 = \frac{1}{4} \lambda \sin u_1 \tag{78}$$

Evidently, for all sufficiently negative λ this equation has solutions. For instance, for $\lambda = -20$, we get $u_1 = 4.10462$, and $u_1 = 4.9063$. This undesirable behavior also arises with finite element approximations and more refined meshes. In Ref. [128] it is shown that the a-posteriori estimates do succeed in identifying the large errors associated with such spurious solutions even though these estimates are justified theoretically only asymptotically for small errors. Hence, if only solution branches are accepted for which the error estimates are below a reasonable tolerance of 5-10%, the spurious solutions should be rejected automatically.

Mesh-Refinement and Continuation

In order to achieve the objective stated at the outset of the previous subsection, adaptive processes appear to be optimal tools. In fact, it is beginning to be a widely accepted observation that for realistic problems it is rarely feasible to design numerical processes which reliably and effectively achieve the desired accuracy in a prescribed error-norm and yet which do not utilize some form of adaptivity.

As the result of the previous subsection shows, the error along any continuation path may vary considerably. Ideally, we would like to ensure that the errors are reasonably constant and below a given tolerance. The only tool for accomplishing this is the use of mesh-refinement (and de-refinement). The effectiveness of adaptive mesh-refinement procedures for certain linear finite-element problems has been discussed, for instance, in Refs. [128], [130], [133], [135], [139]. In [128] it is shown that these adaptive approaches are also highly effective in the nonlinear case.

In its simplest form the process begins with a mesh that meets a prescribed error-tolerance requirement. Then, during the continuation procedure we monitor the error estimators and, at any computed point where the estimate exceeds the tolerance we divide the element(s) with the maximal error-contribution. A more advanced version of the process works also with a lower error tolerance and de-refines the mesh whenever the estimates fall below that lower threshold.

As discussed in Ref. [128], such an adaptive process may require only one-third of the work for a fixed a-priori chosen mesh and involves considerably fewer elements than a fixed mesh for which the error estimates stay below the tolerances.

These results are typical for problems of this type. The error usually varies considerably along any solution curve and it is practically impossible to design a fixed mesh for which it can be guaranteed a priori that the error remains below a prescribed accuracy. Only an adaptive process which modifies the mesh in response to the computed error estimates can accomplish this task. In the example only a mesh-refinement strategy was used but, obviously, it is also desirable to incorporate de-refinement when the estimates fall below a lower threshold.

The results mentioned in the previous subsections are still rather restrictive in their applicability, but there is every reason to believe that they will be as effective also in the case of more general problems in structural mechanics.

Reduction Techniques

In spite of the progress that has been made in the development of the continuation methods discussed here, the solution of large systems of nonlinear equations remains a very costly task. It is not surprising, therefore, that there is a continuing drive to increase the efficiency of these methods.

One particular development which holds considerable promise has been called the reduced basis technique in [140]. In the framework of a continuation procedure for nonlinear structural problems this approach was first proposed in [141] and was developed further in [142], [143] and [144].

Let $\{x(s)\}$, $s \in R^1$, denote the desired solution curve in R^{n+1}. For each parameter value $s = s_o$ the components of the vector $\{x(s_o)\}$ represent coordinates in some global coordinate system. On the other hand, at each point of the solution path there exists a local coordinate system consisting of vectors which represent intrinsic properties of the curve. The situation is shown schematically in Fig. 14. Suppose that the parameter s is the arc length, then the vectors

$$\{y_i\} = \{x^{(i)}(s_o)\}, \quad i = 1,2,... \tag{79}$$

provide the directions of the basis vectors of the local coordinate system. By definition of the arc length we have $\| \{\dot{x}(s_o)\} \|_2 = 1$; moreover, $\| \{\ddot{x}(s_o)\} \|_2$ is the curvature at the particular point, and $\| \{x^{(i)}(s_o)\} \|_2$, $i > 2$, characterize the "torsions" of the curve. Clearly $\{y_o\} = x(s_o)\}$ is the shift of the origin from the global to the local coordinate system.

In the local coordinate system we now propose to approximate the solution $\{x(s)\}$ by

$$\{\pi(\eta)\} = \sum_{i=0}^{\bar{n}} \xi_i(\eta) \{y_i\} \tag{80}$$

with a suitable vector

$$\{\xi(\eta)\} = \begin{Bmatrix} \xi_1(\eta) \\ \cdot \\ \cdot \\ \cdot \\ \xi_{\bar{n}}(\eta) \end{Bmatrix} \tag{81}$$

of "mode-amplitudes". Equation (80) can be viewed as a predictor formula analogous to (68). But unlike in (68) the mode-amplitudes are determined by an application of Galerkin's method to (50). This leads to the system of equations

$$\{G(\xi,\eta)\} = \{0\}, \quad \{\xi\} \in R^{\bar{n}}, \quad \eta \in R^1 \tag{82}$$

with

$$\{G(\xi,\eta)\} = \begin{Bmatrix} \{y_1\}^T\{F(\pi(\xi),\eta)\} \\ \{y_{\bar{n}}\}^T\{F(\pi(\xi),\eta)\} \end{Bmatrix} \tag{83}$$

Hence, G is a nonlinear mapping G: $R^{\bar{n}} \times R^1 \to R^{\bar{n}}$ where $\bar{n}$ is the number of basis vectors (79) we are prepared to compute. In practice, reasonably short segments of the solution curve remain in relatively low dimensional subspaces and, hence, only a few basis vectors of the local coordinate system are usually needed. In fact, in the cited references the total number of basis vectors hardly ever exceeds ten.

Let {x} be a computed solution of the equations (50). Then the procedure consists of the following steps.

(1) Compute the basis vectors $\{y_1\},\ldots,\{y_{\bar{n}}\}$, for instance (but not necessarily) by solving the equations (69).

(2) Reduce the full system $\{F(x,\lambda)\} = \{0\}$ to $\{G(\xi,\eta)\} = \{0\}$ as indicated in (83).

(3) Solve (82) by continuation in $R^{\bar{n}+1}$ for a sequence of parameter values $0 < \eta_1 < \eta_2 < \ldots$. At each value η_i test whether the approximate solution $\{\pi(\eta_i)\}$ remains acceptable; that is, whether a certain error indicator remains below a given tolerance. If it does, take another continuation step with the reduced system.

(4) If the error tolerance is exceeded, say, at $\eta_i = \eta^*$, then compute a point $\{x^*\}$ on the solution curve by solving the full system $\{F(x,\lambda)\} = \{0\}$ with a suitable corrector iteration started from $\{\pi(\eta^*)\}$. If this process is successful return to (1) with the new point, otherwise reduce η^* and try again.

Note that this scheme is based on two continuation procedures; namely, one in $R^{\bar{n}+1}$ and one in R^{n+1}. Clearly, if $\bar{n}$ is much smaller than n, then the continuation steps (3) are comparatively inexpensive. The example problems shown in the cited references indicate that the steps in η between a return to the full system typically are much larger than with a standard continuation process applied to the full system. Hence, the reduced basis technique reduces the total number of the costly corrector iterations in R^{n+1} substantially. These savings are offset, however, by the volume of operations connected with steps (1), (2), and (4). Consequently, the overall performance gains depend crucially on the way these steps are carried out.

In Ref. [144], typical reduction factors in computation time were reported to be of the order of three or four. For details and additional references we refer to the articles cited earlier.

Material Nonlinearities

So far we considered the solution of equations which constitute relations between finite, real valued quantities, such as displacement or deformation variables, and influence parameters, such as load intensities and imperfection amplitudes. Equations of this type are called holonomic in mechanics. The governing equations for conservative mechanical systems belong to this class. The nonlinearities that enter the equations in this case are due to geometrical nonlinear relations between the strains and displacements and/or they are caused by nonlinear elastic properties.

When plasticity, creep and visco-elastic effects come into play, the governing equations no longer will be holonomic because the constitutive equations relating the stress-state to the deformations-state now appear in a so-called rate form; that is, they involve derivative terms. In our present terminology, these terms correspond to path-derivatives of the stress and deformation variables.

This change of form certainly introduces complications into the processes for solving these equations.

Plasticity plays an important role in many buckling problems. It also constitutes a principal aspect of the analysis of extrusion processes. We indicate here only briefly what type of equations may be expected in these cases.

Suppose that the stress-state of the structure is represented by a vector of generalized stresses

$$\{\sigma\} \in R^n \tag{85}$$

and the deformation-state by a vector of generalized displacements

$$\{q\} \in R^n \tag{86}$$

Then the equilibrium equations can be cast in the form

$$\{F(q,\sigma,\lambda)\} = \{0\} \tag{87}$$

where, in general, F is a nonlinear mapping F: $R^n \times R^n \times R^1 \to R^n$, and, as before, λ serves as the load parameter.

In the case of linear elastic behavior we have the constitutive equations

$$\{\sigma\} = [E]\{q\} \tag{88}$$

with an $n \times n$ matrix [E] of elastic constants. Then equations (87) are readily transformed into the familiar form (51) by substitution of (88) into (87). In the case of elastic-plastic behavior the constitutive equations appear in the form

$$\{\dot{\sigma}\} = [C(q,\sigma)]\{\dot{q}\} \tag{89}$$

(see, e.g., [145], [146], [147]) where $\{\dot{\sigma}\}$ and $\{\dot{q}\}$ may be viewed as the path derivatives of $\{\sigma(\eta)\}$ and $\{q(\eta)\}$, respectively. The matrix $[C(q,\sigma)]$ can be written as

$$[C(q,\sigma)] = [E] - [Y(q,\sigma)] \tag{90}$$

Here the plastic part, $[Y(q,\sigma)]$, is very sensitive to changes of the stress-state $\{\sigma\}$. Elements of $[Y(q,\sigma)]$ are non-zero only if the corresponding material parts of the structure experience plastic loading. This indicates that the numerical integration of (89) is a delicate task.

Most engineering approaches use a step-by-step procedure for the solution of (87) and (89) which, in essence, may be characterized by the following scheme.

(1) Let $\{q(0)\}$, $\{\sigma(0)\}$ denote the last computed point. Construct a step η and predictors $\{\pi_1(\eta)\}$, $\{\pi_2(\eta)\}$ for the desired solutions $\{q(\eta)\}$ and $\{\sigma(\eta)\}$, respectively. For instance, the Euler predictor (65) may be used here.

(2) Enter $\{\pi_1(\eta)\}$, $\{\pi_2(\eta)\}$ into the right side of the constitutive equation (89) and integrate this equation numerically. This produces an "improved value for the stress $\{\sigma(\eta)\}$.

(3) Enter $\{\dot{\sigma}(\eta)\}$ into the equilibrium equations (87) which then reduce to the form (51). Solve these equations for $\{q\}$ by means of some suitable corrector iteration started from the predicted point $\{\pi_2(\eta)\}$.

It is possible to improve on the results obtained here by repetition of steps (2) and (3). There exist many variations in the practically used approaches for executing these basic steps. We refer to the survey articles [51], [52], [146], [148], [149], and [150] for further details and discussions. Descriptions of solution procedures in the case of plasticity and the presence of creep effects may also be found in Refs. [36], [92], [145], [151], [152], [153], [154], [155],

[155], [156], [157], [158], [159], and [160].

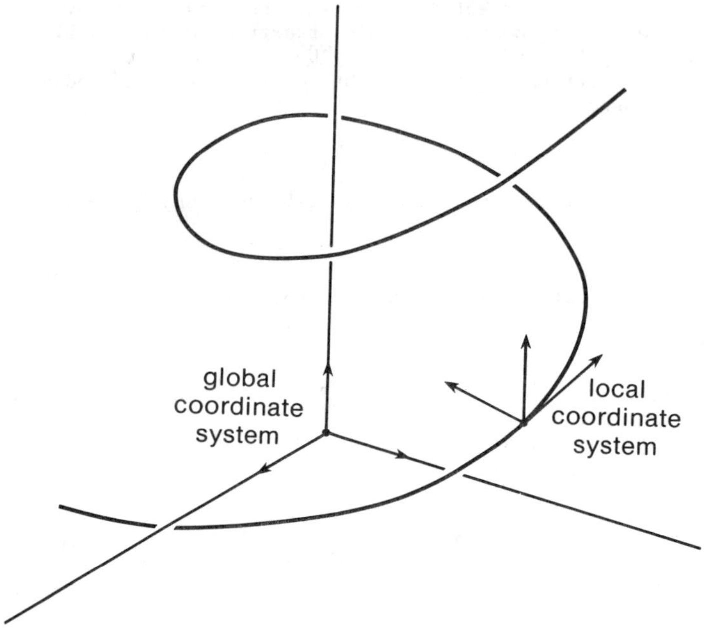

Fig. 14 - The concept of a reduced basis

There appears to be little question that for problems of this nature adaptive parametrizations again should be effective in the solution process. So far, however, the application of such techniques to problems involving plasticity and creep has not been studied widely (see, e.g., [73] and [16]).

REFERENCES

1 Felippa, C. A., "Procedures for Computer Analysis of Large Nonlinear Systems," in Large Engineering Systems, edited by A. Wexler, Pergamon Press, Oxford, 1977.

2 J. T. Oden, "Some Results of Finite Element Applications in Finite Elasticity," Computers and Structures, Vol. 3, 1973, pp. 175-194.

3 J. M. Ortega and W. C. Rheinboldt, Iterative Solution of Nonlinear Equations in Several Variables, Academic Press, New York, 1970.

4 A. M. Ostrowski, Solution of Equations in Euclidean and Banach Spaces, Third Edition, Academic Press, New York, 1973.

5 W. C. Rheinboldt, "Methods for Solving Systems of Nonlinear Equations," CBMS-Reg. Conference Series in Appl. Mathematics, Vol. 14, Society for Ind. and Appl. Math., Philadelphia, Pennsylvania, 1974.

6 H. B. Keller, "Geometrically Isolated, Nonisolated Solutions and Their Approximation," SIAM Journal of Numerical Analysis, Vol. 18, 1981, pp. 822-838.

7 W. C. Rheinboldt, "On Measures of Ill-Conditioning for Nonlinear Equations," Mathematics of Computation, Vol. 30, 1976, pp. 104-111.

8 H. Wozniakowski, "Numerical Stability for Solving Nonlinear Equations," Numerical Mathematics, Vol. 27, 1977, pp. 373-390.

9 L. Rall, Computational Solution of Nonlinear Operator Equations, John Wiley, New York, 1969.

10 H. Schwetlick, Numerische lősung nichtlinearer gleichungen, VEB Deutscher Verlag d. Wiss., Berlin, 1979.

11 W. C. Rheinboldt, "On the Solution of Some Nonlinear Equations Arising in the Application of Finite Element Methods," in Mathematics of Finite Element and Applications II, edited by J. Whiteman, Academic Press, London, 1976, pp. 462-482.

12 A. R. Curtis, M. J. D. Powell, and J. K. Reid, "On the Estimation of Sparse Jacobian Matrices," Journal Inst. Math. Appl., Vol. 13, No. 1, 1974, pp. 117-119.

13 M. P. Kamat, L. T. Watson, and D. J. VandenBrink, An Assessment of Quasi-Newton Sparse Update Techniques for Nonlinear Structural Analysis, Virginia Polytechnic Institute and State University, Computer Science Department, Technical Report CS-80013-R, 1981.

14 J. E. Dennis and J. J. Moré, "Quasi-Newton Methods, Motivation and Theory," SIAM Review, Vol. 19, No. 1, 1977, pp. 46-89.

15 R. Fletcher and M. Powell, "A Rapidly Convergent Descent Method for Minimization," Computer Journal, Vol. 6, 1963, pp. 163-168.

16 C. Broyden, "A New Method for Solving Nonlinear Simultaneous Equations," Computer Journal, Vol. 12, 1969, pp. 94-99.

17 R. Fletcher, "A New Approach to Variable Metric Algorithms," Computer Journal, Vol. 13, 1970, pp. 317-322.

18 D. Goldfarb, "A Family of Variable-Metric Methods Derived by Variational Means," Mathematics of Computation, Vol. 24, 1970, pp. 23-26.

19 D. Shanno, "Conditioning of Quasi-Newton Methods for Function Minimization," Mathematics of Computation, Vol. 24, 1970, pp. 647-656.

20 M. J. D. Powell and Ph. L. Toint, "On the Estimation of Sparse Hessian Matrices," SIAM Journal of Numerical Analysis, Vol. 11, 1979, pp. 1060-1074.

21 W. F. Schmidt, "Extending the Convergence Domain of the Newton-Raphson Method in Structural Analysis," Computers and Structures, Vol. 9, 1978, pp. 265-272.

22 L. K. Schubert, "Modification of a Quasi-Newton Method for Nonlinear Equations with a Sparse Jacobian," Mathematics of Computation, Vol. 24, 1970, pp. 27-30.

23 D. F. Shanno, "On Variable-Metric Methods for Sparse Hessians," Mathematics of Computation, Vol. 34, 1980, pp. 499-514.

24 Ph. L. Toint, "On Sparse and Symmetric Matrix Updating Subject to a Linear Equation," Mathematics of Computation, Vol. 31, 1977, pp. 954-961.

25 Ph. L. Toint, "Some Numerical Results Using a Sparse Matrix Updating Formula in Unconstrained Optimization," Mathematics of Computation, Vol. 32, 1978, pp. 839-851.

26 M. S. Engelman, G. Strang, and K. J. Bathe, "The Application of Quasi-Newton Methods in Fluid Dynamics,," International Journal for Numerical Methods in Engineering, Vol. 17, No. 5, 1981, pp. 707-718.

27 H. Matthies and G. Strang, "The Solution of Nonlinear Finite Element Equations," International Journal for Numerical Methods in Engineering, Vol. 14, 1979, pp. 1613-1626.

28 W. G. Strang, "The Quasi-Newton Method in Finite Element Computations," in Computational Methods in Nonlinear Mechanics, edited by J. T. Oden, North Holland Publishing Company, 1980, pp. 451-456.

29 G. Strang and H. Matthies, Numerical Computations in Nonlinear Mechanics, ASME Publication 79-PVP-1979.

30 K. J. Bathe, "Nonlinear Finite Element Analysis and ADINA," Computers and Structures, Vol. 13, 1981.

31 K. J. Bathe and A. Cimento, "Some Practical Procedures for the Solution of Nonlinear Finite Element Equations," Computer Methods in Applied Mechanics and Engineering, Vol. 22, 1980, p. 59.

32 M. J. Sewell, "On the Connection Between Stability and the Shape of the Equilibrium Surface," Journal of Mechanics and Physics of Solids, Vol. 14, 1966, pp. 203-230.

33 M. J. Sewell, "A General Theory of Equilibrium Paths Through Critical Points, Part I," Proceedings of the Royal Society [A], Vol. 306, 1968, pp. 201-223; Part II, Proceedings of the Royal Society [A], Vol. 306, 1968, pp. 225-238.

34 M. J. Sewell, "Some Mechanical Examples of Catastrophe Theory," Bulletin of the Institute of Mathematics and Appl., Vol. 12, 1976, pp. 163-172.

35 M. J. Sewell, "Some Global Equilibrium Surfaces," International Journal of Mechanical Engineering Education, Vol. 6, 1978, pp. 163-174.

36 W. E. Haisler and D. R. Sanders, "Elastic-Plastic-Creep-Large-Strain Analysis at Elevated Temperature by the Finite Element Method," Computers and Structures, Vol. 10, 1979, pp. 375-381.

37 W. T. Koiter, Over de stabiliteit van het elastisch evenwicht, H. J. Paris Publ., Amsterdam 1945; English translation NASA-TTF-10, 1967, 833 and Air Force Flight Dynamics Laboratory, Wright Patterson Air Force Base, Ohio, AFFDL-TR-70-25, 1970.

38 T. E. Lang and B. J. Hartz, "Finite Element Matrix Formulation of Postbuckling Stability and Imperfection Sensitivity," in High-Speed Computing of Elastic Structures, edited by B. Fraijs de Veubeke, University of Liege, Vol. 2, 1971, pp. 727-758.

39 J. M. T. Thompson, "A General Theory for the Equilibrium and Stability of Discrete Conservative Systems," ZAMP, Vol. 20, 1969, pp. 797-846.

40 J. M. T. Thompson and G. W. Hunt, A General Theory of Elastic Stability, J. Wiley and Sons, Ltd., London, 1973.

41 J. M. T. Thompson and G. W. Hunt, "Toward a Unified Bifurcation Theory," ZAMP, Vol. 26, 1975, pp. 581-603.

42 J. M. T. Thompson and A. C. Walker, "A General Theory for the Branching Analysis of Discrete Structural Systems," International Journal of Solids and Structures, Vol. 15, 1969, pp. 281-288.

43 W. T. Koiter, "Current Trends in the Theory of Buckling," in Proceedings of IUTAM Symposium on Buckling of Structures, edited by B. Budiansky, Springer-Verlag, Berlin, 1976, pp. 1-16.

44 H. B. Keller, "Constructive Methods for Bifurcation and Nonlinear Eigenvalue Problems," in Proceedings of the Third International Symposium on Computing Methods in Applied Sciences and Engineering, Versailles, France, December 1977.

45 W. C. Rheinboldt, "Numerical Analysis of Continuation Methods for Nonlinear Structural Problems," Computers and Structures, Vol. 13, 1981, pp. 103-114.

46 W. C. Rheinboldt and J. V. Burkardt, A Program for a Locally-Parametrized Continuation Process, University of Pittsburgh, Institute for Comp. Math. and Appl., Technical Report ICMA 81-30, Oct. 1981. Published in ACM Transactions on Mathematical Software, Vol. 9, No. 2, June 1983, pp. 215-235.

47 E. Riks, "An Incremental Approach to the Solution of Snapping and Buckling Problems," International Journal of Solids and Structures, Vol. 15, 1979, pp. 529-551.

48 E. Riks, "A Unified Method for the Computation of Critical Equilibrium States of Nonlinear Elastic Systems," Acta Techn. Acad. Sci. Hung., Vol. 87, 1978, pp. 121-141.

49 E. Stein and M. H. Kessel, "Num. Methoden und deren Konvergenz zur statischen Berechnung geometrisch-nichtlinearer Stabwerke im unter- und überkritischen Bereich, Ing. Archiv, Vol. 46, 1977, pp. 323-335.

50 J. A. Stricklin and W. E. Haisler, "Formulations and Solution Procedures for Nonlinear Structural Analysis," Computers and Structures, Vol. 7, 1977, pp. 125-136.

51 J. A. Stricklin, W. E. Haisler, and W. A. Von Riesemann, "Evaluation of Solution Procedures for Material and/or Geometrically Nonlinear Structural Analysis," AIAA Journal, Vol. 11, 1973, pp. 292-299.

52 J. R. Tillerson, J. A. Stricklin, and W. E. Haisler, "Numerical Methods for the Solution of Nonlinear Problems in Structural Analysis," in Numerical Solutions of Nonlinear Structural Problems, edited by R. F. Hartung, AMD-Vol. 6, The American Society of Mechanical Engineers, New York, 1973, pp. 67-101.

53 P. M. Anselone and R. H. Moore, "An Extension of the Newton-Kantorovich Method of Solving Nonlinear Equations with an Application to Elasticity," Journal of Math. Anal. Appl., Vol. 13, 1966, pp. 467-501.

54 J. L. Batoz, A. Chattopadhyay, and G. Dhatt, "Finite Element Large Deflection Analysis of Shallow Shells," International Journal for Numerical Methods in Engineering, Vol. 10, No. 1, 1976, pp. 39-58.

55 P. G. Bergan, "Solution Algorithms for Nonlinear Structural Problems," Computers and Structures, Vol. 12, No. 4, 1980, pp. 497-509.

56 P. G. Bergan, G. Horrigmoe, B. Krakeland, and H. T. Soreide, "Solution Techniques for Nonlinear Finite Element Problems," International Journal for Numerical Methods in Engineering, Vol. 12, No. 11, 1978, pp. 1677-1696.

57 S. Nemat-Nasser and H. D. Shatoff, "Numerical Analysis of Pre- and Post-Critical Response of Elastic Continua at Finite Strains," Computers and Structures, Vol. 3, 1973, pp. 983-999.

58 J. T. Oden, "Some Results of Finite Element Applications in Finite Elasticity," Computers and Structures, Vol. 3, 1973, pp. 175-194.

59 E. Riks, On the Numerical Solution of Snapping Problems in the Theory of Elastic Stability, SUDAAR No. 401, Stanford University, Stanford, California, 1970.

60 E. Riks, "The Application of Newton's Method to the Problem of Elastic Stability," Journal of Applied Mechanics, Vol. 39, 1972, pp. 1060-1066.

61 E. Riks, Basic Scheme Modified Nonlinear Procedure STAGS-A, National Aerospace Laboratories, Tech. Memo. Sc-80-126U, The Netherlands, 1980.

62 A. C. Walker, "A Method of Solution for Nonlinear Simultaneous Algebraic Equations," International Journal for Numerical Methods in Engineering, Vol. 1, 1969, pp. 177-180.

63 G. A. Wempner, "Discrete Approximations Related to Nonlinear Theories of Solids," International Journal of Solids and Structures, Vol. 17, 1971, pp. 1581-1599.

64 D. Benedetti, C. Brebbia, and L. Cedolin, "Geometrical Nonlinear Analysis of Structures by Finite Elements," Meccanica, Vol. 7, No. 1, 1972, pp. 35-44.

65 W. C. Rheinboldt, "Solution Fields of Nonlinear Equations and Continuation Methods," SIAM Journal of Numerical Analysis, Vol. 17, 1980, pp. 221-237.

66 C. B. Haselgrove, "The Solution of Nonlinear Equations and of Differential Equations with Two-Point Boundary Conditions," Computer Journal, Vol. 4, 1961, pp. 255-259.

67 L. O. Chua and A. Ushida, "A Switching Parameter Algorithm for Finding Multiple Solutions of Nonlinear Resistive Circuits," Circuit Theory and Applications, Vol. 4, 1976, pp. 215-239.

68 H. B. Keller, "Global Homotopies and Newton Methods," in Recent Advances in Numerical Analysis, edited by C. de Boor and G. H. Golub, Academic Press, New York, 1978, pp. 73-94.

69 M. Kubicek, "Dependence of Solutions of Nonlinear Equations on a Parameter, Algorithm 502," CACM-TOMS, Vol. 2, 1976, pp. 98-107.

70 R. Menzel and H. Schwetlick, "Zur Lösung parameter-abhangiger nichtlinearer Gleichungen mit singulären Jacobi-Matrizen," Numerische Mathematik, Vol. 30, 1978, pp. 65-79.

71 M. A. Crisfield, "Incremental Iterative Solution Procedures for Nonlinear Structural Analysis," in Proceedings of the International Conference on Numerical Methods for Nonlinear Problems, Swansea, September 1980, pp. 261-290.

72 M. A. Crisfield, "A Fast Incremental/Iterative Solution Procedure that Handles Snap-Through," Computers and Structures, Vol. 13, Nos. 1-3, 1981, pp. 55-62.

73 E. Ramm, "Nonlinear Finite Element Analysis in Structural Mechanics," in Proceedings of the Europe-U.S. Workshop, Ruhr Universität Bochum, edited by W. Wunderlich, E. Stein, and K. J. Bathe, Bochum, West Germany, 1980.

74 E. Riks, "Some Computational Aspects of the Stability Analysis of Nonlinear Structures," presented at the Second International Conference on Finite Elements in Nonlinear Mechanics (FENOMECH) 1981. To appear in Computer Methods in Applied Mechanics and Engineering.

75 Z. Waszczyszyn, Numerical Problems of Nonlinear Stability Analysis of Elastic Structures, Cracow Technical University, Cracow, Poland, Lecture Notes 1980.

76 H. H. Kessel, Theoretische und numerische Behandlung gerader Stäbe mit Endlichen Drehungen, Diss., Forschungs-und Seminar Berichte aus dem Bereich der Mechanik, Univ. Hannover, Report F80/1, February 1980.

77 M. Wessels, Das statische und dynamische Durchschlagsproblem der imperfekten flachen Kugelschale bei elastischer rotations-symmetrischer Verformung, Mitteilungen des Inst. fur Statik der Techn. Univ. Hannover, Report No. 23, 1977.

78 E. Riks, The Incremental Solution of Some Basic Problems in Elastic Stability, National Aerospace Laboratories, Technical Report NLR-TR-74005U, The Netherlands, 1973.

79 R. H. Gallagher, "Perturbation Procedures in Nonlinear Finite Element Structural Analysis," in Computational Mechanics, edited by J. T. Oden, Lecture Notes in Mathematics, Vol. 461, Springer-Verlag, 1975, pp. 75-89.

80 J. W. Hutchinson and W. T. Koiter, "Postbuckling Theory," Applied Mechanics Reviews, Vol. 23, No. 12, 1970, pp. 1353-1366.

81 B. Budiansky, "Theory of Buckling and Postbuckling of Elastic Structures," in Advances in Applied Mechanics, Vol. 14, edited by C. S. Yih, Academic Press, New York, 1974, pp. 1-65.

82 B. Budiansky and J. W. Hutchinson, "Dynamic Buckling of Imperfection Sensitive Structures," in Proceedings of the Eleventh International Congress of Applied Mechanics, Munich, Germany (1964), Springer-Verlag, Berlin, 1966, pp. 636-651.

83 M. J. Sewell, "A Method of Postbuckling Analysis," Journal of Mechanics and Physics of Solids, Vol. 17, 1969, pp. 219-233.

84 J. F. Besseling, "Postbuckling Analysis and Nonlinear Analysis by the Finite Element Method as a Supplement to a Linear Analysis," ZAMM, Vol. 55, No. 4, 1975, pp. T3-T15.

85 J. F. Besseling, Derivatives of Deformation Parameters in Buckling and Postbuckling Analysis, Delft University of Technology, Technical Report WTHD-84, 1977.

86 E. Carnoy, "Postbuckling Analysis of Elastic Structures by the Finite Element Method," Computer Methods in Applied Mechanics and Engineering, Vol. 23, No. 2, 1980, pp. 143-174.

87 R. Casciaro and M. Aristodemo, "Perturbation Analysis of Geometrically Nonlinear Structures," in Finite Elements in Nonlinear Mechanics, edited by P. G. Bergan et al., Tapir Publishing, Trondheim, 1978, pp. 433-452.

88 R. Casciaro, A. DiCarlo and M. Pignatara, A Finite Element Technique for Bifurcation Analysis, Univ. Roma, Ist. di Scienza delle Costruzioni, Tech. Report 11-192, 1976.

89 J. J. Connor and N. Morin, "Perturbation Techniques in the Analysis of Geometrically Nonlinear Shells," in High Speed Computing of Elastic Structures, edited by B. Fraijs de Veubeke, University of Liege, Vol. 2, 1971, pp. 683-705.

90 A. Ecer, "Finite Element Analysis of the Postbuckling Behavior of Structures," AIAA Journal, Vol. 11, No. 11, 1973, pp. 1532-1538.

91 R. T. Haftka, R. H. Mallett and W. Nachbar, "Adaptation of Koiter's Method to Finite Element Analysis of Snap-Through Buckling Behavior," International Journal of Solids and Structures, Vol. 7, No. 10, 1971, pp. 1427-1445.

92 A. Levy and A. B. Pifko, "On Computational Strategies for Problems Involving Plasticity and Creep," International Journal for Numerical Methods in Engineering, Vol. 17, 1981, pp. 747-771.

93 R. H. Mallett and R. T. Haftka, "Progress in Nonlinear Finite Element Analysis Using Asymptotic Solution Techniques," in Advances in Computational Methods in Structural Mechanics and Design, edited by J. T. Oden, UAH Press, The University of Alabama in Huntsville, 1972, pp. 357-374.

94 R. G. Vos, "Finite Element Solution of Nonlinear Structures by Perturbation Technique," in Computational Methods in Nonlinear Mechanics, edited by J. T. Oden et al., The Texas Institute for Computational Mechanics, Austin, Texas, 1974, pp. 787-796.

95 S. T. Mau and R. H. Gallagher, A Finite Element Procedure for Nonlinear Prebuckling and Initial Postbuckling Analysis, NASA CR-1936, 1972.

96 B. O. Almroth, F. A. Brogan and H. B. Marlowe, Collapse Analysis for Shells of General Shape, Air Force Flight Dynamics Laboratory, Wright Patterson Air Force Base, Ohio, Technical Report AFFDL-71-8, August 1972.

97 B. O. Almroth and F. A. Brogan, The STAGS Computer Code, NASA CR-2950, February 1978.

98 T. Matsui and O. Matsuoka, "A New Finite Element Scheme for Instability Analysis of Thin Shells," International Journal for Numerical Methods in Engineering, Vol. 10, 1976, pp. 145-170.

99 H. B. Keller, "Numerical Solution of Bifurcation and Nonlinear Eigenvalue Problems," in Applications of Bifurcation Theory, edited by P. Rabinowitz, Academic Press, New York, 1977, pp. 359-384.

100 W. F. Schmidt, "Adaptive Stepsize Selection for Use with the Continuation Method," International Journal for Numerical Methods in Engineering, Vol. 12, 1978, pp. 677-694.

101 C. Den Heijer and W. C. Rheinboldt, "On Steplength Algorithms for a Class of Continuation Methods," SIAM Journal of Numerical Analysis, Vol. 18, No. 5, 1981, pp. 925-948.

102 J. P. Abbott, "An Efficient Algorithm for the Determination of Certain Bifurcation Points," Journal of Computational and Applied Mathematics, Vol. 4, No. 1, 1978, pp. 19-27.

103 J. C. Paumier, "Une methode numerique pour le calcul des points de retournement. Application a un probleme aux limites non-lineaire," Numerische Mathematik, Vol. 37, 1981, pp. 433-444.

104 G. Pönisch and H. Schwetlich, "Computing Turning Points of Curves Implicitly Defined by Nonlinear Equations Depending on a Parameter," Computing, Vol. 26, 1981, pp. 107-121.

105 W. C. Rheinboldt, "Computation of Critical Boundaries on Equilibrium Manifolds," SIAM Journal of Numerical Analysis, Vol. 19, 1982, pp. 653-669.

106 H. Schwetlick, Effective Methods for Computing Turning Points of Curves Implicitly Defined by Nonlinear Equations, Martin Luther Univ. Halle Wittenberg, Sektion Mathem., Preprint No. 46, 1981.

107 R. Seydel, "Numerical Computation of Branch Points in Nonlinear Equations," Numerische Mathematik, Vol. 33, 1979, pp. 339-352.

108 R. B. Simpson, "A Method for the Numerical Determination of Bifurcation States of Nonlinear Systems of Equations," SIAM Journal of Numerical Analysis, Vol. 12, 1975, pp. 439-451.

109 R. G. Melhem and W. C. Rheinboldt, A Comparison of Methods for Determining Turning Points of Nonlinear Equations, University of Pittsburgh, Institute for Computational Mathematics and Applications, Technical Report ICMA-82-32, January 1982. Published in Computing, Vol. 29, 1982, pp. 201-226.

110 P. H. Rabinowitz (editors), Applications of Bifurcation Theory, Academic Press, New York, 1977.

111 I. Stakgold, "Branching of Solutions of Nonlinear Equations," SIAM Review, Vol. 13, 1971, pp. 289-332.

112 M. M. Vainberg and V. A. Trenogin, Theory of Branching of Solutions of Nonlinear Equations, Noordhoff International Publishing Company, Leyden, 1974.

113 M. J. Sewell, "The Static Perturbation Technique in Buckling Problems," Journal of Mechanics and Physics of Solids, Vol. 13, 1965, pp. 247-265.

114 M. S. Berger and D. Westreich, "A Convergent Iteration Scheme for Bifurcation Theory in Banach-Spaces," Journal of Math. Anal. Appl., Vol. 43, No. 1, 1973, pp. 136-144.

115 D. W. Decker and H. B. Keller, "Multiple Limit Point Bifurcation," Journal of Math. Anal. Appl., Vol. 75, No. 2, 1980, pp. 417-430.

116 D. W. Decker and H. B. Keller, "Solution Branching - A Constructive Technique," in New Approaches to Nonlinear Problems in Dynamics, edited by P. Holmes, SIAM Publication, Philadelphia, Pennsylvania, 1980, pp. 53-69.

117 D. W. Decker and H. B. Keller, "Path Following Near Bifurcation," Comm. Pure and Appl. Math., Vol. 34, No. 2, 1981, pp. 149-175.

118 M. Kubicek and M. Marek, "Evaluation of Limit and Bifurcation Points for Algebraic Equations and Nonlinear Boundary Value Problems," Appl. Math. Comput., Vol. 5, 1979, pp. 253-264.

119 D. Westreich and Y. L. Varol, "Numerical Bifurcation at Simple Eigenvalues," SIAM Journal of Numerical Analysis, Vol. 16, 1979, pp. 538-546.

120 Y. M. J. Demoulin and Y. M. Chen, "An Iteration Method for Studying the Bifurcation Solutions of the Nonlinear Equations, $L(\lambda)u + \varepsilon R(\lambda,u) = 0$," Numerische Mathematik, Vol. 23, No. 1, 1974, pp. 47-61.

121 Y. M. J. Demoulin and Y. M. Chen, "An Iteration Method for Solving Nonlinear Eigenvalue Problems," SIAM Journal of Applied Mathematics, Vol. 28, No. 3, 1975, pp. 588-595.

122 J. P. Keener and H. B. Keller, "Perturbed Bifurcation Theory," Arch. Rat. Mech. Anal., Vol. 50, 1973, pp. 159-175.

123 H. B. Keller, "Nonlinear Bifurcation," J. Diff. Equ., Vol. 7, 1970, pp. 417-434.

124 H. B. Keller and W. F. Langford, "Iterations, Perturbations and Multiplicities for Nonlinear Bifurcation Problems," Arch. Rat. Mech. Anal., Vol. 48, 1972, pp. 83-108.

125 W. C. Rheinboldt, "Numerical Continuation Methods for Finite Element Applications," in Formulations and Computational Algorithms in Finite Element Analysis, edited by J. Bathe, J. T. Oden and W. Wunderlich, M.I.T. Press, Cambridge, Massachusetts, 1977, pp. 599-631.

126 W. C. Rheinboldt, "Numerical Methods for a Class of Finite-Dimensional Bifurcation Problems," SIAM Journal of Numerical Analysis, Vol. 15, 1978, pp. 1-11.

127 G. Moore and A. Spence, "The Calculation of Turning Points of Nonlinear Equations," SIAM Journal of Numerical Analysis, Vol. 17, 1980, pp. 567-576.

128 I. Babuska and W. C. Rheinboldt, Computational Error Estimates and Adaptive Processes for Some Nonlinear Structural Problems, University of Pittsburgh, Institute for Comp. Math. and Appl., Technical Report ICMA-81-28, July 1981. Published in Computer Methods in Applied Mechanics and Engineering, Vol. 34, 1982, pp. 895-937.

129 I. Babuska and A. Miller, A-Posteriori Error Estimates and Adaptive Techniques for the Finite Element Method, University of Maryland, Institute for Physical Science and Technology, Technical Note BN-968, 1981.

130 I. Babuska and W. C. Rheinboldt, "On a System for Adaptive, Parallel Finite Element Computations," in Proceedings of the 1978 Annual Conference, Association for Computing Mech., New York, 1978, pp. 480-489.

131 I. Babuska and W. C. Rheinboldt, "Error Estimates for Adaptive Finite Element Computations," SIAM Journal of Numerical Analysis, Vol. 15, No. 4, 1978, pp. 736-754.

132 I. Babuska and W. C. Rheinboldt, "A-Posteriori Error Estimates for the Finite Element Method," International Journal for Numerical Methods in Engineering, Vol. 12, No. 10, 1978, pp. 1597-1615.

133 I. Babuska and W. C. Rheinboldt, "Adaptive Approaches and Reliability Estimates in Finite Element Analysis," Computer Methods in Applied Mechanics and Engineering, Vols. 17/18, 1979, pp. 519-540.

134 I. Babuska and W. R. Rheinboldt, "On the Reliability and Optimality of the Finite Element Method," Computers and Structures, Vol. 10, Nos. 1/2, 1979, pp. 87-94.

135 I. Babuska and W. C. Rheinboldt, "Reliable Error Estimation and Mesh Adaptation for the Finite Element Method," in Computational Methods in Nonlinear Mechanics, edited by J. T. Oden, North Holland Publishing Co., Amsterdam, 1980, pp. 67-108.

136 I. Babuska and W. C. Rheinboldt, "A-Posteriori Error Analysis of Finite Element Solutions for One-Dimensional Problems," SIAM Journal of Numerical Analysis, Vol. 18, No. 3, 1981, pp. 565-589.

137 R. Gaines, "Difference Equations Associated with Boundary Value Problems for Second-Order Nonlinear Ordinary Differential Equations," SIAM Journal of Numerical Analysis, Vol. 11, 1974, pp. 411-434.

138 H. O. Peitgen, D. Saupe and K. Schmitt, "Nonlinear Elliptic Boundary Value Problems Versus Their Finite Difference Approximations: Numerically Irrelevant Solutions," J. Reine Angew. Math., Vol. 322, 1981, pp. 74-117.

139 P. Zave and W. C. Rheinboldt, "Design of An Adaptive Parallel Finite Element System," ACM-TOMS, Vol. 5, 1979, pp. 1-17.

140 A. K. Noor and J. M. Peters, "Reduced Basis Technique for Nonlinear Analysis of Structures," AIAA Journal, Vol. 18, 1980, pp. 455-462.

141 B. O. Almroth, P. Stern and F. A. Brogan, "Use of Global Functions for Improvement in Efficiency of Nonlinear Analysis," in Proceedings of 22nd Structures, Structural Dynamics and Materials Conference, Atlanta, Georgia, April 6-8, 1981, Part 1, pp. 286-292.

142 A. K. Noor, C. M. Andersen and J. M. Peters, "Reduced Basis Technique for Collapse Analysis of Shells," AIAA Journal, Vol. 19, 1981, pp. 393-397.

143 A. K. Noor, "Recent Advances in Reduction Methods for Nonlinear Problems," Computers and Structures, Vol. 13, 1981, pp. 31-44.

144 B. O. Almroth, P. Stern and F. A. Brogan, "Automatic Choice of Global Shape Functions in Structural Analysis," AIAA Journal, Vol. 16, 1978, pp. 525-528.

145 C. Nyssen, "An Efficient and Accurate Iterative Method Allowing Large Incremental Steps to Solve Elasto-Plastic Problems," Computers and Structures, Vol. 13, 1981, pp. 63-71.

146 J. F. Besseling, "Nonlinear Analysis," in World Congress on Finite Element Methods in Structural Mechanics, edited by J. Robinson, Dorset, England, October 1975.

147 K. Huseyin, Nonlinear Theory of Elastic Stability, Noordhoff International Publishing Co., Leyden, The Netherlands, 1975.

148 H. Armen, "Assumptions, Models and Computational Methods for Plasticity," Computers and Structures, Vol. 10, 1979, pp. 161-174.

149 K. J. Bathe, E. Ramm and E. L. Wilson, "Finite Element Formulation for Large Deformation Dynamic Analysis," International Journal for Numerical Methods in Engineering, Vol. 9, No. 2, 1975, pp. 353-386.

150 J. H. Argyris and M. Kleiber, Incremental Formulation in Nonlinear Mechanics and Large-Strain Elasto-Plasticity, University of Stuttgart, Institute for Statics and Dynamics, Technical Report ISD-211, 1976.

151 K. Axelson and A. Samuelsson, "Finite Element Analysis of Elastic-Plastic Materials Displaying Mixed Hardening," International Journal for Numerical Methods in Engineering, Vol. 14, No. 2, 1979, pp. 211-225.

152 J. Bäcklund and H. Wennerstrom, "Finite Element Analysis of Elasto-Plastic Shells," International Journal for Numerical Methods in Engineering, Vol. 8, No. 2, 1974, pp. 415-424.

153 D. Bushnell, "A Strategy for the Solution of Problems Involving Large Deflections, Plasticity and Creep," International Journal for Numerical Methods in Engineering, Vol. 11, No. 4, 1977, pp. 683-708.

154 M. Capurso, "A General Method for the Incremental Solution of Elastic-Plastic Problems," Meccanica, Vol. 4, 1969, pp. 267-280.

155 O. De Donato and A. Franchi, "A Modified Gradient Method for Finite Element Elasto-Plastic Analysis by Quadratic Programming," Journal of Computer Methods in Applied Mechanics and Engineering, Vol. 2, No. 2, 1973, pp. 107-131.

156 J. W. Hutchinson, "Finite Strain Analysis of Elastic-Plastic Solids and Structures," in Numerical Solution of Nonlinear Structural Problems, edited by R. F. Hartung, AMD-Vol. 6, The American Society of Mechanical Engineers, New York, 1973, pp. 17-29.

157 N. Q. Son, "On the Elastic Plastic Initial Boundary Value Problem and Its Numerical Integration," International Journal for Numerical Methods in Engineering, Vol. 11, 1977, pp. 817-832.

158 Y. Yokoo, T. Nakamura and K. Uetani, "The Incremental Perturbation Method for Large Displacement Analysis of Elastic-Plastic Structures," International Journal for Numerical Methods in Engineering, Vol. 10, 1976, pp. 503-525.

159 O. C. Zienkiewicz, The Finite Element Method, third edition, McGraw-Hill, New York, 1977.

160 O. C. Zienkiewicz and G. C. Cormeau, "Visco-Plasticity and Creep in Elastic Solids - A Unified Numerical Approach," International Journal for Numerical Methods in Engineering, Vol. 8, 1974, pp. 821-845.

161 I. Cormeau, "Numerical Stability in Quasi-Static Elasto-Visco Plasticity," International Journal for Numerical Methods in Engineering, Vol. 9, No. 1, 1975, pp. 109-127.

CHAPTER EIGHT

REANALYSIS, MODAL SYNTHESIS AND DYNAMIC DESIGN

B. P. Wang and W. D. Pikey
University of Virginia
Charlottesville, Virginia

A. R. Palazzolo
Southwest Research Institute
San Antonio, Texas

ABSTRACT

This chapter reviews current methodology for static and dynamic reanalysis, modal synthesis, and dynamic design of large finite element systems. In the case of dynamic reanalysis several approximate methods, as applied to self adjoint systems, are reviewed. Then most of these methods are extended to general, damped systems. For static reanalysis, both exact and approximate methods are reviewed and a new derivation of an exact reanalysis technique is given. Modal synthesis is a field with increasing popularity and utility. Several modal synthesis techniques are summarized and scrutinized. Finally, the application of reanalysis techniques to dynamic design is reviewed. Several numerical examples are included to illustrate the analytical formulations.

INTRODUCTION

The finite element method has made possible the accurate static and dynamic response analysis of large, complex structures (1,2,3). The structural property matrices associated with finite element models are frequently dimensioned in the thousands, as for a complex automobile or piping system models. Ordinarily, the solution of systems of linear equations or eigenvalue problems of this order can be accurately obtained with the techniques presented in computationally oriented linear algebra texts (4,5,6) or in more specialized references (7). During the design of these structures a particular set of critical parameters are usually varied in order to obtain an optimum design. Efficient and accurate methods of evaluating how changes in these parameters affect response variables, or what parameter changes are required to attain prescribed response levels are very beneficial. Of course, to justify their use these methods must be more efficient than a complete reanalysis for each parameter set change and yet must maintain sufficient accuracy. The four topics discussed in this chapter are directed towards achieving this goal.

Considered first is the change in eigenvalues and eigenvectors as certain parts of the structure are modified. This eigensolution reanalysis utilizes the original modal properties to provide efficient estimates of the modified system's eigensolutions. The next topic addresses the calculation of parameter changes required to obtain specified system eigenvalues and/or eigenvectors. This is termed "prescribed eigensolution design". The methods here can be used to improve the agreement of analytical models with modal testing, i.e., to perform system identification. The third area is modal synthesis which may be viewed as a modification problem in which the number of system degrees of freedom changes due to the modifications. Finally, static reanalysis methods are treated; approximate solutions to the equilibrium equation are obtained as chosen parameters are modified.

The efficiency and accuracy of the approximate methods considered improve relative to a complete reanalysis as the modifications become smaller. The modifications either have small magnitudes distributed over large portions of the structure or are localized and of arbirary magnitude.

The related topics concerning optimized eigensolution design, systems with repeated eigenvalues, and modifications which leave certain eigenvalues invariant are not discussed. These topics may be found in the references.

NOMENCLATURE

General Notation

$\underline{diag}$ ( )	=	diagonal matrix
$\underline{I}_k$	=	unit matrix of dimension k
i, j, k, l, m, n,	=	integer indices
$\bar{m}_i$, a_{1i}, a_{2i}	=	1, common eigenvector normalization convention
"o"	=	right superscript, original or unmodified system quantity
T	=	right superscript, matrix transpose
Δ	=	quantity change, unless otherwise indicated
$\hat{\delta}_{ij}$	=	Kronecker delta, = 1 if i=j, = 0 if i $\neq$ j
Π	=	series product expression
Σ	=	series summation expression
___	=	underbar, indicates matrix-vector quantity
Re ( )	=	real part of complex quantity ( )
Im ( )	=	imaginary part of complex quantity ( )
$\underline{A} > 0$		matrix $\underline{A}$ is symmetric, positive definite
$\underline{A} \geq 0$		matrix $\underline{A}$ is symmetric, positive semi-definite
dof		degrees of freedom
det ( )	=	determinant of

Vibrations, Eigensolution Reanalysis, Prescribed Eigensolution Design

$\underline{A}_1$, $\underline{B}_1$	=	system property matrices of state space formulation for mass modification reanalysis
$\underline{A}_2$, $\underline{B}_2$	=	system property matrices of state space formulation for stiffness and damping modification reanalysis
a_{1i}, a_{2i}	=	ith mode normalization constants for $\underline{A}_1$, $\underline{B}_1$ and $\underline{A}_2$, $\underline{B}_2$ formulations, respectively
$\underline{C}^o$	=	unmodified system's classical or proportional damping matrix
$\underline{C}$	=	general damping matrix
$\underline{\Delta C}$	=	damping modification matrix
$\underline{D}$	=	dynamical matrix for regular eigenvalue problem of the state space formulation
d_i	=	ith design parameter of system

F_{ij} = ij element of receptance matrix ($\underline{F}$), for proportionately damped unmodified systems

G_{ij} = ij element of receptance matrix ($\underline{G}$) for undamped, symmetric unmodified systems

$g(\omega_n^2)$, $g(\lambda_n)$ = characteristic equation of the modified system

i = unit imaginary number, $i = \sqrt{-1}$

$j_1, j_2, \ldots j_p$ = sparsity indices in receptance method

$\underline{K}^o$ = unmodified system's symmetric, positive semi-definite stiffness matrix

$\underline{K}$ = general stiffness matrix

$\underline{\Delta K}$ = stiffness modification matrix

L = number of unmodified system lower modes used in reanalysis

$\underline{M}^o$ = unmodified system's symmetric, positive definite mass matrix

$\underline{M}$ = general mass matrix

$\underline{\Delta M}$ = mass modification matrix

$\bar{m}_i$ = ith mode normalization constant for undamped, positive semi-definite systems

N = number of system degrees of freedom

R = higher mode factor, receptance method

$\underline{S}$ = effective modification matrix

Ω_k^2 = kth eigenvalue of an undamped system

ω_k^2 = kth eigenvalue of an undamped modified system

α_k = kth complex eigenvalue of a damped, general system

λ_k = kth complex eigenvalue of a damped, general modified system

$\underline{\phi}_k$ = kth eigenvector of an undamped, system

$\underline{\theta}_k$ = kth eigenvector of an undamped, modified system

$\underline{\Lambda}_k$ = kth complex eigenvector of a damped, general system

$\underline{\psi}_k$ = kth complex eigenvector of a damped, general modified system

$\underline{\delta}_k$ = kth adjoint eigenvector of a damped, general system

$\underline{\tau}_k$ = kth adjoint eigenvector of a damped, general modified system

$\underline{\Gamma}_k$ = kth complex eigenvector - state space formulation

$\underline{\gamma}_k$ = kth left eigenvector, $(\lambda \underline{A}^T + \underline{B}^T)\underline{\gamma} = \underline{0}$

$\underline{\beta}_k$ = kth left eigenvector, $(\lambda \underline{I} - \underline{D}^T)\underline{\beta} = \underline{0}$

$\underline{\xi}_k$ = kth generalized coordinate vector

ϕ_{ij} = ith component of $\underline{\phi}_j$

ξ_{ij} = ith component of $\underline{\xi}_j$

ζ_k = kth mode proportional damping factor

μ_m, μ_c, μ_k = mass, damping and stiffness modification magnitudes in rank 1 matrix-eigensolution reanalysis

Modal Synthesis

$\underline{f}^k_j$ = reaction force vector acting on the junction degrees of freedom (dof) of substructure k

$\underline{G}^k$ = receptance matrix of undamped substructure k

i = subscript indicating substructure interior dof

j = subscript indicating substructure junction (interface) dof

$\underline{K}^n$ = symmetric stiffness matrix of substructure n

$\underline{\Delta K}$ = receptance method connection-modification stiffness matrix

$\underline{M}^n$ = symmetric mass matrix of substructure n

$\underline{\Delta M}$ = receptance method connection-modification mass matrix

$\bar{m}_{kn}$ = kth constrained interface-normal mode normalization constant of substructure n. Also, kth normal mode normalization constant of substructure n.

m_n = number of constrained interface-lower normal modes of substructure n used in synthesis. Also, number of lower normal modes of substructure n used in synthesis

N_n = total number of degrees of freedom of substructure n (interior plus interface)

$\underline{Q}$ = coordinate transformation matrix between the substructures

$\underline{q}_c^k$ = generalized coordinate vector for the constraint modes of substructure k

$\underline{q}_n^k$ = generalized coordinate vector for the fixed interface normal modes of substructure k

$\bar{\underline{q}}$ = vector of "independent" generalized coordinates

R_n = receptance higher mode factor of the nth substructure

r = number of interface degrees of freedom (dof)

$\underline{S}$ = effective connection and modification matrix for the receptance method

$\underline{U}$ = combined system displacement vector

$\underline{U}_i^m$ = displacement vector for the interior dof of the mth undamped substructure

$\underline{U}_j^m$ = displacement vector for the interface dof of the mth undamped substructure

$\underline{\phi}_n^m$ = fixed interface-normal modal matrix for the mth substructure (uncoupled system)

$\underline{\phi}_{nk}^m$ = kth fixed interface-normal mode of the mth substructure (uncoupled system)

$\underline{\Phi}_c^m$ = constraint modal matrix for the mth substructure (uncoupled system)

$\underline{\Phi}^m$ = normal modal matrix for the mth substructure (uncoupled system)

$\underline{\phi}_k^m$ = kth normal mode of the mth substructure (uncoupled system)

ϕ_{ikm} = ith component of the kth normal mode of the mth substructure (uncoupled system)

Ω_{km}^2 = kth constrained-interface eigenvalue of the mth substructure, (uncoupled system). Also, kth eigenvalue of the mth substructure, (uncoupled system)

$\underline{\theta}_k$ = kth eigenvector of the coupled system

$\underline{\theta}_k^m$ = kth eigenvector of the mth substructure (coupled system)

ω_k^2 = kth eigenvalue of the coupled system

Static Reanalysis

$\underline{b}$ = a Boolean matrix which expands $\underline{\Delta \tilde{\tilde{K}}}$ into $\underline{\Delta K}$, $\underline{\Delta K} = \underline{b}^T\, \underline{\Delta \tilde{\tilde{K}}}\, \underline{b}$

B = system bandwidth

d_i = ith design parameter

D = number of design variables

$\underline{K}$ = system stiffness matrix

$\underline{K}_i$ = modified system stiffness matrix with the 1 through ith nonzero columns of $\underline{\Delta K}$ included

$\underline{\Delta K}$ = stiffness modification matrix of system

$\underline{\Delta \tilde{K}}$ = $\underline{\Delta K}$ with all null columns removed

$\underline{\Delta \tilde{K}}_i = \underline{X}_i$ = ith non-null column of $\underline{\Delta K}$

$\underline{\Delta \tilde{\tilde{K}}}$ = $\underline{\Delta \tilde{K}}$ with all null rows removed

$\underline{L}$ = lower triangular matrix

n_c = number of nonnull columns (rows) of $\underline{\Delta K}$

$\underline{P}$ = external load vector

r = number of reduced basis vectors

$\underline{R}$ = transformation matrix

$\underline{U}$ = original system solution

$\overline{\underline{U}}$ = modified system solution

$\underline{U}^{(i)}$ = ith basis vector used in the reduced basis method

$\underline{U}_i$ = modified system solution after the 1 through ith nonnull columns of $\underline{\Delta K}$ are included

$\underline{W}_i^{(k)} = \underline{K}_k^{-1} \underline{X}_i = \underline{K}_k^{-1} \underline{\Delta \tilde{K}}_i$

$\underline{X}_i$ = $\underline{\Delta \tilde{K}}_i$, ith column of $\underline{X}$

$\underline{Y}_i^T$ = ith row of $\underline{Y}^T$

VIBRATION FUNDAMENTALS

This section provides a short review of the types of vibratory systems most commonly discussed in the literature. This material should suffice as background material and as a nomenclature aid to subsequent discussions.

Undamped Symmetric Systems

The undamped symmetric system is the most common type of system encountered in structural vibration problems. Analytically the eigenvalue problem can be represented by

$$(-\Omega_k^2\, \underline{M}^o + \underline{K}^o)\, \underline{\phi}_k = \underline{0} \qquad (N \times 1) \qquad (1)$$

With the modal matrix

$$\underline{\Phi} = [\underline{\phi}_1 \vdots \underline{\phi}_2 \vdots \cdots \vdots \underline{\phi}_L] \qquad (N \times L),\ L \leq N \qquad (2)$$

the orthogonality conditions are

$$(\underline{\Phi}^T \underline{M}^o \underline{\Phi})_{ij} = \underline{\phi}_i^T \underline{M}^o \underline{\phi}_j = \hat{\delta}_{ij} \bar{m}_i \qquad (1 \times 1) \qquad (3)$$

$$(\underline{\Phi}^T \underline{K}^o \underline{\Phi})_{ij} = \underline{\phi}_i^T \underline{K}^o \underline{\phi}_j = \hat{\delta}_{ij} \bar{m}_i \Omega_i^2 \qquad (1 \times 1) \qquad (4)$$

Proportionately Damped Systems

The classical damping model of proportional damping is very popular in structural forced response studies since it results in uncoupled equations of motion. A brief mathematical description is

$$(\alpha_k^2 \underline{M}^o + \alpha_k \underline{C}^o + \underline{K}^o) \underline{\Lambda}_k = \underline{0} \qquad (N \times 1) \qquad (5)$$

Equations (3) and (4) still apply, as well as

$$(\underline{\Phi}^T \underline{C}^o \underline{\Phi})_{ij} = \underline{\phi}_i^T \underline{C}^o \underline{\phi}_j = \hat{\delta}_{ij}\ 2\ \zeta_i \Omega_i \bar{m}_i \qquad (1 \times 1) \qquad (6)$$

$$\alpha_k = -\zeta_k \Omega_k \pm i\ \Omega_k \sqrt{1 - \zeta_k^2} \qquad (1 \times 1) \qquad (7)$$

$$\underline{\Lambda}_k = \underline{\phi}_k \qquad (N \times 1) \qquad (8)$$

$$\underline{C}^o = \underline{M}^o \left(\sum_{k=1}^{N} \underline{\phi}_k \underline{\phi}_k^T 2\zeta_k \Omega_k / \bar{m}_k\right) \underline{M}^o \qquad (N \times N) \qquad (9)$$

General Damped Systems

General damped systems are encountered most often in modeling spinning structures especially in the study of rotor-bearing systems (12,13). Biorthogonality conditions between the system's right (regular) and left (adjoint) eigenvectors appear here. The defining equations are

Regular System: $$(\alpha_k^2 \underline{M} + \alpha_k \underline{C} + \underline{K}) \underline{\Lambda}_k = \underline{0} \qquad (N \times 1) \qquad (10)$$

Adjoint System: $$(\alpha_k^2 \underline{M}^T + \alpha_k \underline{C}^T + \underline{K}^T) \underline{\delta}_k = \underline{0} \qquad (N \times 1) \qquad (11)$$

Generalized Eigenvalue Problem Formulation

$$(\alpha_k \underline{A}_1 + \underline{B}_1) \underline{\Gamma}_k = \underline{0}, \qquad (\alpha_k \underline{A}_1^T + \underline{B}_1^T) \underline{\gamma}_k = \underline{0} \qquad (2N \times 1) \tag{12}$$

$$(\alpha_k \underline{A}_2 + \underline{B}_2) \underline{\Gamma}_k = \underline{0}, \qquad (\alpha_k \underline{A}_2^T + \underline{B}_2^T) \underline{\gamma}_k = \underline{0} \qquad (2N \times 1) \tag{13}$$

$$\underline{A}_1 = \left[\begin{array}{c|c} \underline{M} & \underline{0} \\ \hline \underline{0} & -\underline{K} \end{array}\right], \qquad \underline{B}_1 = \left[\begin{array}{c|c} \underline{C} & \underline{K} \\ \hline \underline{K} & \underline{0} \end{array}\right] \qquad (2N \times 2N) \tag{14}$$

$$\underline{A}_2 = \left[\begin{array}{c|c} \underline{0} & \underline{M} \\ \hline \underline{M} & \underline{C} \end{array}\right], \qquad \underline{B}_2 = \left[\begin{array}{c|c} -\underline{M} & \underline{0} \\ \hline \underline{0} & \underline{K} \end{array}\right] \qquad (2N \times 2N) \tag{15}$$

$$\underline{\Gamma} = [\underline{\Gamma}_1 \,|\, \underline{\Gamma}_2 \,|\cdots|\, \underline{\Gamma}_L] = \left[\begin{array}{c|c|c|c} \alpha_1 \underline{\Lambda}_1 & \alpha_2 \underline{\Lambda}_2 & \cdots & \alpha_L \underline{\Lambda}_L \\ \underline{\Lambda}_1 & \underline{\Lambda}_2 & & \underline{\Lambda}_L \end{array}\right] \qquad (2N \times L) \tag{16}$$

$$\underline{\gamma} = [\underline{\gamma}_1 \,|\, \underline{\gamma}_2 \,|\cdots|\, \underline{\gamma}_L] = \left[\begin{array}{c|c|c|c} \alpha_1 \underline{\delta}_1 & \alpha_2 \underline{\delta}_2 & \cdots & \alpha_L \underline{\delta}_L \\ \underline{\delta}_1 & \underline{\delta}_2 & & \underline{\delta}_L \end{array}\right] \qquad (2N \times L) \tag{17}$$

$$\begin{aligned}(\underline{\gamma}^T \underline{A}_1 \underline{\Gamma})_{ij} &= \underline{\gamma}_i^T \underline{A}_1 \underline{\Gamma}_j = \underline{\delta}_i^T (\alpha_i \alpha_j \underline{M} - \underline{K}) \underline{\Lambda}_j \\ &= \hat{\delta}_{ij}\, \underline{\delta}_i^T (\alpha_i^2 \underline{M} - \underline{K}) \underline{\Lambda}_i = \hat{\delta}_{ij}\, a_{1i} \qquad (1 \times 1)\end{aligned} \tag{18}$$

$$\begin{aligned}(\underline{\gamma}^T \underline{B}_1 \underline{\Gamma})_{ij} &= \underline{\gamma}_i^T \underline{B}_1 \underline{\Gamma}_j = \underline{\delta}_i^T (\alpha_i \alpha_j \underline{C} + (\alpha_i + \alpha_j) \underline{K}) \underline{\Lambda}_j \\ &= \hat{\delta}_{ij}\, \underline{\delta}_i^T (\alpha_i^2 \underline{C} + 2\alpha_i \underline{K}) \underline{\Lambda}_i = -\hat{\delta}_{ij}\, a_{1i} \alpha_i \qquad (1 \times 1)\end{aligned} \tag{19}$$

$$\begin{aligned}(\underline{\gamma}^T \underline{A}_2 \underline{\Gamma})_{ij} &= \underline{\gamma}_i^T \underline{A}_2 \underline{\Gamma}_j = \underline{\delta}_i^T ((\alpha_i + \alpha_j) \underline{M} + \underline{C}) \underline{\Lambda}_j \\ &= \hat{\delta}_{ij}\, \underline{\delta}_i^T (2\alpha_i \underline{M} + \underline{C}) \underline{\Lambda}_i = \hat{\delta}_{ij}\, a_{2i} \qquad (1 \times 1)\end{aligned} \tag{20}$$

$$(\underline{\gamma}^T \underline{B}_2 \underline{\Gamma})_{ij} = \underline{\gamma}_i^T \underline{B}_2 \underline{\Gamma}_j = \underline{\delta}_i^T (- \alpha_i \alpha_j \underline{M} + \underline{K}) \underline{\Lambda}_j$$

$$= \hat{\delta}_{ij} \underline{\delta}_i^T (- \alpha_i^2 \underline{M} + \underline{K}) \underline{\Lambda}_i = - \hat{\delta}_{ij} a_{2i} \alpha_i \qquad (1 \times 1) \qquad (21)$$

$$a_{2i} = a_{1i}/\alpha_i \quad , \quad \alpha_i \neq 0$$

Regular Eigenvalue Problem Formulation

$$\underline{D} = - \underline{A}_1^{-1} \underline{B}_1 = - \underline{A}_2^{-1} \underline{B}_2 = \left[\begin{array}{c|c} - \underline{M}^{-1} \underline{C} & - \underline{M}^{-1} \underline{K} \\ \hline \underline{I}_N & \underline{0} \end{array}\right]$$

$$\underline{D}^{-1} = \left[\begin{array}{c|c} \underline{0} & \underline{I}_N \\ \hline - \underline{K}^{-1} \underline{M} & - \underline{K}^{-1} \underline{C} \end{array}\right] \qquad (2N \times 2N) \qquad (22)$$

$\underline{M}$, $\underline{K}$ - Non Singular

$$(\frac{1}{\alpha_k} \underline{I}_{2N} - \underline{D}^{-1}) \underline{\Gamma}_k = \underline{0}, \; (\frac{1}{\alpha_k} \underline{I}_{2N} - (\underline{D}^{-1})^T) \underline{\beta}_k = \underline{0} \quad (2N \times 1) \qquad (23)$$

$$\underline{\beta}_i^T \underline{\Gamma}_j = \hat{\delta}_{ij} a_{1i} , \quad \underline{\beta}_i^T \underline{D} \underline{\Gamma}_j = \hat{\delta}_{ij} a_{1i} \alpha_i \qquad (1 \times 1) \qquad (24)$$

$$\underline{\beta}_i = \underline{A}_1^T \underline{\gamma}_i \qquad (2N \times 1) \qquad (25)$$

$\underline{M}$ - Non Singular

$$(\alpha_k \underline{I}_{2N} - \underline{D}) \underline{\Gamma}_k = \underline{0}, \qquad (\alpha_k \underline{I}_{2N} - \underline{D}^T) \underline{\beta}_k = \underline{0} \qquad (2N \times 1) \qquad (26)$$

$$\underline{\beta}_i^T \underline{\Gamma}_j = \hat{\delta}_{ij} a_{2i}, \quad \underline{\beta}_i^T \underline{D} \underline{\Gamma}_j = \hat{\delta}_{ij} a_{2i} \alpha_i \qquad (1 \times 1) \qquad (27)$$

$$\underline{\beta}_i = \underline{A}_2^T \underline{\gamma}_i \qquad (2N \times 1) \qquad (28)$$

Symmetric Damped Systems (Lagrangian)

$\underline{M}$: positive definite, $\underline{C}$ and $\underline{K}$: positive semi-definite, $\underline{D} \neq \underline{D}^T$ (29)

$$\underline{\delta}_k = \underline{\Lambda}_k \; (N \times 1), \; \underline{\gamma}_k = \underline{\Gamma}_k, \; \underline{\gamma}_k \neq \underline{\beta}_k \neq \underline{\Gamma}_k \qquad (2N \times 1) \qquad (30)$$

Real $(\alpha_k) \leq 0$, equality holding only if (1) $\underline{C}$ is positive semi-definite or (2) $\underline{K}$ is positive semi-definite or (3) $\underline{C} = \underline{0}$.

Structural Damping

Structural or hysteretic damping is used to account for the frequency-independent energy dissipation which occurs within the material of a structure. A brief mathematical description of the free vibration problem is

$$(\alpha_k^2 \underline{M} + (\underline{K}_1 + i \underline{K}_2)) \underline{\Lambda}_k = \underline{0} \qquad (N \times 1) \tag{31}$$

$$\underline{M} = \underline{M}^T, \ \underline{K}_1 = \underline{K}_1^T, \ \ \underline{K}_2 = \underline{K}_2^T \qquad (N \times N) \tag{32}$$

$$\underline{\Lambda}_j^T \underline{M} \underline{\Lambda}_k = \hat{\delta}_{jk} \tilde{m}_j, \ \ \underline{\Lambda}_j^T (\underline{K}_1 + i \underline{K}_2) \underline{\Lambda}_k = \hat{\delta}_{jk} \tilde{m}_j \alpha_j^2 \qquad (1 \times 1) \tag{33}$$

assuming $\alpha_j^2 \neq \alpha_k^2$

Gyroscopic Systems

A conservative gyroscopic system is encountered in models of spinning structures (14,15). Usually a general damping matrix is added to account for energy dissipation. Neglecting the additional damping, this system type exhibits several interesting modal characteristics.

$$\text{Regular System:} \quad (\alpha_k^2 \underline{M} + \alpha_k \underline{C} + \underline{K}) \underline{\Lambda}_k = \underline{0} \qquad (N \times 1) \tag{34}$$

$$\text{Adjoint System:} \quad (\alpha_k^2 \underline{M}^T + \alpha_k \underline{C}^T + \underline{K}^T) \underline{\delta}_k = \underline{0} \qquad (N \times 1) \tag{35}$$

$$\begin{gathered} \underline{M} > 0, \ \underline{K} \geq 0, \ \underline{C}^T = - \underline{C} \ \text{(skew symmetric)} \\ \text{Real } (\alpha_k) = 0, \ \underline{\delta}_k = \bar{\underline{\Lambda}}_k \ \text{(complex conjugate)} \end{gathered} \tag{36}$$

The second property of equation (36) is useful in checking rotordynamic stability codes. If viscous damping and nonsymmetric forces are ignored and if the rotor is run at spin rate ω, then at spin rate $-\omega$ the resulting eigenvectors should be complex conjugates (reference 16, p. 21).

EIGENSOLUTION REANALYSIS

In the following five subsections, some techniques for obtaining the eigenvalues and eigenvectors of modified structural systems are outlined. Use of the unmodified system's modal characteristics leads to greater computational efficiency when compared with total reanalysis. The results of the first two subsections can only produce approximate eigensolutions, while those of the final three subsections may provide exact results if the unmodified system's modal data are complete.

Perturbation Type 1

This method assumes relatively small modifications so that the eigensolution changes are only of the first order. A Rayleigh's quotient (17) approximation is

$$\omega_n^2 = \Omega_n^2 + \Delta(\Omega_n^2) \simeq \frac{\underline{\phi}_n^T (\underline{K}^o + \underline{\Delta K}) \underline{\phi}_n}{\underline{\phi}_n^T (\underline{M}^o + \underline{\Delta M}) \underline{\phi}_n} = \frac{\bar{m}_n \Omega_n^2 + \underline{\phi}_n^T \underline{\Delta K} \underline{\phi}_n}{\bar{m}_n + \underline{\phi}_n^T \underline{\Delta M} \underline{\phi}_n} \tag{37}$$

which uses the original system's eigenvectors. Stetson and Palma (18) have derived the following formulas for the eigensolution perturbations of an undamped symmetric system,

$$\Delta(\Omega_n^2)/\Omega_n^2 \cong 2\Delta\Omega_n/\Omega_n \cong \underline{\phi}_n^T \, (\underline{\Delta K}/\Omega_n^2 - \underline{\Delta M}) \, \underline{\phi}_n/\bar{m}_n \tag{38}$$

$$\underline{\theta}_n = \underline{\phi}_n + \underline{\Delta\phi}_n = \underline{\phi}_n + \sum_{k=1}^{N} C_{nk} \, \underline{\phi}_k \tag{39}$$

$$C_{nk} = \frac{\Omega_n^2}{\bar{m}_k \, (\Omega_n^2 - \Omega_k^2)} \quad \underline{\phi}_n^T \, (\underline{\Delta K}/\Omega_n^2 - \underline{\Delta M}) \, \underline{\phi}_k, \qquad C_{nn} = 0 \tag{40}$$

Franklin (98) shows that $\{C_{nn} = 0\}$ in equations (39) and (40), is a necessary normalization convention for the modified system eigenvector. The convention is: considering $\underline{\theta}_n$ expanded with $\underline{\phi}_i$ the coefficient of $\underline{\phi}_n$ exactly equals 1.0. This ensures that both $\Delta\underline{\phi}_n$ and $\Delta(\Omega_n^2)$ are identically zero when $\underline{\Delta M}$ and $\underline{\Delta K}$ are null matrices. Lund (19) has applied similar formulas to a study of critical speed sensitivities to parameter variation in rotor-bearing system design. Lancaster (20) has treated the problem of adding a damping modification matrix, $\underline{\Delta C}$, to an initially undamped, symmetric system ($\underline{M}^o$, $\underline{K}^o$).

Assuming a normalization convention, in which $\bar{m}_n=1$, his results are

$$\varepsilon \, \overline{\underline{\Delta C}} = \underline{\Phi}^T \, \underline{\Delta C} \, \underline{\Phi} \tag{41}$$

$$\lambda_n = i\Omega_n + \varepsilon \, (- \overline{\underline{\Delta C}}_{nn}/2) + \varepsilon^2 \, t_n^* \tag{42}$$

$$\underline{\psi}_n = \underline{\phi}_n + \varepsilon \, \underline{\Phi} \, (\underline{R}_n + \varepsilon \, \underline{S}_n) \tag{43}$$

$$R_{kn} = i\Omega_n \, \overline{\underline{\Delta C}}_{kn}/(\Omega_n^2 - \Omega_k^2) \quad , \qquad R_{nn} = 0 \tag{44}$$

$$t_n^* = (\overline{\underline{\Delta C}}_{nn})^2/(i8\Omega_n) - \sum_{j=1}^{N} \overline{\underline{\Delta C}}_{nj} \, R_{jn}/2 \tag{45}$$

$$S_{kn} = \frac{\overline{\underline{\Delta C}}_{kn} \, \overline{\underline{\Delta C}}_{nn} \, (\Omega_k^2 + \Omega_n^2)}{2(\Omega_n^2 - \Omega_k^2)^2} + \frac{i\Omega_n \sum_{j=1}^{N} R_{jn} \, \overline{\underline{\Delta C}}_{kj}}{\Omega_n^2 - \Omega_k^2}, \quad S_{nn} = 0 \tag{46}$$

In equation (41) the constant ε is selected so that $\overline{\underline{\Delta C}}_{ij}$ are approximately the same order of magnitude as $\underline{M}_{ij}^o$ and $\underline{K}_{ij}^o$. Aubrun (21) considers the addition of damping and stiffness modification matrices, $\underline{\Delta C}$ and $\underline{\Delta K}$, to an initially undamped, symmetric system. With an $\bar{m}_n = 1$ normalization convention his perturbed eigenvalue formula is given by

$$\lambda_n = - \underline{\phi}_n^T \, \underline{\Delta C} \, \underline{\phi}_n/2 + i(\Omega_n + \underline{\phi}_n^T \, \underline{\Delta K} \, \underline{\phi}_n/2\Omega_n) \tag{47}$$

Meirovitch and Ryland (22) have treated the case of initially gyroscopic systems. The initial system eigensolutions are shown to be calculable from a real symmetric matrix formulation. The modification consists of the addition of a symmetric damping matrix to the gyroscopic system. Second-order perturbation formulas for the modified system's eigensolution are derived. Finally these eigensolutions are utilized in forced responses analyses.

Romstad, Hutchinson, and Runge (23) have approached this topic in a similar manner to Lancaster. Their results are also expressed as a power series in the small quantity ε as in equations (42) and (43).

Perturbation Type 2

This perturbation technique explicitly involves derivatives of the system property matrices with respect to a selected set of "design" parameters,

$$\underline{d} = (d_1\ d_2\ \cdots\ d_r)^T \qquad (r \times 1) \tag{48}$$

The initial system parameter values are

$$\underline{d}^o = (d_1^o\ d_2^o\ \cdots\ d_r^o)^T \qquad (r \times 1) \tag{49}$$

Eigensolution derivatives with respect to these parameters are used in truncated Taylor series, expanded about the initial design vector, $\underline{d}^o$.

Fox and Kapoor (24) have treated undamped, symmetric systems in this manner. Their results, employing the $\bar{m}_n = 1$ normalization convention, are

$$\underline{M}\ (\underline{d}^o) = \underline{M}^o, \quad \underline{K}\ (\underline{d}^o) = K^o \tag{50}$$

$$\omega_n^2 = \Omega_n^2 + \left.\frac{\partial(\Omega_n^2)}{\partial d_1}\right|_{\underline{d}^o} \Delta d_1 + \cdots + \left.\frac{\partial(\Omega_n^2)}{\partial d_r}\right|_{\underline{d}^o} \Delta d_r \tag{51}$$

$$\frac{\partial(\Omega_n^2)}{\partial d_k} = \underline{\phi}_n^T \left(\frac{\partial}{\partial d_k} \underline{K} - \Omega_n^2 \frac{\partial}{\partial d_k} \underline{M} \right) \underline{\phi}_n \tag{52}$$

$$\underline{\theta}_n = \underline{\phi}_n + \left.\frac{\partial}{\partial d_1} \underline{\phi}_n \right|_{\underline{d}^o} \Delta d_1 + \cdots + \left.\frac{\partial}{\partial d_r} \underline{\phi}_n \right|_{\underline{d}^o} \Delta d_r \tag{53}$$

The nth eigenvector formula is

$$\frac{\partial}{\partial d_k} \underline{\phi}_n = - (\underline{W}_n^2 + 2\,\underline{M}\,\underline{\phi}_n\,\underline{\phi}_n^T\,\underline{M})^{-1} \left(\underline{W}_n \frac{\partial}{\partial d_k} \underline{W}_n + \underline{M}\,\underline{\phi}_n\,\underline{\phi}_n^T \frac{\partial}{\partial d_k} \underline{M}\right)\underline{\phi}_n \tag{54}$$

$$\underline{W}_n = \Omega_n^2\,\underline{M} - \underline{K}, \quad \frac{\partial}{\partial d_k} \underline{W}_n = \frac{\partial(\Omega_n^2)}{\partial d_k} \underline{M} + \Omega_n^2 \frac{\partial}{\partial d_k} \underline{M} - \frac{\partial}{\partial d_k} \underline{K} \tag{55}$$

The complete eigenvector set formula is

$$\frac{\partial}{\partial d_k} \underline{\phi}_n = \sum_{j=1}^{N} a_{nkj}\, \underline{\phi}_j \tag{56}$$

$$a_{nkj} = \underline{\phi}_j^T \left(\frac{\partial}{\partial d_k} \underline{K} - \Omega_n^2 \frac{\partial}{\partial d_k} \underline{M}\right) \underline{\phi}_n / (\Omega_n^2 - \Omega_j^2)$$

$$a_{nkn} = - \underline{\phi}_n^T \left(\frac{\partial}{\partial d_k} \underline{M}\right) \underline{\phi}_n / 2 \tag{57}$$

Equations (51) and (52) produce the same results as the Rayleigh quotient formula, equations (37), when $\partial\underline{M}/\partial d_k = \underline{0}$ and the stiffness matrix is a linear function of the design variables.

A second-order perturbation formula for the eigenvalues of an undamped, symmetric system is derived from the three-term Taylor series expansion (Brogan 25)

$$\omega_n^2 = \Omega_n^2 + \sum_{j=1}^{r} \left.\frac{\partial(\Omega_n^2)}{\partial d_j}\right|_{\underline{d}^o} \Delta d_j + \tfrac{1}{2} \sum_{i=1}^{r} \sum_{j=1}^{r} \left.\frac{\partial^2(\Omega_n^2)}{\partial d_i \partial d_j}\right|_{\underline{d}^o} \Delta d_i\, \Delta d_j \tag{58}$$

where from Rudisill's paper (26)

$$\frac{\partial^2(\Omega^2_n)}{\partial d_i \partial d_j} = \underline{\phi}_n^T \Big(\Big(\frac{\partial^2 \underline{K}}{\partial d_i \partial d_j} - \Omega_n^2 \frac{\partial^2 \underline{M}}{\partial d_i \partial d_j} - \frac{\partial(\Omega^2_n)}{\partial d_i} \frac{\partial \underline{M}}{\partial d_j}$$

$$- \frac{\partial(\Omega_n^2)}{\partial d_j} \frac{\partial \underline{M}}{\partial d_i}\Big) \underline{\phi}_n + \Big(\frac{\partial K}{\partial d_j} - \Omega_n^2 \frac{\partial M}{\partial d_j} - \frac{\partial(\Omega_n^2)}{\partial d_j} \underline{M}\Big) \frac{\partial \phi_n}{\partial d_i} \tag{59}$$

$$+\Big(\frac{\partial \underline{K}}{\partial d_i} - \Omega_n^2 \frac{\partial \underline{M}}{\partial d_i} - \frac{\partial(\Omega_n^2)}{\partial d_i} \underline{M}\Big)\frac{\partial \underline{\phi}_n}{\partial d_j} \Big)$$

Thus the second derivative of an eigenvalue depends on the first derivative of both the eigenvalue and its eigenvector. The simple spring mass model shown in Figure 1 illustrates the increased accuracy obtainable from a second-order perturbation. The results are

$\Omega_1^2 = 0.3820,\ \Omega_2^2 = 2.6180,\ \underline{\phi}_1 = [0.5257 \quad 0.8507]^T,$

$\underline{\phi}_2 = [0.8507 \quad - 0.5257]^T$

$\partial\Omega_1^2/\partial k_1 = 0.2764,\ \partial^2\Omega_1^2/\partial k_1^2 = - 0.1788,\ \ \partial\ \underline{\phi}_1/\partial k_1 = [- 0.1701 \quad 0.1051]^T$

Solution Method	ω_1^2	Error
Exact	0.5000	-
1st Order Perturbation	0.5202	4.04%
2nd Order Perturbation	0.4970	-0.60%

Bhatia (27) has employed this type of perturbation scheme for undamped, symmetric systems in a different way. The modified system modal matrix is defined as

$$\underline{\Theta} = [\underline{\theta}_1 \mid \underline{\theta}_2 \mid \cdots \mid \underline{\theta}_L] \qquad (N \times L) \tag{60}$$

the corresponding modal mass and stiffness matrices are,

$$\bar{\underline{M}} = \underline{\Theta}^T \underline{M}\ \underline{\Theta}\ , \qquad \bar{\underline{K}} = \underline{\Theta}^T\ \underline{K}\ \underline{\Theta} \qquad (L \times L) \tag{61}$$

The partial derivatives of these modal matrices with respect to mass and stiffness design parameters are derived and substituted into first order Taylor series formulas. For any specific parameter set only the condensed (order L) eigenvalue problem

$$(\ \bar{\underline{K}} - \omega_n^2\ \bar{\underline{M}})\ \underline{\xi}_n = \underline{0} \qquad (L \times 1),\ \underline{\theta}_n = \underline{T}\ \underline{\xi}_n \qquad (N \times 1) \tag{62}$$

need be solved. Static condensation (Clough 28) is directly incorporated by the method.

Type 2 perturbation has been developed by several authors for general damped systems. Plaut (29) and Rogers (30) approached this problem using right and left eigenvectors of the generalized eigenvalue problem, equation (13). Their results are outlined below, in which an $a_{2n} = 1.0$ normalization convention is utilized.

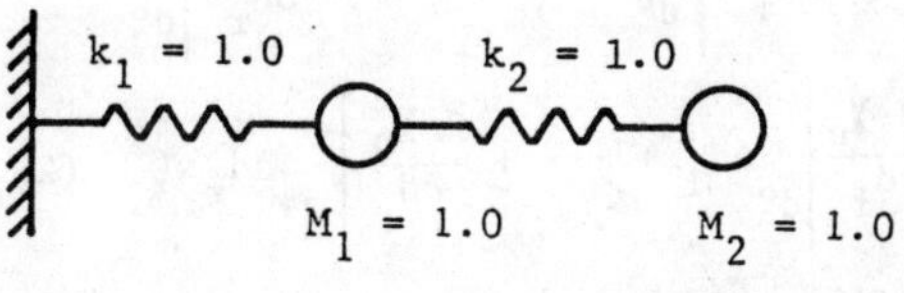

1.

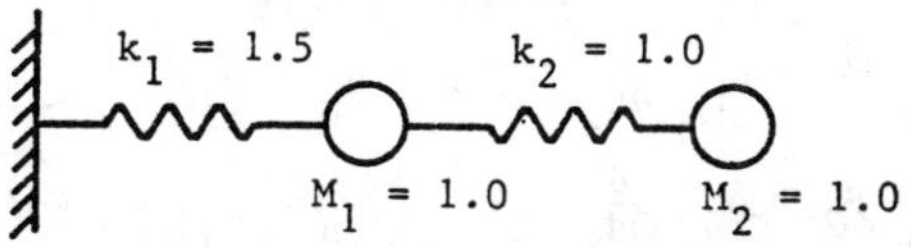

2.

Figure 1. Analysis of modified 2 dof system using perturbation methods
(1) original system
(2) modified system

$$\lambda_n \tilde{=} \alpha_n + \frac{\partial \alpha_n}{\partial d_1}\bigg|_{\underline{d}^o} \Delta d_1 + \cdots + \frac{\partial \alpha_n}{\partial d_r}\bigg|_{\underline{d}^o} \Delta d_r \tag{63}$$

$$\begin{bmatrix} \lambda_n \underline{\psi}_n \\ \hline \underline{\psi}_n \end{bmatrix} \cong \underline{\Gamma}_n + \frac{\partial \underline{\Gamma}_n}{\partial d_1}\bigg|_{\underline{d}^o} \Delta d_1 + \cdots + \frac{\partial \underline{\Gamma}_n}{\partial d_r}\bigg|_{\underline{d}^o} \Delta d_r \quad (2N \times 1) \tag{64}$$

$$\begin{bmatrix} \lambda_n \underline{\tau}_n \\ \hline \underline{\tau}_n \end{bmatrix} \tilde{=} \underline{\gamma}_n + \frac{\partial \underline{\gamma}_n}{\partial d_1}\bigg|_{\underline{d}^o} \Delta d_1 + \cdots + \frac{\partial \underline{\gamma}_n}{\partial d_r}\bigg|_{\underline{d}^o} \Delta d_r \quad (2N \times 1) \tag{65}$$

$$\frac{\partial \alpha_n}{\partial d_k} = - \underline{\delta}_n^T \left(\alpha_n^2 \frac{\partial \underline{M}}{\partial d_k} + \alpha_n \frac{\partial \underline{C}}{\partial d_k} + \frac{\partial \underline{K}}{\partial d_k}\right) \underline{\Lambda}_n \tag{66}$$

$$\frac{\partial \underline{\Gamma}_n}{\partial d_k} = \sum_{j=1}^{2N} c_{nkj} \underline{\Gamma}_j \ , \ \frac{\partial \underline{\gamma}_n}{\partial d_k} = \sum_{j=1}^{2N} f_{nkj} \underline{\gamma}_j \tag{67}$$

$$c_{nkj} = - \underline{\gamma}_j^T \left(\frac{\partial}{\partial d_k} \underline{B}_2 + \alpha_n \frac{\partial}{\partial d_k} \underline{A}_2\right) \underline{\Gamma}_n / (\alpha_n - \alpha_j) \qquad (j \neq n) \tag{68}$$

$$f_{nkj} = - \underline{\gamma}_n^T \left(\frac{\partial}{\partial d_k} \underline{B}_2 + \alpha_n \frac{\partial}{\partial d_k} \underline{A}_2\right) \underline{\Gamma}_j / (\alpha_n - \alpha_j) \qquad (j \neq n) \tag{69}$$

$$c_{nkn} + f_{nkn} = - \underline{\gamma}_n^T \frac{\partial \underline{A}_2}{\partial d_k} \underline{\Gamma}_n \tag{70}$$

Since two vectors, $\underline{\Gamma}_n$ and $\underline{\gamma}_n$, correspond to eigenvalue α_n, an additional modal constraint must be imposed to uniquely solve for c_{nkn} and f_{nkn}. Rogers chooses $\Gamma_{mn} = 1.0$, for some m, which yields

$$c_{nkn} = - \sum_{\substack{j=1 \\ j \neq n}}^{2N} c_{nkj} \Gamma_{mj} \tag{71}$$

Equations (63) - (71) are a generalization of Fox's analysis, equations (50) - (57). Comparing these formulas requires consideration of the mode normalization conventions used. Similar to equation (56), the eigenvector derivative formulas require both full sets of unmodified system right and left eigenvectors. As with undamped symmetric systems (54), an approach, proposed by both Garg (31) and also Rudisill (26), is available which requires only the nth unmodified system eigenvlaue and right eigenvector. Garg's method involves the solution of two sets of 2N+1 real simultaneous equations. Rudisill requires the solution of 2N complex simultaneous equations, but also uses the nth left eigenvector of the unmodified system. With this formulation, or its undamped counterpart, equation (54), only one matrix inversion (triangularization) per eigensolution is computed, independent of the number of d_k.

Bodewig (reference 32, p. 283) has presented a summary and extension of Jacobi's work on method 2 eigensolution perturbation of "neighbor systems." This reference is limited to the regular eigenvalue problem formulation, i.e., $\underline{A}\ \underline{x} = \lambda\ \underline{x}$.

Assumed Modes - Rayleigh Ritz Approach

This technique is discussed by Clough (28), Meirovitch (17), Hurty (33), and Bisplinghoff (34), as applied to both continuous structural members, and discrete system vibrations. The method here involves an expansion of the modified system eigenvectors by a partial set of the original system's eigenvectors. This limits the modified system eigenvectors to the vector subspace formed by the partial set. When the initial system is undamped and symmetric this implies

$$\underline{\psi}_n = \underline{\Phi}\,\underline{\xi}_n = \sum_{i=1}^{L} \xi_{in}\,\underline{\phi}_i \qquad (N \times 1) \tag{72}$$

Substitute this transformation into the modified system's equilibrium equations, written as

$$(\lambda_n^2\,(\underline{M}^o + \underline{\Delta M}) + \lambda_n\,\underline{\Delta C} + (\underline{K}^o + \underline{\Delta K}))\underline{\psi}_n = \underline{0} \qquad (N \times 1) \tag{73}$$

Premultiply by $\underline{\Phi}^T$, use the orthogonality relations of equations (3) and (4), and arrange the results into a state vector, generalized eigenvalue problem form

$$\left\{\lambda_n \begin{bmatrix} \underline{0} & \underline{\text{diag}}\,(\bar{m}_i) + \underline{\Phi}^T\,\underline{\Delta M}\,\underline{\Phi} \\ \underline{\text{diag}}\,(\bar{m}_i) + \underline{\Phi}^T\,\underline{\Delta M}\,\underline{\Phi} & \underline{\Phi}^T\,\underline{\Delta C}\,\underline{\Phi} \end{bmatrix} + \begin{bmatrix} -\underline{\text{diag}}\,(\bar{m}_i) - \underline{\Phi}^T\,\underline{\Delta M}\,\underline{\Phi} & \underline{0} \\ \underline{0} & \underline{\text{diag}}\,(\bar{m}_i\Omega_i^2) + \underline{\Phi}^T\,\underline{\Delta K}\,\underline{\Phi} \end{bmatrix}\right\} \begin{bmatrix} \lambda_n\,\underline{\xi}_n \\ \underline{\xi}_n \end{bmatrix} = \begin{bmatrix} \underline{0} \\ \underline{0} \end{bmatrix} \tag{74}$$

The order of the transformed system (2L) is selected to be significantly smaller than that of a direct solution of equation (73), i.e. 2N. Gunter and Choy (35) report excellent results with this method in calculating the complex eigenvalues of non-conservative rotor bearing systems. Accuracy comparisons of the modified system's eigenvectors and normalization constants, a_{1i} or a_{2i}, were not included.

The assumed modes approach for undamped, symmetric modifications has the form

$$(-\omega_n^2\,(\underline{\text{diag}}\,(\bar{m}_i) + \underline{\Phi}^T\,\underline{\Delta M}\,\underline{\Phi}) + (\underline{\text{diag}}\,(\bar{m}_i\,\Omega_i^2) + \underline{\Phi}^T\,\underline{\Delta K}\,\underline{\Phi}))\,\underline{\xi}_n = \underline{0} \qquad (L \times 1) \tag{75}$$

$$\underline{\theta}_n = \underline{\Phi}\,\underline{\xi}_n \qquad (N \times 1) \tag{76}$$

The ij element of the coefficient matrix in equation (75) is

$$Q_{nij} = \hat{\delta}_{ij}\;\bar{m}_i(\Omega_i^2 - \omega_n^2) + \underline{\phi}_i^T\,(\underline{\Delta K} - \omega_n^2\,\underline{\Delta M})\underline{\phi}_j \qquad (1 \times 1) \tag{77}$$

Then, if the off-diagonal terms are ignored, the condition for nontrivial $\underline{\xi}_n$ is

$$\prod_{i=1}^{L} \{\, \bar{m}_i(\Omega_i^2 - \omega_n^2) + \underline{\phi}_i^T\,\underline{\Delta K}\,\underline{\phi}_i - \omega_n^2\,\underline{\phi}_i^T\,\underline{\Delta M}\,\underline{\phi}_i \} = 0 \qquad (1 \times 1) \tag{78}$$

which shows, by comparison with equation (37), that the assumed modes method is a generalization of Rayleigh's quotient.

Romstad (23) has compared assumed modes (condensed eigenvalue method) to several other reanalysis techniques as applied to column elastic stability problems.

Rank 1 Modification Matrices

This approach is a subclass of assumed modes which results when the modification matrices are restricted to the form,

$$\underset{(1x1)}{\mu} \cdot \underset{(Nx1)}{\underline{P}} \cdot \underset{(1xN)}{\underline{g}^T} \qquad (NxN) \tag{79}$$

where μ is the modification magnitude and the vectors $\underline{P}$ and $\underline{g}$ position the modification. A simple example is the attachment of a spring (k_s) between two system degrees of freedom,

$$\underline{\Delta K} = k_s \cdot \begin{bmatrix} 0 \\ \cdot \\ \cdot \\ \cdot \\ 1 \\ \cdot \\ \cdot \\ \cdot \\ -1 \\ \cdot \\ \cdot \\ \cdot \\ 0 \end{bmatrix} \cdot [0\cdots1\cdots-1\cdots0] = \begin{bmatrix} 0 & \cdot & \cdot & \cdot & 0 \\ \cdot & \cdot & \cdot & \cdot & \cdot \\ \cdot & k_s & \cdots & -k_s & \cdot \\ \cdot & \cdot & & \cdot & \cdot \\ \cdot & \cdot & & \cdot & \cdot \\ \cdot & \cdot & & \cdot & \cdot \\ \cdot & -k_s & \cdots & k_s & \cdot \\ \cdot & \cdot & & \cdot & \cdot \\ 0 & \cdot & & \cdot & 0 \end{bmatrix} \tag{80}$$

Other practical forms of equation (79) may be found in the Static Reanalysis section.

Weissenburger (36,37) initially examined this modification form, although Wilkinson (4) had previously presented its analysis for symmetric matrices, in the regular eigenvalue problem form, $\underline{A}\ \underline{x} = \lambda\ \underline{x}$. Weissenburger's work was concerned with the discrete modification, i.e., mass, spring, dashpot attachment, of continuous structural members such as beams, plates, and rings. The Rayleigh Ritz method (17) and energy principles were used in transforming from the continuous to the discrete model and the modification is then represented in the form of equation (79).

Pomazal (38,39), Hallquist (40,41), and Snyder extended this approach to modified discrete systems. An advantage of the form of equation (79) is that the modified system's characteristic equation becomes an explicity nondeterminantal function, which is easily differentiated for Newton-Raphson iteration. Also, the corresponding eigenvectors are calculated without solving simultaneous homogeneous equations or using inverse iteration. The following subsections summarize the results for various types of vibratory systems. The classification refers to the unmodified system.

Undamped, Symmetric

$$\underline{\Delta K} = \mu_k\ \underline{P}\ \underline{P}^T, \quad \underline{\Delta M} = \mu_m\ \underline{P}\ \underline{P}^T \tag{81}$$

Assumed modes transformation matrix: $\underline{\Phi}$, equation (2)

Premultiplication matrix: $\underline{\Phi}^T$

Modified system characteristic equation:

$$g(\omega_n^2) = \frac{1}{\mu_k - \mu_m \omega_n^2} + \sum_{i=1}^{L} \frac{(\underline{\phi}_i^T\ \underline{P})^2}{\bar{m}_i(\Omega_i^2 - \omega_n^2)} = 0 \tag{82}$$

Modified system eigenvector formula:

$$\underline{\theta}_n = \sum_{i=1}^{L} \frac{(\underline{\phi}_i^T\ \underline{P})}{\bar{m}_i(\Omega_i^2 - \omega_n^2)}\ \underline{\phi}_i \qquad (Nx1) \tag{83}$$

Proportionately Damped, Symmetric

$$\underline{\Delta M} = \mu_m \underline{P} \underline{g}^T, \ \underline{\Delta K} = \mu_k \underline{P} \underline{g}^T, \ \underline{\Delta C} = \mu_c \underline{P} \underline{g}^T \tag{84}$$

Assumed modes transformation matrix: $\underline{\Phi}$, equation (2)

Premultiplication matrix: $\underline{\Phi}^T$

Modified system characteristic equation:

$$g(\lambda_n) = \frac{1}{\mu_m\lambda_n^2 + \mu_c\lambda_n + \mu_k} + \sum_{i=1}^{L} \frac{(\underline{\phi}_i^T \underline{g})\ (\underline{\phi}_i^T \underline{P})}{\bar{m}_i(\lambda_n^2 + 2\zeta_i\Omega_i\lambda_n + \Omega_i^2)} = 0 \tag{85}$$

Modified system eigenvector formula:

$$\underline{\psi}_n = \sum_{i=1}^{L} \frac{(\underline{\phi}_i^T \underline{P})}{\bar{m}_i(\lambda_n^2 + 2\zeta_i\Omega_i\lambda_n + \Omega_i^2)} \underline{\phi}_i \qquad (N\text{x}1) \tag{86}$$

General, Damped

<u>Mass Modification</u>

$\underline{M}$, $\underline{K}$ nonsingular

$\underline{\Delta M} = \mu_m \underline{P} \underline{g}^T$

Assumed modes transformation matrix: $\underline{\Gamma}$, equation (16)

Premultiplication matrix: $\underline{\gamma}^T$, equation (17)

Modified system characteristic equation:

$$g(\lambda_n) = \frac{1}{\mu_m\lambda_n} + \sum_{i=1}^{L} \frac{\alpha_i^2\ (\underline{\Lambda}_i^T \underline{g})\ (\underline{\delta}_i^T \underline{P})}{a_{1i}\ (\lambda_n - \alpha_i)} = 0 \tag{87}$$

Modified system eigenvector formula

$$\underline{\psi}_n = \sum_{i=1}^{L} \frac{\alpha_i\ (\underline{\delta}_i^T \underline{P})}{a_{1i}(\lambda_n - \alpha_i)} \underline{\Lambda}_i \qquad (N \text{ x } 1) \tag{88}$$

<u>Stiffness and Damping Modifications</u>

$\underline{M}$ nonsingular

$$\underline{\Delta K} = \mu_k \underline{P} \underline{g}^T, \quad \underline{\Delta C} = \mu_c \underline{P} \underline{g}^T \tag{89}$$

Assumed modes transformation matrix: $\underline{\Gamma}$, equation (16)

Premultiplication matrix: $\underline{\gamma}^T$, equation (17)

Modified system characteristic equation:

$$g(\lambda_n) = \frac{1}{\mu_c\lambda_n + \mu_k} + \sum_{i=1}^{L} \frac{(\underline{\Lambda}_i^T \underline{g})(\underline{\delta}_i^T \underline{P})}{a_{2i}\ (\lambda_n - \alpha_i)} = 0 \tag{90}$$

Modified system eigenvector formula:

$$\underline{\psi}_n = \sum_{i=1}^{L} \frac{(\underline{\delta}_i^T \underline{P})}{a_{2i}\,(\lambda_n - \alpha_i)} \underline{\Lambda}_i \qquad (N\text{x}1) \qquad (91)$$

To treat the case of an initially damped symmetric system substitute

$$\underline{g} = \underline{P} \quad \text{and} \quad \underline{\delta}_i = \underline{\Lambda}_i \qquad (N\text{x}1) \qquad (92)$$

in equations (87) - (91). For an initially gyroscopic system substitute

$$\underline{\delta}_i = \overline{\underline{\Lambda}}_i \quad \text{(complex conjugate)} \qquad (93)$$

into these equations. Using the general damped case with equations (87) - (91), the complex conjugate unmodified system eigensolution ($\overline{\alpha}_i$, $\overline{a}_{2i}$, $\overline{\underline{\Lambda}}_i$, $\overline{\underline{\delta}}_i$) should be included as an additional term in the summations whenever a complex eigensolution (α_i, a_{2i}, $\underline{\Lambda}_i$, $\underline{\delta}_i$) is used.

Normally only one of the constants, μ_m, μ_c, or μ_k is nonzero for a particular modification. For most problems the total modification may be expressed as a summation of terms like equation (79). The preceeding equations then from the basis of a recurrence scheme where one modification is added at each step. The eigensolutions of the (j-1)th step are used as the "unmodified system" eigensolutions for the jth step. The property matrices must also be updated at each step since they are required in the calculation of the normalization constants ($\overline{m}_i$, a_{1i}, a_{2i}). Care must be taken when the system type changes as the modification terms are added. Hallquist (41) has pointed out that this method is useful when adding element matrices as modifications to a finite element model. This is the case since every real positive semi-definite matrix is orthogonally similar to the diagonal matrix of its eigenvalues, i.e.,

$$\underline{H} = \underline{Y}\,\underline{\sigma}\,\underline{Y}^T = \sum_{i=1}^{N} \sigma_i\, \underline{Y}_i\, \underline{Y}_i^T \qquad (94)$$

where σ_i are the nonzero eigenvalues and $\underline{Y}_i$ the orthonormal eigenvectors, of $\underline{H}$. The addition of $\underline{H}$ is then equivalent to adding n column vector-row vector product matrices (see reference (92) for a discussion.) Using this decomposition Vilmann and Snyder (42) have treated the line modification, i.e., rigid or spring line support, of continuous structural members.

Receptance Approach

This approach is distinguished by it ability to condense the eigenvalue problem according to the sparsity of the modification matrices, to incorporate the effects of truncated higher order modes of the unmodified system, and to treat multiple modifications simultaneously. The method assumes that all eigenvalues are, at least to some degree, changed by the modification, which is the usual case.

The receptance or dynamic flexibility influence coefficient $G_{ij}(\omega)$ is the response coefficient at dof i due to a unit harmonic force of frequency ω applied at dof j. For an undamped symmetric system

$$G_{ij}(\omega) = (\underline{K}^o - \omega^2 \underline{M}^o)^{-1}_{ij} = \sum_{k=1}^{N} \frac{\phi_{ik}\,\phi_{jk}}{\overline{m}_k\,(\Omega_k^2 - \omega^2)} \quad , \ \omega^2 \neq \Omega_k^2 \qquad (95)$$

which results from the orthogonality conditions, equations (3) and (4). Equation (95) allows selected receptances to be calculated without a complete matrix inversion. If the system is constrained ($\Omega_k \neq 0$) equation (95) may be rewritten as

$$G_{ij}(\omega) = X_{sij} + \omega^2 \sum_{k=1}^{N} \frac{\phi_{ik}\,\phi_{jk}}{\bar{m}_k\,\Omega_k^2\,(\Omega_k^2 - \omega^2)} \tag{96}$$

$$X_{sij} = \sum_{k=1}^{N} \frac{\phi_{ik}\,\phi_{jk}}{\bar{m}_k\,\Omega_k^2} = (\underline{K}^{-1})_{ij} \tag{97}$$

= static deflection at dof i due to a unit load at dof j.

The static flexibility influence coefficient X_{sij} attenuates the higher mode contributions to $G_{ij}(\omega)$ by the factor $1/\Omega_k^2$. This leads to a more accurate estimate of $G_{ij}(\omega)$ when only a partial set of normal modes is available.

The use of receptances in a general eigensolution reanalysis method was proposed by Hirai and Yoshimura (43). The effects of local modifications on an original system were considered as closed loop feedback type forces. This reference was restricted to undamped, symmetric original system property and modification matrices. The authors of the present chapter have generalized the method to include initially proportionally damped systems and arbitrary, damped modification matrices. The importance of this extension is emphasized by recalling that inclusion of any discrete damping results in a 2N order eigenvalue problem, ((12) or (13)). The adjoint eigenvector of the modified system, (11), is also shown to be calculable in an efficient manner. An outline of the procedure, which includes Hirai's work as a special case follows.

The modified system equilibrium equation is

$$(\lambda_n^2\,(\underline{M}^o + \underline{\Delta M}) + \lambda_n\,(\underline{C}^o + \underline{\Delta C}) + (\underline{K}^o + \underline{\Delta K}))\underline{\psi}_n = \underline{0} \quad (N\text{x}1) \tag{98}$$

Define the transformation (general receptance) matrix as

$$\underline{F}(\lambda_n) = [\underline{F}_1 \,\vdots\, \underline{F}_2 \,\vdots\, \cdots \,\vdots\, \underline{F}_N] = (\lambda_n^2\,\underline{M}^o + \lambda_n\,\underline{C}^o + \underline{K}^o)^{-1} \quad (N\text{x}N) \tag{99}$$

and the effective modification matrix as

$$\underline{S}(\lambda_n) = (\lambda_n^2\,\underline{\Delta M} + \lambda_n\,\underline{\Delta C} + \underline{\Delta K}) \quad (N\text{x}N) \tag{100}$$

Equation (98) is then expressed by

$$(\underline{I}_N + \underline{S}(\lambda_n)\,\underline{F}\,(\lambda_n))\,\underline{\xi}_n = \underline{0} \quad (N\text{x}1) \tag{101}$$

$$\underline{\psi}_n = \underline{F}(\lambda_n)\,\underline{\xi}_n \quad (N\text{x}1) \tag{102}$$

Designate the p nonnull rows of the sparse matrix $\underline{S}(\lambda_n)$ by the set of ascending integers

$$\underline{J} = (j_1,\, j_2,\, \ldots\, j_p)^T \tag{103}$$

The set $\underline{J}$ is the union of the three, individual sets of nonnull rows (columns) associated with $\underline{\Delta M}$, $\underline{\Delta C}$, and $\underline{\Delta K}$. In turn these individual sets are the unions of the sets of nonnull rows (columns) of their respective element matrices.

Since in general

$$\underline{S}\,\underline{F} = \begin{bmatrix} \tilde{\underline{S}}_1 \\ \hdashline \tilde{\underline{S}}_2 \\ \hdashline \vdots \\ \hdashline \tilde{\underline{S}}_N \end{bmatrix} \underline{F} = \begin{bmatrix} \tilde{\underline{S}}_1\,\underline{F} \\ \hdashline \tilde{\underline{S}}_2\,\underline{F} \\ \hdashline \vdots \\ \hdashline \tilde{\underline{S}}_N\,\underline{F} \end{bmatrix} \quad (N\mathrm{x}N) \tag{104}$$

it follows from equations (101) and (103) that

$$\xi_{kn} = 0 \;, \qquad k \notin (j_1 \;, j_2 \;, \ldots j_p) \tag{105}$$

The effective modification matrix $\underline{S}$, is now restricted so that for each null row the corresponding column in $\underline{S}$ is also null. This condition is not an implication of symmetry or skew symmetry for $\underline{\Delta M}$, $\underline{\Delta K}$, or $\underline{\Delta C}$. The transformed eigenproblem is condensed to the pth order system

$$(\underline{I}_p + \hat{\underline{S}}\,(\lambda_n)\,\hat{\underline{F}}\,(\lambda_n))\,\hat{\underline{\xi}}_n = \underline{0} \qquad (p\mathrm{x}1) \tag{106}$$

$$\hat{\underline{S}}(\lambda_n) = \lambda_n^2\,\hat{\underline{\Delta M}} + \lambda_n\,\hat{\underline{\Delta C}} + \hat{\underline{\Delta K}} \qquad (p\mathrm{x}p) \tag{107}$$

$$\underset{(p\mathrm{x}1)}{\hat{\underline{\xi}}_n} = \begin{bmatrix} \xi_{j_1 n} \\ \xi_{j_2 n} \\ \vdots \\ \xi_{j_p n} \end{bmatrix}, \quad \underset{(p\mathrm{x}p)}{\hat{\underline{\Delta M}}} = \begin{bmatrix} \Delta M_{j_1 j_1} & \Delta M_{j_1 j_2} & \cdots & \Delta M_{j_1 j_p} \\ \Delta M_{j_2 j_1} & \Delta M_{j_2 j_2} & \cdots & \Delta M_{j_2 j_p} \\ \vdots & \vdots & & \vdots \\ \Delta M_{j_p j_1} & \Delta M_{j_p j_2} & \cdots & \Delta M_{j_p j_p} \end{bmatrix}$$

$$\underset{(p\mathrm{x}p)}{\hat{\underline{F}}(\lambda_n)} = \begin{bmatrix} F_{j_1 j_1} & F_{j_1 j_2} & \cdots & F_{j_1 j_p} \\ F_{j_2 j_1} & F_{j_2 j_2} & \cdots & F_{j_2 j_p} \\ \vdots & \vdots & & \vdots \\ F_{j_p j_1} & F_{j_p j_2} & \cdots & F_{j_p j_p} \end{bmatrix} \tag{108}$$

The condensed damping and stiffness modification matrices, $\hat{\underline{\Delta C}}$ and $\hat{\underline{\Delta K}}$ are identical in form to $\hat{\underline{\Delta M}}$ in equation (108), with ΔM replaced with ΔC and ΔK, respectively. From equation (106) the modified system characteristic equation

$$g(\lambda_n) = \det(\underline{I}_p + \hat{\underline{S}}(\lambda_n)\,\hat{\underline{F}}(\lambda_n)) = 0 \tag{109}$$

The condensed transformed eigenvector is obtained as the solution to equation (106), after which the actual modified system eigenvector can be formed using equations (102) and (105)

$$\underline{\psi}_n = \underline{\bar{F}}(\lambda_n)\ \underline{\hat{\xi}}_n = [\underline{F}_{j_1} \mid \underline{F}_{j_2} \mid \cdots \mid \underline{F}_{j_p}]\ \underline{\hat{\xi}}_n \qquad (N\text{x}1) \qquad (110)$$

The modified system's adjoint eigenvector, $\underline{\tau}_n$, is calculated from equations (112) and (113)

$$(\lambda_n^2(\underline{M}^\circ + \underline{\Delta M}^T) + \lambda_n\ (\underline{C}^\circ + \underline{\Delta C}^T) + (\underline{K}^\circ + \underline{\Delta K}^T))\ \underline{\tau}_n = \underline{0} \quad (N\text{x}1) \qquad (111)$$

$$(\underline{I}_p + \underline{\hat{S}}^T(\lambda_n)\ \underline{\hat{F}}(\lambda_n))\ \underline{\hat{v}}_n = \underline{0} \qquad (p\text{x}1) \qquad (112)$$

$$\underline{\tau}_n = \underline{\bar{F}}(\lambda_n)\ \underline{\hat{v}}_n \qquad (N\text{x}1) \qquad (113)$$

The following formulas provide the columns of the condensed general receptance matrix, $\underline{\bar{F}}(\lambda_n)$, in equation (110)

$$\underline{F}_{j_q}(\lambda_n) \cong \sum_{k=1}^{L} \frac{\phi_{j_q k}}{\bar{m}_k(\lambda_n^2 + 2\zeta_k\Omega_k\lambda_n + \Omega_k^2)}\ \underline{\phi}_k \quad , \ R=0 \qquad (114)$$

$$\underline{F}_{j_q}(\lambda_n) \cong \{\underline{I}_N + (\underline{K}^\circ)^{-1}(-\lambda_n^2\ \underline{M}^\circ - \lambda_n\ \underline{C}^\circ) + \ldots$$

$$+ ((\underline{K}^\circ)^{-1}(-\ \lambda_n^2\ \underline{M}^\circ - \lambda_n\ \underline{C}^\circ))^{R-1}\}\ (\underline{K}^\circ)^{-1}_{j_q}$$

$$+ (-\ \lambda_n^2)^R \sum_{k=1}^{L} \frac{\phi_{j_q k}(\lambda_n + 2\zeta_k\Omega_k)^R}{\bar{m}_k(\lambda_n\Omega_k^2)^R(\lambda_n^2 + 2\zeta_k\Omega_k\lambda_n + \Omega_k^2)}\ \underline{\phi}_k \quad , \ R=1,2,\ldots \qquad (115)$$

where $q = 1,2,\ldots p$

L = number of unmodified system normal modes, $\underline{\phi}_k$ used. If L=N, equations (114) and (115) are exact.

$(\underline{K}^\circ)^{-1}_{j_q}$: j_q column of $(\underline{K}^\circ)^{-1}$ = unmodified system static deflection vector due to a unit load applied at dof j_q.

The integer R in equations (114) and (115) is referred to as the higher mode factor. The computational work required to obtain the columns of $\underline{F}$ increases as R increases. The contribution from higher modes, however, becomes more attenuated. This is most easily seen when the unmodified system is undamped ($\zeta_k = 0$); then as R increases, the accuracy of $\underline{F}_{j_q}$ improves for a fixed L. Note that in using equation (115) when R is greater than 2, the powers of the matrix, $(\underline{K}^\circ)^{-1}(-\lambda_n^2\ \underline{M}^\circ - \lambda_n\ \underline{C}^\circ)$ should not be explicitly evaluated and stored. This path would require approximately $N^2 + N^3$ additional operations per term. Since the result is a vector, each additional term of this form involves only a matrix vector product, i.e., N^2 operations (32, p. 234).

To obtain the zeroes of equation (109) Newton Raphson (NR) iteration is applied. Hirai suggested a trial and error approach to solving this equation which is adequate for his treatment of undamped, symmetric systems. The following derivatives are used in the NR iteration

$$\frac{\partial}{\partial\lambda_n}\ \underline{\hat{S}}(\lambda_n) = 2\ \lambda_n\ \underline{\hat{\Delta M}} + \underline{\hat{\Delta C}} \qquad (p\text{x}p) \qquad (116)$$

$$\frac{\partial}{\partial \lambda_n} \hat{\underline{F}}(\lambda_n) = - \bar{\underline{F}}^T(\lambda_n) \, (2\lambda_n \, \underline{M}^o + \underline{C}^o) \, \bar{\underline{F}}(\lambda_n) \qquad (p \times p) \tag{117}$$

along with the standard formula for differentiating the determinant function (44, p. 33). The NR formula is taken from Lancaster (15) as

$$\lambda_n^{(\ell+1)} = \lambda_n^{(\ell)} - \frac{r(\lambda_n^{(\ell)})}{\left.\frac{\partial r}{\partial \lambda_n}\right|_{\lambda_n=\lambda_n^{(\ell)}} - r(\lambda_n^{(\ell)}) \cdot \sum_{j=1}^{t} \frac{1}{\lambda_n^{(\ell)} - \lambda_j}} \tag{118}$$

where the summation in the denominator ensures that the iteration does not converge to one of the t zeroes already obtained (λ_j). The iterated function is defined as

$$r(\lambda_n) = g(\lambda_n) \, h(\lambda_n) = g(\lambda_n) \prod_{k=1}^{L} (\lambda_n^2 + 2\zeta_k \Omega_k \lambda_n + \Omega_k^2) \tag{119}$$

which exhibits improved convergence characteristics over $g(\lambda_n)$, and may be time-scaled to control its magnitude. An approximate initial guess, $\lambda_n^{(1)}$, is obtained from equations (3), (4), and (98) as the solution of

$$\lambda_n^2(\bar{m}_n + \hat{\underline{\phi}}_n^T \hat{\underline{\Delta M}} \, \hat{\underline{\phi}}_n) + \lambda_n \, (2\zeta_n \Omega_n \, \bar{m}_n + \hat{\underline{\phi}}_n^T \, \hat{\underline{\Delta C}} \, \hat{\underline{\phi}}_n) + (\bar{m}_n \Omega_n^2 + \hat{\underline{\phi}}_n^T \, \hat{\underline{\Delta K}} \, \hat{\underline{\phi}}_n) = 0$$

$$\hat{\underline{\phi}}_n = [\phi_{j_1 n} \; \phi_{j_2 n} \; \cdots \; \phi_{j_p n}]^T \qquad (p \times 1) \tag{120}$$

Other applications of the receptance method in modification theory have been discussed by Bishop (45), Whittaker (46), and Done (47, 48).

Numerical Example

The undamped forward, circular synchronous rotor model shown in figure 2 is the original system. This model remains approximately valid when dampers are added. The modifications are the dashpots attached at bearing stations 2 and 9. The system displacement vector is

$$\underline{X} = [x_1 \; \theta_1 \; \cdots \; x_{10} \; \theta_{10}]^T \qquad (20 \times 1) \tag{121}$$

and the modification indices are (equation (103))

$$p = 2 \qquad j_1 = 3 \qquad j_2 = 17$$

The condensed system matrices are

$$\hat{\underline{\Delta M}} = \hat{\underline{\Delta K}} = \begin{bmatrix} 0 & 0 \\ 0 & 0 \end{bmatrix}, \; \hat{\underline{\Delta C}} = \begin{bmatrix} C_b & 0 \\ 0 & C_b \end{bmatrix}, \; \hat{\underline{F}}(\lambda_n) = \begin{bmatrix} F_{3,3} & F_{3,17} \\ F_{17,3} & F_{17,17} \end{bmatrix} \tag{122}$$

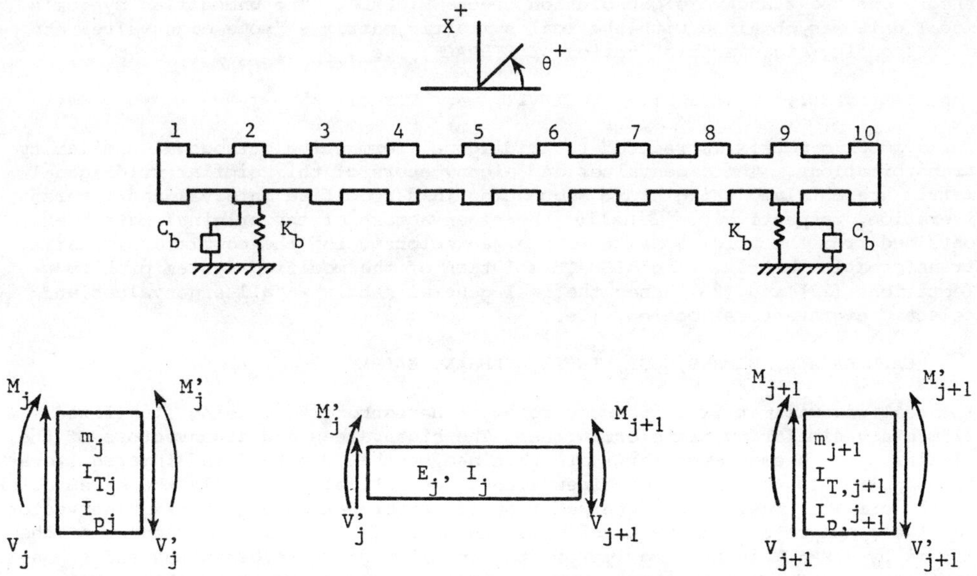

d = 5in. (12.7 cm), L = 108 in. (2.74 m), E = 30 x 10^6 lb./in.^{2}

(206.8 GN/m^2), I = 30.68 in.^{4} (1.277 x 10^3 cm^4),

$m_1 = m_{10}$ = 0.08635 lb. s.^{2} in^{-1} (1.257 k_g)

$m_2 = \ldots = m_9$ = 0.1727 lb. s.^{2} in^{-1} (2.52 k_g)

$I_{p1} = I_{p10}$ = 0.2698 lb. in. s.^{2} (0.03036 k_g m^2)

$I_{p2} = \ldots = I_{p9}$ = 0.5396 lb. in. s.^{2} (0.06095 k_g m^2)

$I_{T1} = I_{T10}$ = 1.1711 lb. in. s.^{2} (0.13196 k_g m^2)

$I_{T2} = \ldots = I_{T9}$ = 2.3422 lb. in. s.^{2} (0.26393 k_g m^2)

K_b = 150,000 lb./in. (26269.0 kN/m)

C_b (100,200,300,400,500) lb.s./in.

(17.51, 32.03, 52.54, 70.05, 87.56) kN. sec./m.

Ω_1 = 291.84 rad./sec., Ω_2 = 575.36, Ω_3 = 682.20

Ω_4 = 1207.83, Ω_5 = 2267.83

Figure 2. Uniform rotor model. Unmodified system, C_b = 0

A CDC Cyber 172 computer was used for the example solution, by both the reanalysis theory and the standard eigensolution code - EISPACK. The unmodified system's modal data was obtained with the real symmetric matrix - "some eigenvalues and corresponding eigenvectors" option of EISPACK, i.e.,

CALL TRED1, BISECT, TINVIT, TRBAK1

The symmetric matrix is reduced to tridiagonal form using orthogonal similarity transformations. The eigenvalues and eigenvectors of this similar tridiagonal matrix are obtained using Sturm sequencing in a specified interval and inverse iteration, respectively. Finally, the eigenvectors of the original matrix are obtained from the tridiagonal matrix eigenvectors using the complete similarity transformation matrix. The EISPACK solution of the modified system problem (equations (22) and (23)) used the real general matrix - "all eigenvalues and selected eigenvectors" option, i.e.,

CALL BALANC, ELMHES, HQR, INVIT, ELMBAK, BALBAK

The real general matrix is reduced to upper Hessenberg form using stabilized elementary similarity transformations. The eigenvalues and eigenvectors of the similar upper Hessenberg matrix are obtained by the QR method and inverse iteration applied to the specified eigenvalues, respectively. Finally the eigenvectors of the original matrix are obtained from the upper Hessenberg matrix eigenvectors and the complete similarity transformation matrix. Initial conditioning of the matrix by EISPACK is made to improve the accuracy of the eigenvalues and eigenvectors. A reference on these subjects is the texts by Goult, Hoskins, Milner, and Pratt (5), and Forsythe (49).

Table 1 compares eigensolution three (3) as calculated by EISPACK and the receptance solutions with higher mode factors of R=0,1,2, for C_b=400. The corresponding error analysis, i.e.,

percent error = 100 x (EISPACK - reanalysis)/EISPACK

is included in Table 2. The mode normalization constants (a_{2i}, equation (20)) used in modal forced response studies are compared in Table 3. Table 4 lists central processor times used to calculate three and five modified system eigensolutions and check orthogonality. These results come from permanent file runs with C_b assuming the five values shown in order to simulate a parametric study. The individual damping case times are obtained using the utility subprogram: CALL SECOND (T). Further decomposition of the total run times include:

EISPACK solution - Property matrices formation 0.6 cp seconds
- Orthogonality check; 0.5 (5 mode), 0.2 (3 mode) cp seconds/damping case

Reanalysis solution - Property matrices formation 0.55 cp seconds
- Original system eigensolution and orthogonality check 0.58 cp seconds
- Modified system orthogonality check 0.50 (5 mode), 0.2 (3 mode) cp secs./damping case

The average number of iterations for convergence, per mode, are enclosed in parentheses in Table 4. Also included is the percentage of time required for reanalysis compared with EISPACK. These percentages are compensated for modified system orthogonality check times. Times 1 and 2 are the total central processor time of the run, and portion of this time during execution, respectively. The assumed modes approach solution time is also listed. That methods results are identical (in accuracy) to the receptance, R=0, predictions. The orthogonality condition matrices, equation (20), for C_b=400 and five modified system eigenvectors are listed in Table 5. The eigenvectors have been normalized here to the a_{2i}=1.0 convention. These matrix elements are complex numbers and only the moduli are shown. A comparison of the initial guess eigenvalues from equation (120) to the calculated eigenvalues is made in Table 6. These initial guesses are used with all three higher mode factors. The eigensolution reanalysis results of this sec-

Table 1 Modified rotor eigensolution 3, C_b = 400 lb.s./in. (70.05 kN. s./m)

MODE NUMBER 3

COMPLEX EIGENVALUE (REAL, IMAGINARY)

EISPACK		R=0		R=1		R=2	
-.4423E+03	.4832E+03	-.4290E+03	.4828E+03	-.4422E+03	.4834E+03	-.4423E+03	.4832E+03

COMPLEX EIGENVECTOR (REAL, IMAGINARY)

	EISPACK		R=0		R=1		R=2	
1	.1000E+01	0.	.1000E+01	0.	.1000E+01	0.	.1000E+01	0.
2	-.2611E-01	.6952E-03	-.2819E-01	.2792E-02	-.2615E-01	.6652E-03	-.2611E-01	.6946E-03
3	.6878E+00	.2068E-01	.6714E+00	.3733E-01	.6875E+00	.2045E-01	.6878E+00	.2067E-01
4	-.2584E-01	.3713E-02	-.2578E-01	.3668E-02	-.2584E-01	.3713E-02	-.2584E-01	.3713E-02
5	.3903E+00	.8827E-01	.3876E+00	.9124E-01	.3902E+00	.8822E-01	.3903E+00	.8827E-01
6	-.2300E-01	.6390E-02	-.2185E-01	.5239E-02	-.2298E-01	.6409E-02	-.2300E-01	.6390E-02
7	.1530E+00	.1567E+00	.1533E+00	.1565E+00	.1530E+00	.1567E+00	.1530E+00	.1567E+00
8	-.1589E-01	.4620E-02	-.1650E-01	.5193E-02	-.1590E-01	.4612E-02	-.1589E-01	.4620E-02
9	.2136E-01	.1944E+00	.1182E-01	.2037E+00	.2119E-01	.1943E+00	.2136E-01	.1944E+00
10	-.5676E-02	.1596E-02	-.6330E-02	.2226E-02	-.5691E-02	.1583E-02	-.5676E-02	.1595E-02
11	.2136E-01	.1944E+00	.1182E-01	.2037E+00	.2119E-01	.1943E+00	.2136E-01	.1944E+00
12	.5676E-02	-.1596E-02	.6330E-02	-.2226E-02	.5691E-02	-.1583E-02	.5676E-02	-.1595E-02
13	.1530E+00	.1567E+00	.1533E+00	.1565E+00	.1530E+00	.1567E+00	.1530E+00	.1567E+00
14	.1589E-01	-.4620E-02	.1650E-01	-.5193E-02	.1590E-01	-.4612E-02	.1589E-01	-.4620E-02
15	.3903E+00	.8827E-01	.3876E+00	.9124E-01	.3902E+00	.8822E-01	.3903E+00	.8827E-01
16	.2300E-01	-.6390E-02	.2185E-01	-.5239E-02	.2298E-01	-.6409E-02	.2300E-01	-.6390E-02
17	.6878E+00	.2068E-01	.6714E+00	.3733E-01	.6875E+00	.2045E-01	.6878E+00	.2067E-01
18	.2584E-01	-.3713E-02	.2578E-01	-.3668E-02	.2584E-01	-.3713E-02	.2584E-01	-.3713E-02
19	.1000E+01	.9176E-12	.1000E+01	.1192E-11	.1000E+01	-.1616E-11	.1000E+01	-.2568E-11
20	.2611E-01	-.6952E-03	.2819E-01	-.2792E-02	.2615E-01	-.6652E-03	.2611E-01	-.6946E-03

Table 2 Error analysis. Modified rotor eigensolution 3, C_b = 400 lb.s./in. (70.05 kN.s./m)

PERCENT ERRORS

COMPLEX EIGENVALUE...(R)REAL (I)IMAGINARY

R=0,(R)	R=1,(R)	R=2,(R)	R=0,(I)	R=1,(I)	R=2,(I)
3.00178	.00540	-.00070	.08209	-.04118	-.00013

COMPLEX EIGENVECTOR...(R)REAL (I)IMAGINARY

	R=0,(R)	R=1,(R)	R=2,(R)	R=0,(I)	R=1,(I)	R=2,(I)
1	0.00000	0.00000	0.00000	0.00000	0.00000	0.00000
2	-7.95109	-.14137	.00159	-301.64435	4.31010	.08853
3	2.38342	.04005	-.00046	-80.53948	1.07550	.02254
4	.22689	-.00310	.00007	1.22460	.01315	.00081
5	.68814	.01712	-.00020	-3.36135	.05766	.00141
6	4.99887	.10241	-.00124	18.00924	-.30247	-.00654
7	-.21493	-.02425	.00039	.12717	-.02082	-.00053
8	-3.77888	-.05916	.00069	-12.40482	.17472	.00331
9	44.64934	.79146	-.00973	-4.77661	.07291	.00152
10	-11.52057	-.26967	.00363	-39.47649	.80887	.01838
11	44.64934	.79146	-.00973	-4.77661	.07291	.00152
12	-11.52057	-.26967	.00363	-39.47649	.80887	.01838
13	-.21493	-.02425	.00039	.12717	-.02082	-.00053
14	-3.77888	-.05916	.00069	-12.40482	.17472	.00331
15	.68814	.01712	-.00020	-3.36135	.05766	.00141
16	4.99887	.10241	-.00124	18.00924	-.30247	-.00654
17	2.38342	.04005	-.00046	-80.53948	1.07550	.02254
18	.22689	-.00310	.00007	1.22460	.01315	.00081
19	.00000	.00000	-.00000	-29.89478	276.10119	379.83403
20	-7.95109	-.14137	.00159	-301.64435	4.31010	.08853

Table 3 Mode normalization constant comparison. Modified rotor eigensolutions (1-5), C_b = 400 lb. s./in. (70.05 kN.s./m)

MODE NORMALIZATION CONSTANTS (REAL,IMAGINARY)

	EISPACK		R=0		R=1		R=2	
1	.4286E+04	.1438E+03	.4217E+04	.6902E+02	.4286E+04	.1435E+03	.4286E+04	.1438E+03
2	-.3762E+01	.3791E+03	-.1578E+02	.3859E+03	-.3831E+01	.3788E+03	-.3754E+01	.3791E+03
3	-.5993E+01	.3441E+03	-.1237E+02	.3469E+03	-.6042E+01	.3440E+03	-.5992E+01	.3441E+03
4	.2161E+03	.1329E+04	.1900E+03	.1327E+04	.2135E+03	.1329E+04	.2158E+03	.1329E+04
5	-.1158E+04	.2478E+04	-.1021E+04	.2560E+04	-.1134E+04	.2494E+04	-.1153E+04	.2481E+04

PERCENT ERRORS...(R)REAL...(I)IMAGINARY

	R=0,(R)	R=1,(R)	R=2,(R)	R=0,(I)	R=1,(I)	R=2,(I)
1	1.60806	.00432	.00001	52.00097	.19822	.00078
2	-319.52647	-1.83713	.22190	-1.80298	.08367	-.00005
3	-106.48426	-.82285	.02405	-.79153	.02747	.00026
4	12.05893	1.20134	.12998	.18757	.01543	.00188
5	11.83046	2.03174	.36618	-3.31714	-.65110	-.13324

Table 4. Efficiency comparison for eigensolution reanalysis example. Times in CP seconds. ( ) Average number of iterations per mode. Three (3) modified system modes calculated.

C_b	EISPACK	Assumed Modes	R = 0	R = 1	R = 2
100	4.10	0.58 9.7%	0.96 (4.0) 19.5%	0.96 (4.0) 19.5%	0.99 (4.0) 20.3%
200	3.93	0.60 10.7%	0.95 (4.0) 20.1%	1.08 (5.0) 23.6%	1.02 (4.3) 22.0%
300	4.01	0.58 10.0%	1.04 (4.7) 22.0%	1.11 (5.3) 23.9%	1.10 (5.0) 23.6%
400	4.01	0.59 10.2%	1.03 (4.7) 21.8%	1.24 (6.3) 27.3%	1.14 (5.3) 24.7%
500	3.96	0.58 10.1%	1.15 (5.7) 25.3%	1.37 (7.3) 31.1%	1.27 (6.3) 28.5%
Time 1	22.04	5.2 20%	7.78 32.2%	8.46 35.5%	8.12 33.8%
Time 2	20.67	3.8 14.3%	6.37 27.3%	7.02 30.6%	6.71 29.0%

Five (5) Modified System Modes Calculated

C_b	EISPACK	Assumed Modes	R = 0	R = 1	R = 2
100	4.62	1.02 12.6%	1.67 (3.8) 28.4%	1.75 (4.0) 30.3%	1.71 (3.8) 29.4%
200	4.57	1.07 14.0%	1.73 (4.0) 30.2%	1.88 (4.8) 33.9%	1.82 (4.2) 32.4%
300	4.60	1.05 13.4%	1.78 (4.4) 31.2%	1.93 (5.0) 34.9%	1.97 (4.8) 35.9%
400	4.50	1.03 13.3%	1.79 (4.4) 32.3%	2.06 (5.6) 39.0%	2.01 (5.0) 37.8%
500	4.57	1.02 12.8%	1.91 (5.0) 34.6%	2.22 (6.4) 42.3%	2.13 (5.6) 40.1%
Time 1	24.82	7.48 22%	11.56 40.6%	12.58 45.2%	12.23 43.6%
Time 2	23.50	6.1 17%	10.13 36.3%	11.13 41.1%	10.84 39.7%

Table 5. Modified System Modal Orthogonality Matrices, $(\underline{\gamma}^T \underline{A}_2 \underline{\Gamma})_{ij}$, for C_b = 400. lb.s./in. (70.0 kN.s./m)

	i \ j	1	2	3	4	5
EISPACK	1	.1000 E + 01	.1251 E - 11	.2518 E - 11	.3287 E - 11	.6452 E - 12
	2		.1000 E + 01	.2553 E - 11	.2373 E - 11	.5349 E - 11
	3			.1000 E + 01	.1779 E - 11	.9740 E - 12
	4		Symmetric		.1000 E + 01	.1399 E - 11
	5					.1000 E + 01
R = 0	1	.1000 E + 01	.6973 E - 13	.2092 E - 13	.5385 E - 13	.2252 E - 13
	2		.1000 E + 01	.1814 E - 11	.1392 E - 12	.6646 E - 13
	3			.1000 E + 01	.1901 E - 12	.5764 E - 13
	4		Symmetric		.1000 E + 01	.1026 E - 12
	5					.1000 E + 01
R = 1	1	.1000 E + 01	.7428 E - 12	.6141 E - 04	.2208 E - 12	.9401 E - 04
	2		.1000 E + 01	.1102 E - 11	.2486 E - 03	.4798 E - 12
	3			.1000 E + 01	.2963 E - 12	.7143 E - 03
	4		Symmetric		.1000 E + 01	.1168 E - 12
	5					.1000 E + 01
R = 2	1	.1000 E + 01	.3955 E - 11	.1052 E - 05	.3444 E - 11	.1795 E - 04
	2		.1000 E + 01	.5528 E - 11	.2598 E - 04	.6713 E - 11
	3			.1000 E + 01	.2032 E - 11	.1358 E - 03
	4		Symmetric		.1000 E + 01	.9414 E - 11
	5					.1000 E + 01

Table 6. Comparison of modified system eigenvalues with initial guess formula, eg. 120. C_b = 400 lb. sec./in. (70.0 kN.s./m) (real, imaginary)

mode i	Eq. 120	R = 0	R = 1	R = 2	EISPACK
1	- 36.42, 289.56	- 27.08, 310.71	- 26.82, 310.80	- 26.81, 310.80	- 26.81, 310.80
2	- 431.41, 380.69	- 435.14, 379.35	- 455.30, 376.50	- 455.14, 376.06	- 455.14, 376.06
3	- 408.31 546.52	- 428.99, 482.79	- 442.24, 483.38	- 442.27, 483.18	- 442.26, 483.18
4	- 8.02, 1207.81	- 4.29, 1203.81	- 4.56, 1203.83	- 4.58, 1203.84	- 4.58, 1203.84
5	- 70.60, 2266.73	- 59.26, 2240.80	- 62.30, 2243.54	- 62.83, 2244.03	- 62.96, 2244.13

tion employed L=5 original system - undamped modes as shown in Table 7. The convergence criterion used with equation (118) was,

$$\left| \mathrm{Re}(\lambda_n^{(\ell+1)}) - \mathrm{Re}(\lambda_n^{(\ell)}) \right| < \varepsilon \quad \text{and} \quad \left| \mathrm{Im}(\lambda_n^{(\ell+1)}) - \mathrm{Im}(\lambda_n^{(\ell)}) \right| < \varepsilon, \tag{123}$$

$$\varepsilon = 10^{-10}$$

Further observations for this example may be of interest.

1) A 10% modification problem, $p/N = 2/20 = 0.1$. See equation (103).
2) Approximate eigensolution accuracy improves substantially with increasing higher mode factor, R.
3) R = 1 or 2 are good compromises between accuracy and efficiency.
4) Although R=0 provides acceptable eigenvalues the corresponding eigenvectors and normalization constants are sometimes poor, for C_b = 400 lb.S./in. (70.0 kN S./m).
5) As C_b increases so does the reanalysis time
6) Decreasing the convergence factor (ε, equation (123)) especially improves eigenvector accuracy and orthogonality.
7) For any given method the eigenvector orthogonality check alone is not a reliable indicator of eigensolution accuracy when a partial set of modes is considered.
8) Decreasing the number of modified system modes required increases the efficiency of reanalysis as compared with EISPACK. The 3 and 5 mode calculation times in Table 4 represent 15% and 25% of the possible modes.
9) The R=2 results show better efficiency than R=1 since fewer iterations occur.

PRESCRIBED EIGENSOLUTION DESIGN

Often the goal of design is to construct a system which responds with certain eigenvalues and eigenvectors. This section presents several methods for accomplishing this. To achieve a specified frequency, the first technique results in global changes of the system. With the second technique only particular system elements need be altered.

Global Modification Approach

The contents of this subsection follow closely the work of Lancaster (15). The procedure consists of prescribing a complete set of modal characteristics and then calculating the associated property matrices. This concept is similar to the spectral representation of a matrix.

For an undamped, symmetric system suppose the modal quantities

$$\underline{\Phi} = [\underline{\phi}_1 \,\vdots\, \underline{\phi}_2 \,\vdots\, \cdots \,\vdots\, \underline{\phi}_N], \ \underline{\mathrm{diag}}\ (\Omega_i^2), \ \underline{\mathrm{diag}}\ (\bar{m}_i) \qquad (N\mathrm{x}N) \tag{124}$$

are prescribed, with $\underline{\phi}_i$ linearly independent. The corresponding property matrices are then calculated from

$$\underline{M}^{-1} = \sum_{i=1}^{N} \underline{\phi}_i \, \underline{\phi}_i^T/\bar{m}_i, \quad \underline{K} = \underline{M} \cdot \sum_{i=1}^{N} \Omega_i^2 \, \underline{\phi}_i \, \underline{\phi}_i^T/\bar{m}_i \cdot \underline{M} \qquad (N\mathrm{x}N) \tag{125}$$

Berman and Flannelly (50) have used relations similar to equation (125) in studying system parameter identification from modal testing, and also eigensolution reanalysis.

Two sets of property matrix changes may be calculated that will change the diagonal eigenvalue matrix in a prescribed fashion, yet leave the eigenvectors invariant, these are

Table 7 The five lowest undamped rotor modes

	$\underline{\phi}_1$	$\underline{\phi}_2$	$\underline{\phi}_3$	$\underline{\phi}_4$	$\underline{\phi}_5$
X_1	.10000E+01	.10000E+01	.10000E+01	.10000E+01	.10000E+01
θ_1	-.35113E+00	-.19690E-01	-.36244E-01	-.79009E-01	-.12919E+00
X_2	-.32092E+01	.77312E+00	.57883E+00	.99445E-01	-.36444E+00
θ_2	-.35021E+00	-.17377E-01	-.32902E-01	-.67798E-01	-.86634E-01
X_3	-.72603E+01	.57919E+00	.22506E+00	-.53118E+00	-.82261E+00
θ_3	-.31346E+00	-.16070E-01	-.26063E-01	-.33757E-01	.14839E-01
X_4	-.10486E+02	.37155E+00	-.39367E-01	-.66045E+00	-.13816E+00
θ_4	-.21537E+00	-.18800E-01	-.17539E-01	.12271E-01	.84746E-01
X_5	-.12265E+02	.12922E+00	-.18446E+00	-.28985E+00	.76367E+00
θ_5	-.76547E-01	-.21295E-01	-.62558E-02	.45216E-01	.47868E-01
X_6	-.12265E+02	-.12922E+00	-.18446E+00	.28985E+00	.76367E+00
θ_6	.76547E-01	-.21295E-01	.62558E-02	.45216E-01	-.47868E-01
X_7	-.10486E+02	-.37155E+00	-.39367E-01	.66045E+00	-.13816E+00
θ_7	.21537E+00	-.18800E-01	.17539E-01	.12271E-01	-.84746E-01
X_8	-.72603E+01	-.57919E+00	.22506E+00	.53118E+00	-.82261E+00
θ_8	.31346E+00	-.16070E-01	.26063E-01	-.33757E-01	-.14839E-01
X_9	-.32092E+01	-.77312E+00	.57883E+00	-.99445E-01	-.36444E+00
θ_9	.35021E+00	-.17377E-01	.32902E-01	-.67798E-01	.86634E-01
X_{10}	.10000E+01	-.10000E+01	.10000E+01	-.10000E+01	.10000E+01
θ_{10}	.35113E+00	-.19690E-01	.36244E-01	-.79009E-01	.12919E+00

$$1)\quad \underline{\Delta M} = \underline{0}, \quad \underline{\Delta K} = \underline{M} \cdot \sum_{i=1}^{N} \Delta(\Omega_i^2)\, \underline{\phi}_i\, \underline{\phi}_i^T/\bar{m}_i \cdot \underline{M} \qquad (N\text{x}N) \tag{126}$$

$$2)\quad \underline{\Delta K} = \underline{0}, \quad \underline{\Delta M} = -\, \underline{M} \cdot \sum_{i=1}^{N} \frac{\Delta(\Omega_i^2)}{\bar{m}_i(\Omega_i^2 + \Delta(\Omega_i^2))}\, \underline{\phi}_i\, \underline{\phi}_i^T \cdot \underline{M} \qquad (N\text{x}N) \tag{127}$$

For a general damped system (equations 10,11) 2N complex eigenvalues, eigenvectors, and adjoint eigenvectors are selected

$$\alpha_i \;\; i=1,2,\ldots 2N, \;\; [\underline{\Lambda}_1 \,\vdots\, \underline{\Lambda}_2 \,\vdots\, \cdots \,\vdots\, \underline{\Lambda}_{2N}], \;\; [\underline{\delta}_1 \,\vdots\, \underline{\delta}_2 \,\vdots\, \cdots \,\vdots\, \underline{\delta}_{2N}] \quad (N\text{x}2N) \tag{128}$$

For real property matrices to result, the jth eigensolution when complex, must be accompanied by its complex conjugate eigensolution. Additionally the 2N x 2N matrix $\underline{\Gamma}$ (equation 16) must be nonsingular and the selected eigenvectors must satisfy

$$\sum_{i=1}^{2N} \underline{\Lambda}_i\, \underline{\delta}_i^T = \underline{0} \qquad (N\text{x}N) \tag{129}$$

The property matrices are then expressed as

$$\underline{M}^{-1} = \sum_{i=1}^{2N} \alpha_i\, \underline{\Lambda}_i\, \underline{\delta}_i^T \;, \quad \underline{C} = -\, \underline{M} \cdot \sum_{i=1}^{2N} \alpha_i^2\, \underline{\Lambda}_i\, \underline{\delta}_i^T \cdot \underline{M} \qquad (N\text{x}N) \tag{130}$$

$$\underline{K} = -\, \underline{C} \sum_{i=1}^{2N} \alpha_i^2\, \underline{\Lambda}_i\, \underline{\delta}_i^T \cdot \underline{M} - \underline{M} \sum_{i=1}^{2N} \alpha_i^3\, \underline{\Lambda}_i\, \underline{\delta}_i^T \cdot \underline{M} \qquad (N\text{x}N) \tag{131}$$

and if $\underline{K}^{-1}$ is known to exist, apriori, an alternative to equation (131) is

$$\underline{K}^{-1} = -\sum_{i=1}^{2N} \underline{\Lambda}_i\, \underline{\delta}_i^T/\alpha_i \qquad (N\text{x}N) \tag{132}$$

These property matrices automatically satisfy $a_{2i} = 1.0$, (equation 20).

The following two-degree-of-freedom system was analyzed by Hurty (33, pg. 333) and Klosterman (51, pg 104). These authors calculated the modal characteristics of a specific set of 2 x 2 property matrices $\underline{M}$, $\underline{K}$, and $\underline{C}$. The modal properties were determined to be

$$\alpha_{1,2} = -\,0.06624 \pm i\, 1.9872 \;,$$

$$\underline{\Lambda}_{1,2} = \underline{\delta}_{1,2} = \begin{bmatrix} 0.30212 \mp i\, 0.30177 \\ -\,0.01598 \mp i\, 0.03276 \end{bmatrix},$$

$$\alpha_{3,4} = -\,0.52972 \pm i\, 9.1862$$

$$\underline{\Lambda}_{3,4} = \underline{\delta}_{3,4} = \begin{bmatrix} 0.002804 \mp i\, 0.01478 \\ -\,1.22951 \pm i\, 1.22917 \end{bmatrix}$$

Lancaster's equations are then checked by recovering $\underline{M}$, $\underline{K}$, and $\underline{C}$ from these modal properties. From equations (129-131)

$$\underline{M} = \begin{bmatrix} 1.38182 & 0.00972 \\ 0.00972 & 0.01808 \end{bmatrix} , \quad \underline{C} = \begin{bmatrix} 0.17969 & 0.05989 \\ 0.05989 & 0.01996 \end{bmatrix}$$

$$\underline{K} = \begin{bmatrix} 5.45440 & -0.00084 \\ -0.00084 & 1.52716 \end{bmatrix} , \quad \sum_{i=1}^{2N} \underline{\Lambda}_i \underline{\delta}_i^T = \begin{bmatrix} 0.31 \times 10^{-7} & 1.86 \times 10^{-6} \\ 1.86 \times 10^{-6} & 0.32 \times 10^{-4} \end{bmatrix}$$

which are nearly identical to Hurty and Klosterman's original matrices. The modal normalization constants, a_{2i}, are 1.0. Also equation (129) would be satisfied exactly only if more significant figures were used in the eigensolutions.

Local Modification, Perturbation Method

This technique prescribes eigensolution perturbations about an original or base system's eigensolutions. A subset of the system's physical parameters are selected to effect the perturbations. Stetson's (18) approach inverts reanalysis equations (38-40). The original system and modification matrices are undamped and symmetric, e.g., equations (1-4). The assumption is made that changes to the system may be expressed as linear combinations of p independent stiffness ($\Delta\hat{k}_\ell$) and q independent inertia ($\Delta\hat{m}_\ell$) parameters, in the form,

$$\Delta K_{ij} = \sum_{\ell=1}^{p} a_{i\ell} a_{j\ell} \Delta\hat{k}_\ell \quad , \quad \Delta M_i = \sum_{\ell=1}^{q} b_{i\ell} \Delta\hat{m}_\ell \tag{133}$$

The ith eigenvector perturbation is expanded by

$$\underline{\Delta\phi}_i = \sum_{\ell=1}^{N} C_{i\ell} \underline{\phi}_\ell \quad , \quad C_{ii} = 0 \qquad (N\mathrm{x}1) \tag{134}$$

The remaining $C_{i\ell}$ are determined from equations (3) and (134) as

$$C_{i\ell} = \underline{\phi}_\ell^T \underline{M}^\circ \Delta \underline{\phi}_i / \bar{m}_\ell \qquad \ell \neq i \tag{135}$$

To be consistent with the reanalysis procedure the same eigenvector normalization must be used. The prescribed eigenvector $\underline{\theta}_i$ is first divided by its expansion coefficient of $\underline{\phi}_i$. This yields the modified system eigenvector, $\underline{\theta}_i'$, with a $\underline{\phi}_i$ expansion coefficient of unity. The eigenvector change, $\underline{\Delta\phi}_i$, is calculated as the difference $\underline{\theta}_i' - \underline{\phi}_i$. The succeeding equations will show that although an eigenvalue change may be prescribed, an eigenvector change can only be effected by prescribing its decomposition coefficients, $C_{i\ell}$. Hence, a total prescription of $\underline{\Delta\phi}_i$ would require the knowledge of all N base system modes, $\underline{\phi}_k$. With just a partial set of $\underline{\phi}_k$ only the contribution of this set to $\underline{\Delta\phi}_i$ by equations (134) and (135) is specified. Define the constants

$$A_{i\ell k} = (2\bar{m}_\ell \Omega_i^2)^{-1} \sum_{n=1}^{N} \sum_{j=1}^{N} a_{nk} a_{jk} \phi_{ni} \phi_{j\ell},$$

$$B_{i\ell k} = -(2\bar{m}_\ell)^{-1} \sum_{n=1}^{N} b_{nk} \phi_{ni} \phi_{n\ell} \tag{136}$$

$$\Delta_{i\ell} = C_{i\ell}(\Omega_i^2 - \Omega_\ell^2)/(2\Omega_i^2) \quad i \neq \ell \quad , \quad = \Delta\Omega_i/\Omega_i \qquad i=\ell \tag{137}$$

The perturbation equations are then

$$
\left[\begin{array}{cccc:cccc}
A_{111} & A_{112} & \cdots & A_{11p} & B_{111} & B_{112} & \cdots & B_{11q} \\
A_{121} & A_{122} & \cdots & A_{12p} & B_{121} & B_{122} & \cdots & B_{12q} \\
\vdots & \vdots & & \vdots & \vdots & \vdots & & \vdots \\
A_{1N1} & A_{1N2} & \cdots & A_{1Np} & B_{1N1} & B_{1N2} & \cdots & B_{1Nq} \\ \hdashline
A_{211} & A_{212} & \cdots & A_{21p} & B_{211} & B_{212} & \cdots & B_{21q} \\
\vdots & \vdots & & \vdots & \vdots & \vdots & & \vdots \\
A_{2N1} & A_{2N2} & \cdots & A_{2Np} & B_{2N1} & B_{2N2} & \cdots & B_{2Nq} \\ \hdashline
A_{311} & A_{312} & \cdots & A_{31p} & B_{311} & B_{312} & \cdots & B_{31q} \\
\vdots & \vdots & & \vdots & \vdots & \vdots & & \vdots \\
A_{NN1} & A_{NN2} & \cdots & A_{NNp} & B_{NN1} & B_{NN2} & \cdots & B_{NNq}
\end{array}\right]_{N^2x(p+q)}
\left[\begin{array}{c}
\Delta\hat{k}_1 \\ \Delta\hat{k}_2 \\ \vdots \\ \Delta\hat{k}_p \\ \hdashline \Delta\hat{m}_1 \\ \Delta\hat{m}_2 \\ \vdots \\ \Delta\hat{m}_q
\end{array}\right]_{(p+q)x1}
=
\left[\begin{array}{c}
\Delta_{11} \\ \Delta_{12} \\ \vdots \\ \Delta_{1N} \\ \hdashline \Delta_{21} \\ \vdots \\ \Delta_{2N} \\ \hdashline \Delta_{31} \\ \vdots \\ \Delta_{NN}
\end{array}\right]_{(N^2x1)}
\begin{array}{l} \text{mode 1} \\ \\ \text{mode 2} \\ \\ \text{etc.} \end{array}
\qquad (138)
$$

This equation is easily interpreted when $\Delta\hat{k}_\ell$ and $\Delta\hat{m}_\ell$ are provided and $\Delta\Omega_i$ and $\underline{\Delta\phi_i}$ are calculated, resulting in $\Delta_{i\ell}$ and equations (134) and (137). This case would be an eigensolution reanalysis. Note that usually only a small portion of equation (138), depending on the number of perturbed eigensolutions and available $\underline{\phi_i}$, is actually calculated and stored. When the eigensolution perturbations, $\Delta\Omega_i$ and $\underline{\Delta\phi_i}$, are prescribed the corresponding $\Delta_{i\ell}$ are first calculated from equations (135) and (137). The number of $\Delta_{i\ell}$ depends on the numbers of available $\underline{\phi_i}$ and the physical parameters which are allowed to vary. For a square system of equations to result the numbers of $\Delta_{i\ell}$ and variable physical parameters $(\Delta\hat{k}_\ell, \Delta\hat{m}_\ell)$ must be equal. The nonvariable physical parameters are set to zero and just the equations in (138) which correspond to specified $\Delta_{i\ell}$ are then considered. The resulting condensed system of equations is now solved for the variable $\Delta\hat{m}_\ell$ and $\Delta\hat{k}_\ell$. Obviously the unspecified $\Delta_{i\ell}$ are not controllable with these calculated parameter changes. Use of this method requires a consistent normalization convention for the original and prescribed eigenvectors.

The simple spring mass model of Figure 3 has eigensolutions

$$
\Omega_1=0.5412\Omega_2,\ \underline{\phi_1}=\begin{bmatrix}0.500\\0.7071\\0.500\end{bmatrix},\ \bar{m}_1=m, \quad \Omega_2=(2k/m)^{\frac{1}{2}},\ \underline{\phi_2}=\begin{bmatrix}0.7071\\0.0\\-0.7071\end{bmatrix},\ \bar{m}_2=m, \quad \Omega_3=1.307\Omega_2,\ \underline{\phi_3}=\begin{bmatrix}0.500\\-0.7071\\0.500\end{bmatrix},\ \bar{m}_3=m, \quad \underline{\phi_i}^T\underline{\phi_i}=1
$$

initially. The desired eigensolution modifications are

$$
\Delta\Omega_1=0,\quad \underline{\theta_1}=\begin{bmatrix}0.4243\\0.7071\\0.5657\end{bmatrix},\quad \underline{\theta_1'}=\begin{bmatrix}0.4264\\0.7107\\0.5685\end{bmatrix},\quad \underline{\Delta\phi_1}=\begin{bmatrix}-0.0736\\0.0036\\0.0685\end{bmatrix}
$$

where $\underline{\theta_1}^T\underline{\theta_1} = 1$ and $\underline{\theta_1}$ is divided by 0.995 to obtain $\underline{\theta_1'}$. These modifications are to be realized by just varying m_1 and m_3. Since only two system parameters are allowed to vary, just two $\Delta_{i\ell}$ can be specified. The condition that $\Delta\Omega_1 = 0$ specifies Δ_{11}. The second mode contribution to $\underline{\Delta\phi_1}$, i.e., Δ_{12}, is selected as the remaining $\Delta_{i\ell}$. The constant associated with Δ_{12} is from equation (135), $C_{12} = -0.1005$. Equation (138) then requires

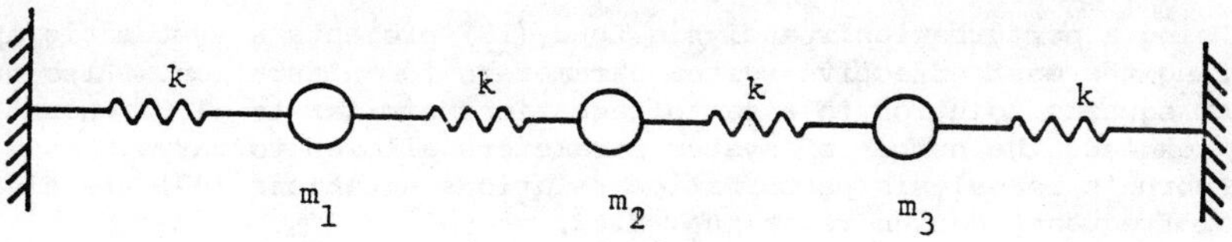

Figure 3. Prescribed eigensolution design example using the local modification - perturbation approach. Original system $m_1 = m_2 = m_3 = m$

$$\begin{bmatrix} B_{111} & B_{113} \\ B_{121} & B_{123} \end{bmatrix} \begin{bmatrix} \Delta\hat{m}_1 \\ \Delta\hat{m}_3 \end{bmatrix} = \begin{bmatrix} \Delta_{11} \\ \Delta_{12} \end{bmatrix} \tag{139}$$

which yields $m_1' = 0.657$ m and $m_3' = 1.343$ m. Replacing the original masses with these produces the first eigensolution

$$\omega_1 = 0.5348\Omega_2, \qquad \underline{\theta}_1 = \begin{bmatrix} 0.4316 \\ 0.7004 \\ 0.5685 \end{bmatrix}, \qquad \underline{\theta}_1^T \underline{\theta}_1 = 1$$

Using a perturbation reanalysis Lund (19) presents a systematic approach of selecting the most effective system parameters for alteration. Also suggested is a least squares solution to a set of equations similar to (138) when the number of $\Delta_{i\ell}$ exceeds the number of system parameters allowed to vary.

Aubrun's reanalysis perturbation relations equations (47) are also damped natural frequency design relations, i.e.,

$$\mathrm{Re}(\lambda_n) = -1/2 \sum_{\ell=1}^{r} \Delta\hat{c}_\ell \sum_{i=1}^{N} \sum_{j=1}^{N} W_{ij\ell}\, \phi_{in}\, \phi_{jn}$$

$$\mathrm{Im}(\lambda_n) = \Omega_n + (2\Omega_n)^{-1} \sum_{\ell=1}^{s} \Delta\hat{k}_\ell \sum_{i=1}^{N} \sum_{j=1}^{N} Z_{ij\ell}\, \phi_{in}\, \phi_{jn} \tag{140}$$

where the modification matrix elements were expressed as linear combinations of independent damping and stiffness parameters as

$$\Delta C_{ij} = \sum_{\ell=1}^{r} W_{ij\ell}\, \Delta\hat{c}_\ell, \quad \Delta K_{ij} = \sum_{\ell=1}^{s} Z_{ij\ell}\, \Delta\hat{k}_\ell \tag{141}$$

Equations 140 are a system of simultaneous linear equations for the $\Delta\hat{c}_\ell$ and $\Delta\hat{k}_\ell$, which are selected to vary to obtain the desired λ_n. The number of selected parameter changes must be equal to the number of prescribed $\mathrm{Re}(\lambda_n)$ and $\mathrm{Im}(\lambda_n)$ for an exact solution.

Local Modification, Receptance Method

This method inverts the eigenvalue reanalysis receptance method of the previous section. For design the natural frequency λ_n is specified in the modified system's condensed characteristic equation (109). The condensation now results from the selection of which system parameters are changed to obtain the desired λ_n. Each prescribed complex natural frequency yields two real equations, i.e.

$$\mathrm{Re}(g(\lambda_n, \underline{d})) = 0, \qquad \mathrm{Im}(g(\lambda_n, \underline{d})) = 0 \tag{142}$$

where $\underline{d}$ is a qx1 vector of unknowns, which are the independent stiffness, mass, or damping parameters selected to obtain the λ_n. Since two equations result for each λ_n the number of λ_n prescribed must be equal to q/2, so that an exact solution for $\underline{d}$ exists. The complex receptance $\hat{\underline{F}}$ in equation (109) are evaluated for each prescribed λ_n with equations (99), (114), or (115).

Consider the rotor problem previously discussed (Figure 2) with both dampers (C_1, C_2) independently variable. By its symmetry identifying either damper with station 2 or 9 is immaterial. These dampers must yield the natural frequency λ^*, while ranging in values from 50 to 500 lb. sec./in. (8.76 to 87.6 kN s./m) From equation (142) the condensed characteristic equation separates into two real equations as,

$$\det\left\{\begin{bmatrix}1 & 0\\ 0 & 1\end{bmatrix} + \begin{bmatrix}\lambda^* C_1 & 0\\ 0 & \lambda^* C_2\end{bmatrix}\begin{bmatrix}F_{3,3}(\lambda^*) & F_{3,17}(\lambda^*)\\ F_{17,3}(\lambda^*) & F_{17,17}(\lambda^*)\end{bmatrix}\right\} = 0 \tag{143}$$

$$1)\ a_1C_1C_2 + a_2C_1 + a_3C_2 = -1 \quad , \quad 2)\ b_1C_1C_2 + b_2C_1 + b_3C_2 = 0 \tag{144}$$

where

$$a_1 + ib_1 = (\lambda^*)^2(F_{3,3}\ F_{17,17} - F_{3,17}^2),\ a_2 + ib_2 = \lambda^* F_{3,3},$$

$$a_3 + ib_3 = \lambda^* F_{17,17}$$

The region ∂_1 in Figure 4 contains all possible λ_1 for the system with (C_1, C_2) restricted as mentioned. The rectangular region σ_1 is the desired eigenvalue placement area. The intersection of ∂_1 and σ_1 (shaded areas in Figure 4) is then the acceptable area for λ^* placement from a parameter limitation and a design prescription standpoint. Prescribe the eigenvalue $\lambda^* = -20 + i304$. This produces the following condensed receptance matrices, $\hat{\underline{F}}(\lambda^*)$, from equations (114) and (115) using L=5 base system modes, $\{(a,b) \to a + ib\}$

$$10^{-5} \times \begin{bmatrix}(0.4081,\ 0.6005) & (-0.495,\ 0.555)\\ (-0.495,\ 0.555) & (0.4081,\ 0.6005)\end{bmatrix},$$

$\underline{R = 0}$,

$$10^{-5} \times \begin{bmatrix}(0.4179,\ 0.6005) & (-0.4975,\ 0.5547)\\ (-0.4975,\ 0.5547) & (0.4179,\ 0.6005)\end{bmatrix}$$

$\underline{R = 1}$,

Equation (144) yields the solution sets:

R=0; $(C_1=160.9,\ C_2=459.2)$, R = 1; $(C_1 = 163.9,\ C_2 = 455.2)$ lb. s./in
$(C_1=28.2,\ C_2=80.4)$, $(C_1 = 28.7,\ C_2 = 79.7)$ kN s./m

The system's first natural frequency with these damper sets is

R=0; $(\lambda_1 = -19.85 + i\ 304.035)$, R = 1; $(\lambda_1 = -19.999 + i\ 304.000)$

from EISPACK. Note that increasing the higher mode factor R in equations (114) yields damper values nearer to the desired pair.

Normally, the region ∂_1 is not known beforehand and consequently σ_1 must be "searched" to obtain the λ^* which possess acceptable parameter sets. For instance, a mesh with selected grid points could be used to cover σ_1. This search does not require the actual solution of eigenvalue problems. For a given value λ^* in σ_1, C_1 and C_2 can be solved for from the set of nonlinear equations (144). If one of the solution (C_1, C_2) is either complex or out of the specified range (50, 500), then we know λ^* is not realizable within the design constraints (i.e. selection of C_1, C_2). For example, $\lambda^* = -20 + i\ 309$ is not realizable. Usually many λ^* would be utilized in this search, which re-emphasizes the importance of the higher mode - complex receptance formulas, equations (114) and (115). Aubrun's perturbation formulas, equation (140) will not yield a solution (C_1, C_2) to this specific example since only dampers are used for the design.

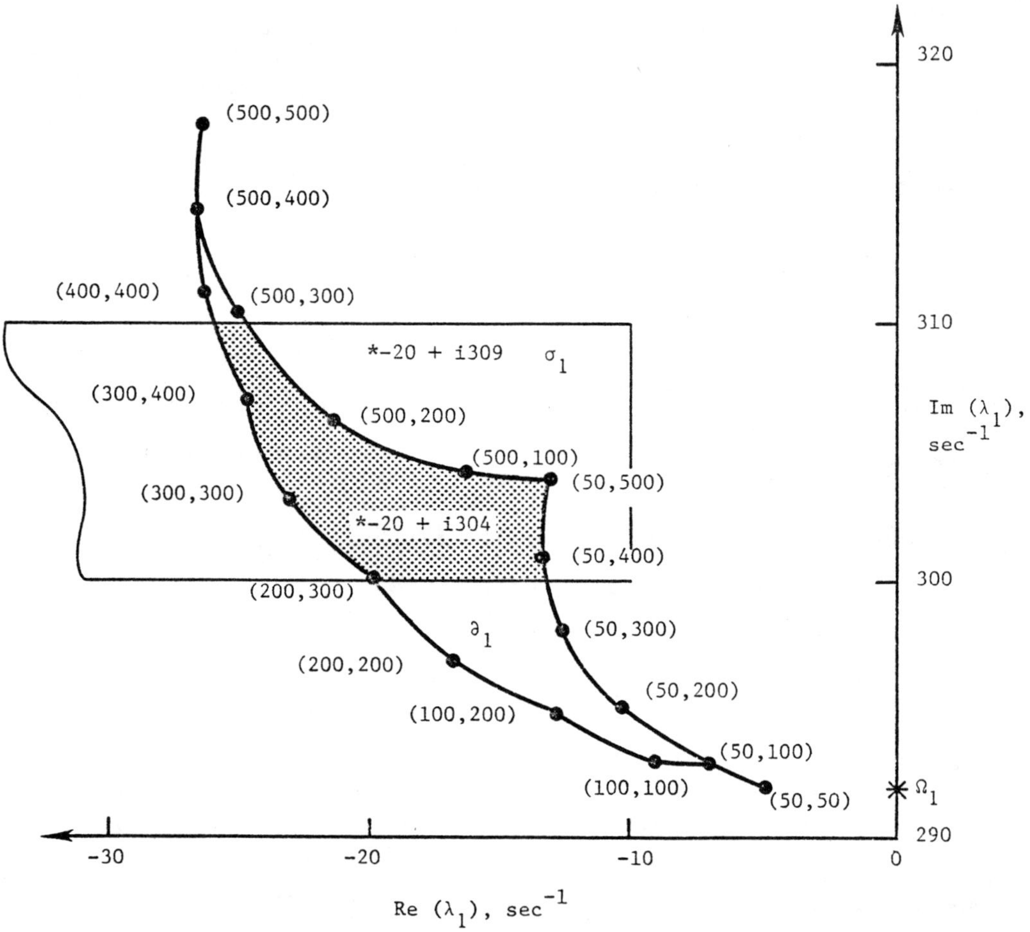

Figure 4. Eigensolution design, rotor example. Parentheses indicate corresponding damping set (C_1, C_2) values. (To convert to SI units multiply by 0.175 kN.s./m)

The receptance approach to undamped design was proposed by Hirai (43). This chapter's authors have extended the method to initially proportionately damped systems with general, damped design modifications.

MODAL SYNTHESIS

Sometimes in the development of a large structural system the separate components or substructures are built at different times and geographical locations. Then a task for the vibration analyst may be to determine the vibration characteristics of the assembled structure. The effect of physical modifications to some components on the vibration characteristics may also be of interest. Consider, for example, the space shuttle, whose main engine assembly is shown in Figure 5. Modifications to one of the pump rotors may effect the modal characteristics of the whole assembly (oxygen pump, hot gas manifold, hydrogen pump, main combustion chamber, nozzle, etc.). An efficient, approximate technique of calculating these changes in the system's modal characteristics would then be a useful aid to the designers. Modal synthesis provides a means to attain these goals.

Component Mode Method

Since the publication of the first paper on a generalized component mode - modal synthesis technique by Hurty (52), many investigations have furthered its development (51, 54-78). A brief review of this subject was reported by Craig and Chang (77) and Craig (78). Additional modal synthesis references are (79 - 85).

Essentially this modal synthesis method involves two main steps: the description of component deformation modes and the coupling of the components. An extensive discussion of various mode sets that can be used to define the component deformation was given by Hintz (65). Three common formulations are fixed interface (Hurty (52, 53), Craig and Bampton (55), Bajan and Feng (56)), free interface (Hou (59)), and branch mode (Benfield and Hruda (60)).

A goal of this synthesis method is to produce an approximate transformed set of system equilibrium equations of reduced dimension. To accomplish this an approximation utilizing a partial change of basis for each components physical coordinates is introduced. The exact form of this transformation is subject to the assumed boundary conditions existing at the component's interconnections (junction points) with neighboring components. The total transformation between the system's physical and generalized coordinates is then represented by a block diagonal transformation matrix.

A displacement compatability requirement is established by considering various junction degrees of freedom. These physical coordinates, although associated with distinct components, must undergo identical motions. Transforming these conditions to generalized coordinates yields a reduced "independent" generalized coordinate vector for the system. Finally, the transformation matrix between this vector and the total-system, physical coordinate vector is inserted into the overall equilibrium equation. The resulting generalized equation of motion has a dimension nearly equal to the total number of component modes used in the component transformations. This number is usually far less than the total number of degrees of freedom in the system.

Component modes assuming fixed intercomponent interfaces are either fixed interface normal modes or constraint modes. The fixed interface normal modes are computed by standard methods assuming that the component's junction coordinates are fixed in space. A constraint mode is defined as the displacement vector of the component's interior (noninterface) degrees of freedom resulting from the unit displacement of a junction coordinate while all remaining junction coordinates are held fixed. This combined set of vectors, if complete, form a set of basis vectors for the vector space associated with the component's displacement vector. The constraint modes actually result from the static condensation method (28, 86) being applied to the elimination of the component's interior degrees of freedom.

Component modes for the free interface assumption are either normal modes or rigid body modes. These modes are calculated with standard techniques assum-

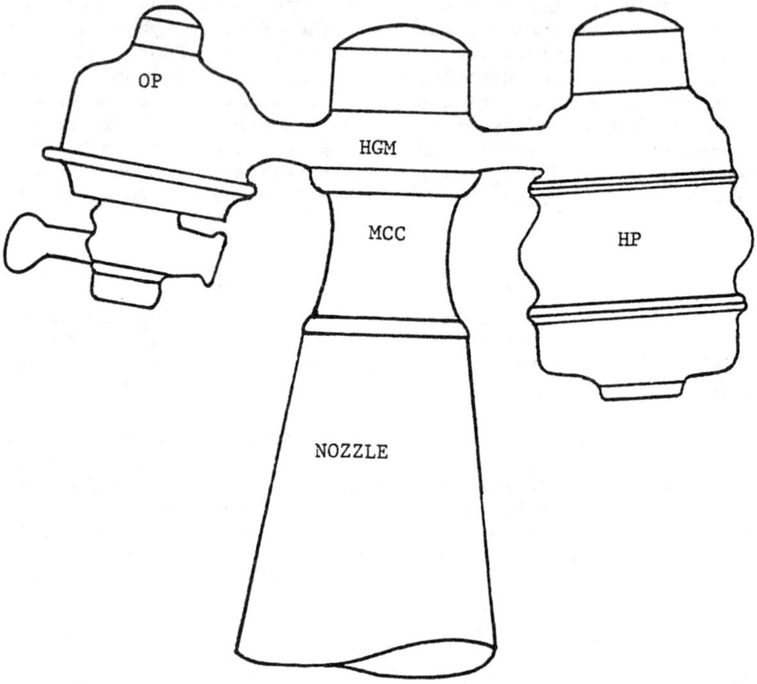

Figure 5. Space shuttle main engine assembly

ing a complete decoupling between the component and its neighboring components.

Branch component modes may be normal-flexible, normal-rigid body, or constraint modes. This results from the branch model consisting of a free component interface and an adjacent fixed component interface at an intercomponent junction.

The following simple example illustrates some of the general steps of the component mode method with a fixed intercomponent interface model. A structure consists of two substructures, labeled 1 and 2, sharing a common interface. The structure's equilibrium equation is given by equation (145).

$$\left[\begin{array}{c:c:c:c}
\underset{(N_1-r)\,x(N_1-r)}{\underline{M}^1_{ii}} & \underset{(N_1-r)\,xr}{\underline{M}^1_{ij}} & \underset{(N_1-r)\,x(N_2-r)}{\underline{0}} & \underset{(N_1-r)\,xr}{\underline{0}} \\ \hdashline
\underset{rx(N_1-r)}{\underline{M}^1_{ji}} & \underset{rxr}{\underline{M}^1_{jj}} & \underset{rx(N_2-r)}{\underline{0}} & \underset{rxr}{\underline{0}} \\ \hdashline
\underset{(N_2-r)\,x(N_1-r)}{\underline{0}} & \underset{(N_2-r)\,xr}{\underline{0}} & \underset{(N_2-r)\,x(N_2-r)}{\underline{M}^2_{ii}} & \underset{(N_2-r)\,xr}{\underline{M}^2_{ij}} \\ \hdashline
\underset{rx(N_1-r)}{\underline{0}} & \underset{rxr}{\underline{0}} & \underset{rx(N_2-r)}{\underline{M}^2_{ji}} & \underset{rxr}{\underline{M}^2_{jj}}
\end{array}\right]
\left[\begin{array}{c}
\underset{(N_1-r)\,x1}{\ddot{\underline{U}}^1_i} \\ \hdashline
\underset{rx1}{\ddot{\underline{U}}^1_j} \\ \hdashline
\underset{(N_2-r)\,x1}{\ddot{\underline{U}}^2_i} \\ \hdashline
\underset{rx1}{\ddot{\underline{U}}^2_j}
\end{array}\right] + \tag{145}$$

$$\left[\begin{array}{c:c:c:c}
\underset{(N_1-r)\,x(N_1-r)}{\underline{K}^1_{ii}} & \underset{(N_1-r)\,xr}{\underline{K}^1_{ij}} & \underset{(N_1-r)\,x(N_2-r)}{\underline{0}} & \underset{(N_1-r)\,xr}{\underline{0}} \\ \hdashline
\underset{rx(N_1-r)}{\underline{K}^1_{ji}} & \underset{rxr}{\underline{K}^1_{jj}} & \underset{rx(N_2-r)}{\underline{0}} & \underset{rxr}{\underline{0}} \\ \hdashline
\underset{(N_2-r)\,x(N_1-r)}{\underline{0}} & \underset{(N_2-r)\,xr}{\underline{0}} & \underset{(N_2-r)\,x(N_2-r)}{\underline{K}^2_{ii}} & \underset{(N_2-r)\,xr}{\underline{K}^2_{ij}} \\ \hdashline
\underset{rx(N_1-r)}{\underline{0}} & \underset{rxr}{\underline{0}} & \underset{rx(N_2-r)}{\underline{K}^2_{ji}} & \underset{rxr}{\underline{K}^2_{jj}}
\end{array}\right]
\left[\begin{array}{c}
\underset{(N_1-r)\,x1}{\underline{U}^1_i} \\ \hdashline
\underset{rx1}{\underline{U}^1_j} \\ \hdashline
\underset{(N_2-r)\,x1}{\underline{U}^2_i} \\ \hdashline
\underset{rx1}{\underline{U}^2_j}
\end{array}\right]
=
\left[\begin{array}{c}
\underset{(N_1-r)\,x1}{\underline{0}} \\ \hdashline
\underset{rx1}{\underline{f}^1_j} \\ \hdashline
\underset{(N_2-r)\,x1}{\underline{0}} \\ \hdashline
\underset{rx1}{\underline{f}^2_j}
\end{array}\right]$$

or

$$\underline{M}\,\ddot{\underline{U}} + \underline{K}\,\underline{U} = \underline{f}(t) \qquad (N_1+N_2)x1 \tag{146}$$

Though the structure is <u>externally</u> unforced, the substructure's interface <u>reaction</u>

forces, $\underline{f}_j^1$ and $\underline{f}_j^2$, are present to provide the substructure coupling. The right subscripts i and j refer to interior and interface (junction) degrees of freedom (dof), respectively. There exist r interface dof linking the substructures. Each substructure's displacement vector is approximately expanded with its fixed interface normal modes and constraint modes as in equation (147).

$$\begin{bmatrix} \underline{U}_i^1 \\ (N_1-r)\times 1 \\ \underline{U}_j^1 \\ r\times 1 \\ \underline{U}_i^2 \\ (N_2-r)\times 1 \\ \underline{U}_j^2 \\ r\times 1 \end{bmatrix} = \begin{bmatrix} \underline{\Phi}_n^1 & \underline{\Phi}_c^1 & \underline{0} & \underline{0} \\ (N_1-r)\times m_1 & (N_1-r)\times r & (N_1-r)\times m_2 & (N_1-r)\times r \\ \underline{0} & \underline{I}_r & \underline{0} & \underline{0} \\ r\times m_1 & r\times r & r\times m_2 & r\times r \\ \underline{0} & \underline{0} & \underline{\Phi}_n^2 & \underline{\Phi}_c^2 \\ (N_2-r)\times m_1 & (N_2-r)\times r & (N_2-r)\times m_2 & (N_2-r)\times r \\ \underline{0} & \underline{0} & \underline{0} & \underline{I}_r \\ r\times m_1 & r\times r & r\times m_2 & r\times r \end{bmatrix} \begin{bmatrix} \underline{q}_n^1 \\ m_1\times 1 \\ \underline{q}_c^1 \\ r\times 1 \\ \underline{q}_n^2 \\ m_2\times 1 \\ \underline{q}_c^2 \\ r\times 1 \end{bmatrix} \tag{147}$$

or

$$\underline{U} = \underline{W}\,\underline{q} \qquad (N_1 x N_2)x1 \tag{148}$$

The n and c subscripts in equation (147) refer to normal mode and constraint mode, respectively. The generalized coordinates are represented by the symbol q. The matrix $\underline{\Phi}_n^\ell$ contains as columns the lowest m_ℓ <u>fixed interface</u> normal modes of the ℓth substructure's interior degrees of freedom, where m_ℓ usually satisfies $m_\ell \ll (N_\ell - r)$. The sth column of $\underline{\Phi}_c^\ell$ is the displacement vector of the ℓth substructure's interior dof due to a unit displacement of $(\underline{U}_j^\ell)_s$, while fixing the remaining interface coordinates. By this definition the sth column of $\underline{\Phi}_c^\ell$ is the solution of

$$\underline{K}_{ii}^\ell\,(\underline{\Phi}_c^\ell)_s = -\,(\underline{K}_{ij}^\ell)_s \quad , \quad (N_\ell - r)x1,\ s = 1,2,\ldots r \tag{149}$$

where subscript s denotes "column s of". Displacement compatability at the substructure interface requires

$$\underline{U}_j^2 = \underline{Q}\,\underline{U}_j^1 \qquad (rx1) \tag{150}$$

where $\underline{Q}$ is a block-diagonal transformation matrix. The submatrices of $\underline{Q}$ are the orthogonal direction cosine matrices <u>(87)</u> which transform displacement components in substructure one's local coordinate system to substructure two's local coordinate system. The matrix $\underline{Q}$ is itself orthogonal, i.e., $\underline{Q}^{-1} = \underline{Q}^T$. Alternatively, equation (150) may be expressed as

$$\underline{A}\,\underline{U} = \underline{0} \qquad (rx1) \quad , \quad \underline{A} = \begin{bmatrix} \underline{0} & \underline{Q} & \underline{0} & -\underline{I}_r \\ r\times(N_1-r) & r\times r & r\times(N_2-r) & r\times r \end{bmatrix} \tag{151}$$

Substitution of equation (148) into (151) yield

$$\underline{A}\,\underline{W}\,\underline{q} = \underline{0} \qquad (r\mathrm{x}1) \qquad (152)$$

This compatability condition among the generalized coordinates is employed to express $\underline{q}_c^2$ in terms of the remaining generalized coordinates. The final transformation between the physical and "independent" generalized coordinates is then given by equation (153).

$$\begin{bmatrix} \underline{U}_i^1 \\ (N_1-r)\mathrm{x}1 \\ \hline \underline{U}_j^1 \\ r\mathrm{x}1 \\ \hline \underline{U}_i^2 \\ (N_2-r)\mathrm{x}1 \\ \hline \underline{U}_j^2 \\ r\mathrm{x}1 \end{bmatrix} = \left[\begin{array}{c|c|c} \underline{\Phi}_n^1 & \underline{\Phi}_c^1 & \underline{0} \\ (N_1-r)\mathrm{x}m_1 & (N_1-r)\mathrm{x}r & (N_1-r)\mathrm{x}m_2 \\ \hline \underline{0} & \underline{I}_r & \underline{0} \\ r\mathrm{x}m_1 & r\mathrm{x}r & r\mathrm{x}m_2 \\ \hline \underline{0} & \underline{\Phi}_c^2\,\underline{Q} & \underline{\Phi}_n^2 \\ (N_2-r)\mathrm{x}m_1 & (N_2-r)\mathrm{x}r & (N_2-r)\mathrm{x}m_2 \\ \hline \underline{0} & \underline{Q} & \underline{0} \\ r\mathrm{x}m_1 & r\mathrm{x}r & r\mathrm{x}m_2 \end{array}\right] \begin{bmatrix} \underline{q}_n^1 \\ m_1\mathrm{x}1 \\ \hline \underline{q}_c^1 \\ r\mathrm{x}1 \\ \hline \underline{q}_n^2 \\ m_2\mathrm{x}1 \end{bmatrix} \qquad (153)$$

or

$$\underline{U} = \underline{T}\,\underline{\bar{q}}$$

Inserting equation (153) into equation (146) yields

$$\underline{\bar{M}}\,\ddot{\underline{\bar{q}}} + \underline{\bar{K}}\,\underline{\bar{q}} = \underline{\bar{f}}(t) \qquad (m_1 + m_2 + r)\mathrm{x}1 \qquad (154)$$

where

$$\underline{\bar{M}} = \underline{T}^T\,\underline{M}\,\underline{T} = \left[\begin{array}{c|c|c} \underline{\bar{M}}_{11} & \underline{\bar{M}}_{12} & \underline{0} \\ m_1\mathrm{x}m_1 & m_1\mathrm{x}r & m_1\mathrm{x}m_2 \\ \hline \underline{\bar{M}}_{12}^T & \underline{\bar{M}}_{22} & \underline{\bar{M}}_{23} \\ r\mathrm{x}m_1 & r\mathrm{x}r & r\mathrm{x}m_2 \\ \hline \underline{0} & \underline{\bar{M}}_{23}^T & \underline{\bar{M}}_{33} \\ m_2\mathrm{x}m_1 & m_2\mathrm{x}r & m_2\mathrm{x}m_2 \end{array}\right] \qquad (m_1+m_2+r)\mathrm{x}(m_1+m_2+r) \qquad (155)$$

$\underline{\bar{M}}_{11} = \underline{diag}(\bar{m}_{k1})$; $\underline{\bar{M}}_{33} = \underline{diag}(\bar{m}_{k2})$; $\underline{\bar{M}}_{23} = \underline{Q}^T((\underline{\Phi}_c^2)^T \underline{M}_{ii}^2 + \underline{M}_{ji}^2)\,\underline{\Phi}_n^2$

$$\underline{\bar{M}}_{22} = (\underline{\Phi}_c^1)^T(\underline{M}_{ii}^1\underline{\Phi}_c^1 + \underline{M}_{ij}^1) + (\underline{M}_{ij}^1)^T\underline{\Phi}_c^1 + \underline{M}_{jj}^1 + \underline{Q}^T((\underline{\Phi}_c^2)^T\underline{M}_{ii}^2\underline{\Phi}_c^2 + \underline{M}_{jj}^2 + (\underline{\Phi}_c^2)^T\underline{M}_{ij}^2 + (\underline{M}_{ij}^2)^T\underline{\Phi}_c^2)\underline{Q}$$

$$\underline{\bar{M}}_{12} = (\underline{\Phi}_n^1)^T(\underline{M}_{ii}^1\ \underline{\Phi}_c^1 + \underline{M}_{ij}^1)$$

$$\underline{\bar{K}} = \underline{T}^T\ \underline{K}\ \underline{T} = \left[\begin{array}{c|c|c} \underline{\bar{K}}_{11} & \underline{0} & \underline{0} \\ m_1 x m_1 & m_1 x r & m_1 x m_2 \\ \hline \underline{0} & \underline{\bar{K}}_{22} & \underline{0} \\ r x m_1 & r x r & r x m_2 \\ \hline \underline{0} & \underline{0} & \underline{\bar{K}}_{33} \\ m_2 x m_1 & m_2 x r & m_2 x m_2 \end{array}\right] \quad (m_1+m_2+r)x(m_1+m_2+r) \tag{156}$$

$$\underline{\bar{K}}_{11} = \underline{\text{diag}}\ (\bar{m}_{k1}\Omega_{k1}^2);\ \underline{\bar{K}}_{33} = \underline{\text{diag}}\ (\bar{m}_{k2}\Omega_{k2}^2)$$

$$\underline{\bar{K}}_{22} = \underline{K}_{jj}^1 + (\underline{\Phi}_c^1)^T\underline{K}_{ij}^1 + \underline{Q}^T(\underline{K}_{jj}^2 + (\underline{\Phi}_c^2)^T\underline{K}_{ij}^2)\underline{Q}$$

$$\underline{\bar{f}} = \underline{T}^T\ \underline{f} = \left[\begin{array}{c} \underline{0} \\ m_1 x 1 \\ \hline \underline{f}_j^1 + \underline{Q}^T\ \underline{f}_j^2 \\ r x 1 \\ \hline \underline{0} \\ m_2 x 1 \end{array}\right] = \underline{0} \qquad (m_1+m_2+r)x1 \tag{157}$$

$$(-\Omega_{k\ell}^2\ \underline{M}_{ii}^\ell + \underline{K}_{ii}^\ell)\underline{\phi}_{nk}^\ell = \underline{0} \quad , \quad (\underline{\Phi}_n^\ell)^T\underline{M}_{ii}^\ell\ \underline{\Phi}_n^\ell = \underline{\text{diag}}(\bar{m}_{k\ell}) \tag{158}$$

Newton's third law applied at the interface is (see equation (150)):

$$\underline{f}_j^2 = -\ \underline{Q}\ \underline{f}_j^1 \quad \text{or} \quad \underline{f}_j^1 = -\ \underline{Q}^{-1}\ \underline{f}_j^2 = -\ \underline{Q}^T\underline{f}_j^2 \qquad (rx1) \tag{159}$$

which explains the results of equation (157). The approximate eigensolutions of the total structure are then obtained from equations (153) and (154), by solving

$$(-\omega_k^2\ \underline{\bar{M}} + \underline{\bar{K}})\underline{\xi}_k = \underline{0} \qquad (m_1+m_2+r)x1 \tag{160}$$

$$\underline{\theta}_k^T = [(\underline{\theta}_i^1)^T \mid (\underline{\theta}_j^1)^T \mid (\underline{\theta}_i^2)^T \mid (\underline{\theta}_j^2)^T]_k = \underline{\xi}_k^T\ \underline{T}^T \qquad 1x(N_1+N_2) \tag{161}$$

Since neither $\underline{\bar{M}}$ nor $\underline{\bar{K}}$ is generally diagonal, an eigenvalue solver code for symmetric matrices may not be applied directly to equation (160). Instead, as suggested by Clough (28), a transformation between $\underline{\xi}_k$ and a secondary generalized coordinate vector is necessary. The transformation matrix may be the Cholesky decomposition matrix for $\underline{\bar{M}}$ or $\underline{\bar{K}}$, if these matrices are positive definite. Alternatively, the transformation matrix may consist of the eigensolutions of either $\underline{\bar{M}}$ or $\underline{\bar{K}}$. Special consideration should be given to the near-diagonal nature of $\underline{\bar{K}}$ in both cases. When both $\underline{\bar{M}}$ and $\underline{\bar{K}}$ are singular the QZ algorithm as outlined in (ref. 5, pg. 155) is used.

The direct solution of the coupled system has order (N_1+N_2-r), while from equation (160) the component mode synthesis approximation has order (m_1+m_2+r). As mentioned by Bathe and Wilson (7), component mode synthesis is actually a Ritz analysis.

The spring mass model in Figure 6 is used to illustrate the formulation of equation (145) which, in this case, is given by equation (162).

$$\begin{bmatrix} m_1 & 0 & 0 & 0 & 0 & 0 & 0 \\ 0 & m_2 & 0 & 0 & 0 & 0 & 0 \\ 0 & 0 & m_3 & 0 & 0 & 0 & 0 \\ 0 & 0 & 0 & m/2 & 0 & 0 & 0 \\ 0 & 0 & 0 & 0 & m_6 & 0 & 0 \\ 0 & 0 & 0 & 0 & 0 & m_7 & 0 \\ 0 & 0 & 0 & 0 & 0 & 0 & m/2 \end{bmatrix} \begin{bmatrix} \ddot{X}_1 \\ \ddot{X}_2 \\ \ddot{X}_3 \\ \ddot{X}_4 \\ \ddot{X}_6 \\ \ddot{X}_7 \\ \ddot{X}_5 \end{bmatrix}$$

$$+ \begin{bmatrix} k_1+k_2 & -k_2 & 0 & 0 & 0 & 0 & 0 \\ -k_2 & k_2+k_3 & -k_3 & 0 & 0 & 0 & 0 \\ 0 & -k_3 & k_3+k_4 & -k_4 & 0 & 0 & 0 \\ 0 & 0 & -k_4 & k_4 & 0 & 0 & 0 \\ 0 & 0 & 0 & 0 & k_5+k_6 & -k_6 & -k_5 \\ 0 & 0 & 0 & 0 & -k_6 & k_6+k_7 & 0 \\ 0 & 0 & 0 & 0 & -k_5 & 0 & k_5 \end{bmatrix} \begin{bmatrix} X_1 \\ X_2 \\ X_3 \\ X_4 \\ X_6 \\ X_7 \\ X_5 \end{bmatrix} = \begin{bmatrix} 0 \\ 0 \\ 0 \\ -F \\ 0 \\ 0 \\ F \end{bmatrix} \quad (162)$$

Rank 1 Tie Matrix Method

This alternate approach to modal synthesis was proposed by Hallquist and Synder (40, 88, 89). The method sequentially connects coordinates of initially uncoupled substructures with springs, rigid links, or dashpots. Each "tie" is made by adding a rank 1 matrix (see the subsection Rank 1 Modification Matrix) to the system equilibrium equations. For a spring tie this matrix has a form similar to equation (80). Although the method is developed to connect many generally damped substructures the simple case of two undamped, symmetric subsystems is presented here for illustration. The uncoupled and connected equilibrium equations for two subsystems are given by equations (163) and (164), respectively.

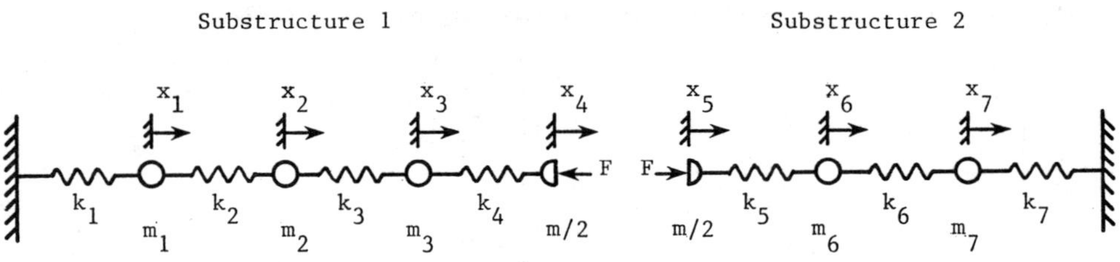

Figure 6. Two component modal synthesis example model

$$\left\{\begin{bmatrix} -\Omega_{\ell 1}^2\,\underline{M}^1 & \underline{0} \\ N_1 x N_1 & N_1 x N_2 \\ \hline \underline{0} & -\Omega_{\ell 2}^2\,\underline{M}^2 \\ N_2 x N_1 & N_2 x N_2 \end{bmatrix} + \begin{bmatrix} \underline{K}^1 & \underline{0} \\ N_1 x N_1 & N_1 x N_2 \\ \hline \underline{0} & \underline{K}^2 \\ N_2 x N_1 & N_2 x N_2 \end{bmatrix}\right\} \begin{bmatrix} \underline{\phi}_\ell^1 \\ N_1 x 1 \\ \hline \underline{\phi}_\ell^2 \\ N_2 x 1 \end{bmatrix} = \begin{bmatrix} \underline{0} \\ N_1 x 1 \\ \hline \underline{0} \\ N_2 x 1 \end{bmatrix} \tag{163}$$

$$\left\{\begin{bmatrix} -\omega_i^2\,\underline{M}^1 & \underline{0} \\ \hline \underline{0} & -\omega_i^2\,\underline{M}^2 \end{bmatrix} + \begin{bmatrix} \underline{K}^1 & \underline{0} \\ \hline \underline{0} & \underline{K}^2 \end{bmatrix} + \right.$$

$$\left.\begin{bmatrix} \mu_k\,\underline{P}\,\underline{P}^T \\ (N_1+N_2) x (N_1+N_2) \end{bmatrix}\right\} \begin{bmatrix} \underline{\theta}_i^1 \\ N_1 x 1 \\ \hline \underline{\theta}_i^2 \\ N_2 x 1 \end{bmatrix} = \begin{bmatrix} \underline{0} \\ N_1 x 1 \\ \hline \underline{0} \\ N_2 x 1 \end{bmatrix} \tag{164}$$

In equation (164) μ_k and $\underline{P}$ are the interconnecting spring's magnitude and positioning vector, respectively. A Ritz- assumed modes transformation is now substituted into equation (164), i.e.,

$$\begin{bmatrix} \underline{\theta}_i^1 \\ N_1 x 1 \\ \hline \underline{\theta}_i^2 \\ N_2 x 1 \end{bmatrix} = \begin{bmatrix} \underline{\Phi}^1 & \underline{0} \\ N_1 x m_1 & N_1 x m_2 \\ \hline \underline{0} & \underline{\Phi}^2 \\ N_2 x m_1 & N_2 x m_2 \end{bmatrix} \begin{bmatrix} \underline{\xi}_i^1 \\ m_1 x 1 \\ \hline \underline{\xi}_i^2 \\ m_2 x 1 \end{bmatrix} , \quad \text{or } \underline{\theta}_i = \underline{\Phi}\,\underline{\xi}_i \tag{165}$$

where $\underline{\Phi}^1$ and $\underline{\Phi}^2$ are the partial modal matrices of subsystems 1 and 2, respectively. Subsystem modal orthogonality is applied and the assumption that ($\omega_i^2 \neq \Omega_{\ell n}^2$ (ℓ=1, ... m_n), n=1,2) is made. The resulting coupled system characteristic equation and eigenvector formula are,

$$g(\omega_i^2) = \frac{1}{\mu_k} + \sum_{n=1}^{2} \sum_{\ell=1}^{m_n} \frac{((\underline{\phi}_\ell^n)^T \underline{P}^n)^2}{\bar{m}_{\ell n}(\Omega_{\ell n}^2 - \omega_i^2)} = 0 \tag{166}$$

$$\underline{\theta}_i^n = \sum_{\ell=1}^{m_n} \frac{(\underline{\phi}_\ell^n)^T \underline{P}^n}{\bar{m}_{\ell n}(\Omega_{\ell n}^2 - \omega_i^2)} \underline{\phi}_\ell^n \qquad n=1,2 \tag{167}$$

$$\underline{P}^T = [(\underline{P}^1)^T \;\; 1xN_1 \;\vdots\; (\underline{P}^2)^T \;\; 1xN_2] \tag{168}$$

These formulas are obvious generalizations of equations (82) and (83). When a rigid link connection is made between the subsystems the term $1/\mu_k$ is set to zero in equation (166). As in reanalysis, equation (166) may be solved for ω_i^2 using Newton Raphson iteration. Multiple ties and/or subsystems may be solved by placing equations (166)-(168) into a recurrence scheme along with equations (82) and (83). Eigensolutions of the preceeding tie or internal connection are then the "unmodified" or "uncoupled" eigensolutions for the next tie or internal connection, etc. The rigid link tie vector between dof 4 and 5 in Figure 6 is,

$$\underline{P}^T = [0 \;\; 0 \;\; 0 \;\; 1 \;\vdots\; -1 \;\; 0 \;\; 0] \tag{169}$$

Receptance Method

The authors of this study have extended the form of the receptance approach presented in the earlier sections to treat modal synthesis problems. The succeeding example treats the coupling of two undamped, positive semi-definite substructures. The uncoupled substructures equilibrium equations are given by equation (163), and the corresponding equations for the coupled system is given by equation (170).

$$\left\{ \begin{bmatrix} -\omega_i^2 \underline{M}^1 & \underline{0} \\ N_1 x N_1 & N_1 x N_2 \\ \hline \underline{0} & -\omega_i^2 \underline{M}^2 \\ N_2 x N_1 & N_2 x N_2 \end{bmatrix} + \begin{bmatrix} \underline{K}^1 & \underline{0} \\ N_1 x N_1 & N_1 x N_2 \\ \hline \underline{0} & \underline{K}^2 \\ N_2 x N_1 & N_2 x N_2 \end{bmatrix} + \begin{bmatrix} \underline{\Delta K} - \omega_i^2 \underline{\Delta M} \\ (N_1+N_2)x(N_1+N_2) \end{bmatrix} \right\} \begin{bmatrix} \underline{\theta}_i^1 \\ N_1 x1 \\ \hline \underline{\theta}_i^2 \\ N_2 x1 \end{bmatrix} = \begin{bmatrix} \underline{0} \\ N_1 x1 \\ \hline \underline{0} \\ N_2 x1 \end{bmatrix} \tag{170}$$

The receptance transformation matrix is defined by equation (171)

$$\underline{\theta}_i = \begin{bmatrix} \underline{\theta}_i^1 \\ N_1 x1 \\ \hline \underline{\theta}_i^2 \\ N_2 x1 \end{bmatrix} = \begin{bmatrix} (\underline{K}^1 - \omega_i^2 \underline{M}^1)^{-1} & \underline{0} \\ N_1 x N_1 & N_1 x N_2 \\ \hline \underline{0} & (\underline{K}^2 - \omega_i^2 \underline{M}^2)^{-1} \\ N_2 x N_1 & N_2 x N_2 \end{bmatrix} \begin{bmatrix} \underline{\xi}_i^1 \\ N_1 x1 \\ \hline \underline{\xi}_i^2 \\ N_2 x1 \end{bmatrix}$$

$$= \begin{bmatrix} \underline{G}^1(\omega_i^2) & \underline{0} \\ N_1 x N_1 & N_1 x N_2 \\ \underline{0} & \underline{G}^2(\omega_i^2) \\ N_2 x N_1 & N_2 x N_2 \end{bmatrix} \begin{bmatrix} \underline{\xi}_i^1 \\ N_1 x 1 \\ \underline{\xi}_i^2 \\ N_2 x 1 \end{bmatrix} = \underline{G}(\omega_i^2)\underline{\xi}_i \tag{171}$$

Substitution of equation (171) into (170) yields,

$$(\underline{I}_{(N_1+N_2)} + \underline{S}(\omega_i^2)\underline{G}(\omega_i^2))\underline{\xi}_i = \underline{0} \ , \quad \underline{S}(\omega_i^2) = \underline{\Delta K} - \omega_i^2 \ \underline{\Delta M} \tag{172}$$

The non-null row (or column) numbers of $\underline{S}$ are in ascending order,

$$j_1, \ j_2, \ \cdots \ j_p \tag{173}$$

Due to this sparsity of $\underline{S}$, equation (172) becomes condensed to the form,

$$(\underline{I}_p + \hat{\underline{S}}(\omega_i^2)\hat{\underline{G}}(\omega_i^2))\hat{\underline{\xi}}_i = \underline{0} \ \ (\text{px}1), \quad \hat{\underline{S}} = \hat{\underline{\Delta K}} - \omega_i^2 \ \hat{\underline{\Delta M}} \tag{174}$$

$$\underset{(\text{pxp})}{\hat{\underline{\Delta K}}} = \begin{bmatrix} \Delta K_{j_1 j_1} & \Delta K_{j_1 j_2} & \cdots & \Delta K_{j_1 j_p} \\ \Delta K_{j_2 j_1} & \Delta K_{j_2 j_2} & \cdots & \Delta K_{j_2 j_p} \\ \vdots & \vdots & \ddots & \vdots \\ \Delta K_{j_p j_1} & \Delta K_{j_p j_2} & \cdots & \Delta K_{j_p j_p} \end{bmatrix},$$

$$\underset{(\text{pxp})}{\hat{\underline{\Delta M}}} = \begin{bmatrix} \Delta M_{j_1 j_1} & \Delta M_{j_1 j_2} & \cdots & \Delta M_{j_1 j_p} \\ \Delta M_{j_2 j_1} & \Delta M_{j_2 j_2} & \cdots & \Delta M_{j_2 j_p} \\ \vdots & \vdots & \ddots & \vdots \\ \Delta M_{j_p j_1} & \Delta M_{j_p j_2} & \cdots & \Delta M_{j_p j_p} \end{bmatrix},$$

$$\hat{\underline{G}}(\omega_i^2) = \begin{bmatrix} G_{j_1 j_1} & G_{j_1 j_2} & \cdots & G_{j_1 j_p} \\ G_{j_2 j_1} & G_{j_2 j_2} & \cdots & G_{j_2 j_p} \\ \vdots & \vdots & \ddots & \vdots \\ G_{j_p j_1} & G_{j_p j_2} & \cdots & G_{j_p j_p} \end{bmatrix} \quad (p\times p) \tag{175}$$

The coupled system's characteristic equation and eigenvector formula are then,

$$g(\omega_i^2) = \det(\underline{I}_p + \hat{\underline{S}}(\omega_i^2)\hat{\underline{G}}(\omega_i^2)) = 0, \quad \underline{\theta}_i = [\underline{G}_{j_1} \,\vdots\, \underline{G}_{j_2} \,\vdots \cdots \vdots\, \underline{G}_{j_p}]\hat{\underline{\xi}}_i \tag{176}$$

where $\underline{G}_j$ is the jth column of $\underline{G}(\omega_i^2)$. The receptance formulas in equations (114) and (115) reduce in this case to,

$$\underline{G}_\ell^n \cong \sum_{k=1}^{m_n} \frac{\phi_{\ell kn}}{\bar{m}_{kn}(\Omega_{kn}^2 - \omega_i^2)} \cdot \underline{\phi}^n{}_k \quad , R_n = 0 \quad n = 1,2 \tag{177}$$

$$\underline{G}_\ell^n \cong \{\underline{I}_{N_n} + \omega_i^2(\underline{K}^n)^{-1}\underline{M}^n + \cdots + (\omega_i^2(\underline{K}^n)^{-1}\underline{M}^n)^{R_n-1}\}(\underline{K}^n)_\ell^{-1}$$
$$+ (\omega_i^2)^{R_n} \sum_{k=1}^{m_n} \frac{\phi_{\ell kn}}{\bar{m}_{kn}(\Omega_{kn}^2)^{R_n}(\Omega_{kn}^2 - \omega_i^2)} \cdot \underline{\phi}^n_k \quad , R_n=1,2,\ldots \quad n = 1,2 \tag{178}$$

where n=1,2 refers to substructures 1 and 2, respectively. The zeroes of equation (176) may be obtained by any search technique such as interval halving or Newton Raphson iteration. Similar to equation (117) the receptance derivative is,

$$\frac{\partial(\underline{G}^n)_{k\ell}}{\partial(\omega_i^2)} = (\underline{G}^n)_k^T \underline{M}^n (\underline{G}^n)_\ell \quad (1\text{x}1) \tag{179}$$

where $(\underline{G}^n)_k$ is the kth column of $\underline{G}^n$. This technique using equations (177) and (178), requires at least a slight alteration of the natural frequencies, i.e. $\omega_i^2 \neq \Omega_{kn}^2$.

Each substructure has associated with it a higher mode factor, R_n, in the receptance formulas (177) and (178). When a substructure (n) is unconstrained just R_n=0 can be immediately applied, since $\underline{K}^n$ is singular. To circumvent this limitation a technique suggested by Clough (ref. 28, pg. 255), applicable to Stodola eigenvalue iteration for unconstrained structures, is used. Small spring constraints are attached to the unconstrained substructure, so that $\underline{K}^n$ is invertible, but near singular. This should at minimum allow a R_n=1 improvement to the receptance calculation.

Alternate to analytic computation, receptances are experimentally measurable, equation (95) and may be recorded over a broad range of excitation frequencies, ω. The characteristic equation in equation (176) can then be solved with test data and information about the connection and internal modification parameter values.

Consider the coupling of the spring mass model in Figure 6 with a spring, k. The coordinates are first renumbered as follows:

$$\text{Substructure 1, } (x_1\ x_2\ x_3\ x_4) \Longrightarrow (U_1^1\ U_2^1\ U_3^1\ U_4^1)$$

$$\text{Substructure 2, } (x_5\ x_6\ x_7) \Longrightarrow (U_1^2\ U_2^2\ U_3^2)$$

The matrix $\underline{\Delta M}$ is zero and the sparsity indices are $p=2$, $j_1=4$, $j_2=5$. From equation (176) the characteristic eq. is,

$$\det\left\{\begin{bmatrix}1 & 0\\ 0 & 1\end{bmatrix} + \begin{bmatrix}k & -k\\ -k & k\end{bmatrix}\begin{bmatrix}G_{44} & G_{45}\\ G_{54} & G_{55}\end{bmatrix}\right\} = \det\left\{\begin{bmatrix}1 & 0\\ 0 & 1\end{bmatrix} + \begin{bmatrix}k & -k\\ -k & k\end{bmatrix}\begin{bmatrix}G_{44}^1 & 0\\ 0 & G_{11}^2\end{bmatrix}\right\} = 0$$

When a natural frequency has been obtained from this equation (ω_i^2), the corresponding coupled system eigenvector is calculated from equations (174) and (176) as,

$$\hat{\xi}_{1i} = 1 \quad , \quad \hat{\xi}_{2i} = (1 + kG_{44}^1)/(kG_{11}^2)\Big|_{\omega_i^2}$$

$$(\underline{\theta}_i^1)^T = [G_{14}^1\ G_{24}^1\ G_{34}^1\ G_{44}^1]\Big|_{\omega_i^2} \quad , \quad (\underline{\theta}_i^2)^T = \hat{\xi}_{2i}[G_{11}^2\ G_{21}^2\ G_{31}^2]\Big|_{\omega_i^2}$$

Example

The spring mass model in Figure 7 is used to illustrate the three modal synthesis techniques discussed. Four substructure 1 and two substructure 2 normal modes were included. The characteristic equation solutions of the tie matrix and receptance approaches were similar to equations (118) and (119). The corresponding convergence criterion was

$$\left| (\omega_i^2)^{(\ell+1)} - (\omega_i^2)^{(\ell)} \right| < \varepsilon, \quad \varepsilon = 10^{-10}$$

Substructure eigensolutions were calculated using the diagonal mass matrix-square root as an initial transformation (ref. 28, pg. 253), then calling the EISPACK symmetric matrix option. The exact solution of the coupled system was solved identically. A symmetric matrix formulation for the component mode method, equation (160), was constructed using the eigensolutions of the non-diagonal matrix $\underline{M}$. Four constraint modes were employed by the component mode method.

Utilizing the tie matrix technique, initially the left junction is joined with a rigid tie (Figure. 7c). This forms a 17 dof system with $m_1+m_2-1=5$ eigen-

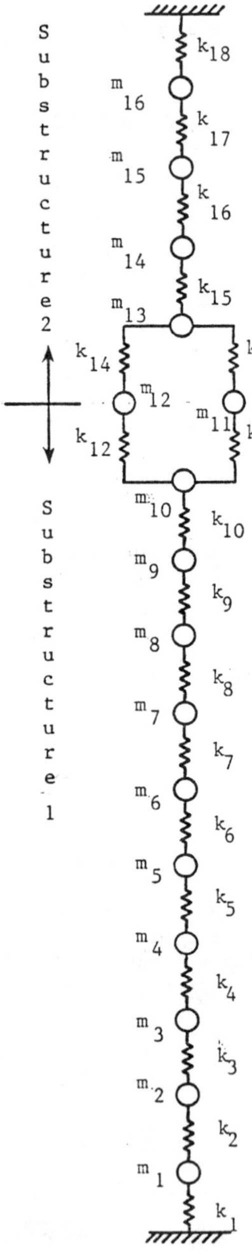

1.

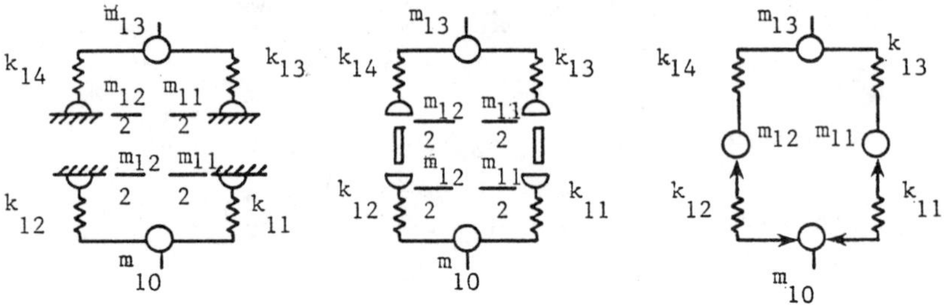

2. 3. 4.

$m_1 = 5m$ $m_2 = 4.5m$ $m_3 = 4.0m$ $m_4 = 4.0m$

$m_5 = 4.0m$ $m_6 = 3.5m$ $m_7 = 3.5m$ $m_8 = 3.5m$

$m_9 = 3.0m$ $m_{10} = 3.0m$ $m_{11} = 2.5m$ $m_{12} = 2.0m$

$m_{13} = 1.5m$ $m_{14} = 5.0m$ $m_{15} = 1.0m$ $m_{16} = 3.0m$

$k_1 = 30K$ $k_2 = 30K$ $k_3 = 27K$ $k_4 = 27K$

$k_5 = 27K$ $k_6 = 24K$ $k_7 = 24K$ $k_8 = 22.5K$

$k_9 = 22.5K$ $k_{10} = 22.5K$ $k_{11} = 21K$ $k_{12} = 19.5K$

$k_{13} = 21K$ $k_{14} = 19.5K$ $k_{15} = 18K$ $k_{16} = 15K$

$k_{17} = 12K$ $k_{18} = 18K$

$m = 0.25$ lb, sec.^{2}/in. (43.8 kg)

$K = 1000$ lb./in. (175.1 kN/m)

▯ = rigid tie

Figure 7 (1) Actual model for modal synthesis example. (2), (3), (4) Interface schemes for the component mode, tie matrix, and receptance methods solutions. Incorporating these eigensolutions as "unmodified system" data, the right junction is connected next as a reanalysis-modification step, equations (82) and (83). The final system then has $m_1+m_2-2=4$ eigensolutions. The receptance method sparsity index, p, was 3 for the example.

A comparison of the various approaches for the second mode eigensolution is shown in Tables 8 and 9. The quantities listed are the coupled system's second natural frequency, ω_2, modal mass normalization constant $\underline{m}_2 = \underline{\theta}_2^t \, \underline{M} \, \underline{\theta}_2$, and the mode shape $\underline{\theta}_2$. These results exhibit the same general accuracy trend shown by the four lowest modes of the coupled system. For this example the tie matrix method has the poorest accuracy, while the receptance (R=3) method, the best. The accuracy of the component mode method is generally between the receptance R=1 and R=2 categories. Orthogonality of the coupled system eigenvectors was not a reliable indicator of the actual eigenvector accuracy, as in the eigensolution reanalysis example. Since only a partial set of the coupled system's eigenvectors were calculated this result was expected.

To illustrate the unconstrained substructure situation, k_{18} was set to zero, disengaging substructure 2 in figures 7c, d. The receptance R=1,2 approaches were solved by setting $k_{18}=\min(k_i)/1200=10.0$ ℓb./in. (1.75 kN/m) The number of included substructure normal modes were identical to the previous example. The results for the second eigensolution are shown in Tables 10 and 11. Double precision arithmetic on the CDC Cyber 172 (approximately 29 significant figures) was necessary in obtaining the receptance, R=2 results. The variables which changed during the iteration were the only ones declared in double precision. The accuracy levels of the component mode and receptance, R=2, approaches were nearly identical in comparing the four lowest, coupled substructure eigensolutions. In the constrained and unconstrained examples the higher mode factor, R_n, for both substructures were identical.

STATIC REANALYSIS

This section summarizes and compares several methods of static reanalysis. Efficient reanalysis is essential to optimal design where many configurations are considered. The two types of approaches discussed are termed the approximate and exact methods, respectively. This classification connotes whether the modified structure's reanalysis solution is approximate or exact. Both methods take advantage of information obtained during the unmodified system's solution.

The approximate methods can be further classified as: perturbation (Taylor series) method, iteration method, and reduced basis method. These are generally applicable to small magnitude modifications distributed over a large portion of the structural system. In constrast, the exact methods are applicable to localized modifications with arbitrary magnitudes. This application requires though that the structural configuration and the validity of the finite element model are not affected.

The underlying principles of the exact methods involve the conception of parallel elements, initial stress, and pseudo loads. Pure algebraic formulas such as the Sherman-Morrison formula (90) and its generalization, the Woodbury formula (90) can also be directly used to develop exact modification methods. In this section, a direct method based on the Woodbury formula due to Argyris and Roy (91), a successive modification method proposed by Kavlie and Powell (92) and the pseudo load method developed by the authors are discussed. The last method although similar to that of Argyris and Roy is derived by only using the system's linearity.

In addition to reanalysis the pseudo load approach provides closed (or semi-closed) form relationships between static response variables and the design parameters. This enables the design (i.e. select design parameters) for prescribed responses.

Approximate Methods

Taylor Series Expansion (93)

The static responses can be expanded in Taylor series as functions of the design parameters, for example,

Table 8 Second mode eigensolutions for modal synthesis example. Constrained substructures.

EIGENSOLUTION 2

	EISPACK (EXACT)	TIE MATRIX	RECEPTANCE R=0	RECEPTANCE R=1	RECEPTANCE R=2	RECEPTANCE R=3	COMPONENT MODE
				NATURAL FREQUENCIES (RAD/SEC)			
	.62510E+02	.64830E+02	.62928E+02	.62541E+02	.62512E+02	.62510E+02	.62583E+02
				MASS NORMALIZATION CONSTANTS			
	.53248E+02	.43655E+02	.47205E+02	.52614E+02	.53185E+02	.53242E+02	.51548E+02
				MODE SHAPE			
1	.10000E+01	.10000E+01	.10000E+01	.10000E+01	.10000E+01	.10000E+01	.10000E+01
2	.18372E+01	.18607E+01	.17868E+01	.18313E+01	.18366E+01	.18371E+01	.18135E+01
3	.24683E+01	.25245E+01	.23367E+01	.24534E+01	.24667E+01	.24681E+01	.24151E+01
4	.27422E+01	.27882E+01	.25771E+01	.27244E+01	.27404E+01	.27420E+01	.26895E+01
5	.26192E+01	.25756E+01	.24974E+01	.26072E+01	.26180E+01	.26191E+01	.25915E+01
6	.20544E+01	.18373E+01	.20043E+01	.20498E+01	.20540E+01	.20544E+01	.20368E+01
7	.11970E+01	.82260E+00	.11416E+01	.11906E+01	.11963E+01	.11969E+01	.11572E+01
8	.10049E+00	-.32167E+00	-.44415E-01	.86434E-01	.99195E-01	.10037E+00	.53064E-01
9	-.10113E+01	-.12907E+01	-.11539E+01	-.10193E+01	-.10117E+01	-.10113E+01	-.99050E+00
10	-.19913E+01	-.19661E+01	-.18334E+01	-.19763E+01	-.19899E+01	-.19912E+01	-.18997E+01
11	-.24015E+01	-.21437E+01	-.21895E+01	-.23824E+01	-.23997E+01	-.24013E+01	-.23734E+01
12	-.23812E+01	-.21182E+01	-.22256E+01	-.23650E+01	-.23797E+01	-.23810E+01	-.23532E+01
13	-.25324E+01	-.20014E+01	-.22665E+01	-.25107E+01	-.25304E+01	-.25322E+01	-.24652E+01
14	-.26428E+01	-.15569E+01	-.23813E+01	-.26172E+01	-.26403E+01	-.26426E+01	-.26182E+01
15	-.19148E+01	-.96906E+00	-.17882E+01	-.19032E+01	-.19137E+01	-.19147E+01	-.19021E+01
16	-.84883E+00	-.28616E+00	-.86488E+00	-.85271E+00	-.84937E+00	-.84890E+00	-.83857E+00

Table 9 Error analysis for second mode eigensolutions. Constrained substructures.

PERCENT ERRORS, EIGENSOLUTION 2

	TIE MATRIX	RECEPTANCE R=0	RECEPTANCE R=1	RECEPTANCE R=2	RECEPTANCE R=3	COMPONENT MODE
			NATURAL FREQUENCIES			
	-3.71233	-.66890	-.05012	-.00422	-.00038	-.11707
			MASS NORMALIZATION CONSTANTS			
	18.01604	11.34843	1.19039	.11801	.01167	3.19327
			MODE SHAPE			
1	0.00000	0.00000	0.00000	0.00000	0.00000	0.00000
2	-1.28008	2.74274	.32154	.03452	.00359	1.28817
3	-2.27594	5.33264	.60482	.06327	.00644	2.15428
4	-1.67959	6.01997	.64801	.06532	.00647	1.92168
5	1.66391	4.64860	.45974	.04428	.00428	1.05734
6	10.56766	2.44169	.22644	.02330	.00247	.85690
7	31.27763	4.62505	.53112	.05944	.00638	3.32718
8	420.10481	144.19861	13.98665	1.28748	.11857	47.19399
9	-27.63220	-14.10543	-.79476	-.04508	-.00269	2.05524
10	1.26845	7.92926	.75664	.07032	.00662	4.59951
11	10.73500	8.82866	.79748	.07480	.00712	1.17161
12	11.04276	6.53274	.67648	.06315	.00595	1.17369
13	20.96665	10.49850	.65762	.07834	.00750	2.65454
14	41.06877	9.89527	.96886	.09521	.00950	.93152
15	49.39054	6.60940	.60650	.05617	.00522	.65934
16	66.28746	-1.89059	-.45714	-.06417	-.00818	1.20833

Table 10 Second mode eigensolutions for modal synthesis example. Unconstrained substructure 2.

EIGENSOLUTION 2

	EISPACK (EXACT)	TIE MATRIX	RECEPTANCE R=0	RECEPTANCE R=1	RECEPTANCE R=2	COMPONENT MODE
			NATURAL FREQUENCIES (RAD/SEC)			
	.52865E+02	.64195E+02	.54302E+02	.52999E+02	.52884E+02	.52870E+02
			MASS NORMALIZATION CONSTANTS			
	.74196E+02	.46037E+02	.60581E+02	.72911E+02	.74029E+02	.73639E+02
			MODE SHAPE			
1	.10000E+01	.10000E+01	.10000E+01	.10000E+01	.10000E+01	.10000E+01
2	.18836E+01	.19860E+01	.18071E+01	.18769E+01	.18830E+01	.18769E+01
3	.26460E+01	.28791E+01	.24388E+01	.26283E+01	.26445E+01	.26309E+01
4	.31345E+01	.32887E+01	.28526E+01	.31109E+01	.31324E+01	.31190E+01
5	.32986E+01	.30076E+01	.30390E+01	.32765E+01	.32963E+01	.32893E+01
6	.30990E+01	.19924E+01	.28877E+01	.30788E+01	.30965E+01	.30917E+01
7	.25838E+01	.74598E+00	.23095E+01	.25558E+01	.25802E+01	.25693E+01
8	.17533E+01	-.37471E+00	.12969E+01	.17117E+01	.17485E+01	.17358E+01
9	.73235E+00	-.10234E+01	.23693E+00	.69289E+00	.72761E+00	.73304E+00
10	-.35686E+00	-.13173E+01	-.44261E+00	-.37408E+00	-.36042E+00	-.33656E+00
11	-.94623E+00	-.13764E+01	-.96267E+00	-.95952E+00	-.94951E+00	-.94351E+00
12	-.94058E+00	-.13731E+01	-.10101E+01	-.95457E+00	-.94373E+00	-.93787E+00
13	-.14569E+01	-.13557E+01	-.12290E+01	-.14475E+01	-.14573E+01	-.14421E+01
14	-.25272E+01	-.12883E+01	-.19151E+01	-.24664E+01	-.25207E+01	-.25217E+01
15	-.32230E+01	-.11673E+01	-.27933E+01	-.31822E+01	-.32163E+01	-.32173E+01
16	-.39051E+01	-.10322E+01	-.37455E+01	-.38963E+01	-.38990E+01	-.38953E+01

Table 11 Error analysis for second mode eigensolutions. Unconstrained substructure 2.

PERCENT ERRORS, EIGENSOLUTION 2

	TIE MATRIX	RECEPTANCE R=0	RECEPTANCE R=1	RECEPTANCE P=2	COMPONENT MODE
			NATURAL FREQUENCIES		
	-21.43304	-2.71650	-.25439	-.03688	-.00916
			MASS NORMALIZATION CONSTANTS		
	37.95168	18.35012	1.73185	.22482	.74991
			MODE SHAPE		
1	C.00000	0.00000	0.00000	0.00000	0.00000
2	-5.43836	4.06129	.35252	.02928	.35229
3	-8.81086	7.82842	.66679	.05623	.57016
4	-4.91930	8.99273	.75288	.06684	.49325
5	8.82206	7.86853	.66766	.06815	.27998
6	35.70802	6.62029	.65343	.08318	.23717
7	71.12835	10.61669	1.08274	.13920	.56008
8	121.37128	26.03288	2.37288	.27487	1.00225
9	239.73586	67.64760	5.38760	.64715	-.09462
10	-269.13884	-24.02884	-4.82428	-.99659	5.68930
11	-45.45761	-1.73678	-1.40470	-.34658	.28779
12	-45.98081	-7.39585	-1.48764	-.33488	.28790
13	6.94671	15.63979	.64232	-.02881	1.01741
14	49.02453	24.21988	2.40644	.25846	.21608
15	63.78156	13.33142	1.26616	.20692	.17673
16	73.56909	4.08738	.22506	.15634	.25030

$$\underline{\bar{U}} = \underline{U} + \sum_{i=1}^{D} \frac{\partial \underline{U}}{\partial d_i} \Delta d_i + \sum_{i=1}^{D} \sum_{j=1}^{D} \frac{\partial^2 \underline{U}}{\partial d_i \partial d_j} \Delta d_i \Delta d_j \tag{180}$$

+ higher order terms

The derivative terms are evaluated by differentiating the system's static equilibrium equation,

$$\underline{K}\ \underline{U} = \underline{P} \tag{181}$$

assuming that the external load vector's, $\underline{P}$, change is negligible when a design parameter changes. The first two derivatives are expressed by,

$$\frac{\partial \underline{U}}{\partial d_i} = - \underline{K}^{-1} \frac{\partial \underline{K}}{\partial d_i} \underline{U} \tag{182}$$

$$\frac{\partial^2 U}{\partial d_i \partial d_j} = - \underline{K}^{-1} \left(\frac{\partial^2 \underline{K}}{\partial d_i \partial d_j} \underline{U} + \frac{\partial \underline{K}}{\partial d_i} \frac{\partial \underline{U}}{\partial d_j} + \frac{\partial \underline{K}}{\partial d_j} \frac{\partial \underline{U}}{\partial d_i} \right) \tag{183}$$

Note that in practice $\underline{K}$ is not inverted, instead the triangularized form of $\underline{K}$ obtained from the unmodified system's solution is used to solve for the vectors in equations (182) and (183). In addition, to maximize the computational efficiency, advantage should be taken of the sparsity of the derivatives of $\underline{K}$. Ordinarily only the first order terms of equation (180) are retained.

Storaasli and Sobieszczanski (94) have applied the first order Taylor series method to a 5000 dof fuselage midsection model. Less than 16% error was observed for single element variation of -100% (i.e. element removal) to +500%, and for -50% to 50% change for multi-elements. The incorporation of second order terms would undoubtedly increase this solution accuracy, but at the expense of increased computational burden.

Iteration Method

The equilibrium equation of the modified system may be written as,

$$\underline{K}\ \underline{\bar{U}} = \underline{P} - \underline{\Delta K}\ \underline{\bar{U}} \tag{184}$$

From this form an iterative solution approach is derived in the following recursive form,

$$\underline{K}\ \underline{\bar{U}}^{(i+1)} = \underline{P} - \underline{\Delta K}\ \underline{\bar{U}}^{(i)} \tag{185}$$

Back substitution is employed to solve for $\underline{\bar{U}}^{(i+1)}$, utilizing the triangularized form of $\underline{K}$ from the unmodified system's solution. The iteration is started using,

$$\underline{\bar{U}}^{(o)} = \underline{U} = \text{unmodified system response} \tag{186}$$

Noor and Lowder (93) suggested a method comprised of the Taylor series and iteration formulas. First $\underline{U}^{(o)}$ is computed via a Taylor series method, i.e.

$$\overline{\underline{U}}^{(o)} = \underline{U} + \sum_{i=1}^{D} \frac{\partial \underline{U}}{\partial d_i} \Delta d_i \tag{187}$$

Then $\overline{\underline{U}}^{(o)}$ is used to initiate the iterative process in eq. 185, for i>0. Usually one or two iteration cycles are reported sufficient to obtain good results.

Reduced Basis Method

Fox and Miura (95) introduced a procedure analogous to assumed modes to reduce the dimension of the modified structure's static equilibrium problem. A set of known system deflection vectors $\underline{U}^{(1)}$, $\underline{U}^{(2)}$, ..., $\underline{U}^{(r)}$ are assumed to span the solution space. Since r<<n = number of dof, this is obviously an approximation. The approximate solution of the modified system then follows as,

$$\overline{\underline{U}} = \sum_{j=1}^{r} C_j \underline{U}^{(j)} , \qquad \underline{C} = [C_1 \; C_2 \ldots C_r]^T \tag{188}$$

$$\underline{\tilde{K}} \; \underline{C} = \underline{\tilde{P}} \qquad (r\times 1) \tag{189}$$

$$\underline{\tilde{K}} = \underline{R}^T (\underline{K} + \underline{\Delta K}) \; \underline{R} \qquad (r\times r) \tag{190}$$

$$\underline{\tilde{P}} = \underline{R}^T \; \underline{P} \qquad (r\times 1), \; \underline{R} = [\underline{U}^{(1)} \vdots \ldots \vdots \underline{U}^{(r)}] \; (n\times r) \tag{191}$$

Fox and Miura indicated this is equivalent to applying the Ritz-Galerkin principle in the subspace spanned by the set of vectors $\underline{U}^{(1)} \ldots \underline{U}^{(r)}$. Although suggestions were provided, a systematic approach to calculating the basis vectors and deciding the value of r was not indicated. Noor and Lowder (93) suggested the use of the following as basis vectors,

$$\underline{U}^{(1)} = \underline{U} \; , \quad \underline{U}^{(i+1)} = \frac{\partial \underline{U}}{\partial d_i} \qquad i=1,2,\ldots D \tag{192}$$

where D is the number of design parameters. Excellent results were obtained.

Exact Methods

Successive Modification Methods (SMM)

This method, developed by Kavlie and Powell (92), incorporates the modification matrix, $\underline{\Delta K}$, a single non-null column at a time. The basis of this approach is the Sherman-Morrison formula (see Householder (90)) for the inverse of a modified matrix, i.e.

$$(\underline{A} + \underline{X} \; \underline{Y}^T)^{-1} = \underline{A}^{-1} - (\underline{A}^{-1} \; \underline{X})(\underline{Y}^T \; \underline{A}^{-1})/(1 + \underline{Y}^T \; \underline{A}^{-1} \; \underline{X}) \tag{193}$$

where $\underline{X}$ and $\underline{Y}$ are column vectors representing the modification to $\underline{A}$.

The system's static equilibrium equations, before and after structural modifications are,

$$\underline{K} \; \underline{U} = \underline{P}, \quad (\underline{K} + \underline{\Delta K}) \; \overline{\underline{U}} = \underline{P} \qquad (n\times 1) \tag{194}$$

Consider the special case when just column j of $\underline{\Delta K}$ is non-null. Designate this column as $\underline{X} = \underline{\tilde{\Delta K}}$. Then

$$\underline{\Delta K} = \underline{X}\,\underline{Y}^T = \underline{\tilde{\Delta K}}\,\underline{Y}^T, \quad \underline{Y}^T = [0 \;\ldots\; 0 \;\underset{\uparrow \text{column } j}{1}\; 0 \;\ldots\; 0] \tag{195}$$

and equation (193) implies

$$(\underline{K} + \underline{\Delta K})^{-1} = \underline{K}^{-1} - \underline{K}^{-1}\,\underline{X}\,\underline{Y}^T\,\underline{K}^{-1}/(1 + \underline{Y}^T\,\underline{K}^{-1}\,\underline{X}) \tag{196}$$

To apply equation (196) directly would explicitly require $\underline{K}^{-1}$. Alternatively, post multiplying this equation by $\underline{P}$ yields

$$\bar{\underline{U}} = \underline{U} - \underline{W}\,\underline{Y}^T\,\underline{U}/(1 + \underline{Y}^T\,\underline{W}), \qquad \underline{K}\,\underline{W} = \underline{X} \tag{197}$$

where $\underline{W}$ is calculated by back substitution using the triangularized form of $\underline{K}$ from the unmodified system's solution.

For the more general case place the n_c non-null columns of $\underline{\Delta K}$ in the columns of the nxn_c matrix $\underline{X}$. The non-null column numbers of $\underline{\Delta K}$ are designated by the set of ascending integers,

$$j_1\; j_2\; \cdots\; j_{n_c} \tag{198}$$

With these definitions the ith row of the $n_c xn$, Boolean matrix $\underline{Y}^T$ which expands $\underline{X}$ into $\underline{\Delta K}$ is null except for the number one (1) in column j_i. The stiffness modification matrix is then given by,

$$\underset{(nxn)}{\underline{\Delta K}} = \underset{(nxn_c)}{\underline{X}}\;\; \underset{(n_c xn)}{\underline{Y}^T} = \underline{\tilde{\Delta K}}\;\underline{Y}^T \tag{199}$$

For example consider a 10 dof system with modifications to $\underline{K}$ in columns 2, 5, 7 and 9, then

$$n_c = 4,\; j_1 = 2,\; j_2 = 5,\; j_3 = 7,\; j_4 = 9$$

$$\underline{\Delta K} = [\underline{0} \mid \underline{\Delta K}_2 \mid \underline{0} \mid \underline{0} \mid \underline{\Delta K}_5 \mid \underline{0} \mid \underline{\Delta K}_7 \mid \underline{0} \mid \underline{\Delta K}_9 \mid \underline{0}]$$

$$\underline{X} = [\underline{\Delta K}_2 \mid \underline{\Delta K}_5 \mid \underline{\Delta K}_7 \mid \underline{\Delta K}_9] = [\underline{X}_1 \mid \underline{X}_2 \mid \underline{X}_3 \mid \underline{X}_4] = \underline{\tilde{\Delta K}}$$

$$\underline{Y}^T = \begin{bmatrix} 0 & 1 & 0 & 0 & 0 & 0 & 0 & 0 & 0 & 0 \\ 0 & 0 & 0 & 0 & 1 & 0 & 0 & 0 & 0 & 0 \\ 0 & 0 & 0 & 0 & 0 & 0 & 1 & 0 & 0 & 0 \\ 0 & 0 & 0 & 0 & 0 & 0 & 0 & 0 & 1 & 0 \end{bmatrix} = \begin{bmatrix} \underline{Y}_1^T \\ \hline \underline{Y}_2^T \\ \hline \underline{Y}_3^T \\ \hline \underline{Y}_4^T \end{bmatrix}$$

Then if more than one column of $\underline{K}$ is modified, the successive modification method of Kavlie and Powell is employed. This assumes the following recursive form;

$$\underline{U}_i = \underline{U}_{i-1} - \underline{W}_i^{(i-1)} \underline{Y}_i^T \underline{U}_{i-1}/(1 + \underline{Y}_i^T \underline{W}_i^{(i-1)}) \qquad (200)$$

$$\underline{W}_i^{(k)} = \underline{K}_k^{-1} \underline{X}_i \quad , \qquad \underline{U}_o = \underline{U} \qquad (201)$$

where $\underline{U}_i$ is the system's displacement vector after the first i non-null columns of $\underline{\Delta K}$ are considered. Note that $\underline{W}_i^{(k)}$ is the system's displacement vector at the stage when k non-null columns of $\underline{\Delta K}$ are included, with $\underline{X}_i$ as the external load vector. These vectors are calculated by the formulas

$$\underline{W}_i^{(k)} = \underline{W}_i^{(k-1)} - \underline{W}_k^{(k-1)} \underline{Y}_k^T \underline{W}_i^{(k-1)}/(1 + \underline{Y}_k^T \underline{W}_k^{(k-1)}) \qquad (202)$$

$$\underline{K}\, \underline{W}_i^{(o)} = \underline{X}_i \qquad , \qquad i = 1,2, \ldots n_c \qquad (203)$$

where $\underline{W}_i^{(o)}$ is calculated by back substitution using the triangularized form of $\underline{K}$ from the unmodified system's solution. Equations (200) through (203) follow directly from the version of the Sherman-Morrison formula given by equation (197). A flow diagram for the 10 dof-n_c=4 system is shown in Figure 8.

Kavlie and Powell provide operation counts for this method, and emphasize that any reanalysis scheme should be carefully scrutinized as to when it is more efficient than complete reanalysis.

Direct Modification Method

This method was developed by Argyris, et. al. (91). The derivation is based on the Woodbury formula (ref., 90),

$$(\underline{A} + \underline{E}\, \underline{C}\, \underline{F}^T)^{-1} = \underline{A}^{-1} - \underline{A}^{-1} \underline{E}\, (\underline{C}^{-1} + \underline{F}^T \underline{A}^{-1} \underline{E})^{-1} \underline{F}^T \underline{A}^{-1} \qquad (204)$$

however a derivation from physical arguments is also included. For reanalysis of the static equilibrium equation substitute

$$\underline{A} = \underline{K}, \quad \underline{E} = \underline{b}^T, \quad \underline{F} = \underline{b}^T, \quad \underline{C} = \underline{\approx{\Delta K}} \qquad (205)$$

$$\underline{\Delta K} = \underline{b}^T \underline{\approx{\Delta K}}\, \underline{b} = \underline{E}\, \underline{C}\, \underline{F}^T \qquad (206)$$

into equation (204) where $\underline{b} = \underline{Y}^T$ (see equation (199)). This yields

$$(\underline{K} + \underline{\Delta K})^{-1} = (\underline{K} + \underline{b}^T \underline{\approx{\Delta K}}\, \underline{b})^{-1} = \underline{K}^{-1} - \underline{K}^{-1} \underline{b}^T (\underline{\approx{\Delta K}}^{-1} + \underline{b}\, \underline{K}^{-1} \underline{b}^T)^{-1} \underline{b}\, \underline{K}^{-1} \qquad (207)$$

Post multiply equation (207) by $\underline{P}$ and use equation (194). This gives

$$\underline{\Delta U} = \underline{\bar{U}} - \underline{U} = -\, (\underline{L}^T)^{-1} \underline{Z}\, \underline{Q}^{-1} (\underline{Q}^{-1} + \underline{\approx{\Delta K}})^{-1} \underline{\approx{\Delta K}}\, \underline{b}\, \underline{U} \qquad (208)$$

where from the unmodified system solution the Cholesky decomposition of $\underline{K}$ is,

$$\underline{K} = \underline{L}\, \underline{L}^T \qquad (209)$$

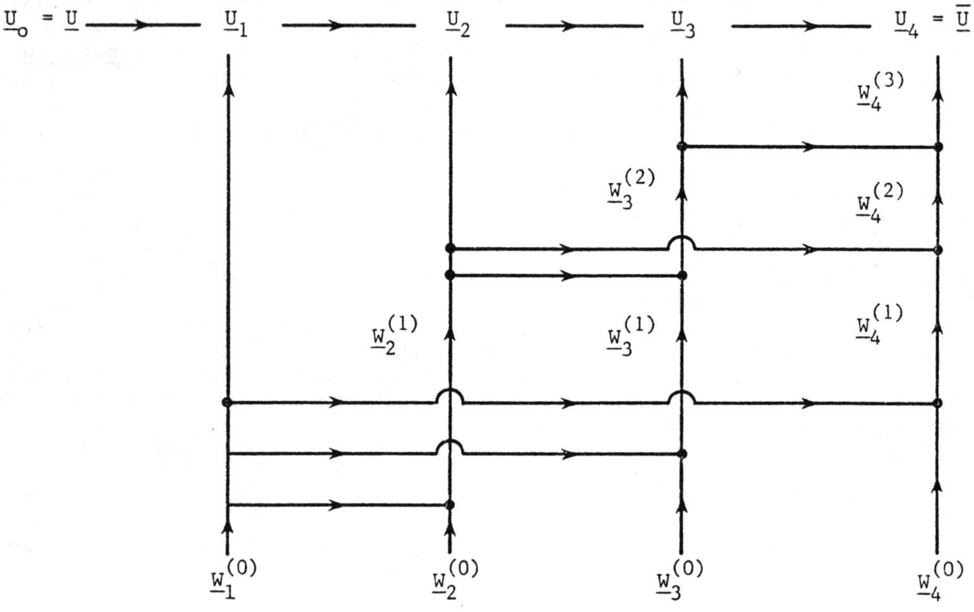

Figure 8. Flow diagram for static reanalysis (SMM), 10 dof - n_c = 4 system

and $\underline{L}\ \underline{Z} = \underline{b}^T, \quad \underline{Q} = \underline{Z}^T\underline{Z}$ (210)

Computationally, the following procedure was suggested,

(1) Compute $\underline{\tilde{r}}' = \underline{\Delta\tilde{\tilde{K}}}\ \underline{b}\ \underline{U}$, (2) Evaluate $\underline{Q}$ and $\underline{Z}$,

(3) Triangularize $\underline{Q}$; $\underline{Q} = \underline{L}_Q\ \underline{L}_Q^T$ and evaluate $\underline{Q}^{-1}$,

(4) Triangularize $(\underline{Q}^{-1} + \underline{\Delta\tilde{\tilde{K}}})$; $(\underline{Q}^{-1} + \underline{\Delta\tilde{\tilde{K}}} = \underline{L}_s\ \underline{L}_s^T$,

(5) Compute $\underline{g}$ and $\underline{\tilde{r}}''$ from $\underline{L}_s\ \underline{L}_s^T\ \underline{g} = \underline{\tilde{r}}'$ and $\underline{L}_Q\ \underline{L}_Q^T\ \underline{\tilde{r}}'' = \underline{g}$,

(6) Compute $\underline{\tilde{r}}''' = \underline{Z}\ \underline{\tilde{r}}''$, finally

(7) Solve $\underline{L}^T\ (\underline{\bar{U}} - \underline{U}) = -\ \underline{\tilde{r}}'''$.

Argyris emphasized that the preceeding algorithm is more efficient than complete reanalysis only when n_c is approximately less than 0.75B. Also mentioned is that Argyris's approach is generally more efficient than Kavlie and Powell's as expressed by equation (200)-(203).

Pseudo Load Method

This method is proposed by the present authors. It is hypothesized that the modifications actually behave as "closed-loop" deflection dependent loadings, forcing the unmodified system. Furthermore, suppose that for a localized modification, the added pseudo loading only is dependent on a small portion of the displacements. The modified system solution employs the available information from the solution of the unmodified system. This permits the modified system displacements to be expressed as functions of the displacements associated with only that portion of the system where modifications occur. Partitioning the modified system displacement vector and equating the modification related displacements yields a reduced set of equations. The following analytically summarizes the preceeding concepts.

Substitute equation (199) into equation (184)

$$\underline{K}\ \underline{\bar{U}} = \underline{P} - \underline{X}\ \underline{Y}^T\ \underline{\bar{U}} \qquad (n\text{x}1) \qquad (211)$$

$$\underline{\bar{U}} = \underline{U} - \underline{K}^{-1}\ \underline{X}\ \underline{Y}^T\ \underline{\bar{U}} \qquad (n\text{x}1) \qquad (212)$$

Employ the previous notation of equation (197). Equation (212) is expressed as

$$\underline{\bar{U}} = \underline{U} - \underline{W}\ \underline{Y}^T\ \underline{\bar{U}} \qquad (n\text{x}1) \qquad (213)$$

The Boolean matrix $\underline{Y}^T$ condenses $\underline{\bar{U}}$ to the form,

$$\underline{\hat{\bar{U}}} = \underline{Y}^T\ \underline{\bar{U}} \qquad (n_c\text{x}1) \qquad (214)$$

This condensed displacement vector contains only the coordinates which correspond to non-null columns of $\underline{\Delta K}$, i.e. $\bar{U}_{j_i}$, i=1,2,...n_c. Equation (213) becomes,

$$\underline{\bar{U}} = \underline{U} - \underline{W}\ \underline{\hat{\bar{U}}} \qquad (n\text{x}1) \qquad (215)$$

By shifting rows (j_i, i=1,2,...,n_c) in $\underline{\bar{U}}$, $\underline{U}$ and $\underline{W}$ to the top in equation (215), it is seen that

$$\begin{bmatrix} \hat{\bar{\underline{U}}} \\ n_c x1 \\ \hdashline \bar{\underline{U}}_r \\ (n-n_c) \\ x1 \end{bmatrix} = \begin{bmatrix} \hat{\underline{U}} \\ n_c x1 \\ \hdashline \underline{U}_r \\ (n-n_c) \\ x1 \end{bmatrix} - \begin{bmatrix} \hat{\underline{W}} \\ n_c x n_c \\ \hdashline \underline{W}_r \\ (n-n_c) \\ x n_c \end{bmatrix} \begin{bmatrix} \hat{\bar{\underline{U}}} \\ n_c x1 \end{bmatrix} \qquad (nx1) \tag{216}$$

The condensed displacement vector is then calculable from

$$(\underline{I}_{n_c} + \hat{\underline{W}})\ \hat{\bar{\underline{U}}} = \hat{\underline{U}} \qquad (n_c x1) \tag{217}$$

After which the remaining displacements are found using

$$\bar{\underline{U}}_r = \underline{U}_r - \underline{W}_r\ \hat{\bar{\underline{U}}} \qquad (n-n_c)x1 \tag{218}$$

The computation of $\underline{W}$ in equation (213) proceeds by solving the separate sets of equations $\underline{K}\ \underline{W}_i = \underline{X}_i$, $i=1\ldots n_c$. These sets are solved by back substitution utilizing the triangularized form of $\underline{K}$ from the unmodified system's solution.

The pseudo load method appears to resemble the direct modification method. Compared with the successive modification method, this method treats all modifications simultaneously. In addition, the derivation of the pseudo load method is simple and direct. The unmodified system's displacement vector and triangularized form of $\underline{K}$ may be obtained from any appropriate finite element code. A simple truss problem is included to illustrate the pseudo load method.

The geometric and material properties of the truss members are shown in Figure 9. Employing the direct stiffness method (ref. 96) with the appropriate boundary conditions provides the static equilibrium equation,

$$0.125 \times 10^6 \begin{bmatrix} 5 & 1 & 0 & 0 \\ 1 & 5 & 0 & -4 \\ 0 & 0 & 5 & -1 \\ 0 & -4 & -1 & 5 \end{bmatrix} \begin{bmatrix} U_1 \\ U_2 \\ U_3 \\ U_4 \end{bmatrix} = \begin{bmatrix} 0 \\ 1000 \\ 0 \\ 0 \end{bmatrix}, \quad \underline{K}\ \underline{U} = \underline{P} \tag{219}$$

The Cholesky decomposition of $\underline{K}$ is $\underline{K} = \underline{L}\ \underline{L}^T$;

$$\underline{L}\ \underline{L}^T = 0.125 \times 10^6 \begin{bmatrix} (5)^{\frac{1}{2}} & 0 & 0 & 0 \\ (5)^{-\frac{1}{2}} & (24/5)^{\frac{1}{2}} & 0 & 0 \\ 0 & 0 & (5)^{\frac{1}{2}} & 0 \\ 0 & -(10/3)^{\frac{1}{2}} & -(5)^{-\frac{1}{2}} & (22/15)^{\frac{1}{2}} \end{bmatrix}$$

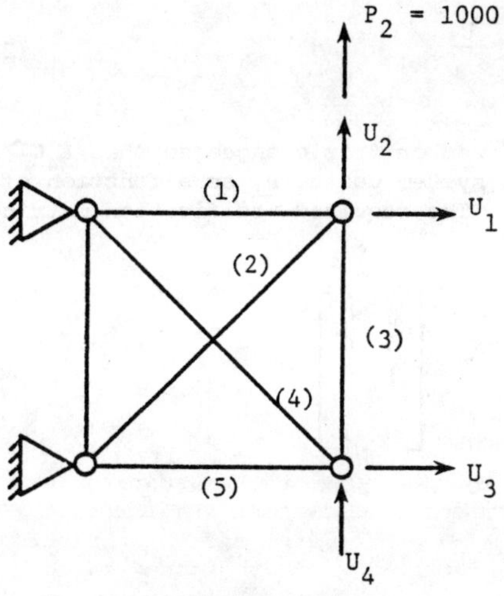

$L_1 = L_3 = L_5 = 20$ in. (50.8cm)

$L_2 = L_4 = 20\sqrt{2}$ in. (71.84cm)

$A_1 = A_3 = A_5 = 1.0 \text{ in}^2$ (6.45cm^2)

$A_2 = A_4 = \sqrt{2} / 2 \text{ in}^2$ (4.56cm^2)

$E = 1.0 \times 10^7 \text{ lb/in}^2$ (68.95 GN/m^2)

Figure 9. Truss used to illustrate the pseudo load method of static reanalysis

$$
\times \begin{bmatrix} (5)^{\frac{1}{2}} & (5)^{-\frac{1}{2}} & 0 & 0 \\ 0 & (24/5)^{\frac{1}{2}} & 0 & -(10/3)^{\frac{1}{2}} \\ 0 & 0 & (5)^{\frac{1}{2}} & -(5)^{-\frac{1}{2}} \\ 0 & 0 & 0 & (22/15)^{\frac{1}{2}} \end{bmatrix}
$$

The solution of $\underline{U}$ proceeds in the standard fashion,

$$
\underline{P} = \underline{L}\,\underline{L}^T\,\underline{U} \Rightarrow \underline{P} = \underline{L}\,\underline{Y} \quad , \quad \underline{Y} = \underline{L}^T\,\underline{U}
$$
$$
\underline{U} = (2/11) \times 10^{-3}\ [-6 \quad 30 \quad 5 \quad 25] \tag{220}
$$

Now suppose that the cross-sectional area of member 4 is changed so that $A_4 \Rightarrow A'_4 = \sqrt{2}/2\ (1 + \alpha)$. The responses of the modified system due to $\underline{P}$, as a function of α, can be calculated by the pseudo load method. The required modification matrices and indices for the problem are,

$$
\underline{\Delta K} = \begin{bmatrix} 0 & 0 & 0 & 0 \\ 0 & 0 & 0 & 0 \\ 0 & 0 & e & -e \\ 0 & 0 & -e & e \end{bmatrix}, \quad \underline{X} = \begin{bmatrix} 0 & 0 \\ 0 & 0 \\ e & -e \\ -e & e \end{bmatrix}, \quad \underline{Y} = \begin{bmatrix} 0 & 0 \\ 0 & 0 \\ 1 & 0 \\ 0 & 1 \end{bmatrix},
$$

$$
\hat{\underline{\bar{U}}} = \begin{bmatrix} \bar{U}_3 \\ \bar{U}_4 \end{bmatrix}, \quad \underline{\bar{U}}_r = \begin{bmatrix} \bar{U}_1 \\ \bar{U}_2 \end{bmatrix}
$$

$$
e = 0.125 \times 10^6 \cdot \alpha \quad , \quad n_c = 2, \quad j_1 = 3, \quad j_2 = 4
$$

Using the decomposed form of $\underline{K}$, the matrix $\underline{W}$ is,

$$
\underline{W} = [\underline{W}_1 \mid \underline{W}_2] = \frac{\alpha}{11} \begin{bmatrix} 1 & -1 \\ -5 & 5 \\ 1 & -1 \\ -6 & 6 \end{bmatrix}
$$

The modified system responses are from equations (217) and (218)

$$
\bar{U}_3 = ((1 + 6\alpha/11)U_3 + \alpha\, U_4/11)/(1 + 7\alpha/11) \tag{221}
$$

$$
\bar{U}_4 = (6\alpha U_3/11 + (1 + \alpha/11)U_4)/(1 + 7\alpha/11) \tag{222}
$$

$$
\bar{U}_1 = U_1 - \alpha(\bar{U}_3 - \bar{U}_4)/11 \tag{223}
$$

$$
\bar{U}_2 = U_2 - 5\alpha(-\bar{U}_3 + \bar{U}_4)/11 \tag{224}
$$

Results like equations (221) and (222) are generally very useful since they provide (1) an efficient basis for performing a parametric study of the static response, and (2) means for prescribed static responses. The second use is illustrated by prescribing either $\bar{U}_3$ or $\bar{U}_4$ in equations (221) or (222) and then calculating the required factor α, i.e. from equation (221),

$$\alpha = 11(U_3 - \bar{U}_3)/(7\ \bar{U}_3 - 6\ U_3 - U_4) \tag{225}$$

For example if it is desired for $\bar{U}_3 = 0.9\ U_3$, then from equation (225), $\alpha = -0.234$, and from equations (221)-(224),

$$\underline{\bar{U}} = [-\ 6.5 \quad 32.5 \quad 4.5 \quad 28.0] \times (2/11) \times 10^{-3}$$

If from equation (225), $\alpha < -1.0$, then the prescribed value of $\bar{U}_3$ is not realizable by only modifying member 4.

The generalization of the preceeding discussion to many design variables, least squares solutions, etc. will be a subject for further research.

SUMMARY AND CONCLUSIONS

In this study, various methods of eigensolution reanalysis and design, modal synthesis, and static reanalysis and design were examined. Employing generalized receptances and pseudo loads, several new techniques were developed.

The main concern in applying the approximate methods presented are solution accuracy and efficiency. These quantities vary depending upon 1) time required to determine precisely how a modification(s) affects the system's property matrices, 2) size and extent of the modification(s), 3) size of the unmodified system, and 4) whether the solution technique is iterative or non-interative. Accuracy and efficiency obviously behave as occupants of a seesaw. As accuracy increases efficiency decreases, and vice versa. The optimum balance between these two opposing characteristics should be determined by judging how critical is the accuracy of the computed results in the corresponding design stage. Experience with the various methods is perhaps the best guide to their application. For this reason more numerical experiments are now planned (ref. 97).

The use of an auxiliary function in equation (119) to improve convergence properties is somewhat semi-empirical. Further analysis concerning its use should be reported in reference (97). In any case, the eigenvalues produced by one of the non-receptance methods (i.e. assumed modes) should be sufficient as starting values to insure convergence in equation (118), with $r(\lambda_n)$ replaced by $g(\lambda_n)$. Employing a higher mode factor would then improve the accuracy of the initial method's eigenvalues and yield the corresponding eigenvectors.

The static reanalysis techniques assume that the external load vector ($\underline{P}$) is invariant while the stiffness matrix of the structure is modified. This assumption should be applied with caution since structural modifications will in all cases change the distributed dead weight load of the structure.

The modal synthesis techniques are indispensable for analyzing very large structural systems. Though many formulations have been proposed, the practical application of modal synthesis is not wide spread. This primarily results from the absence of this capability from most generic finite element codes. The addition of a general modal synthesis procedure to a good finite element code will be well received by the user community.

ACKNOWLEGEMENT

This study was supported by the Office of Naval Research.

REFERENCES

1 Zienkiewicz, O. C., The Finite Element Method, 3rd. ed., McGraw-Hill, London, 1977.

2 Desai, C. S., and Abel, J. F., Introduction to the Finite Element Method, 1st. ed., Van Nostrand Reinhold, New York, 1972.

3 Oden, J. T., Finite Elements of Nonlinear Continua, 1st. ed., McGraw-Hill, New York, 1972.

4 Wilkinson, J. H., The Algebraic Eigenvalue Problem, 1st. ed., Clarendon Press, Oxford, 1965.

5 Goult, R. J., Hoskins, R. F., Milner, J. A., and Pratt, M. J., Computational Methods in Linear Algebra, 1st. ed., Wiley, New York, 1974.

6 Faddeeva, V. N., Computational Methods of Linear Algebra, 1st ed., Dover, New York, 1959.

7 Bathe, K. J., and Wilson, E. L., Numerical Methods in Finite - Element Analysis, 1st. ed., Prentice Hall, New Jersey, 1976.

8 Clough, R. W., and Wilson, E. L., "Dynamic Analysis of Large Structural Systems with Local Nonlinearities," Computer Methods in Applied Mechanics and Engineering, Vol. 17/18, 1979, pp. 107-129.

9 Morris, N. F., "The Use of Modal Superposition in Nonlinear Dynamics," Computers and Structures, Vol. 7, 1977, pp. 65-72.

10 Nickell, R. E., "Nonlinear Dynamics by Mode Superposition," Computer Methods in Applied Mechanics and Engineering, Vol. 7, 1976, pp. 107-129.

11 Arora, J. S., "Survey of Structural Reanalysis Techniques," Journal of the Structural Division, ASCE, Vol. 102, No. ST4, April 1976, pp. 783-803.

12 Pilkey, W. D., and Chang, P. Y., Modern Formulas for Statics and Dynamics, 1st ed., McGraw-Hill, New York, 1978.

13 Lund, J. W., "Stability and Damped Critical Speeds of a Flexible Rotor in Fluid Film Bearings," Journal of Engineering for Industry Trans. ASME, May 1974, pp. 509-517.

14 Frazer, R. A., Duncan, W. J., and Collar, A. R., Elementary Matrices, 1st ed., Macmillan, New York, 1947, pp. 277-279.

15 Lancaster, P., Lambda-matrices and Vibrating Systems, 1st ed., Pergamon Press, Toronto, 1966.

16 Choy, K. C., Dynamic Analysis of Flexible Rotor-Bearing Systems Using a Modal Approach, Ph.D. Dissertation, University of Virginia, 1977.

17 Meirovitch, L., Analytical Methods in Vibrations, 1st ed., Macmillan, New York, 1967.

18 Stetson, K. A., and Palma, G. E., "Inversion of First Order Perturbation Theory and Its Application to Structural Design," AIAA Journal, Vol. 14, No. 4, April 1976, pp. 454-460.

19 Lund, J. W., "Sensitivity of the Critical Speeds of a Rotor to Changes in the Design," Journal of Mechanical Design, Trans. ASME, Vol. 102, January 1980, pp. 115-121.

20 Lancaster, P., "Free Vibrations of Lightly Damped Systems by Perturbation Methods," Quarterly Journal of Mechanics and App. Math., Vol. 13, 1960, pp. 138-155.

21 Aubrun, J. N., "Theory of the Control of Structures by Low Authority Controllers," AIAA Conference on Large Space Platforms: Future Needs and Capabilities, Los Angeles, CA., Sept. 27-29, 1978, paper No. 78-1689 (also, J. Guid. & Control, Vol. 3, No. 5, 1980, pp. 444-451).

22 Meirovitch, L., and Ryland II, G., "Response of Slightly Damped Gyroscopic Systems," Journal of Sound and Vibration, Vol. 67, No. 1, 1979, pp. 1-19.

23 Romstad, K. M., Hutchinson, J. R., and Runge, K. H., "Design Parameter Variation and Structural Response," Inter. Jour. for Numerical Method in Engin., Vol. 5, 1973, pp. 337-349.

24 Fox, R. L., and Kapoor, M. P., "Rates of Change of Eigenvalues and Eigenvectors," AIAA Journal, Vol. 6, No. 12, 1968, pp. 2426-29.

25 Brogan, W. L., Modern Control Theory, 1st. ed., Quantum, New York, 1974.

26 Rudisill, C. S., "Derivatives of Eigenvalues and Eigenvectors for a General Matrix," AIAA Journal, Vol. 12, No. 5, May 1974, pp. 721-722.

27 Bhatia, K. G., "Rapid Iterative Reanalysis for Automated Design," TN D-7357, NASA Tech. Note, October 1973.

28 Clough, R. W., and Penzien, J., Dynamics of Structures, 1st. ed.,

McGraw-Hill, New York, 1975.

29 Plaut, R. H., "Derivatives of Eigenvalues and Eigenvectors in Non Self Adjoint Systems," AIAA Journal, Vol. 11, No. 2, February 1973, pp. 250-251.

30 Rogers, L. C., "Derivatives of Eigenvalues and Eigenvectors," AIAA Journal, Vol. 8, No. 5, May 1970, pp. 943-944.

31 Garg, S., "Derivatives of Eigensolutions for a General Matrix," AIAA Journal, Vol. 11, No. 8, August 1973, pp. 1191-1194.

32 Bodewig, E., Matrix Calculus, 1st ed., North Holland Pub. Co., Amsterdam, 1956.

33 Hurty, W. C., and Rubinstein, M. F., Dynamics of Structures, 1st ed., Prenctice Hall, New Jersey, 1964.

34 Bisplinghoff, R. L., Ashley, H., and Halfman, R. L., Aero-elasticity, Addison-Wesley, 1955.

35 Gunter, E. J., Choy, K. C., and Allaire, P. E., "Modal Analysis of Turborotors Using Planar Modes-Theory," Journal of the Franklin Institute, Vol. 305, No. 4, 1978, pp. 221-243.

36 Weissenburger, J. T., The Effects of Local Modifications on the Eigenvalues and Eigenvectors of Linear Systems, Ph.D. Dissertation, Sever Instit. of Technology, Washington University, 1966, U. M. 6607529.

37 Weissenburger, J. T., "Effect of Local Modifications on the Vibration Characteristics of Linear Systems," Journal of Applied Mechanics, Trans. ASME, Vol. 35, 1968, pp. 327-332.

38 Pomazal, R. J., The Effect of Local Modifications on the Eigenvalues and Eigenvectors of Damped Linear Systems, Ph.D. Dissertation, Michigan Technological University, 1969, U. M. 7013559.

39 Pomazal, R. J., "Local Modifications of Damped Linear Systems," AIAA Journal, Vol. 9, No. 11, 1971, pp. 2216-21.

40 Hallquist, J. O., Modification and Synthesis of Large Dynamic Structural Systems, Ph.D. Dissertation, Michigan Technological University, 1974, U. M. 7514397.

41 Hallquist, J. O., "An Efficient Method for Determining the Effects of Mass Modifications in Damped Systems," Journal of Sound and Vibration, Vol. 44, No. 3, 1976, pp. 449-459.

42 Vilmann, C. R., and Snyder, V. W., "Line Modification of Continuous Vibratory Systems," Journal of the Structural Division, ASCE, Vol. 104, No. ST12, December 1978, pp. 1819-1826.

43 Hirai, I., Yoshimura, T., and Takamura, K., "On a Direct Eigenvalue Analysis for Locally Modified Structures," Inter. Journal for Numerical Methods in Eng., Vol. 6, 1973, pp. 441-42.

44 Ayres, F., Theory and Problems of Matrices, 1st ed., McGraw-Hill-Schaum's Outline Series, New York, 1962.

45 Bishop, R. E. D., The Mechanics of Vibration, 1st ed., Cambridge at the University Press, 1960, pp. 159 and 225.

46 Whittaker, E. T., A Treatise on the Analytical Dynamics of Particles and Rigid Bodies, Cambridge University Press, 1965, Ch. 7.

47 Done, G. T. S., and Hughes, A. D., "The Response of a Vibrating Structure as a Function of Structural Parameters," Journal of Sound and Vibration, Vol. 38, No. 2, 1975, pp. 255-266.

48 Done, G. T. S., Hughes, A. D., and Webby, J., "The Response of a Vibrating Structure as a Function of Structural Parameters - Application and Experiment," Journal of Sound and Vibration, Vol. 49, No. 2, 1976. pp. 149-159.

49 Forsythe, G. E., Malcolm, M. A., and Moler, C. B., Computer Methods for Mathematical Computations, 1st ed., Prentice-Hall, 1977.

50 Berman, A., and Flannelly, W., "Theory of Incomplete Models of Dynamic Structures," AIAA Journal, Vol. 9, No. 8, August 1971, pp. 1481-1487.

51 Klosterman, A. L., On the Experimental Determination and Use of Modal Representations of Dynamic Characteristics, Ph.D. Dissertation, University of Cincinnati, 1971.

52 Hurty, H. C., "Vibration of Structural Systems by Component Mode Synthesis," Proc. ASCE, Vol. 85, No. 4, August 1960, pp. 51-69.

53 Hurty, H. C., "Dynamic Analysis of Structural Systems Using Component Modes," AIAA Journal, Vol. 3, No. 4, April 1965, pp. 678-685.

54 Bamford, R. M., "A Modal Combination Program for Dynamic Analysis of Structures," Tech. Memo 33-290, Jet Propulsion Laboratory, Pasadena, California, July 1967.

55 Craig, R. R., Jr., and Bampton, M. C. C., "Coupling of Substructures for Dynamic Analyses," AIAA Journal, Vol. 6, No. 7, July 1968, pp. 1313-19.

56 Bajan, R. L., and Feng, C. C., "Free Vibration Analysis by the Modal Substitution Method," AAS Symposium on Space Projections from the Rocky Mountain Region, American Astronautical Society Paper, No. 68-8-1, Denver, CO., July 1968.

57 Bajan, R. L., Feng, C. C., and Jaszlics, I. J., "Vibration Analysis of Complex Structural Systems by Modal Substitution," Proceedings of the 30th Shock and Vibration Symposium, Monterey, California, October 1968.

58 Goldman, R. L., "Vibration Analysis by Dynamic Partitioning," AIAA Journal, Vol. 7, No. 6, June 1969, pp. 1152-1154.

59 Hou, S., "Review of Modal Synthesis Techniques and a New Approach," The Shock and Vibration Bulletin, No. 40, Pt. 4, Naval Research Laboratory, Washington, D. C., December 1969, pp. 25-39.

60 Benfield, W. A., and Hruda, R. F., "Vibration Analysis of Structures by Component Mode Substitution," AIAA Journal, Vol. 9, No. 7, July 1971, pp. 1255-61.

61 MacNeal, R. H., "A Hybrid Method of Component Mode Synthesis," Journal of Computers and Structures, Vol. 1, No. 4, December 1971, pp. 581-601.

62 Goldenberg, S., and Shapiro, M., "A Study of Modal Coupling Procedures," NASA CR-1152252, 1972, Gruman Aerospace Corp., NASA Contract No. NAS-10535-8.

63 Rubin, S., "An Improved Component-Mode Representation," AIAA/ASME/SAE 15th Structures, Structural Dynamics, and Materials Conference, AIAA Paper No. 74-386, Las Vegas, Nevada, April 1974.

64 Kuhar, E. J., and Stahle, C. V., "A Dynamic Transformation Method for Modal Synthesis," AIAA Journal, Vol. 12, No. 5, May 1974, pp. 672-678.

65 Hintz, R. M., "Analytical Methods in Component Modal Synthesis," AIAA Journal, Vol. 13, No. 8, August 1975, pp. 2007-2016.

66 Craig, R. R., Jr., and Chang, C. J., "Substructure Coupling with Reduction of Interface Coordinates--Fixed-Interface Methods," No. 75-1, January 1975, TICOM, The Univ. of Texas at Austin, Austin, TX.

67 Craig, R. R., Jr., and Chang, C. J., "Free-Interface Methods of Substructure Coupling for Dynamic Analysis," AIAA J., Vol. 14, 1976, pp. 1633-1635.

68 Klosterman, A. L., "A Combined Experimental and Analytical Procedure for Improving Automotive System Dynamics," Automotive Engineering Congress, Society of Automotive Engineers, Paper No. 720093, Detroit, MI., Jan. 1972.

69 Klosterman, A. L., and McClelland, W. A., "Combining Experimental and Analytical Techniques for Dynamic System Analysis," Tokyo Seminar on Finite Element Analysis, Nov. 1973.

70 Kana, D. D., and Huzar, S., "Synthesis of Shuttle Vehicle Damping Using Substructure Test Results," Interim Report for NASA Contract No. NAS8-27569, June 1972, Southwest Research Institute, San Antonio, TX.

71 Kana, D. D., and Huzar, S., "Synthesis of Shuttle Vehicle Damping Using Substructure Test Results," Journal of Spacecraft and Rockets, Vol. 10, No. 12, Dec. 1973, pp. 790-797.

72 Hasselman, T. K., "Damping Synthesis from Substructure Tests," AIAA/ASME/SAE 15th Structures, Structural Dynamics and Materials Conference, AIAA Paper No. 74-387, Las Vegas, NV., April 1974.

73 Neubert, V. H., and Raney, J. P., eds., Synthesis of Vibrating Systems, The American Society of Mechanical Engineers, Nov. 1971, Bk. No. H00072.

74 Ryan, R. S., ed., Symposium on Substrucutre Testing and Synthesis, NASA Marshall Space Flight Center, August 1972.

75 Hurty, W. C., "Introduction to Modal Synthesis Techniques," Synthesis of Vibrating Systems, ASME, Nov. 1971.

76 Benfield, W. A., Bodley, C. S., and Morosow, G., "Modal Synthesis Methods," Symposium on Substructure Testing and Synthesis, NASA, August 1972.

77 Craig, R. R., and Chang, C. J., "A Review of Substructure Coupling Methods for Dynamic Analysis," NASA CP-2001, Vol. 2, pp. 292-407.

78 Craig, R. R., "Methods of Component Mode Synthesis," Shock and Vibration Digest, Vol. 9, No. 11, Nov. 1977.

79 Hasselman, T. K., and Kaplan, A., "Dynamic Analysis of Large Systems by Complex Mode Synthesis," Journal of Dynamic System, Measurement, and Control, Trans. ASME, Sept. 1974, pp. 327-333.

80 Kung, W. C., and Hohenemser, K. H., "Eigenvalue Analysis for Coupled Large Linear Damped Structures," Computer Methods in Applied Mechanics and Eng-

ineering, Vol. 12, 1977, pp. 69-75.

81 Leung, Y. T., "An Accurate Method of Dynamic Substructuring with Simplified Computation," International Journal for Numerical Methods in Engineering, Vol. 14, 1979, pp. 1241-56.

82 Arora, J. S., and Nguyen, D. T., "Dynamic Substructural Analysis with Substructures," Tech. Report No. 46, Dec. 1, 1978, Division of Materials Engineering, College of Engineering, The University of Iowa, Iows City, Iowa.

83 Stavrinidis, C., "Theory and Practice of Modal Synthesis Techniques," Finite Element Methods in the Commerical Environment, Edited by J. Robinson, Robinson and Associates, 1978, Ch. 15.

84 Imbert, J. F., "A Survey of Current Capability for Dynamic Analysis of Complex Structures," Finite Element Methods in the Commercial Environment, Edited by J. Robinson, Robinson and Associates, 1978, Ch. 20.

85 Craig, R. R., "Substructure Coupling for Dynamic Analysis," Advances in Civil Engineering Through Engineering Mechanics, ASCE, 1977, pp. 389-392.

86 Guyan, R. J., "Reduction of Stiffness and Mass Matrices," AIAA Journal, Vol. 3, No. 2, Feb. 1965, p. 380.

87 Palazzolo, A. B., "Formalism for the Rotation Matrix of Rotations About an Arbitrary Axis," American Journal of Physics, Vol. 44, No. 1, Jan. 1976, pp. 63-67.

88 Halquist, J. O., and Synder, V., "Synthesis of Two Discrete Vibratory Systems Using Eigenvalue Modification," AIAA Journal, Vol. 12, No. 2, Feb. 1973, pp. 247-249.

89 Hallquist, J. O., and Synder, V. W., "On the Connection of Viscously Damped Continuous Vibratory Systems," Journal of Sound and Vibration, Vol. 32, No. 1, 1974, pp. 131-142.

90 Householder, A. S., The Theory of Matrices in Numerical Analysis, 1st ed., Dover Publications, Inc., New York, 1964.

91 Argyris, J. H., Brönlund, O. E., and Roy, J. R., "A Direct Modification Procedure for the Displacement Method," AIAA Journal, Vol. 9, No. 9, Sept. 1971, pp. 1861-1864.

92 Kavlie, D., and Powell, G., "Efficient Reanalysis of Modified Structures," Journal of the Structural Division, ASCE, Vol. 97, No. ST1, Jan. 1971, pp. 377-392.

93 Noor, A. K., and Lowder, H. E., "Approximate Techniques of Structural Reanalysis," International Journal of Computers and Structures, Vol. 4, No. 4, 1974, pp. 801-812.

94 Storaasli, O. O., and Sobieszczanski, J., "On the Accuracy of the Taylor Approximation for Structure Resizing," AIAA Journal, Vol. 12, No. 2, Feb. 1974, pp. 231-233.

95 Fox, R. L., and Miura, H., "An Approximate Analysis Technique for Design Calculations," AIAA Journal, Vol. 9, No. 1, Jan. 1971, pp. 177-179.

96 Martin, H. C., Introduction to Matrix Methods of Structural Analysis, 1st ed., McGraw-Hill, New York, 1966.

97 Palazzolo, A. B., Ph. D. Dissertation, University of Virginia, Charlottesville, Virginia 1980.

98 Franklin, J. N., Matrix Theory, 1st ed., Prentice-Hall, N. J., 1968.

CHAPTER NINE

SOLUTION ERRORS IN FINITE ELEMENT ANALYSIS

S. Utku and R. J. Melosh
Duke University
Durham, North Carolina

ABSTRACT

The development of the finite element method so far indicates that it is a discretization technique especially suited for positive definite, self-adjoint, elliptic sysytems, or systems with such components. The application of the method leads to the discretized equations in the form of $\dot{\underset{\sim}{u}}=\underset{\sim}{f}(\underset{\sim}{u})$, where $\underset{\sim}{u}$ lists the response of the discretized system at n pre-selected points called nodes. Instead of explicit expressions, vector function $\underset{\sim}{f}$ and its Jacobian $\underset{\sim}{f}_{,u}$ are available only numerically for a numerically given $\underset{\sim}{u}$. The solution of $\dot{\underset{\sim}{u}}=\underset{\sim}{f}(\underset{\sim}{u})$ is usually obtained by a digital computer. Due to the finiteness of the computer wordlength, the numerical solution $\underset{\sim}{u}_c$ is in general different from $\underset{\sim}{u}$. Let $\underset{\sim}{u}(\underset{\sim}{x},t)$ denote the actual response of the system in continuum at points corresponding to those of $\underset{\sim}{u}$. In the literature, $\underset{\sim}{u}(\underset{\sim}{x},t)-\underset{\sim}{u}$ is called the discretization errors, $\underset{\sim}{u}-\underset{\sim}{u}_c$ the round-off errors, and the sum of the two, that is, $\underset{\sim}{u}(\underset{\sim}{x},t)-\underset{\sim}{u}_c$ is called the solution errors. In this chapter, a state-of-the-art survey is given on the identification, growth, relative magnitudes, estimation, and control of the components of the solution errors.

INTRODUCTION

In this section the definitions of the notation and the terminology used in the chapter are given, and the scope and the organization of the material discussed are outlined.

Notation

The finite element method is being widely used in many disciplines for many diversified problems with different objectives. Therefore, it is very difficult to give a mathematically precise definition of the method which is satisfactory for everyone. Yet in order to deal with the problem of errors it is necessary to have a mathematical definition. For the sake of discussions in this chapter, a definition will be given in the next subsection.

The notation used in this chapter is slightly different from the rest of the book such that brackets are reserved for functions being operated by a continuum operator, e.g., $M[\psi]$ indicates that the operator M is operating on function ψ. Matrices are denoted by non-italic letters with symbol tilde (~) underneath, which is the standard notation for typesetters to make the symbol boldface type. If the matrix is a single column, the symbol underlined by the tilde is a lower case letter, otherwise it is an upper case letter. For example, an nxm matrix may be denoted as $\underset{\sim}{A}$, its i th column is $\underset{\sim}{a}_i$, and its (i,j) element is $a_{i,j}$. The time derivatives are shown with dots above, and other derivatives are denoted by a comma in the subscript. For example, if $\phi=\phi(x_1,x_2,\cdots,x_n,t)$, it is denoted as $\phi(\underset{\sim}{x},t)$, its derivative with respect to time t is shown as $\dot{\phi}$, the derivative with respect to x_i is $\phi_{,x_i}$. The Jacobian of ϕ may be shown as $\underset{\sim}{h}=\phi_{,\underset{\sim}{x}}$, and its Hessian may be shown as $\underset{\sim}{G}=\underset{\sim}{h}_{,\underset{\sim}{x}}=\phi_{,\underset{\sim}{x}\underset{\sim}{x}}$.

Definitions

Finite Element Method

Observing that the method was first introduced by the structural engineers in solving the boundary value problems of elasticity, here it is assumed that the method is a discretization technique for positive definite, self-adjoint, and elliptic systems for which an equivalent variational formulation is available. Then the finite element method is a Rayleigh-Ritz method using an admissible trial solution where the undetermined parameters are the local values of the response at pre-selected finite number of points (nodes), and the coordinate functions are the suitably chosen generalized pyramid functions (1) of class p where $p\geq m-1$ and m is the highest order differentiation appearing in the functional of the variational formulation (2,3). Unless otherwise stated, this definition will be used in this chapter.

Let $\underset{\sim}{x}$ denote the coordinates of a point in the spatial solution domain, and let $u(\underset{\sim}{x},t)$ denote the actual response quantity at this point at time t. Let $\underset{\sim}{x}_i$, $i=1,\cdots,n$ denote the coordinates of the nodes. The list of actual responses at these nodes at time t is denoted by $\underset{\sim}{u}(\underset{\sim}{x},t)=[u(\underset{\sim}{x}_1,t),u(\underset{\sim}{x}_2,t),\cdots,u(\underset{\sim}{x}_n,t)]^T$. Let $\underset{\sim}{u}(t)=[u_1(t),u_2(t),\cdots,u_n(t)]^T$ denote the finite element approximation of $\underset{\sim}{u}(\underset{\sim}{x},t)$, i.e., the undetermined parameters. Let $\underset{\sim}{\psi}(\underset{\sim}{x}) = [\psi_1(\underset{\sim}{x}),\psi_2(\underset{\sim}{x}),\cdots,\psi_n(\underset{\sim}{x})]^T$ denote the chosen generalized pyramid functions, i.e., the coordinate functions. Since for pyramid functions $\psi_j(\underset{\sim}{x}_j)=1$, then $\Psi(\underset{\sim}{x},t)=\underset{\sim}{u}(t)^T\underset{\sim}{\psi}(\underset{\sim}{x})$ is a trial function such that $\Psi(\underset{\sim}{x}_j,t)$ is an approximation of $u(\underset{\sim}{x}_j,t)$. Suppose $\underset{\sim}{\psi}(\underset{\sim}{x})$ is such that the essential boundary conditions are satisfied by $\Psi(\underset{\sim}{x},t)$ for any $\underset{\sim}{u}(t)$; then Ψ is admissible. Let Φ denote the variational functional. The use of Ψ in Φ, and the application of the Rayleigh-Ritz procedure leads to

$$\dot{\underset{\sim}{u}}=\underset{\sim}{f}(\underset{\sim}{u}) \tag{1}$$

Consider the power series expansion of $\underset{\sim}{f}$ at a point $\underset{\sim}{u}_\circ$

$$\underset{\sim}{f}(\underset{\sim}{u}) = \underset{\sim}{f}(\underset{\sim}{u}_\circ) + \underset{\sim}{f}_{,\underset{\sim}{u}}(\underset{\sim}{u}_\circ)\ (\underset{\sim}{u}-\underset{\sim}{u}_\circ) + \cdots \tag{2}$$

The algorithms of the finite element method are such that, given the numerical value of $\underset{\sim}{u}_\circ$, the numerical values of the vector function $\underset{\sim}{f}$, and its Jacobian $\underset{\sim}{f}_{,\underset{\sim}{u}}$, i.e., $\underset{\sim}{f}(\underset{\sim}{u}_\circ)$ and $\underset{\sim}{f}_{,\underset{\sim}{u}}(\underset{\sim}{u}_\circ)$ are readily available, perhaps, after considerable computation.

In the case of time independent boundary value problems with system loads p, in Eqs.(1 and 2), $\dot{\underset{\sim}{u}}=\underset{\sim}{o}$, $\underset{\sim}{u}_\circ=\underset{\sim}{o}$, $\underset{\sim}{f}(\underset{\sim}{o})=-\underset{\sim}{p}$, and $\underset{\sim}{f}_{,\underset{\sim}{u}}(\underset{\sim}{o}) = \underset{\sim}{K}+\lambda\underset{\sim}{G}$ where $\underset{\sim}{K}$ is the stiffness matrix, $\underset{\sim}{G}$ is the geometric matrix, and λ is the scalar representing the scale of the initial stress magnitudes (or some other similar quantities). With these, from Eqs.(1 and 2), the response of the discretized system may be formally written as $\underset{\sim}{u}=[\underset{\sim}{K}+\lambda\underset{\sim}{G}]^{-1}\underset{\sim}{p}$, so long as the problem is a linear one. The formal solution implies that further numerical operations are needed in order to obtain the solution numerically.

In general, given the initial conditions, the solution of Eq.(1) is obtained numerically in the finite element method. Due to the finiteness of the computer wordlength, the numerical solution $\underset{\sim}{u}_c(t)$ of Eq.(1) is different from its exact solution $\underset{\sim}{u}(t)$.

Various Errors

Consider the actual physical system for which the numerical solution $\underset{\sim}{u}_c(t)$ is obtained. Suppose one makes very careful measurements of the response quantities with extreme accuracy. Let e represent the difference between the measured quantities and the corresponding computed quantities $\underset{\sim}{u}_c(t)$ at a given time. Vector $\underset{\sim}{e}$ is called the total error, its ith component e_i is the ith total error at time t. The total error is the sum of various errors defined below.

Mathematical modeling error. The analysis which yielded $\underset{\sim}{u}_c(t)$ is based on a mathematical formulation abstracted from the actual physical system. During this abstraction, for the sake of mathematical convenience, many simplifying assumptions are made relative to the geometry of the solution domain, system parameters, and functional structure and magnitude of the response quantities. The quantity $\underset{\sim}{u}(\underset{\sim}{x},t)$, defined previously as the actual responses at the nodes at time t, is the response of the mathematical model. The difference between the measured quantities of the physical system and the corresponding $\underset{\sim}{u}(\underset{\sim}{x},t)$ at a given time is the mathematical modeling error at that time. The Newtonian Mechanics, the Beam Theory, and the Thin Shell Theory are examples of mathematical models of actual physical systems. Very little mathematical modeling error results, if the assumptions of the mathematical model are reasonable for the actual system represented by that model. Otherwise the modeling errors may be unacceptably large. For example, in order to use the Newtonian Mechanics, the velocities should be far smaller than the relativistic values. Likewise, for the Beam Theory the height-to-span ratio, and for the Thin Shell Theory the thickness-times-curvature must be sufficiently small. In this chapter, it is assumed that the mathematical models are proper for the physical systems, and the mathematical modeling errors are negligible.

Discretization errors. These are caused by representing the infinitely many degrees-of-freedom response of the mathematical model by the finite number of degrees-of-freedom in the discretized system. With the notation defined earlier, the discretization error at time t is $\underset{\sim}{u}(t)-\underset{\sim}{u}(\underset{\sim}{x},t)$ (4).

Round-off errors. These are caused by the limitation of digital computers in representing real numbers. Due to the finiteness of the computer wordlengths, only a finite subset of the infinitely many real numbers can be represented in these machines. None of the irrational numbers, and very few of the rational numbers can be represented. With the notation defined earlier, the round-off error at time t is $\underset{\sim}{u}_c(t)-\underset{\sim}{u}(t)$ (4).

Solution errors. The total error less the mathematical modeling error is called the solution error. In fact, these errors are the sum of the discretization and round-off errors, i.e., $\underset{\sim}{u}_c(t)-\underset{\sim}{u}(\underset{\sim}{x},t)$ constitute the solution errors at time t (4).

Equation Errors Versus Solution Errors

From an analysis point of view, the errors defined above may be further identified by their simpler constituents as shown below.

Equation errors. The discretized equations, i.e., those in (1), are in fact the approximations of the governing equation of the mathematical model at specific points (the nodes) at time t. In fact, the equation sign in (1) indicates only an approximation. Let $\underset{\sim}{r}$ denote the residue to make the equation an exact equation, such that (1) may be rewritten as

$$\dot{\underset{\sim}{u}}(\underset{\sim}{x},t) = \underset{\sim}{f}(\underset{\sim}{u}(\underset{\sim}{x},t)) - \underset{\sim}{r} \tag{3}$$

Vector $\underset{\sim}{r}$ is called the equation error at time t. There are three basic components of the equation error: $\underset{\sim}{r}_d$, $\underset{\sim}{r}_r$, and $\underset{\sim}{r}_i$. Vector $\underset{\sim}{r}_d$ is called the equation discretization error, and it represents all errors in representing the governing equations at the nodes by means of the finite elements. Vector $\underset{\sim}{r}_r$ is called the equation round-off error which lists all errors caused by representing the discrete equations only by the numbers available to the digital computer. Vector $\underset{\sim}{r}_i$ is called the inherited errors at time t, and it represents the effects of all equation errors of the earlier times (4).

Solution errors. The definition of this error is given above. In terms of the equation errors, the solution errors at time τ may be redefined as the sum of the effects of all equation errors at times $t \leq \tau$, and the manipulation errors (see below for definition).

Transformation of Equation Errors into Solution Error

The mechanisms by which the equation errors are transformed into the response to become the solution errors are of two different kinds as explained below.

Intrinsic characteristics of the system. Note that (3) is basically a set of ordinary differential equations which may or may not have stable solutions. In a non-stable system, errors such as $\underset{\sim}{r}$, propagate with ever increasing magnitudes, whereas in a stable system they propagate with decreasing magnitudes. The stability is an intrinsic characteristic of the system. The eigenvalues of the Jacobian of $\underset{\sim}{f}$, i.e., those of $\underset{\sim}{f}_{,\underset{\sim}{u}}$, represent such characteristics - a fact which has been known for a long time (5). With the eigenvalues of $f_{,\underset{\sim}{u}}$, it is possible to predict the manner in which the equation errors are transformed into the solution errors.

Manipulation. As stated earlier for (1), the solution of (3) is likewise obtained numerically by using one of the many solution algorithms and a digital computer. During the solution process, depending upon the solution algorithm, not only an unpredictable amount of round-off errors are committed but also the intrinsic characteristics of the system may be altered. The effect of these in the solution error is called the manipulation error (6). It is possible to have large manipulation errors in an intrinsically stable system due to a wrong choice of the solution algorithm.

Terminology Related with the Error Measures

As discussed earlier, in the finite element method, one is interested in the accuracy of the computed response quantities $\underset{\sim}{u}_c(t)$ at the nodes at any time t. In terms of the actual response of the mathematical model at the same nodes and time, $\underset{\sim}{u}(\underset{\sim}{x},t)$, the solution error $\underset{\sim}{e}$ may be expressed as

$$\underset{\sim}{e} = \underset{\sim}{e}(t) = \underset{\sim}{u}(\underset{\sim}{x},t) - \underset{\sim}{u}_c(t) \tag{4}$$

The knowledge of $\underset{\sim}{e}$ enables one to compute the actual response $\underset{\sim}{u}(\underset{\sim}{x},t)$ from the computed response $\underset{\sim}{u}_c(t)$. Since $\underset{\sim}{u}(\underset{\sim}{x},t)$ is not available in general, the computation of $\underset{\sim}{e}$ by other means is necessary. This is a very hard proposition. In practice, rather than $\underset{\sim}{e}$, an estimate of $\underset{\sim}{e}$, or an estimate of a related quantity is sought. Some of the related quantities are defined below.

Local errors. In an n-node discrete system

$$\underset{\sim}{e} = [e_1, e_2, \cdots, e_n]^T \tag{5}$$

where the jth component, e_j, is the error in the computed response at node j. This quantity, i.e., e_j, is called the local error at node j.

Error magnitudes. Many times, especially in the case of round-off errors, the magnitude of an error is easier to compute than its actual value. The magnitude of the jth local error e_j is shown by $|e_j|$. The vector listing the magnitudes of the components of $\underset{\sim}{e}$ is shown by $|\underset{\sim}{e}|$. Namely

$$|\underset{\sim}{e}| = [|e_1|, |e_2|, \cdots, |e_n|]^T \tag{6}$$

Error norms. Often, rather than $\underset{\sim}{e}$, one attempts to compute some norm of $\underset{\sim}{e}$ which is shown as $\|\underset{\sim}{e}\|$ and is a positive scalar. There are various ways of defining the norms of $\underset{\sim}{e}$, however, each must obey the following rules: the positivity rule (that is, $\|\underset{\sim}{e}\| > 0$, and $\|\underset{\sim}{e}\| = 0$ only if $\underset{\sim}{e} = \underset{\sim}{o}$), the homogeneity rule (that is, for any scalar λ, $\|\lambda e\| = |\lambda| \, \|e\|$), and the triangle inequality (that is, if

$\tilde{e}=\tilde{e}_1+\tilde{e}_2$, then, $\| \tilde{e}_1 \| + \| \tilde{e}_2 \| \geq \| \tilde{e} \|$). The most widely used norms are the p-norms:

$$\| \tilde{e} \|_p = (|e_1|^p + |e_2|^p + \cdots + |e_n|^p)^{1/p} \quad \text{for } p=1,2, \text{ or } \infty \tag{7}$$

Also used are the Euclid-norms:

$$\| \tilde{e} \|_E = \| \tilde{e} \|_2 \tag{8}$$

and the positive-definite-quadratic-form-norms:

$$\| \tilde{e} \|_q = (\frac{1}{2} \tilde{e}^T \tilde{A} \tilde{e})^{1/2} \tag{9}$$

where $\tilde{A}$ is a constant n th order real, symmetric, and positive definite matrix. From the definitions of the norms, it can be shown that

$$| e_j | \leq \| \tilde{e} \| \quad \text{for any } j \tag{10}$$

Therefore, any norm of the solution error can be used as an upper bound for the magnitude of any of its local errors [if (9) is used, $\tilde{A}$ is such that $a_{jj}>1$].

Absolute error. The quantity defined in (4) is also called the absolute solution error. Sometimes, it may be more feasible to deal with the relative errors (defined below) than the absolute errors.

Relative error. In those systems where the response appears to be growing with ever increasing magnitudes, it may be more meaningful to deal with the ratio of the error to the response. Let e_j denote the jth local solution error, and let u_{c_j} denote the computed response at the same point. The quantity e_{r_j}

$$e_{r_j} = e_j/u_{c_j} \quad , \quad u_{c_j}\neq 0, \quad \text{for any } j=1,\cdots,n \tag{11}$$

is called the relative local error. Similarly the quantity $\| \tilde{e} \| / \| \tilde{u}_c \|, (\tilde{u}_c \neq \tilde{0})$, is called the relative solution-error-norm.

Scope

Many of the concepts defined in the preceding subsection are common in all discretization techniques. In the discussions of this chapter these concepts are used to the extent that they are useful in explaining the errors in the finite element solutions. Naturally, the ones which play a more important role in the finite element method are emphasized more. The scope of the discussions is thus limited by the relevance to the finite element method. The objective is to survey the state-of-the-art of various aspects of the error phenomena, such as the quantification of its basic components, the understanding of their propagation, and the estimation of the errors present in the computed response. The problem of how to select the mesh and the interpolation functions in order to minimize the errors is treated in Chapter 3.

Organization

Having defined the notation and the terminology of this chapter in the present section, the equation errors are studied, the factors effecting their magnitudes are reviewed, their relative importance is discussed, and their quantification is given in the next section. The third section deals with the role of the intrinsic system properties in transmitting the equation errors into the solution errors. The discussion of the manipulation errors is given in the fourth section, and the survey of the current research is given in the fifth section. The sixth section discusses the state-of-the-art of practical error estimation. Finally, in the seventh section, the conclusions deduced from the discussions of this chapter are listed. Following the list of references, a bibliography is provided containing publications relevant to this chapter, as a starting point to many others.

EQUATION ERRORS

The application of the finite element method to the mathematical model of the actual physical system yields the discrete equations of the type of (1) which only approximates the conditions of the mathematical model at the nodes. The sources of the approximation are the use of the finite set of real numbers representable in a digital computer, the use of finite number of nodal points, and the application of the finite element method not to the mathematical model but to an approximation of it. In the preceding section, the errors caused by these sources are defined as the round-off errors, the discretization errors, and the inherited errors of the equation, respectively. Only after adding these error quantities to the equations, (1) becomes an exact equation as shown in (3). In the following paragraphs these errors are studied, the factors effecting their magnitudes are reviewed, and their relative importance is discussed.

Equation Round-off Errors

As discussed earlier, the finite element method provides, instead of the explicit expressions for (1), the numerical values of $\underset{\sim}{f}(\underset{\sim}{u}_\circ)$ and $\underset{\sim}{f}_{,\underset{\sim}{u}}(\underset{\sim}{u}_\circ)$, that is, the numerical values of the vector function $\underset{\sim}{f}$ and its Jacobian $\underset{\sim}{f}_{,\underset{\sim}{u}}$ at $\underset{\sim}{u}=\underset{\sim}{u}_\circ$. For example, in the equilibrium problems of elasticity, when $\underset{\sim}{u}_\circ$ is a geometrically compatible deflection state, $\underset{\sim}{f}(\underset{\sim}{u}_\circ)$ is the list of unbalanced forces at the nodes, and $\underset{\sim}{f}_{,\underset{\sim}{u}}(\underset{\sim}{u}_\circ)$ is the stiffness matrix associated with the directions of the components of $u_\circ$. In order to obtain $\underset{\sim}{f}(\underset{\sim}{u}_\circ)$ and $\underset{\sim}{f}_{,\underset{\sim}{u}}(\underset{\sim}{u}_\circ)$, the elemental matrices are calculated and assembled in a digital computer, always using the finite real number set of the digital computer during the arithmetic operations. Obviously, the computed matrices are different from the intended $\underset{\sim}{f}(\underset{\sim}{u}_\circ)$ and $\underset{\sim}{f}_{,\underset{\sim}{u}}(\underset{\sim}{u}_\circ)$, and the effect of the difference on (1) is the equation round-off error. The exact computation of this error is not possible; however, with the following rules, an estimate can be made.

Most of the modern digital computers use <u>floating-point arithmetic</u>, and the numbers used in this arithmetic are represented as floating-point numbers. The representation of a floating-point number consists of an <u>exponent</u> and a <u>mantissa</u> of t number of binary bits long. The exponent is such that the mantissa is a quantity between 0.5 and 1.0, therefore, the exponent portion may be taken as the upper bound estimate of the magnitude of the actual number. Let a_1 denote the actual number, $|a_1|$ its magnitude, and $fl(a_1)$ its machine representation; then, the round-off error, ε, involved in the representation may be expressed as

$$\varepsilon = fl(a_1) - a_1 \qquad \text{then} \qquad |\varepsilon| \le |a_1|\ 2^{-t} \tag{12}$$

where t is the number of binary bits assigned for the mantissa. Let a_1 and b_1 denote two real numbers, a_1+b_1 and a_1b_1 their actual sum and product, and $fl(a_1+b_1)$ and $fl(a_1b_1)$ denote the corresponding machine results. It can be shown that the following hold

$$\varepsilon = fl(a_1+b_1) - (a_1+b_1) \qquad \text{then} \qquad |\varepsilon| \le (|a_1|+|b_1|)2^{-t} \tag{13}$$

and

$$\varepsilon = fl(a_1b_1) - a_1b_1 \qquad \text{then} \qquad |\varepsilon| \le |a_1|\ |b_1|2^{-t} \tag{14}$$

Similar inequalities may be written for the round-off errors in matrix operations. Let $\underset{\sim}{a}$ and $\underset{\sim}{b}$ denote two vectors of order n, and $fl(\underset{\sim}{a}^T\underset{\sim}{b})$ denote the result of $\underset{\sim}{a}^T\underset{\sim}{b}$ product carried out in a t-bit mantissa machine. Then

$$\varepsilon = fl(\underset{\sim}{a}^T\underset{\sim}{b}) - \underset{\sim}{a}^T\underset{\sim}{b} \qquad \text{then} \qquad |\varepsilon| \le n\ \|\underset{\sim}{a}\|\ \|\underset{\sim}{b}\|\ 2^{-t} \tag{15}$$

Similarly, if $\underset{\sim}{A}$ and $\underset{\sim}{B}$ denote two pxn and nxq matrices, and $fl(\underset{\sim}{A}\underset{\sim}{B})$ is the result obtained for $\underset{\sim}{A}\underset{\sim}{B}$ product in a t-bit mantissa machine, one may write

$$\tilde{F} = fl(\tilde{A}\tilde{B}) - \tilde{A}\tilde{B} \qquad \text{then} \qquad \| \tilde{F} \| \leq \| \tilde{A} \| \, \| \tilde{B} \| \, n \, 2^{-t} \tag{16}$$

where $\|\tilde{A}\|$, $\|\tilde{B}\|$, and $\|\tilde{F}\|$ are the Euclid norms or subordinate matrix norms of $\tilde{A}$, $\tilde{B}$, and $\tilde{F}$, respectively (7).

From these it is clear that in order to minimize the equation round-off errors one should use large t (i.e., machines with longer wordlength, or double-precision arithmetic), smaller magnitude quantities (so that the norms appearing in the estimates of $|\varepsilon|$ be small), and smaller size matrices (so that n appearing in the definitions of $|\varepsilon|$ be small).

Using (13), with $a_1>0$, and $b_1=-c_1$ with $c_1>0$, the relative error in the computed quantity $fl(a_1-c_1)$ may be expressed as

$$|\varepsilon|/|fl(a_1-c_1)| \leq 2^{-t}\,(|a_1|+|c_1|)/|fl(a_1-c_1)| \tag{17}$$

which shows that the computed quantity $fl(a_1-c_1)$ may be overwhelmed by the round-off error if $|a_1-c_1|$ is sufficiently small. Unfortunately, in the finite element method, this type of differencing occurs very often, such as computing the differences (and in the case of shells, the differences of the differences) of the nodal coordinates of element vertices. It is clear that, given a machine (i.e., given a mantissa length t), there is always a limit to the mesh refinement beyond which the computed quantities may be 100% erroneous.

The equation round-off errors, $\tilde{r}_r$, may be held negligibly small by using sufficiently large t (i.e., longer wordlength machines and double-precision arithmetic) with not too refined finite element meshes. This is the current practice in the finite element technology.

Equation Discretization Errors

As shown in the previous section, in the finite element method the actual response $u(\tilde{x},t)$ is approximated by the trial solution $\Psi(\tilde{x},t)$ which is

$$\Psi(\tilde{x},t) = \tilde{u}(t)^T \tilde{\psi}(\tilde{x}) \tag{18}$$

where

$$\tilde{\psi}(\tilde{x}) = [\psi_1(\tilde{x}),\ \psi_2(\tilde{x}),\ \cdots,\ \psi_n(\tilde{x})]^T \tag{19}$$

and

$$\tilde{u}(t) = [u_1(t),\ u_2(t),\ \cdots,\ u_n(t)]^T \tag{20}$$

where $u_j(t)$ is to represent $u(\tilde{x}_j,t)$, i.e., the response at the jth node, and $\psi_j(\tilde{x})$ is the jth pyramid function. Note that (18) implies that, for the pyramid functions,

$$\psi_j(\tilde{x}_j) = 1 \qquad \text{for} \qquad j=1,2,\cdots,n \tag{21}$$

Let $\mathcal{D}_j$ denote the spatial domain defined by the finite elements meeting at node j. The jth generalized pyramid function is such that

$$\psi_j(\tilde{x}) = 0 \quad \text{if } \tilde{x} \text{ is on or outside the boundary of domain } \mathcal{D}_j \tag{22}$$

and $\psi_j(\tilde{x})$ is a known interpolated value such that

$$|\psi_j(\tilde{x})| \leq 1 \qquad \text{if } \tilde{x} \text{ is inside the domain } \mathcal{D}_j \tag{23}$$

Let $\Delta\Psi=\Delta\Psi(\tilde{x})=\Delta\Psi(\tilde{x},t)$ denote the difference between the actual and the assumed responses:

$$\Delta\Psi = u(\tilde{x},t) - \Psi(\tilde{x},t) \tag{24}$$

In the finite element method the pyramid functions are selected such that $\Psi(\tilde{x},t)$

is of class $p \geq m-1$, m being the highest order differentiation appearing in functional Φ of the variational formulation of the problem, and

$$\lim_{n\to\infty} \Delta\Psi \to 0 \quad \text{for all } \underset{\sim}{x} \text{ in the solution domain} \tag{25}$$

is guaranteed (which means that, given t, $\Psi(\underset{\sim}{x},t)$ is the power series expansion of $u(\underset{\sim}{x},t)$ about $\underset{\sim}{x}$, up to a selected order).

The functional Φ of the variational formulation involves the derivatives of $u(\underset{\sim}{x},t)$ up to order m, and integrals in the solution domain. Formally one may write

$$\Phi[u(\underset{\sim}{x},t)] = \Phi[\Psi(\underset{\sim}{x},t)+\Delta\Psi(\underset{\sim}{x},t)] + \Delta\Phi[\Psi(\underset{\sim}{x},t)+\Delta\Psi(\underset{\sim}{x},t)] \tag{26}$$

where $\Delta\Phi$ represents the errors caused by the possibilities that (a) the sum of the spatial domains represented by the finite elements may be different than the actual spatial domain, (b) the essential boundary conditions of the problem may not be satisfied by $\Psi(\underset{\sim}{x},t)$ at points which are not nodal points, and (c) the additional boundary conditions of the problem, if there are any, may not be satisfied by $\Psi(\underset{\sim}{x},t)$ at all. Because of $\Delta\Phi$ and $\Delta\Psi$, the application of the Rayleigh-Ritz procedure to $[u(\underset{\sim}{x},t)]$ and $\Phi[\Psi(\underset{\sim}{x},t)]$ will, in general, yield different equations of the type of (1). The ones obtained from $\Phi[u(\underset{\sim}{x},t)]$ would be the exact ones, and the ones obtained from $\Phi[\Psi(\underset{\sim}{x},t)]$ would be the approximate ones. Let the difference between these two sets of equations denoted by $\underset{\sim}{r}_d$. Vector $\underset{\sim}{r}_d$ constitutes the equation discretization errors. Note that

$$\lim_{n\to\infty} \underset{\sim}{r}_d \to \underset{\sim}{0} \tag{27}$$

For a given n, it is possible to express $\underset{\sim}{r}_d$ in terms of the higher order derivatives of the response and the mesh sizes, by taking advantage of the remainder theorem of the power series expansions. If the response of the actual system is sufficiently smooth (that is, if the higher order derivatives are not varying rapidly in the finite elements), by using the approximate solution itself, $\underset{\sim}{r}_d$ may be approximately evaluated by such expressions. This is being done in the finite difference methods (8,9). Its extension to the finite element method is pr-posed (10,11). From these expressions it is possible to obtain relations such as

$$\| \underset{\sim}{r}_d \| = O(h^p) \tag{28}$$

where h is the typical mesh size of the mesh used, and p is a power usually larger than one. Such expressions are useful in assessing the rate with which the equation discretization errors will vanish with decreasing mesh size. The power p is related with the degree of the interpolation rule used in the pyramid functions [see the comment in parenthesis below (25)].

There has been some interest among the investigators to express the equation discretization errors (12,13), or their components in the element level (14,15).

From the above discussion, it is clear that the equation discretization errors decrease with decreasing mesh size, and the rate with which the reduction takes place increases by the use of higher order interpolation rules, i.e., higher order elements. For further information on the effects of mesh and interpolation rule, the reader is referred to Chapter 3.

Inherited Errors in the Equations

As discussed earlier, instead of the explicit expressions for (1), the finite element method provides the numerical values of $\underset{\sim}{f}(\underset{\sim}{u}_o)$ and $\underset{\sim}{f}_{,\underset{\sim}{u}}(\underset{\sim}{u}_o)$ at a given $\underset{\sim}{u}=\underset{\sim}{u}_o$. If $\underset{\sim}{u}_o$ is a prescribed state (such as the initial state), then in $\underset{\sim}{f}(\underset{\sim}{u}_o)$ and $\underset{\sim}{f}_{,\underset{\sim}{u}}(\underset{\sim}{u}_o)$ only the round-off and the equation discretization error effects exist. However, in many problems, such as the nonlinear equilibrium problems, and linear or nonlinear propagation problems, one needs the computation of the response at many time stations. In such problems, $\underset{\sim}{u}_o$ is the computed response (at one of the time stations), and therefore, it contains errors inherited from the preceding analysis. Let $\underset{\sim}{r}_i$ represent the effect of such inherited errors present in $\underset{\sim}{u}_o$ on the discrete equations. Vector $\underset{\sim}{r}_i$ is called the equation inherited errors. The magnitude of the equation inherited errors depends on the magnitude of the inherited errors in $\underset{\sim}{u}_o$. The inherited errors in $\underset{\sim}{u}_o$ are the sum of the effects of all earlier discretization and round-off errors. Depending upon the intrinsic system characteristics and also the manipulation techniques used in the analysis, the earlier discretization and round-off errors may contribute to the errors in $\underset{\sim}{u}_o$ with increasing or decreasing magnitudes. If they contribute with increasing magnitudes, the inherited errors $\underset{\sim}{r}_i$ in the discrete equations may easily overwhelm the other two error components, i.e., $\underset{\sim}{r}_d$ and $\underset{\sim}{r}_r$, discussed earlier.

In order to control the inherited equation errors, one must first control the equation round-off errors and the equation discretization errors, and then control the propagation of their effects in the response. Given the equation errors, the computation of their effects in the solution, and the propagation of such effects are discussed in the next two sections. From such discussions it is clear that, one may do very little other than selecting appropriate solution algorithms, in controlling the error propagation. Therefore the crux of the matter in controlling the inherited errors is to minimize, as much as possible, the equation round-off and the equation discretization errors.

TRANSFORMATION OF EQUATION ERRORS INTO SOLUTION ERRORS BY SYSTEM CHARACTERISTICS

Consider the exact discretized equations given in (3). In the previous section the constituents of the equation errors, $\underset{\sim}{r}$, are discussed. Let $\underset{\sim}{u}'(t)$ denote the exact solution of (3) in the absence of $\underset{\sim}{r}$, i.e., the solution of (3) when $\underset{\sim}{r}=\underset{\sim}{o}$. The quantity $\underset{\sim}{h}$, defined as

$$\underset{\sim}{h} = \underset{\sim}{u}'(t) - \underset{\sim}{u}(\underset{\sim}{x},t) \qquad (29)$$

is the effect of the equation errors on the response. In fact, $\underset{\sim}{h}$ is the solution error in the absence of the manipulation errors, and it may be considered as the transformation of the equation errors as the solution errors. In this section the relationships between $\underset{\sim}{r}$ and $\underset{\sim}{h}$ are discussed, and the role of the intrinsic system characteristics in these relationships is shown.

Let $\underset{\sim}{u}(\underset{\sim}{x},t_o)=\underset{\sim}{u}'(t_o)=\underset{\sim}{u}_o$ denote the response at time t_o. Noting that the equation error $\underset{\sim}{r}$ is also a function of response $\underset{\sim}{u}$, the power series expansion of the right hand side of (3) about $\underset{\sim}{u}_o$ may be written as

$$\underset{\sim}{f}(\underset{\sim}{u}(\underset{\sim}{x},t_o))-\underset{\sim}{r} = \{\underset{\sim}{f}(\underset{\sim}{u}_o)-\underset{\sim}{r}(\underset{\sim}{u}_o)\}+[\underset{\sim}{f}_{,\underset{\sim}{u}}(\underset{\sim}{u}_o)-\underset{\sim}{r}_{,\underset{\sim}{u}}(\underset{\sim}{u}_o)]\{\underset{\sim}{u}(\underset{\sim}{x},t_o)-\underset{\sim}{u}_o\}+\underset{\sim}{t}_f+\underset{\sim}{t}_r \qquad (30)$$

where $\underset{\sim}{t}_f$ and $\underset{\sim}{t}_r$ are the remainders of the expansions of $\underset{\sim}{f}$ and $\underset{\sim}{r}$, respectively. Defining

$$\underset{\sim}{f}(\underset{\sim}{u}_o) - \underset{\sim}{r}(\underset{\sim}{u}_o) = -\underset{\sim}{p} \qquad (31)$$

$$\underset{\sim}{f}_{,\underset{\sim}{u}}(\underset{\sim}{u}_o) - \underset{\sim}{r}_{,\underset{\sim}{u}}(\underset{\sim}{u}_o) = \underset{\sim}{K} \qquad (32)$$

$$\underset{\sim}{u}(\underset{\sim}{x},t_o) - \underset{\sim}{u}_o = \Delta\underset{\sim}{u} \qquad (33)$$

and

$$\delta\underset{\sim}{p} = -\underset{\sim}{r}(\underset{\sim}{u}_o) \qquad (34)$$

$$\delta\underset{\sim}{K} = \underset{\sim}{r}_{,\underset{\sim}{u}}(\underset{\sim}{u}_o) \qquad (35)$$

$$\Delta\underset{\sim}{u}' = \underset{\sim}{u}' - \underset{\sim}{u}_o \qquad (36)$$

one may write

$$\underset{\sim}{f}(\underset{\sim}{u}_o) = -(\underset{\sim}{p} + \delta\underset{\sim}{p}) \qquad (37)$$

$$\underset{\sim}{f}_{,\underset{\sim}{u}}(\underset{\sim}{u}_o) = \underset{\sim}{K} + \delta\underset{\sim}{K} \qquad (38)$$

$$\Delta\underset{\sim}{u}' = \Delta\underset{\sim}{u} + \underset{\sim}{h} \qquad (39)$$

where $\underset{\sim}{h}$ is as defined in (29). In the finite element method one computes numerically the vector function $\underset{\sim}{f}$ and its Jacobian at $\underset{\sim}{u}_o$ (i.e., the unbalanced forces and the stiffness matrix). Namely, $\underset{\sim}{p}+\delta\underset{\sim}{p}$ and $\underset{\sim}{K}+\delta\underset{\sim}{K}$ are computed instead of their true values $\underset{\sim}{p}$ and $\underset{\sim}{K}$, respectively. As a result, instead of true incremental response $\Delta\underset{\sim}{u}$, one computes $\Delta\underset{\sim}{u}+\underset{\sim}{h}$, where $\underset{\sim}{h}$ represents the induced errors.

Effect of System Characteristics in Equilibrium Problems

For equilibrium problems with no time dependent system components, $\dot{\underset{\sim}{u}}$ is absent in the governing equations, thus (3) becomes for $t=t_o$

$$\underset{\sim}{o} = \underset{\sim}{f}(\underset{\sim}{u}(\underset{\sim}{x},t_o)) - \underset{\sim}{r} \tag{40}$$

Using the expansion given in (30), this may be rewritten as

$$[\underset{\sim}{f}_{,\underset{\sim}{u}}(\underset{\sim}{u}_o)-\underset{\sim}{r}_{,\underset{\sim}{u}}(\underset{\sim}{u}_o)]\{\underset{\sim}{u}(\underset{\sim}{x},t_o)-\underset{\sim}{u}_o\} = -\{\underset{\sim}{f}(\underset{\sim}{u}_o)-\underset{\sim}{r}(\underset{\sim}{u}_o)\} - \underset{\sim}{t}_f \tag{41}$$

where it is assumed that $\underset{\sim}{t}_r=\underset{\sim}{o}$ (i.e., the equation errors are varying linearly with the response at the vicinity of $\underset{\sim}{u}_o$). By using the definitions in (31), (32), and (33) this becomes

$$\underset{\sim}{K}\,\Delta\underset{\sim}{u} = \underset{\sim}{p} - \underset{\sim}{t}_f \tag{42}$$

In the finite element method, since the equation errors are not numerically available, instead of $\underset{\sim}{K}$ and $\underset{\sim}{p}$, one uses $\underset{\sim}{K}+\delta\underset{\sim}{K}$ and $\underset{\sim}{p}+\delta\underset{\sim}{p}$ in (42), and as a result, $\Delta\underset{\sim}{u}$ becomes $\Delta\underset{\sim}{u}+\underset{\sim}{h}$:

$$[\underset{\sim}{K}+\delta\underset{\sim}{K}]\{\Delta\underset{\sim}{u}+\underset{\sim}{h}\} = \{\underset{\sim}{p}+\delta\underset{\sim}{p}\} - \underset{\sim}{t}_f \tag{43}$$

In (42) and (43), $\underset{\sim}{K}$ and $\underset{\sim}{K}+\delta\underset{\sim}{K}$ represent the actual and the approximate systems, $\underset{\sim}{p}$ and $\underset{\sim}{p}+\delta\underset{\sim}{p}$ represent the actual and the approximate system loads, and $\underset{\sim}{t}_f$ represent the nonlinear terms of the system.

Linear Equilibrium Problems

In these problems, due to the linearity of the vector function $\underset{\sim}{f}$ with respect to the response $\underset{\sim}{u}$, one has

$$\underset{\sim}{t}_f = \underset{\sim}{o} \tag{44}$$

With this, (42) and (43) become

$$\underset{\sim}{K}\,\Delta\underset{\sim}{u} = \underset{\sim}{p} \tag{45}$$

and

$$[\underset{\sim}{K}+\delta\underset{\sim}{K}]\{\Delta\underset{\sim}{u}+\underset{\sim}{h}\} = \{\underset{\sim}{p}+\delta\underset{\sim}{p}\} \tag{46}$$

Subtracting side-by-side, and then formally solving for $\underset{\sim}{h}$ leads to

$$\underset{\sim}{h} = [\underset{\sim}{K}+\delta\underset{\sim}{K}]^{-1}\{\delta\underset{\sim}{p}-\delta\underset{\sim}{K}\Delta\underset{\sim}{u}\} \tag{47}$$

which is the relation showing how the errors in the equations transform into the errors in the solution. Here, the errors are the absolute errors, and $\underset{\sim}{K}+\delta\underset{\sim}{K}$ stands for the system characteristics.

One gains more insight if one seeks the answer of the following question: Given some norm of the relative errors in the equations, what is the corresponding relative error in the solution? Through manipulation of (45) and (46), the following may be obtained (16):

$$\|\underset{\sim}{h}\|/\|\Delta\underset{\sim}{u}\| \leq \|\underset{\sim}{K}\|\,\|\underset{\sim}{K}^{-1}\|\,[(\|\delta\underset{\sim}{p}\|/\|\underset{\sim}{p}\|)+\alpha(\|\delta\underset{\sim}{K}\|/\|\underset{\sim}{K}\|)] \tag{48}$$

where

$$\alpha = (1 - \|\underset{\sim}{K}\| \|\underset{\sim}{K}^{-1}\| \ \|\delta\underset{\sim}{K}\| / \|\underset{\sim}{K}\|)^{-1} \tag{49}$$

In these equations $\|\underset{\sim}{h}\| / \|\Delta\underset{\sim}{u}\|$ is the norm of the relative errors in the incremental response, and $\|\delta\underset{\sim}{p}\| / \|\underset{\sim}{p}\|$ and $\|\delta\underset{\sim}{K}\| / \|\underset{\sim}{K}\|$ are the norms of the relative errors in the equations. The factor $\|\underset{\sim}{K}\| \|\underset{\sim}{K}^{-1}\|$ is the conditioning number of the system, which is a system property as shown below. Using p=2 subordinate vector norms for the matrices, it can be shown that (17)

$$\|\underset{\sim}{K}\| \ \|\underset{\sim}{K}^{-1}\| = \lambda_1 / \lambda_n \tag{50}$$

where λ_1 is the largest, and λ_n is the smallest eigenvalue of $[\underset{\sim}{K}^H\underset{\sim}{K}]^{1/2}$ (here, H shows the hermitian transpose). It can be shown that the eigenvalues of $\underset{\sim}{K}$ and $[\underset{\sim}{K}^H\underset{\sim}{K}]^{1/2}$ are identical when $\underset{\sim}{K}$ is real symmetric and positive definite. Clearly, the transformation of the equation errors into solution errors depends on the system eigenvalues. When λ_1/λ_n is a large number, one should try to reduce the equation errors more vigorously. For example, in the linear equilibrium problems of cantilevered structures it can be shown that λ_1/λ_n is very large, and therefore, one must have very small equation errors in order to have acceptably accurate solutions.

Eigenvalue Problems

In these problems, in addition to (44), there are no system loads. Therefore

$$\underset{\sim}{p} = \delta\underset{\sim}{p} = \underset{\sim}{o} \tag{51}$$

and

$$\underset{\sim}{K} = \underset{\sim}{A} - \lambda\underset{\sim}{B} \tag{52}$$

$$\delta\underset{\sim}{K} = \delta\underset{\sim}{A} - \lambda\delta\underset{\sim}{B} \tag{53}$$

where λ is a system parameter. In elasticity problems, λ may be a constant showing the scale factor of initial stress magnitudes at $\underset{\sim}{u}_o$ state, or it may be a constant related with the free vibration frequencies. With (51), (52), and (53), (42) and (43) become

$$\underset{\sim}{A} \ \Delta\underset{\sim}{u} = \lambda \ \underset{\sim}{B} \ \Delta\underset{\sim}{u} \tag{54}$$

and

$$[\underset{\sim}{A}+\delta\underset{\sim}{A}]\{\Delta\underset{\sim}{u}+\underset{\sim}{h}\} = \lambda \ [\underset{\sim}{B}+\delta\underset{\sim}{B}]\{\Delta\underset{\sim}{u}+\underset{\sim}{h}\} \tag{55}$$

Because of the equation errors $\delta\underset{\sim}{A}$ and $\delta\underset{\sim}{B}$, the eigenvalues and the eigenvectors of the exact equations (54) are different then those of (55). The difference is the solution errors corresponding to the equation errors $\delta\underset{\sim}{A}$ and $\delta\underset{\sim}{B}$. The relationship between $\underset{\sim}{A}$ and $\underset{\sim}{B}$, and the errors in the eigenvalues and the eigenvectors are extensively discussed in (18). As an example, consider the case where both $\underset{\sim}{A}$ and $\underset{\sim}{B}$, and $\underset{\sim}{A}+\delta\underset{\sim}{A}$ and $\underset{\sim}{B}+\delta\underset{\sim}{B}$ are real and symmetric, and $\underset{\sim}{B}$ and $\underset{\sim}{B}+\delta\underset{\sim}{B}$ are positive definite (which is the case in most of the problems of linear structural mechanics). Then, both of the eigenvalue problems defined in (54) and (55) are non-defective, and they possess real eigenvalues. Let $(\lambda_i, \underset{\sim}{v}_i)$, $i=1,\cdots,n$ denote the eigenpairs of the exact system in (54). Let $(\mu, \underset{\sim}{s})$ denote an eigenpair of the approximate problem in (55). Suppose $\underset{\sim}{v}_i$, for all i, are normalized with $\underset{\sim}{B}$ such that $\underset{\sim}{V}^{-1}\underset{\sim}{B} \ \underset{\sim}{V} = \underset{\sim}{I}$, then from (54) one writes that $\underset{\sim}{A} = \underset{\sim}{V} \operatorname{diag}(\lambda_i) \ \underset{\sim}{V}^{-1}$. From (55), noting that $(\mu, \underset{\sim}{s})$ is an eigenpair, one writes

$$[\underset{\sim}{A}-\mu\underset{\sim}{B}] \ \underset{\sim}{s} = \underset{\sim}{d} \qquad \text{where} \qquad \underset{\sim}{d} = [\mu\delta\underset{\sim}{B}-\delta\underset{\sim}{A}] \ \underset{\sim}{s} \tag{56}$$

The use of $\underset{\sim}{A} = \underset{\sim}{V} \operatorname{diag}(\lambda_i) \ \underset{\sim}{V}^{-1}$ and $\underset{\sim}{B} = \underset{\sim}{V} \ \underset{\sim}{V}^{-1}$ in (56), after some manipulations yield (19)

$$\min (\lambda_i-\mu) \leq \kappa \; \|d\|/\|s\| \qquad \text{where} \quad \kappa = \|V\|\,\|V^{-1}\| \tag{57}$$

which establishes an upper bound for the error in the computed eigenvalue μ in terms of the system characteristics and the equation errors. Similar bounds may be computed for the errors in the computed eigenvectors and Rayleigh (or Schwarz) quotients (18).

Nonlinear Equilibrium Problems

The exact and the approximate discrete equations of these problems are as in (42) and (43). Given the numerical values of u, the finite element method provides $f(u)$ and $f_{,u}$ numerically. This, therefore, naturally leads to the use of the Newton-Raphson methods for the solution of (40); since in these methods, one only needs the evaluation of f and its Jacobian $f_{,u}$ at the successive estimates of the equilibrium state $u=u_o+\Delta u$, i.e., at states $u_1, u_2, \cdots, u_k \simeq u$ (for sufficiently large k). The recurrence formula defining the estimates of the successive states may be obtained from (41) as

$$u_{k+1} = u_k - [f_{,u}(u_k)-r_{,u}(u_k)]^{-1}\{f(u_k)-r(u_k)\}, \text{ for } k=0,1,\cdots \tag{58}$$

with u_o known. Defining

$$f_{,u}(u_k) = [K+\delta K]_k \tag{59}$$

$$f(u_k) = -\{p+\delta p\}_k \tag{60}$$

and noting that, in general, the equation error r is not available, and the finite element method provides only $[K+\delta K]_k$ and $\{p+\delta p\}_k$, (58) becomes

$$u'_{k+1} = u_k + h_{k+1} = u_k + [K+\delta K]_k^{-1}\{p+\delta p\}_k \;, \quad \text{for } k=0,1,\cdots \tag{60}$$

with $h_o=0$ and u_o known. Vector h_{k+1} represent the solution errors due to the equation errors $[\delta K]_k$ and $\{\delta p\}_k$ defined as

$$[\delta K]_k = -r_{,u}(u_k) \qquad \text{and} \qquad \{\delta p\}_k = -r(u_k) \tag{61}$$

Suppose when k=m, $\{p+\delta p\}_m$ is acceptably small so that u'_m can be used as an approximation of the true equilibrium state $u_m=u+\Delta u$. Then, for k=m, using the definitions (59), (60), and (61), one may write from (58) and (60)

$$u_m = u_{m-1} + [K]_{m-1}^{-1}\{p\}_{m-1} \tag{62}$$

and

$$u_m + h_m = u_{m-1} + [K+\delta K]_{m-1}^{-1}\{p+\delta p\}_{m-1} \tag{63}$$

Subtracting side-by-side one may write

$$h_m = [K+\delta K]_{m-1}^{-1}\{p+\delta p\}_{m-1} - [K]_{m-1}^{-1}\{p\}_{m-1} \tag{63a}$$

which indicates that the solution error in the mth estimate is caused by δK and δp of the m-1st step, and it is of the type of (47). Thus, the discussions for the linear equilibrium problems given in this section apply also for the nonlinear equilibrium problems.

Effect of System Characteristics in Propagation Problems

The governing exact discrete equations of these problems are as in (3) for which the following holds

$$u(x,t_o) = u_o \qquad \text{known} \tag{64}$$

The power series expansion of the right hand side of (3) as in (30) leads to

$$\{\dot{u}(x,t)-\dot{u}_o\} = [f,_u - r,_u]_{u_o}\{u(x,t)-u_o\} + t_f \tag{65}$$

where it is assumed that $t_r = 0$, and the use is made of $u(x,t_o)=u_o=f(u_o)-r(u_o)$. The initial conditions for this propagation problem of $u(x,t)-u_o$ are

$$\{u(x,t) - u_o\}_{t=t_o} = 0 \tag{65a}$$

In the finite element method, in the case of the absence of the equation errors r, (65) becomes

$$\{\dot{u}'(t)-\dot{u}_o\} = [f,_u]_{u_o}\{u'(t)-u_o\} + t_f \tag{66}$$

and the initial conditions of the propagation problem of $u'(t)-u_o$ are

$$\{u'(t)-u_o\}_{t=t_o} = h_o \tag{67}$$

where the relationship between $u(x,t)$ and $u'(t)$ is as in (29). In (67), h_o may be interpreted as the inherited error at time t_o. At times t in the immediate vicinity of t_o, vector t_f is of second order, and it may be neglected in (66) in order to linearize the problem. Let $v(t) \simeq u'(t)-u_o$ denote the dependent variable of the linearized problem. Then for (66) and (67) one may write

$$\dot{v} = [K+\delta K]_o\, v \qquad \text{with} \qquad v(t_o) = h_o \tag{68}$$

where $[K+\delta K]_o = [f,_u]_{u_o}$ is the coefficient matrix provided by the finite element method. From (68), it may be seen that the propagation of the inherited error h_o is a function of the eigenvalues of $[K+\delta K]_o$. If all of the eigenvalues are with negative real parts, then h_o will propagate with decreasing magnitudes. However, even one eigenvalue with a positive real part will cause the propagation of the inherited error h_o with increasing magnitudes. When $[K+\delta K]_o$ is real and symmetric then all of the eigenvalues are real, and there are n mutually orthogonal eigenvectors. Let (μ_i, s_i), $i=1,\cdots,n$ denote the eigenpairs of $[K+\delta K]_o$. Suppose the eigenvectors are normalized such that $S^T S = I$. Then one can also write that $[K+\delta K]_o = A = S^T \mathrm{diag}(\mu_i) S$. Considering the transformation $v=S\xi$, the problem in (68) may be rewritten as $\dot{\xi}=\mathrm{diag}(\mu_i)\xi$ with the initial conditions of $\xi(t_o)=S^T h_o$; the solution of which is $\xi = \mathrm{diag}(e^{\mu_i t}) S^T h_o$. By transforming back, one may write for the solution of (68) as $v=S\ \mathrm{diag}(e^{\mu_i t}) S^T h_o$. This shows clearly that the positive real parts in the eigenvalues μ_i will cause the propagation of h_o with increasing magnitudes. This, of course, has been known for a long time, as a result of studies dealing with system stabilities (5).

In an intrinsicly unstable system, the errors will tend to grow like the response itself. In such cases, rather than the absolute error, the relative error is a more meaningful quantity. In other words, for unstable systems, instead of h, one may consider $[h_1/u'_1,\ h_2/u'_2,\ \cdots\ ,\ h_n/u'_n]^T$, provided that $u'_i \neq 0$, $i=1,\cdots,n$.

From the above discussion, it is clear that the system characteristics play a very important role, especially in the propagation problems, in the growth of the errors.

MANIPULATION ERRORS

In the previous section, the manner in which the equation errors r are transformed into the solution errors, and the effect of the intrinsic system characteristics on this transformation are discussed, assuming that no further errors are incorporated into the response as the discrete equations (1) are solved numerically. Since in the finite element method the solution of (1) is obtained in a digital computer by means of some solution algorithm, unfortunately, additional errors are incorporated into the solution. These additional errors are defined as the manipulation errors (see the Introduction Section).

There are two sources of the manipulation errors: finiteness of the computer wordlengths, and the solution algorithms. The first causes further round-off errors during manipulations, and the second may cause the alteration of the growth patterns of the equation errors. Let $\underset{\sim}{g}$ denote the manipulation errors, then

$$\underset{\sim}{g} = \underset{\sim}{u}_c(t) - \underset{\sim}{u}'(t) \tag{69}$$

where $\underset{\sim}{u}_c(t)$ is the computed response, and $\underset{\sim}{u}'(t)$ is the exact solution of the approximate equations (1). Denoting the exact solution of the mathematical model by $\underset{\sim}{u}(\underset{\sim}{x},t)$ and using (29), one may write

$$\underset{\sim}{u}(\underset{\sim}{x},t) - \underset{\sim}{u}_c(t) = \underset{\sim}{g} + \underset{\sim}{h} \tag{70}$$

which is the total solution error.

In this section, the manipulation errors are discussed for each of the class of problems dealt with in the preceding section.

Manipulation Errors in Equilibrium Problems

In these problems, since $\dot{\underset{\sim}{u}}$ does not exist in the equations, the approximate discrete equations (1) become

$$\underset{\sim}{f}(\underset{\sim}{u}') = \underset{\sim}{o} \tag{71}$$

The power series expansion of $\underset{\sim}{f}$ about $\underset{\sim}{u}_o$ may be written as

$$\underset{\sim}{o} = \underset{\sim}{f}(\underset{\sim}{u}_o) + [\underset{\sim}{f},_{\underset{\sim}{u}}(\underset{\sim}{u}_o)]\{\underset{\sim}{u}'-\underset{\sim}{u}_o\} + \underset{\sim}{t}_f \tag{72}$$

where $\underset{\sim}{t}_f$ represents the remainder of the expansion. Given the numerical values of $\underset{\sim}{u}_o$, the finite element method provides the numerical values of $\underset{\sim}{f}(\underset{\sim}{u}_o)$ and $\underset{\sim}{f},_{\underset{\sim}{u}}(\underset{\sim}{u}_o)$ as

$$\underset{\sim}{f}(\underset{\sim}{u}_o) = -\{\underset{\sim}{p}+\delta\underset{\sim}{p}\}_o \tag{73}$$

and

$$\underset{\sim}{f},_{\underset{\sim}{u}}(\underset{\sim}{u}_o) = [\underset{\sim}{K}+\delta\underset{\sim}{K}]_o \tag{74}$$

where the components $\delta\underset{\sim}{p}$ and $\delta\underset{\sim}{K}$ are the unknown equation errors already in the computed matrices.

Linear Equilibrium Problems

In these problems the remainder term $\underset{\sim}{t}_f$ in the power series expansion is zero, then from (72), (73), and (74) one may write

$$[\underset{\sim}{K}+\delta\underset{\sim}{K}]_o\{\underset{\sim}{u}'-\underset{\sim}{u}_o\} = \{\underset{\sim}{p}+\delta\underset{\sim}{p}\}_o \tag{75}$$

where $\underset{\sim}{u}_o$, $[\underset{\sim}{K}+\delta\underset{\sim}{K}]_o$, and $\{\underset{\sim}{p}+\delta\underset{\sim}{p}\}_o$ are known, and $\underset{\sim}{u}'$ is unknown. One may obtain the solution of (75) in a digital computer by using one of the available algorithms. The solution algorithms for this problem may be classified as the direct methods (i.e., the factorization techniques) where the number of arithmetic operations is known a priori, and the indirect methods (i.e., the iteration techniques) where the number of arithmetic operations is not known a priori. In the finite element method the factorization techniques are being used more often.

In the factorization techniques, one first finds the factors of $[\underset{\sim}{K}+\delta\underset{\sim}{K}]_o$ as either $\underset{\sim}{L}\underset{\sim}{U}$, where $\underset{\sim}{L}$ is unit lower triangular and $\underset{\sim}{U}$ is upper triangular, or as $\underset{\sim}{Q}\underset{\sim}{R}$, where $\underset{\sim}{Q}$ is unitary and R is upper triangular. In the finite element method, usually the $\underset{\sim}{L}\underset{\sim}{U}$ algorithms are preferred (since, generally, $[\underset{\sim}{K}+\delta\underset{\sim}{K}]_o$ is real, symmetric and banded, for which the factorization leads to $\underset{\sim}{U}^T\underset{\sim}{U}$ with banded $\underset{\sim}{U}$):

$$[\underset{\sim}{K}+\delta\underset{\sim}{K}]_o = \underset{\sim}{L}\ \underset{\sim}{U} \tag{76}$$

This is called the decomposition phase of the algorithm. Using (76), the equation in (75) may be rewritten as

$$\underset{\sim}{L}\ \underset{\sim}{U}\ \{\underset{\sim}{u}'-\underset{\sim}{u}_\circ\} = \{\underset{\sim}{p}+\delta\underset{\sim}{p}\}_\circ \tag{77}$$

Then, in the forward pass phase of the algorithm, from

$$\underset{\sim}{L}\ \underset{\sim}{z} = \{\underset{\sim}{p}+\delta\underset{\sim}{p}\}_\circ \tag{78}$$

the auxiliary quantities $\underset{\sim}{z}$ are easily solved due to the special structure of $\underset{\sim}{L}$. Finally, in the backward pass phase, from

$$\underset{\sim}{U}\ \{\underset{\sim}{u}'-\underset{\sim}{u}_\circ\} = \underset{\sim}{z} \tag{79}$$

the solution of (75), $\underset{\sim}{u}'-\underset{\sim}{u}_\circ$, is easily obtained with the special structure of $\underset{\sim}{U}$. However, at every phase of the algorithm, the round-off errors are introduced into the computed quantities. In actuality, instead of (76), (78), (79), and (75), one has, respectively,

$$[\underset{\sim}{K}+\delta\underset{\sim}{K}]_\circ = \underset{\sim}{L}\ \underset{\sim}{U} - \Delta\underset{\sim}{K} \tag{80}$$

$$\underset{\sim}{L}\ \underset{\sim}{z} = \{\underset{\sim}{p}+\delta\underset{\sim}{p}\}_\circ + \underset{\sim}{b} \tag{81}$$

$$\underset{\sim}{U}\ \{\underset{\sim}{u}_c-\underset{\sim}{u}_\circ\} = \underset{\sim}{z} - \underset{\sim}{c} \tag{82}$$

and

$$([\underset{\sim}{K}+\delta\underset{\sim}{K}]_\circ + \Delta\underset{\sim}{K})(\underset{\sim}{u}_c-\underset{\sim}{u}_\circ) = \{\underset{\sim}{p}+\delta\underset{\sim}{p}\}_\circ + \Delta\underset{\sim}{p} \quad \text{where} \quad \Delta\underset{\sim}{p} = \underset{\sim}{b} + \underset{\sim}{L}\ \underset{\sim}{c} \tag{83}$$

In these equations $\Delta\underset{\sim}{K}$, $\underset{\sim}{b}$, and $\underset{\sim}{c}$ are the round-off error effects associated with the decomposition, the forward pass, and the backward pass, respectively. It may be observed from (83) that $\Delta\underset{\sim}{K}$ and $\Delta\underset{\sim}{p}$ are the counterparts of $\delta\underset{\sim}{K}$ and $\delta\underset{\sim}{p}$, and they are caused by the manipulation. The contribution of $\Delta\underset{\sim}{K}$ and $\Delta\underset{\sim}{p}$ on the solution $\underset{\sim}{u}_c$ is the manipulation error $\underset{\sim}{g}$. Note that the transformation of $\Delta\underset{\sim}{K}$ and $\Delta\underset{\sim}{p}$ into $\underset{\sim}{g}$ is the same as the transformation of $\delta\underset{\sim}{K}$ and $\delta\underset{\sim}{p}$ into $\underset{\sim}{h}$. This type of transformation is already discussed in the previous section.

Among the iterative methods, Gauss-Seidel iteration (with over-relaxation and under-relaxation options) is most often used. In this method, (75) is first scaled with $\text{diag}[(k_{ii}+k_{ii})^{-1}]$ such that

$$\text{diag}[(k_{ii}+\delta k_{ii})^{-1}][\underset{\sim}{K}+\delta\underset{\sim}{K}]_\circ = -\underset{\sim}{L} + \underset{\sim}{I} - \underset{\sim}{U} \tag{84}$$

and

$$\text{diag}[(k_{ii}+\delta k_{ii})^{-1}]\{\underset{\sim}{p}+\delta\underset{\sim}{p}\}_\circ = \underset{\sim}{q} \tag{85}$$

where $\underset{\sim}{L}$ and $\underset{\sim}{U}$ are the zero lower triangular and the zero upper triangular matrices, respectively. Defining

$$\underset{\sim}{v}' = \underset{\sim}{u}' - \underset{\sim}{u}_\circ \tag{86}$$

(75) may be rewritten as

$$\underset{\sim}{v}' = \underset{\sim}{q} + \underset{\sim}{L}\ \underset{\sim}{v}' + \underset{\sim}{U}\ \underset{\sim}{v}' \tag{87}$$

and the Gauss-Seidel iteration without relaxation is

$$\underset{\sim}{v}'_{k+1} = \underset{\sim}{q} + \underset{\sim}{L}\ \underset{\sim}{v}'_{k+1} + \underset{\sim}{U}\ \underset{\sim}{v}'_k \quad , \quad \text{for } k=0,1,\cdots \quad \text{with } \underset{\sim}{v}'_0=\underset{\sim}{o} \tag{88}$$

In actuality, due to the round-off errors during the manipulation, instead of (84), (85), (86), and (88), one has, respectively,

$$\text{diag}[(k_{ii}+\delta k_{ii})^{-1}][\underset{\sim}{K}+\delta\underset{\sim}{K}]_\circ = -\underset{\sim}{L} + \underset{\sim}{I} - \underset{\sim}{U} - \text{diag}[(k_{ii}+\delta k_{ii})^{-1}]\Delta\underset{\sim}{K} \tag{89}$$

$$\text{diag}[(k_{ii}+\delta k_{ii})^{-1}]\{\underset{\sim}{p}+\delta\underset{\sim}{p}\}_\circ = \underset{\sim}{q} + \underset{\sim}{d} \tag{90}$$

$$\mathbf{v} = \mathbf{u}_c - \mathbf{u}_\circ \tag{91}$$

$$\mathbf{v} = \mathbf{q} + \mathbf{d} + \mathbf{L}\,\mathbf{v} + \mathbf{U}\,\mathbf{v} - \text{diag}[(k_{ii}+\delta k_{ii})^{-1}]\ \Delta\mathbf{K}\ \mathbf{v} \tag{92}$$

and

$$\mathbf{v}_{k+1} = \mathbf{q} + \mathbf{d} + + \mathbf{L}\,\mathbf{v}_{k+1} + \mathbf{U}\,\mathbf{v}_k + \mathbf{d}_k \quad \text{for } k=0,1,\cdots \quad \text{with } \mathbf{v}_0=\mathbf{o} \tag{93}$$

By back substitution one may write for (75)

$$([\mathbf{K}+\delta\mathbf{K}]_\circ + \Delta\mathbf{K})(\mathbf{u}_c-\mathbf{u}_\circ) = \{\mathbf{p}+\delta\mathbf{p}\}_\circ + \Delta\mathbf{p} \tag{94}$$

where

$$\Delta\mathbf{p} = \text{diag}(k_{ii}+ k_{ii})(\mathbf{d} + \sum_k \mathbf{d}_k) \tag{95}$$

In (94) $\Delta\mathbf{K}$ and $\Delta\mathbf{p}$ represent the errors caused by the manipulation (their effect in the computed response $\mathbf{u}_c$, i.e., $\mathbf{g}$, is the manipulation error). The transformation of $\Delta\mathbf{K}$ and $\Delta\mathbf{p}$ into $\mathbf{g}$ is the same as the transformation of $\delta\mathbf{K}$ and $\delta\mathbf{p}$ into $\mathbf{h}$. This is already discussed in the previous section.

The approximate solution obtained for (75) by means of a digital computer and a solution algorithm is essentially the exact solution of (83) or (94). Thus, the knowledge of $\Delta\mathbf{K}$ and $\Delta\mathbf{p}$ would enable one to obtain the exact solution $\mathbf{u}'$ of (75) by (69), just as the knowledge of $\delta\mathbf{K}$ and $\delta\mathbf{p}$ would enable one to obtain the exact solution $\mathbf{u}(\mathbf{x},t)$ of (40) by (29). However, the computation of $\Delta\mathbf{K}$ and $\Delta\mathbf{p}$ is a much harder problem than the computation of $\delta\mathbf{K}$ and $\delta\mathbf{p}$. The main difficulty is in the apparent randomness of the rounding-off processes. Other factors determining the magnitudes of $\Delta\mathbf{K}$ and $\Delta\mathbf{p}$ are those discussed for (12)-(17), and also the type of the algorithm. A good account of possibilities and difficulties for mostly used algorithms is given in (20). In general the magnitudes of $\Delta\mathbf{K}$ and $\Delta\mathbf{p}$ are smaller if $[\mathbf{K}+\delta\mathbf{K}]_\circ$ is of small order, banded, symmetric, positive definite, and has a small conditioning number. Obviously, the algorithms which take advantage of these properties when they exist, produce smaller magnitude $\Delta\mathbf{K}$ and $\Delta\mathbf{p}$.

Eigenvalue Problems

These problems are the special case of the linear equilibrium problems discussed in the preceding sub-section. For this class of problems, in (72),

$$\mathbf{t}_f = \mathbf{o} \tag{96}$$

$$\mathbf{f}(\mathbf{u}_\circ) = \mathbf{o} \tag{97}$$

$$[\mathbf{f}_{,\mathbf{u}}(\mathbf{u}_\circ)] = [\mathbf{A}+\delta\mathbf{A}] - \lambda\ [\mathbf{B}+\delta\mathbf{B}] \tag{98}$$

and thus, it becomes

$$[\mathbf{A}+\delta\mathbf{A}]\{\mathbf{u}'-\mathbf{u}_\circ\} = \lambda\ [\mathbf{B}+\delta\mathbf{B}]\{\mathbf{u}'-\mathbf{u}_\circ\} \tag{99}$$

which is a general algebraic eigenvalue problem. In (99), $\delta\mathbf{A}$ and $\delta\mathbf{B}$ represent the equation errors, and the finite element method produces the numerical values of $[\mathbf{A}+\delta\mathbf{A}]$ and $[\mathbf{B}+\delta\mathbf{B}]$.

Since usually $n>4$, the solution of these problems is essentially obtained by a digital computer and iterative solution algorithms. During the iterations, many round-off errors take place, and the solutions thus obtained are approximate for (99) but basically exact for a modified problem such as

$$[\mathbf{A}+\delta\mathbf{A} + \Delta\mathbf{A}]\{\mathbf{u}_c-\mathbf{u}_\circ\} = \lambda\ [\mathbf{B}+\delta\mathbf{B} + \Delta\mathbf{B}]\{\mathbf{u}_c-\mathbf{u}_\circ\} \tag{100}$$

where $\Delta\mathbf{A}$ and $\Delta\mathbf{B}$ represent the modifications caused by the manipulations. The effect of $\Delta\mathbf{A}$ and $\Delta\mathbf{B}$ on the computed eigenvalues and eigenvectors are the manipulation errors. Note that in (100) $\Delta\mathbf{A}$ and $\Delta\mathbf{B}$ play the same role as $\delta\mathbf{A}$ and $\delta\mathbf{B}$.

Therefore, the discussions of the previous section related with the effects of δA and δB on the computed eigenpairs also apply to those of ΔA and ΔB. The problem of quantifying ΔA and ΔB is usually a harder problem than that of δA and δB. The main difficulty lies again in the apparent randomness of the rounding-off processes. Other factors determining the magnitudes of ΔA and ΔB are those discussed for (12)-(17), and also the type of the solution algorithm. A good account of possibilities and difficulties for more often used algorithms is given in (20). In general the magnitudes of ΔA and ΔB are smaller if $[A+\delta A]$ and $[B+\delta B]$ are of small order, banded, real, symmetric, and positive definite. Obviously, the algorithms which take advantage of these, when they exist, produce smaller magnitude ΔA and ΔB.

Nonlinear Equilibrium Problems

The discrete governing equations and their power series expansions for these problems are as in (71) and (72). In these problems the remainder in (72) is not zero. The usual method of solving these problems is the Newton-Raphson iteration as given in (60), since, given a u_k, the finite element method provides $f(u_k)$ and $f_{,u}(u_k)$ as $-\{p+\delta p\}_k$ and $[K+\delta K]_k$, respectively. One may see from (60) that, in order to obtain the response at the (k+1)st step, one has to solve a set of linear equations of the type of (75). This indicates that the computed response contains also the manipulation errors, and it is essentially the exact solution of a set of modified equations as in (94). Let u'_k denote the response at step k without the manipulation errors, g_k denote the manipulation errors such that u'_k+g_k is the computed response u_{ck}, and $[\Delta K]_k$ and $\{\Delta p\}_k$ denote the modifications caused in the equations by the manipulation. Thus, instead of

$$u'_{k+1} = u'_k + [K+\delta K]_k^{-1}\{p+\delta p\}_k \quad , \text{ for } k=0,1,\cdots \quad \text{with } u'_0=0 \tag{101}$$

one has

$$u'_{k+1} + g_{k+1} = u'_k + [K+\delta K + \Delta K]_k^{-1}\{p+\delta p + \Delta p\}_k \quad , \quad k=0,1,\cdots \ \& \ u'_0=0 \tag{102}$$

Suppose when k=m, the residue $\{p+\delta p\}_m$ is sufficiently small so that $u_{ck+1}=u'_{k+1}+g_{k+1}$ can be used as the solution representing the equilibrium state. Then, subtracting (101) and (102) side-by-side, and using m for k+1, one may write

$$g_m = [K+\delta K + \Delta K]_{m-1}^{-1}\{p+\delta p + \Delta p\}_{m-1} - [K+\delta K]_{m-1}^{-1}\{p+\delta p\}_{m-1} \tag{103}$$

which indicates that the manipulation error at the mth step is caused by ΔK and Δp of the m-1st step, and the relationship is of the type of (63). Thus, it is established that the manipulation errors have a similar effect on the solution as the discretization. It is important to note that the manipulation errors of steps preceding the m-1st reflect on the solution as inherited errors, and their effects are in δK and δp.

There are various variants of the basic Newton-Raphson algorithm, and they are all being widely used. As the algorithm changes, the quantities ΔK, Δp, and m all change. In other words, the manipulation errors are very much algorithm dependent. The assessment of ΔK and Δp is a very difficult problem mainly because of the apparent randomness of the rounding-off processes. The factors discussed for (12)-(17) also directly effect the magnitudes of ΔK and Δp.

Manipulation Errors in Propagation Problems

In these problems the equations are as in (1), with the known initial conditions $u(x,t_o)$, i.e.,

$$\dot{u}'(t) = f(u'(t)) \qquad \text{for } t > t_o \tag{104}$$

and

$$u(x,t_o) = u'_o \quad \text{known} \quad \text{at } t = t_o \tag{105}$$

In the numerical solutions of these equations, the time variable t is considered by its discrete values t_k such that

$$t_{k+1} = t_k + h_k \qquad k=0,1,\cdots \tag{106}$$

where t_k is the time at the kth discrete station, and h_k is the time increment at station k. In many algorithms h_k is taken as constant, that is,

$$h_k = h \quad , \quad k=0,1,\cdots \tag{107}$$

and in many other algorithms it can be varied from station to station. The numerical solutions provide the values of the response only at the discrete time stations, chronologically, starting with $\underset{\sim}{u}'_o$, as $\underset{\sim}{u}_c(t_k)$, k=0,1,···, instead of $\underset{\sim}{u}'(t_k)$, k=0,1,··· . The difference $\underset{\sim}{g}_k=\underset{\sim}{g}(t_k)$, k=0,1,···, defined as

$$\underset{\sim}{g}_k = \underset{\sim}{u}_c(t_k) - \underset{\sim}{u}'(t_k) \tag{108}$$

is due to the manipulations with a finite machine and an approximate algorithm. Of course, at the kth station, one also has the solution errors due to discretization, $\underset{\sim}{h}(t_k)=\underset{\sim}{h}_k$:

$$\underset{\sim}{h}_k = \underset{\sim}{u}'(t_k) - \underset{\sim}{u}(\underset{\sim}{x},t_k) \tag{109}$$

Suppose the solution of (104) is already marched out up to the kth station, and the response for station k+1 is to be computed. As far as this computation is concerned, the quantity $\underset{\sim}{e}_k$ defined as

$$\underset{\sim}{e}_k = \underset{\sim}{h}_k + \underset{\sim}{g}_k \tag{110}$$

(i.e., the <u>total solution error</u> at station k) is the inherited error. The numerical solution at time station k+1, i.e., $\underset{\sim}{u}_c(t_{k+1})$, will not only contain the propagated version of the inherited error $\underset{\sim}{e}_k$, but also the round-off errors $\underset{\sim}{e}_k^r$ of the arithmetic operations of the step and the truncation errors $\underset{\sim}{e}_k^t$ of the step due to the approximate nature of the algorithm. Let $\underset{\sim}{A}_k$ denote the mechanism by which the inherited errors $\underset{\sim}{e}_k$ at time t_k propagate to time t_{k+1}. With this, one may write

$$\underset{\sim}{e}_{k+1} = \underset{\sim}{A}_k \, \underset{\sim}{e}_k + \underset{\sim}{e}_k^r + \underset{\sim}{e}_k^t \tag{111}$$

Clearly, $\underset{\sim}{e}_k^r$ and $\underset{\sim}{e}_k^t$ are algorithm dependent. It is shown below that $\underset{\sim}{A}_k$ is also algorithm dependent. Therefore, $\underset{\sim}{A}_k$, $\underset{\sim}{e}_k^t$, and $\underset{\sim}{e}_k^r$, k=0,1,···, represent the effect of the manipulations.

In the finite element method, given $\underset{\sim}{u}_c(t_k)$, one has the numerical values of the vector function $\underset{\sim}{f}$ and its Jacobian $\underset{\sim}{f}_{,\underset{\sim}{u}}$ for $\underset{\sim}{u}_c(t_k)$, rather than the explicit expressions of the equations in (104). Let $\underset{\sim}{f}_k$ and $\underset{\sim}{f}_{,k}$ denote the values of $\underset{\sim}{f}$ and $\underset{\sim}{f}_{,\underset{\sim}{u}}$ at $\underset{\sim}{u}_c(t_k)$. Namely

$$\underset{\sim}{f}_k = \underset{\sim}{f}(\underset{\sim}{u}_c(t_k)) = -\{\underset{\sim}{p}+\delta\underset{\sim}{p}\}_{t=t_k} \tag{112}$$

and

$$\underset{\sim}{f}_{,k} = \underset{\sim}{f}_{,\underset{\sim}{u}}(\underset{\sim}{u}_c(t_k)) = [\underset{\sim}{K}+\delta\underset{\sim}{K}]_{t=t_k} \tag{113}$$

Many of the algorithms with which one may march out the numerical solution may be expressed as

$$\underset{\sim}{u}_c(t_{k+1}) = \underset{\sim}{u}_c(t_{k-q}) + (q+1)\, h \text{ (weighted average of } \underset{\sim}{f}_i,\ i=k,\cdots) \tag{114}$$

where q is a non-negative integer, and h is the time increment (if the time increments are variable, h represents some averaged value). If q=0, and $\underset{\sim}{f}_i$ values used in the "weighted average" belong to $u_c(t)$ with $t_k \le t \le t_{k+1}$, the algorithms are called the <u>single-step methods</u> (such as the Euler method, the Runge-Kutta methods), whereas, if q>0, and $\underset{\sim}{f}_i$ values used in the "weighted average" are those of the time stations, they are called the <u>multi-step methods</u> (various predictor, and predictor-corrector methods). For multi-step methods, (114) may be rewritten as

$$u_c(t_{k+1}) = u_c(t_{k-q}) + (q+1)\, h \sum_{i=0}^{r} \beta_i f_{k+s-i} \tag{115}$$

where s is either zero or one, and $r \geq 0$. If s=0, the methods are called open-type or predictor. If s=1, the methods are called closed-type or corrector. It may be observed that the multi-step methods are not self-starting (i.e., initially one needs the response at several time stations in order to use them), and the corrector methods require the use of a predictor (since the corrector requires f_{k+1} for the prediction of $u_c(t_{k+1})$.

Each of the above methods employs different amounts of arithmetic operations, and each has different truncation errors. One may compute different responses $u_c(t_{k+1})$ for the k+1st station by using different methods, all using the same data at the kth station. The derivation of the equations of the type of (114) for various methods is such that, as a by-product, one also obtains expressions for their truncation errors (basically, by matching the interpolating polynomials with the power series expansions, and using the remainder theorem). The expressions for the truncation errors are of the type

$$e_r^t = \rho\, O(h^p) \tag{116}$$

where ρ lists the values of the higher order derivatives at some unknown time, h is the time increment at station k, and p is a positive integer. The expressions for the truncation errors indicate concisely how fast the truncation errors will vanish with decreasing size of time increments. Unfortunately, the expressions for round-off errors cannot be expressed as easily, although some upper bound values may be stated for the components of e_k^r. It is interesting to note that, as p increases in (116), the truncation errors of the method vanishes rapidly with decreasing mesh size, however, meanwhile, the magnitudes of the round-off errors grow. The methods with large p are called higher-order methods.

As mentioned in the discussion of (111), the third element of the manipulation errors, i.e., matrix A_k, is also method dependent, in addition to the fact that A_k also depends on the intrinsic properties of the system as represented by the Jacobian matrix $f_{,k}$. This can be shown by a simple example. Suppose a single step method is being used, and h is sufficiently small. Then (114) may be rewritten as

$$u_c(t_{k+1}) \cong u_c(t_k) + h\, f_{,k}\, u_c(t_k) \tag{117}$$

where it is assumed that f_i values in the interval of $t_k - t_{k+1}$ do not change, and they may be approximated by $f_i \simeq f_{,i} u_c(t_i)$ [see the discussions leading to the linearized equations (68)]. One may rewrite (117) as

$$u_c(t_{k+1}) \cong A_k\, u_c(t_k) \tag{118}$$

where

$$A_k = I + h\, f_{,k} = I + h\, [K+\delta K]_{t=t_k} \tag{119}$$

Since (118) shows the propagation of the solution at t_k into that of t_{k+1}, matrix A_k in (118) is the same as the one in (111). Matrix A_k is clearly system dependent through the Jacobian $f_{,k}$, and algorithm dependent through the time increment h and the way it is related to $f_{,k}$. One may observe from (118) that, if the eigenvalues of A_k are inside the unit circle centered at the origin of the complex plane, the propagation process will be with decreasing magnitudes, otherwise, it will be with increasing magnitudes. Matrix A_k is a matrix polynomial of the Jacobian $f_{,k}$, therefore, the eigenvalues of A_k are one plus the h multiple of those of $f_{,k}$. From this, it can be shown that, if $f_{,k}$ is such that the system is unstable, i.e., there is at least one eigenvalue of $f_{,k}$ with a positive real part, then there will be at least one eigenvalue of A_k outside the unit circle, regardless of the value of the time increment h. On the other hand, even if the system is stable, i.e., none of the eigenvalues of $f_{,k}$ is with real positive part, by improper choice of the time increment h, one may have some of the eigenvalues of A_k to fall outside the unit circle. In other words, the algorithm may render a stable system into an unstable one.

In the multi-step methods, the structure of $\underset{\sim}{A}_k$ depends on the algorithm more than it depends in the single-step methods. Here, too, $\underset{\sim}{A}_k$ is a matrix polynomial of $\underset{\sim}{f}_{,k}$, where the degree of the polynomial is greater than one, and the polynomial coefficients depend on not only h but also β_i, $i=0,1,\cdots$, the coefficients of the algorithm. Let $p(\underset{\sim}{f}_{,k})=\underset{\sim}{A}_k$ denote the matrix polynomial. If the eigenvalues of $\underset{\sim}{f}_{,k}$ are μ_i, $i=1,2,\cdots,n$; then the eigenvalues of $\underset{\sim}{A}_k$ are $p(\mu_i)$, $i=1,2,\cdots,n$. Clearly, even if all μ_i are with negative real parts, i.e., the system is stable, $p(\mu_i)$ may be such that they may fall outside the unit circle centered at the origin of the complex plane by either the wrong choice of h, or by wrong choice of the algorithm, or both, and thus cause instabilities by enlarging the magnitudes of the inherited errors without bound.

CURRENT RESEARCH ON ERROR PREDICTION

In the preceding sections, various errors which may take place in the finite element analysis are defined, the factors affecting their magnitudes and growth are discussed. The finite element method, in essence, is the computation of the vector function $\underset{\sim}{f}$ and its Jacobian $\underset{\sim}{f}_{,u}$, related to (1). The errors in the computed response, in one way or another, are all associated with the errors in the numerical values of $\underset{\sim}{f}$ and $\underset{\sim}{f}_{,u}$. These errors are essentially due to discretization and the manipulation, since the inherited errors are the propagated versions of the discretization and manipulation errors committed earlier. In other words, the building blocks of the solution errors are the errors in the numerical values of the Jacobian $\underset{\sim}{f}_{,u}$, i.e., $\delta\underset{\sim}{K}^d$, $\delta\underset{\sim}{K}^r$, $\Delta\underset{\sim}{K}$, and the vector function $\underset{\sim}{f}$, i.e., $-\delta\underset{\sim}{p}^d$, $-\delta\underset{\sim}{p}^r$, $\Delta\underset{\sim}{p}$ (where d and r for discretization and round-off, and δ for equation-phase and Δ for solution-phase). In the finite element method, instead of $\underset{\sim}{f}$ and $\underset{\sim}{f}_{,u}$, one deals with $\underset{\sim}{f}-\delta\underset{\sim}{p}-\delta\underset{\sim}{p}^d-\delta\underset{\sim}{p}^r-\Delta\underset{\sim}{p}$ and $\underset{\sim}{f}_{,u}+\delta\underset{\sim}{K}^d+\delta\underset{\sim}{K}^r+\Delta\underset{\sim}{K}$ ($\delta\underset{\sim}{p}$ representing the inherited error). The knowledge of the blocks enables one to compute the solution error.

In the following paragraphs, a short review of the published works on the solution errors in the finite element method is given. The references are only to indicate the trends, and are by no means complete.

Computation of the Equation Round-Off Errors $\delta\underset{\sim}{p}^r$, $\delta\underset{\sim}{p}$, $\delta\underset{\sim}{K}^r$, $\Delta\underset{\sim}{K}$

The quantities $\delta\underset{\sim}{p}^r$, $\delta\underset{\sim}{p}$, $\delta\underset{\sim}{K}^r$, and $\Delta\underset{\sim}{K}$ are the basic blocks of the manipulation error analysis. Yet in the recent finite element literature almost no work is available dealing with either a priori or a posteriori evaluation of these quantities. Probably this is partly due to the difficult nature of the problem, and partly due to the existence of a rather easy and yet effective measure for controlling the magnitudes of the round-off errors (discussed in the next section). However, in the finite difference literature one may find many interesting investigations on this matter (21). Once these equation errors are evaluated, the computation of their effects in both the equilibrium and also the propagation problems can easily be done as outlined earlier. The methods of such computations have been extensively studied in the texts of the numerical analysis (20), (21), (22).

Computation of the Equation Discretization Errors $\delta\underset{\sim}{K}^d$, $\delta\underset{\sim}{p}^d$

The quantities $\delta\underset{\sim}{K}^d$ and $\delta\underset{\sim}{p}^d$ are the basic blocks of the discretization error analysis. Once they are numerically available, the computation of their effects in the response can easily be computed as discussed earlier. The methods of such computations have been extensively studied in the texts of numerical analysis (20), (21), (22), (23). The adaptation of these methods for the finite element analysis has been proposed (10), (11).

A Priori Computation of $\delta\underset{\sim}{K}^d$ and $\delta\underset{\sim}{p}^d$

The quantities $\delta\underset{\sim}{K}^d$ and $\delta\underset{\sim}{p}^d$ are governed essentially by the remainder theorem of the power series expansions. Since the evaluation of the higher order derivatives of the response quantities at unknown points is required for their definition, a priori estimation of these quantities is impossible unless the response is such that the higher order derivatives appearing in the expressions for $\delta \underset{\sim}{K}^d$ and δp^d are all zero. There have been very few efforts in the finite element literature dealing with the expressions for these quantities (12), (13), (14), (15).

A Posteriori Computation of $\delta \underset{\sim}{K}^d$ and $\delta \underset{\sim}{p}^d$

A posteriori computation of the equation discretization errors $\delta \underset{\sim}{K}^d$ and δp^d is quite possible (10), (11). This has been done in the finite difference method for a long time (22), (23). In the finite element method, the investigators are looking into this problem only recently (14), (15), (24), (25).

Computation of Some Norm of the Solution Discretization Error

In the recent literature, this is the most active area in the error problem of the finite element method. Most work has been confined to the linear equilibrium problems with positive definite and self-adjoint operators. Many investigators, motivated by the problem of convergence in the finite element method, tried to obtain an upper bound value for some norm of the solution discretization errors in the form of Kh^p, where K and p are constants, and h is a typical mesh size. The true solution of the discretized problem, $\Psi(\underset{\sim}{x},t)$, is as defined in (18). The true solution of the mathematical model is $u(\underset{\sim}{x},t)$. Let D denote the spatial domain of the problem. Then, for the Euclid norm of the solution discretization error at time t, $\pi(t)$, may be expressed as

$$\pi_E(t) = \| u(\underset{\sim}{x},t) \|_E = \sqrt{\int_D (u(\underset{\sim}{x},t)-\Psi(\underset{\sim}{x},t))^2 \, d\underset{\sim}{x}} \qquad (120)$$

Let π denote any norm of the solution discretization error at time t. Given a mesh with typical mesh size h, if one writes

$$\pi \leq K\, h^p \qquad (121)$$

what is the minimum value of p for which (121) is true? Is K a true constant? The answers of these questions may be found in (26), (27), (28), (29), (30), (31), (32), (33), (34), (35), (36), (37).

In the linear elasticity problems, many investigators dealt with the energy norms [i.e., the positive-definite-quadratic-form-norm as in (9), defined over domain D] of the finite element solutions. They showed that, depending upon the type of the functional used, the energy norms may constitute a minimizing or maximizing sequence with mesh refinement (1), (38), (21), (39), (3). The fact that, by changing the functional, one can obtain the upper and lower bounds of the energy norms is important especially in the eigenvalue problems where the energy norms are quite closely related with the eigenvalues, and in the equilibrium problems with a single concentrated load where the energy norms are the scaled values of the displacement in the direction of the single concentrated load.

The studies dealing with the bounding of norms of the discretization errors have no doubt shed light to the convergence problem of the finite element method. However, they are of limited help in assessing the errors in the computed response quantities $\underset{\sim}{u}_c(t)$.

STATE OF THE ART OF ERROR ESTIMATION

Because of the difficulties in quantitative estimation through numerical analysis, the current practice in assessing the solution errors in the computed response quantities is through computer experimentation, and it is mostly confined to the linear equilibrium problems. In these experiments, the same problem is solved repeatedly, each time halving the mesh size. Then for each point in the crude mesh (or for selected mesh points) the response is plotted against the mesh size. The study of these plots enables one to assess the errors as discussed below.

Solution Errors Due To Manipulation

Due to their apparently random character, the effect of the round-off errors is reflected on the response-mesh size curves erratically. These curves assume a randomly oscillating form when the solution errors due to round-off are large [Fig. 2.41 of (40) is a good example]. Once such a behavior is identified, the errors can be controlled by using larger mesh sizes, or longer mantissa lengths, or both.

Algorithmic portions of the manipulation errors usually manifest themselves by extremely large computed response quantities. When they are identified, their control is first attempted by varying the parameters of the algorithm (such as decreasing the time increment in propagation problems, or readjusting the relaxation parameter in iterative methods, etc.). If this fails, one usually changes the algorithm, hoping that the new one will work.

Solution Errors Due To Discretization

Since these errors decrease with decreasing mesh size, the response-mesh size curves assume a converging appearance with decreasing mesh size, if no other error exists in the response quantities. If the convergence is monotonic, one may use the Richardson's extrapolation technique to find the value of the response corresponding to zero mesh size (41), (42), (43), (44). This technique is based on two assumptions: (i) The error is caused by only the discretization, (ii) The discretization error decreases monotonically with decreasing mesh size. These assumptions are valid assumptions if the manipulation errors are rendered negligible as discussed above, and if the finite element representations are as defined in the introduction. The application of the Richardson's extrapolation type techniques for the finite element method has already appeared in the literature (29), (45), (46).

In the Richardson's extrapolation, at a point, one assumes

$$u_c - u = H\, h^p \qquad (122)$$

where u_c is the computed response, u its value without discretization errors, h is the typical mesh size, and K and p are the constants to be determined as a result of computer experimentation. Since (122) contains three constants to be determined (i.e., u, K, and p), one needs at least three experiments with typical mesh-sizes h_1, h_2, and h_3, to yield the responses at the point, u_{c1}, u_{c2}, and u_{c3}, respectively. By writing (122) for (u_{ci}, h_i), i=1,2,3, one obtains three equations from which K, p, and u may be solved.

CONCLUSIONS

From the discussions of this chapter, the following conclusions may be drawn:

1. The errors in the computed results originate from two sources: the round-off errors in the numerical representations, and the discretization errors caused by representing the infinite degrees of freedom reponse by finite degrees of freedom. These errors may be represented as the equation errors.
2. Depending upon the system characterisitics, the equation errors reflect to the solution by changing their magnitudes.
3. The algorithms used in obtaining the solution from the equations contribute further to the solution errors in two ways: by causing more round-off errors, and by altering the system characteristics.
4. The combined system-algorithm characteristics play a very important role in error propagation, especially in the propagation problems.
5. The Jacobian $\tilde{f}_{,\tilde{u}}$ computed by means of the finite element method possesses very favorable system characteristics (such as symmetry, positive definiteness, and bandedness) for error reduction, provided that one uses those solution algorithms which take advantage of these favorable properties.
6. Very little has been done in assessing the equation errors in the finite ele-

ment method, although the mechanisms by which these reflect on the solution are very well understood.

7. The works trying to obtain bounds for the norms of the discretization errors in terms of typical mesh sizes are very useful in understanding the convergence problem, but they are of limited help in assessing the errors in a meaningful way.

8. Although it is possible, no components exist in the present finite element software to handle the error problem.

9. In order to assess the errors by computer experiments, the same problem should be solved at least three times by gradually refining the finite element mesh. Then, the response-mesh size plots should be produced for each mesh point of the crudest mesh, if possible.

10. In the response-mesh size plots the erratic appearance signals the presence of excessive round-off errors.

11. The Richardson's extrapolation technique may be applied successfully to the response-mesh size curves to find the response for infinitely small meshsize, if the discretization is the only reason for the errors, and if the results are obtained by means of conforming elements.

ACKNOWLEDGMENTS

The authors wish to acknowledge the help of Mr. Mohamed M. Essawi, a graduate teaching assistant in the Civil Engineering Department of Duke University, in collecting the references.

REFERENCES

1 Synge, J. L., The Hypercircle Method in Mathematical Physics, Cambridge University Press, Ltd., Cambridge, 1957.

2 Melosh, R. J., "Basis for Derivation of Matrices for the Direct Stiffness Method", AIAA Journal, Vol. 1, No. 7, July 1963, pp. 1631-1637.

3 Utku, S., "Stiffness Matrices for Thin Triangular Elements of Nonzero Gaussian Curvature", AIAA Journal, Vol. 5, No. 9, Sept. 1967, pp. 1659-1667.

4 Crandall, S. H., Engineering Analysis, A Survey of Numerical Procedures, McGraw-Hill Book Co., New York, 1956, Chapter 3.

5 Poincare, H., "Sur l'equilibre d'une Mass Fluide animee d'un Movement de Rotation", Acta Mathematica, No. 7, Sept. 1885, pp. 259-380. [Oeuvre de Henri Poincare, Tome 7, Gauthier-Villars et Cie., Paris, 1951, pp. 40-140].

6 Melosh, R. J., "Inherited Error in Finite Element Analyses of Structures", Computers & Structures, Vol. 3, Pergamon Press, 1973, pp. 1205-1217.

7 Wilkinson, J. H., The Algebraic Eigenvalue Problem, Clarendon Press, Oxford, 1965, pp. 56-58.

8 Collatz, L., The Numerical Treatment of Differential Equations, 3rd Ed., Springer-Verlag, New York, 1966, [1st Ed., 1951, in German], pp. 348-353.

9 Crandall, S. H., Engineering Analysis, A Survey of Numerical Procedures, McGraw-Hill Book Co., New York, 1956, pp. 163-171, and 265-269.

10 Utku, S., "Error Computation in Numerical Solutions of Linear Boundary Value Problems", Proceedings of the Second International Conference on Mathematical Modeling, University of Missouri, Rolla, Mo., July 1979, pp. 285-294.

11 Utku, S., and El-Essawi, M. M., "Error Computation in Finite Element Methods", Proceedings of the Seventh Conference on Electronic Computation, ASCE, New York, August 1979, pp. 584-592.

12 Walz, J. E., Fulton, R.E., Cyrus, N.J., "Accuracy and Convergence of Finite Element Approximations", AFFDL-TR-68-150, Wright-Patterson Air Force Base, Ohio, 1968, pp. 995-1027

13 Walz, J.E., Fulton, R.E., Cyrus, N.J., and Eppink, R. T., Accuracy of Finite Element Approximations to Structural Problems , TN-D-5728, NASA, Washington D.C., March 1970, pp. 1-53.

14 Gray, W. G., and Pinder, G. F., "On the Relationship Between the Finite Element and Finite Difference Methods", International Journal for Numerical Methods in Engineering, Vol. 10, 1976, pp. 893-923.

15 Jamet, P.,"Estimation of the Interpolation Error for Quadrilateral Finite Elements Which Can Degenerate into Triangles", SIAM J. Numer. Anal., Vol. 14,

No. 5, Oct. 1977, pp. 925-930.
16 Wilkinson, J. H., The Algebraic Eigenvalue Problem, Clarendon Press, Oxford, 1965, pp. 189-191.
17 Wilkinson, J. H., The Algebraic Eigenvalue Problem, Clarendon Press, Oxford, 1965, pp. 87-89.
18 Wilkinson, J. H., The Algebraic Eigenvalue Problem, Clarendon Press, Oxford, 1965, Chapter 3.
19 Wilkinson, J. H., The Algebraic Eigenvalue Problem, Clarendon Press, Oxford, 1965, pp. 170-171.
20 Wilkinson, J. H., The Algebraic Eigenvalue Problem, Clarendon Press, Oxford, 1965.
21 Crandall, S. H., Engineering Analysis, A Survey of Numerical Procedures, McGraw-Hill Book Co., New York, 1956.
22 Carnahan, B., Luther, H. A., and Wilkes, J. O., Applied Numerical Methods, John Wiley & Sons, Inc., New York, 1969.
23 Collatz, L., The Numerical Treatment of Differential Equations, 3rd Ed., Springer-Verlag, New York, 1966 [1st Ed. in German, 1951].
24 Babuska, I., and Rheinboldt, W. C., "Error Estimates for Adaptive Finite Element Computations", SIAM J. Numer. Anal., Vol. 15, No. 4, Aug. 1978, pp. 736-754.
25 Babuska, I., and Rheinboldt, W.C., "On the Reliability and Optimality of the Finite Element Method", Computers & Structures, Vol. 10, 1979, pp. 87-94.
26 McLay, R. W., "Completeness and Convergence Properties of Finite Element Displacement Functions - A General Treatment", AIAA Paper No. 67-143, AIAA Fifth Aerospace Sciences Meeting, N.Y., Jan. 1967.
27 Tong, P., and Pian, T. H. H., "The Convergence of Finite Element Method in Solving Linear Elastic Problems", Int. J. Solids & Structures, Vol. 3, 1967, pp. 865-879.
28 Johnson, M. W., and McLay, R. W., "Convergence of the Finite Element Method in the Theory of Elasticity", Transactions of the ASME, June 1968, pp. 274-278.
29 Lynn, P. P., and Boresi, A. P., "Kinds of Convergence and Improved Convergence of Conforming Finite Element Solutions in Plate Bending", Nuclear Engineering and Design, No. 11, 1970, pp. 159-176.
30 Fix, G., and Strang, G., "Fourier Analysis of the Finite Element Method in Ritz-Galerkin Theory", Studies in Applied Math., Vol. 48, No. 3, 1969, pp. 265-273.
31 Fried, I., "Accuracy of Finite Element Eigenproblems", J. of Sound and Vibration, Vol. 18(2), 1971, pp. 289-295.
32 Schultz, M. H., "L^2 Error Bounds for the Rayleigh Ritz Galerkin Method", SIAM J. Numer. Anal., Vol. 8, No. 4, Dec. 1971, pp. 737-749.
33 Babuska, I., "Error Bounds for Finite Element Method", Numer. Math., No. 16, 1971, pp. 322-333.
34 Zlamal, M., "Some Recent Advances in the Mathematics of Finite Elements", The Mathematics of Finite Elements and Applications, Whiteman Edtr., Academic Press, 1973, pp. 59-81.
35 Barnhill, R. E., and Whiteman, J. R., "Error Analysis of Finite Element Methods with Triangles for Elliptic Boundary Value Problems", The Mathematics of Finite Elements and Applications, Whiteman Edtr., Academic Press, 1973, pp. 83-112.
36 Ciarlet, P. G., "Orders of Convergence in Finite Element Methods", The Mathematics of Finite Elements and Applications, Whiteman Edtr., Academic Press, 1973, pp. 113-129.
37 Babuska, I., and Kellogg, R. B., "Nonuniform Error Estimates for the Finite Element Method", SIAM J. Numer. Anal., Vol. 12, No. 6, 1975, pp. 868-875.
38 Prager, W., and Synge, J. L., "Approximations in Elasticity Based on the Concept of Function Spaces", Quart. Appl. Math., Vol. 5, 1947, pp. 241-269.
39 Fraeijs de Veubeke, B. M., Matrix Methods of Structural Analysis, Pergamon Press, Ltd., Oxford, 1964.
40 Utku, S., Instructor's Manual for Part II of Elementary Structural Analysis by Norris, Wilbur, and Utku, 3rd Ed., McGraw-Hill Book Co., New York, 1976, pp. 91-97.
41 Richardson, L. F., "The Approximate Arithmetic Solution by Finite Differences of Physical Problems", Trans. Roy. Soc. London, A210, 1910, pp. 307-357.
42 Richardson, L. F., and Gaunt, J. A., "The Deferred Approach to the Limit,"

Trans. Roy. Soc. London, A226, 1927, pp. 299-361.

43 Crandall, S. H., Engineering Analysis, A Survey of Numerical Procedures, McGraw-Hill Book Co., New York, 1956, pp. 171-173, 269-270.

44 Carnahan, B., Luther, H.A., and Wilkes, J. O., Applied Numerical Methods, John Wiley & Sons, Inc., New York, 1969, pp. 78, 90, 364.

45 Lynn, P. P., and Dhillon, B. S., "Convergence of Eigenvalue Solutions in Conforming Plate Bending Finite Elements," Int. J. for Numerical Methods in Eng., Vol. 4, 1972, pp. 217-234.

46 Ramey, G. E., and Krishnamurthy, N., "Error Estimates for Conforming Finite Element Solutions," Computers & Structures, Vol. 4, 1974, pp. 1207-1222.

BIBLIOGRAPHY

1 Babuska, I., "Error Bounds for Finite Element Method," Numer. Math., Vol. 16, 1971, pp. 322-333.

2 Babuska, I., and Aziz, A.K., "Survey Lectures on the Mathematical Foundations of the Finite Element Method", The Mathematical Foundations of the Finite Element Method with Applications to Partial Differential Equations, A. K. Aziz, Edtr., Academic Press, New York, 1972, pp.3-359.

3 Babuska, I., "The Finite Element Method with Lagrangian Multipliers", Numer. Math., Vol. 20, 1973, pp. 179-192.

4 Babuska, I., and Kellogg, R. B., "Nonuniform Error Estimates for the Finite Element Method", SIAM J. Numer. Anal., Vol. 12, No. 6, 1975, pp. 868-875.

5 Babuska, I., "The Self-Adaptive Approach in the Finite Element Method", The Mathematics of Finite Elements and Applications II, J. R. Whiteman, Edtr., Academic Press, London, 1975, pp. 125-142.

6 Babuska, I., and Rheinboldt, W. C., "Error Estimates for Adaptive Finite Element Computations", SIAM J. Numer. Anal., Vol. 15, No. 4, Aug. 1978, pp. 736-754.

7 Babuska, I., and Rheinboldt, W. C., "On the Reliability and Optimality of the Finite Element Method", Computers & Structures, Vol. 10, 1979, pp. 87-94.

8 Babuska, I., "Reliable Error Estimation and Mesh Adaptation for the Finite Element Method", Computational Methods in Nonlinear Mechanics, J. T. Oden, Edtr., North Holland, Amsterdam, 1980, pp. 67-108.

9 Barnhill, R. E., and Whiteman, J. R., "Error Analysis of Finite Element Methods with Triangles for Elliptic Boundary Value Problems", The Mathematics of Finite Elements and Applications, Whiteman, Edtr., Academic Press, 1973, pp. 83-112.

10 Barnhill, R. E., amd Whiteman, J. R., "Error Analysis of Galerkin Methods for Dirichlet Problems Containing Boundary Singularities", J. Inst. Math. Appl., Vol. 15, 1975, pp. 121-125.

11 Barnhill, R. E., and Wilcox, C. H., "Computable Error Bounds for Finite Element Approximations to the Drichlet Problem," University of Utah Report, 1977.

12 Barnhill, R. E., Brown, J. H., McQueen, N., and Mitchell, A. R., "Computable Finite Element Error Bounds for Poisson's Equation", Int. J. Numer. Meth. Eng., Vol. 11, No. 3, pp. 593-597. (Also letters to editor in Vol. 12, 1978, p.1629).

13 Barnhill, R. E., Brown, J. H., and Mitchell, A. R.,"A Comparison of Finite Element Error Bounds for Poisson's Equation", Technical Report, BICOM 80/1, Institute of Computational Mathematics, Brunel University, 1980.

14 Bazeley, G. P., Cheung, Y. K., Irons, B. M., Zienkiewicz, O. C., "Triangular Elements in Plate Bending - Conforming and Nonconforming Solutions," Proceedings of the Conference on Matrix Methods in Structural Mechanics, Wright Patterson Air Force Base, Ohio, Oct. 1965, AFFDL-TR-66-80, pp. 547-576.

15 Bramble, J. H., and Hilbert, S. R., "Estimation of Linear Functionals on Sobolev Spaces with Application to Fourier Transforms and Spline Interpolation", SIAM J. Numer. Anal., Vol. 7, 1970, pp. 113-124.

16 Bramble, J. H., and Zlamal, M., "Triangular Elements in Finite Element Method", Math. Comput., Vol. 24, 1970, pp. 809-820.

17 Brezzi, F., "On the Existence, Uniqueness and Approximation of Saddle-Point Problems Arising From Lagrangian Multipliers", Rev. Francaise Automat. Informat. Recherche Operationnelle Ser. Rouge Anal. Numer., R-2, 1974, pp. 129-151.

18 Carnahan, B., Luther, H. A., and Wilkes, J. O., Applied Numerical Methods, John Wiley & Sons, Inc., New York, 1969.

19 Ciarlet, P. G., and Raviart, P.-A., "Interpolation Theory Over Curved Elements, with Applications to Finite Element Methods", Comput. Methods Appl. Mech. Engrg., Vol. 1, 1972, pp. 217-249.

20 Ciarlet, P. G., "Orders of Convergence in Finite Element Methods", The Mathematics of Finite Elements and Applications, Whiteman, Edtr., Academic Press, 1973, pp. 113-129.

21 Collatz, L. The Numerical Treatment of Differential Equations, 3rd Ed., Springer-Verlag, New York, 1966, [1st Ed., 1951, in German]

22 Courant, R., "Variational Methods for the Solution of Problems of Equilibrium and Vibrations", Bull. Amer. Math. Soc., Vol. 49, 1943, pp. 1-23.

23 Crandall, S. H., Engineering Analysis, A Survey of Numerical Procedures, McGraw-Hill Book Co., New York, 1956.

24 Crouzeix, M., and Raviart, P. -A., "Conforming and Nonconforming Finite Element Methods for Solving Stationary Stokes Equations I", Rev. Francaise Automat. Informat. Recherche Operationnelle Ser. Rouge Anal. Numer., R-3, 1973, pp. 33-76.

25 Falk, R. S., "Error Estimates for the Approximation of a Class of Variational Inequalities", Math. Comput., Vol. 28, 1974, pp. 963-971.

26 Fix, G. J., and Strang, G., "Fourier Analysis of the Finite Element Method in Ritz-Galerkin Theory", Studies in Applied Math., Vol. 48, No. 3, 1969, pp. 265-273.

27 Fraeijs de Veubeke, B. M., Matrix Methods of Structural Analysis, Pergamon Press, Ltd., Oxford, 1964.

28 Fraeijs de Veubeke, B. M., "A Conforming Finite Element for Plate Bending", Int. J. Solids and Structures, Vol. 4, 1968, pp. 95-108.

29 Fried, I., "Accuracy of Finite Element Eigenproblems", J. of Sound and Vibration, Vol. 18(2), 1971, pp. 289-295.

30 Gabay, D., and Mercier, B., " A Dual Algorithm for the Solution of Nonlinear Variational Problems via Finite Element Approximation", Comput. Math. Appl., 1976.

31 Glowinski, R., and Marrocco, A., "Sur l'Approximation par Elements Finis d'Ordre un$_2$ et la Resolution par Penalisation-Dualite, d'un Classe de Problemes de Dirichlet Non Lineaires", Rev. Francaise Automat. Informat. Recherche Operationnelle Ser. Rouge Anal. Numer., R-2, 1975, pp. 41-76.

32 Glowinski, R., Lions, J. -L., Tremolieres, R., Analyse Numerique des Inequations Variationnelles, Theorie Generale, Premieres Applications, Vol. 1, Dunod, Paris, 1976.

33 Glowinski, R., Lions, J. -L., Tremolieres, R., Analyse Numerique des Inequations Variationnelles, Applications aux Phenomenes Stationnaires et d'Evolution, Vol. 2, Dunod, Paris, 1976.

34 Gray, W. G., and Pinder, G. F., "On the Relationship Between the Finite Element and Finite Difference Methods", International Journal for Numerical Methods in Engineering, Vol. 10, 1976, pp. 893-923.

35 Gregory, J. A., "Error Bounds for Linear Interpolation on Triangles", The Mathematics of Finite Elements and Applications II, MAFELAP, J. R. Whiteman, Edtr., Academic Press, London, 1976.

36 Jamet, P., "Estimation of the Interpolation Error for Quadrilateral Finite Elements Which Can Degenerate into Triangles", SIAM J. Numer. Anal., Vol. 14, No. 5, Oct. 1977, pp. 925-930.

37 Johnson, M. W., and McLay, R.W., "Convergence of the Finite Element Method in the Theory of Elasticity", J. Appl. Mech., Ser. E., Vol. 35, 1968, pp. 274-278.

38 Lesaint, P., "Finite Element Methods for Symmetric Hyperbolic Equations", Numer. Math., Vol. 21, 1973, pp. 244-255.

39 Lynn, P. P., and Boresi, A. P., "Kinds of Convergence and Improved Convergence of Conforming Finite Element Solutions in Plate Bending", Nuclear Engineering and Design, No. 11, 1970, pp. 159-176.

40 Lynn, P. P., and Dhillon, B. S., "Convergence of Eigenvalue Solutions in Conforming Plate Bending Finite Elements", Int. J. for Numerical Methods in Eng., Vol. 4, 1972, pp. 217-234.

41 McLay, R. W., "Completeness and Convergence Properties of Finite Element Displacement Functions - A General Treatment", AIAA Paper No. 67-143, AIAA Fifth Aerospace Sciences Meeting, N.Y., Jan. 1967.

42 Melosh, R. J., "Basis for Derivation of Matrices for the Direct Stiffness Method", AIAA Journal, Vol. 1, No. 7, July 1963, pp. 1631-1637.

43 Melosh, R. J., "Inherited Error in Finite Element Analyses of Structures," Computers & Structures, Vol. 3, Pergamon Press, 1973, pp. 1205-1217.

44 Nitsche, J. A., "Ein Kriterium fur die Quasi-Optimalitat des Ritzchen Verfahrens", Numer. Math., Vol. 11, 1968, pp. 346-348.

45 Oden, J. T., and Lee, J. K., "Theory of Mixed and Hybrid Finite Element Approximations in Linear Elasticity",(IUTAM/IUM Symposium on Applications of Methods of Functional Analysis to Problems of Mechanics), Lecture Notes in Mathematics Springer-Verlag, Berlin, 1975.

46 Oden, J. T., and Reddy, J. N., An Introduction to the Mathematical Theory of Finite Elements, Wiley Interscience, New York, 1976.

47 Pian, T. H. H., and Tong, P., "A Variational Principle and the Convergence of a Finite Element Method Based on Assumed Stress Distribution", International Journal of Solids and Structures , Vol. 5, 1969, pp. 463-472.

48 Poincare, H., "Sur l'Equilibre d'une Mass Fluide Animee d'un Movement de Rotation", Acta Mathematica, No. 7, Sept. 1885, pp. 259-380 [Oeuvre de Henri Poincare, Tome 7, Gauthier-Villars et Cie., Paris, 1951, pp. 40-140].

49 Prager, W., and Synge, J. L., "Approximations in Elasticity Based on the Concept of Function Spaces", Quart. Appl. Math., Vol. 5, 1947, pp. 241-269.

50 Ramey, G. E., and Krishnamurthy, N., "Error Estimates for Conforming Finite Element Solutions", Computers & Structures, Vol. 4, 1974, pp. 1207-1222.

51 Raviart, P. -A., Methode des Elements Finis, Lecture Notes (D. E. A. Analyse Numerique), Laboratoire d'Analyse Numerique, Universite Pierre et Marie Curie (Paris VI), 1972.

52 Richardson, L. F., "The Approximate Arithmetic Solution by Finite Differences of Physical Problems", Trans. Roy. Soc. London, A210, 1910, pp. 307-357.

53 Richardson, L. F., and Gaunt, J. A., "The Deferred Approach to the Limit", Trans. Roy. Soc. London, A226, 1927, pp. 299-361.

54 Schultz, M. H., "L^2 Error Bounds for the Rayleigh Ritz Galerkin Method", SIAM J. Numer. Anal., Vol. 8, No. 4, Dec. 1971, pp. 737-749.

55 Scott, R., "Finite Element Convergence for Singular Data", Numer. Math., Vol. 21, 1973, pp. 317-327.

56 Scott, R., "Optimal L^∞ Estimates for the Finite Element Method on Irregular Meshes", Math. Comput., Vol. 30, 1976, pp. 681-697.

57 Synge, J. L., The Hypercircle Method in Mathematical Physics, Cambridge University Press, Ltd., Cambridge, 1957.

58 Strang, G., and Berger, A., "The Change in Solution Due to Change in Domain", Proceedings of the A. M. S. Symposium on Partial Differential Equations, Berkeley, Academic Press, New York, 1971.

59 Strang, G., "Variational Crimes in the Finite Element Method", The Mathematical Foundations of the Finite Element Method with Applications to Partial Differential Equations, A. K. Aziz, Edtr., Academic Press, New York, 1972, pp. 689-710.

60 Strang, G., "Piecewise Polynomials and the Finite Element Method", Bull. Amer. Math. Soc., Vol. 79, 1973, pp. 1128-1137.

61 Strang, G, and Fix, G. J., An Analysis of the Finite Element Method, Prentice-Hall, Englewood Cliffs, New Jersey, 1973.

62 Tong, P., and Pian, T. H. H., "The Convergence of Finite Element Method in Solving Linear Elasticity Problems", Int. J. Solids & Structures, Vol. 3, 1967, pp. 865-879.

63 Utku, S., "Stiffness Matrices for Thin Triangular Elements of Nonzero Gaussian Curvature", AIAA Journal, Vol. 5, No. 9, Sept. 1967, pp. 1659-1667.

64 Utku, S., Instructor's Manual for Part II of Elementary Structural Analysis by Norris, Wilbur and Utku, 3rd Ed., McGraw-Hill Book Co., New York, 1976, pp. 91-97.

65 Utku, S., "Error Computation in Numerical Solutions of Linear Boundary Value Problems", Proceedings of the Second International Conference on Mathematical Modeling, University of Missouri, Rolla, Mo., July 1979, pp. 285-294.

66 Utku, S., and El-Essawi, M. M., "Error Computation in Finite Element Methods", Proceedings of the Seventh Conference on Electronic Computation, ASCE, New York, August 1979, pp. 584-592.

67 Wachspress, E. L., A Rational Finite Element Basis, Academic Press, New York, 1975.

68 Walz, J. E., Fulton, R. E., Cyrus, N. J., "Accuracy and Convergence of Finite Element Approximations", AFFDL-TR-68-150, Wright-Patterson Air Force Base,

Ohio, 1968, pp. 995-1027.

69 Watz, J. E., Fulton, R. E., Cyrus, N. J., and Eppink, R. T., "Accuracy of Finite Element Approximations to Structural Problems," TN-D-5728, NASA, Washington D. C., March, 1970, pp. 1-53.

70 Wilkinson, J. H., The Algebraic Eigenvalue Problem, Clarendon Press, Oxford, 1965.

71 Zlamal, M., "On the Finite Element Method", Numer. Math., Vol. 12, pp. 394-409.

72 Zlamal, M., "Some Recent Advances in the Mathematics of Finite Elements", The Mathematics of Finite Elements and Applications, Whiteman, Edtr., Academic Press, 1973, pp. 59-81.

CHAPTER TEN

STATUS AND TRENDS IN FINITE ELEMENT SOFTWARE

E. Schrem
Head, Software Development Section
Institute for Statics and Dynamics
University of Stuttgart
West Germany

ABSTRACT

The main subject of this chapter is large general purpose software systems. Their characteristic properties are defined and general considerations for their assessment and evaluation are presented. The prospects of their further development (including pre- and postprocessors) are estimated. The impact of progress in computer technology is discussed; in particular, low-cost computers, supercomputers, peripheral equipment and software tools. Software for nonlinear analysis is discussed together with special purpose software where particular attention is given to automated design, adaptive mesh refinement, and utilization of microprocessors. Joint software development activities in Europe are presented as examples of present software projects.

LARGE GENERAL PURPOSE SOFTWARE SYSTEMS

Characteristic Properties

During the past fifteen years finite element computer programs have popped up like mushrooms after a warm rain. Depending on the criteria for identifying a program, estimates of their total number vary between 600 and several thousand. Since 1970 several more or less comprehensive tables, data sheets, and bibliographies about finite element software have been compiled; the most important ones are Refs. [1, 6, 50]. Nevertheless, it can be safely assumed that ninety nine percent of all finite element applications are performed with less than thirty different programs. Among the particularly successful ones, the large general purpose software systems constitute an important subset due to the following properties:

1. Generality. A rich variety of functions and element types are provided such that virtually any actual linear analysis problem for any conceivable structure or continuum can be solved. In addition to linear static analysis, which still covers by far the majority of finite element applications, there are also integrated auxiliary features; in particular, dynamic analysis, heat transfer, and some important subdomains of nonlinear analysis.
2. Size. The source code comprises 100,000 to 600,000 Fortran statements as the result of a development effort that ranges from fifty to several hundred man years.

3. Wide international distribution. Each software system has between fifty and several hundred installations worldwide (e.g., ASKA is installed in Europe, United States, Japan, Comecon Countries, South America, Israel, India, and South Africa; NASTRAN has a similar distribution, including Australia; ASAS is installed in Europe, North America, and Australia).

4. Large user community. There are thousands of users in industry, data centers, consulting firms, research organizations, and universities.

5. Comprehensive support. In addition to the printed documentation (user manuals, training manuals, sample problems and test cases, programmer manuals) the following services are available: training courses, user meetings, hotline consulting, assistance by data centers and consulting organizations.

6. Portability. The code is generally written in Standard Fortran IV with only a few and carefully designed interfaces to the support functions of the host computer system. This facilitates the installation on a large variety of computer systems (e.g., ASKA is presently running on thirteen different computer systems manufactured by IBM, Amdahl, CDC, Univac, Honeywell, ICL, Burroughs, DEC, PRIME, PERKIN-ELLMER, and CRAY; ASAS is installed on a similar variety of computer systems).

7. Maintenance. There exist well-established formal mechanisms for program maintenance, including integration and quality assurance of software extensions, that are generally structured in several levels [2, 3, 4]. New versions are released at regular intervals (about one in one to two years) through these mechanisms.

Widely known examples of large general purpose finite element software systems are NASTRAN, ASKA, ASAS, ANSYS, MARC, STRUDL, SESAM, TPS10, and STARDYNE. It is not easy to terminate such an enumeration with the right program name because only the programs at the beginning of the list meet all seven characteristic properties without restriction, whereas towards the end of the list at least one property is not fully present (e.g., geographic distribution or portability). The list of large general purpose systems with a more limited distribution is even longer and will not be given explicitly in order to avoid the injustice of omission in borderline cases (this dilemma is passed to the authors of Chapter 12). Due to historical reasons, many companies in aerospace and nuclear engineering have developed in-house finite element programs of respectable size which are still in use (and sometimes there are also a few out-of-house installations).

It should also be mentioned that in many cases the basic name of a program system conveys little information without a specification of the version and the supporting organization. This is particularly the case for NASTRAN (where MSC/NASTRAN is by far the most important one outside the United States) and for STRUDL. This effect is mainly due to a combination of low price and unsatisfactory software support by the original distributing organization (SAP is the most drastic example: since price and support are almost zero, there are dozens of finite element software packages based upon SAP). Nowadays it is commonly recognized that the free distribution of software system without further software support will have this undesirable effect of mushrooming variants with uneconomical duplication of effort. As a result, the original policies of public funding of software development that incurred free distribution with zero support have fallen into a severe crisis.

Assessment and Evaluation

Due to their size and complexity, it is extremely difficult to evaluate and compare the features of large general purpose finite element computer programs. The International Symposium on Structural Mechanics Software in 1974 [1, 5] provided a valuable service to the profession by collecting a large amount of data about structural analysis software packages. Also, the information compiled by Fredriksson and Mackerle [6, 50] represents an important source of reference material. However, some caution is appropriate in comparing the features of various programs in tabular form, particularly when the information has been given directly or indirectly by the program developers. First of all, it is not possible to formulate in a standardized questionnaire all relevant features of a generalized purpose system in a way that permits an unbiased and unambiguous comparison with other similarly complex software systems. Furthermore, there is a strong temptation for the software developers to assure features by entering a "yes" in the questionnaire, all the more because there is no space for listing any "but".

As an extreme example, a friend of the author programmed, by himself, a finite element package of considerable size and generality. He was in a position to claim to be able to solve any static analysis problem, if necessary by adding some program modifications; thus he was able to solve quite impressive problems. The author is not aware of a single instance where the assurances proved to be a complete failure. This extreme "single programmer/single user approach" can be found quite frequently in university environments. With the advent of more powerful software tools (programming languages, database management, libraries of mathematical software, and low-price hardware) in the more distant future this approach will have to be taken more seriously as an alternative to the concept of very large monolithic general purpose software. Flexibility and economics of (small) size are quite strong arguments, but there are very serious unsolved problems with regard to software reliability, quality assurance, and transfer of technology to a larger user community.

Sporadically, assessments and comparative studies of major finite element software systems appear in the open literature. The comprehensive studies by Fredriksson and Mackerle (Linkoping University/AEC) [6, 50] and by Sollogoub, Wahl, and Dreyer (CTICM/CNEXO) [7] are particularly prominent ones due to their rich background material, and due to the obvious endeavours of the referees to be critical, objective, and evaluative. Since adequately performed comparative assessments are quite expensive, their publication can help to avoid unproductive parallel work. However, it is important to note that comparative lists of features become rapidly obsolete (often enough during the time in which a comprehensive study is in progress) because considerable effort is still spent for the continuous further development of the successful general purpose software systems. As a consequence, all serious authors refer to the original sources of information for getting an up-to-date picture of the situation. Also it should be mentioned that a universally valid, relative grading of large software systems is a safely failing enterprise.

Recently there appeared an exceptionally well-written paper by Taig [8] on selection criteria for structural analysis software. A particularly valuable argument in this paper expresses the fact that in the evaluation process the structure of the basic program deserves just as much attention as the analysis features themselves. This is of paramount importance in order to be able to add pre- and postprocessing software and to have ready access to intermediate data. The interfaces must be carefully designed and "remain stable as the program evolves to avoid obsolescence or, worse still, inaccuracy in the future." Taig also emphasizes the importance of continuity with respect to software development and support over a very long period of time.

Experience of other users can be invaluable, in particular if two criteria are met: first a good working knowledge of the software package in question (and, ideally, of a few more, too), and second, no direct responsibility for the selection of that particular system. On the other hand, users with a heavy commitment for the selection and further development of a particular software system can easily express just as enthusiastic views as the developers themselves. As a brief glance into any issue of Finite Element News makes immediately apparent, there is now a contest between software suppliers to coin the most impressive superlatives about their products.

TRENDS AND PROSPECTS

Software Development

During the last decade, assessments of the state-of-the-art and of further trends of finite element software have been a major topic of three excellent international conferences [9, 1, 5, 10]. Without exception, the large general purpose software systems have been in heavy use since the early seventies [11] and have left their teething troubles far behind. As a consequence, trend prediction in this field [47, 48, 49] has become a less perilous enterprise than it was ten years ago. This might explain why three papers [4, 12, 13] recently arrived independently at strikingly consistent views. Since at least two of these are easily accessible we will refrain from reiterating the topics in full length.

With respect to the "bread and butter" applications in industry, the features of general purpose software systems are already well established and tried in the field. The element libraries have become fairly standardized and the analysis procedures (solution of linear equations, eigenvalue extraction, numerical integration) are efficient and accurate. In this case we can observe a very strong convergence of features as each software system is continually improved in order to keep up with its competitors [12, 13]. The impact of academic research (including "unconventional" element models, adaptive discretization techniques, and structural optimization) upon the large software systems is almost nil, mainly because new results of research with a general field of application have become quite rare.

From a software engineering viewpoint the situation is far from being satisfactory. Although it is now commonplace that a large software system should be built upon a sound database concept and a good decomposition into functional modules, the knowledge of how this should be done for finite element software developed only gradually, with the growing experience gathered during the work on the existing systems. This is the main reason why in the important case of substructure analysis [14], "few systems are well structured ... and some are extremely cumbersome to use in the substructure mode" [8]. Reprogramming or patching the existing systems is of little help because the software engineering concepts affect the code throughout. An entirely new software system is the only feasible solution.

How good basic software tools can facilitate the development of finite element software has been demonstrated, at least in principle, by a relatively small team at the University of Illinois [15, 16, 43] which developed, on the basis of POLO II, an impressively comprehensive finite element software package. This encourages the previously expressed conjecture that some day the "single programmer finite element system" might become feasible.

Another promising concept is the programming system approach [3, 17, 18, 19, 20]. Enough work has already been completed to know that this is a feasible and quite attractive basis for developing new finite element software (at least from a purely technical point of view). The production software based upon a modern programming system can certainly compete with the established general purpose software systems with respect to computational efficiency. Programming is much simpler and software reliability and maintainability are considerably superior. Due to the open-ended concept the programs are easy to modify and extend.

Nevertheless, it is a striking fact that not a single new large finite element software system has successfully entered the market since the early seventies. It was observed some years ago [36] that in order to be adopted by members of the profession, new programs must be able to solve problems which cannot be solved by the established ones. However, up to the present day there are no important new problem areas in sight that could not also be implemented in the existing software systems (admittedly, not always in the most elegant way). The considerable financial risks in the development of a new finite element software system have been described recently in a quite impressive and convincing way [20a].

The marketing efforts required to launch a new large finite element software system would also incur investments that might easily surpass the development cost (which is in the multimillion dollar range) because users have learned to insist on guarantees for continuity in terms of software support and further development over five to ten years. These are expensive activities which are financially self-supporting only when a large user basis already exists (estimates arrive at a minimum of twenty installations, or the equivalent of heavy use in five to ten large corporations). This is also the reason why most large corporations have abandoned the further use of finite element software developed in-house in favor of using one of several of the commonly available software systems. Nevertheless, the investments of industry in the adaptation of out-of-house software to the particular requirements (user training and support, pre- and postprocessing, hardware configuration, and extension of analysis features) are very high [21]; in many cases they surpass the previous annual investments in in-house core systems. This certainly does not facilitate a shift to a new software system. The very large development costs and marketing risks will certainly preclude the advent of new large general purpose systems, at least during the next five years.

Pre- and Postprocessors

The situation is entirely different in the area of pre- and postprocessing, in which quite intensive software development efforts have to be expected in the future. Apart from considerable in-house developments in industry, there are also numerous software packages offered on the market, mainly by software houses, hardware manufacturers, and universities. The size of the packages is increasing continually; some are rapidly approaching the margin of 100,000 FORTRAN statements.

It is important to note that the boundary between kernel system and pre- and postprocessors is fuzzy by its nature. All large general purpose systems support pre- and postprocessing to some degree. Important design goals for kernel systems are portability, problem generality and coherence of features. Therefore, any software solution that involves hardware dependence (graphics) or loss of problem generality (specialization due to a higher degree of problem orientation) is necessarily the domain of satellite systems. This is the reason why the concept of kernel/satellite software appears to be universally accepted in finite element software.

A good satellite system which supports the user optimally in the model description and result interpretation has to possess a very high degree of problem orientation. Therefore, a "general purpose pre- and postprocessing system" entails a natural contradiction of design goals, all the more, because it is also the task of the satellite systems to integrate and adapt a broad variety of peripheral equipment (in particular for graphics). Little wonder that we have a much more complex situation than with the kernel systems (see Chapter 11 for the full story). This provides also a fair chance on the market for relatively small software development organizations. There is also a strong motivation for large user groups (e.g., structural analysis departments in industry) and for hardware manufacturers to develop their own pre- and postprocessors which, in most cases, can be interfaced with a large number of different kernel systems. Together with cheaper and more powerful peripheral equipment the coming years will bring considerable cost reductions due to improved, problem-oriented pre- and postprocessing.

IMPACT OF PROGRESS IN COMPUTER TECHNOLOGY

Since Chapter 16 discusses in detail the impact of new computing systems on finite element technology, we will restrict ourselves to the aspects that appear to be relevant from the viewpoint of a developer of large general purpose software systems.

Low-Cost Computers

Since minicomputers appeared on the market it has been an intriguing question as to how they could be utilized in finite element analysis. Whereas they have been in use for pre- and postprocessing from the very beginning, it was obvious that they were not suited for large general purpose software due to their limited central storage capacity and their slow floating point arithmetic. The earliest investigations of the prospects of minicomputers go back to 1968 [25]. A conclusion was reached which is all the more valid today: It is wasted effort to spend large investments on software development to accomodate serious hardware restrictions. Such software will be superseded within a few years due to the rapid progress of hardware technology.

The situation changed as soon as minicomputers with larger address spaces and faster arithmetic appeared [22, 23] that at the same time promised considerably better cost-effectiveness than the existing large mainframes [24, 44]. In particular, the new computers with 32-bit word length, very large address spaces, and fast hardware or firmware floating-point operations (the DEC VAX 11/780 and the PRIME computers are presently the most familiar ones in our field) promised to change quite drastically the market for large-scale finite element software [25, 13]. With respect to storage capacity and computing power, these new machines resemble the big mainframes of the early seventies more than the minicomputers of that time. Therefore, the large general purpose packages can be installed on them with relatively little effort. For instance, at ISD we installed the static analysis part of ASKA on a PRIME 550 within two weeks (after a few enhancements of the basic system utilities that required another six man weeks). With regard to library management, binding, and loading, the PRIME computers are presently superior to any other computer system on which ASKA is installed.

These computer systems provide the economic benefits of mass fabrication and LSI technology to the end user. They could be characterized as low-cost computers although a realistically powerful finite element analysis system still requires investments for hardware in the range of 200,000 to 450,000 dollars. This is mainly due to the need for large backing storage and other peripheral equipment (e.g., for graphics). However, the entrance ticket for finite element analysis on a minicomputer system will soon be as low as 60,000 dollars with the option of continually upgrading the hardware configuration according to the growth of the analysis work.

The opportunity of running the same finite element software system on a large machine (often via teleprocessing) and on a local minicomputer provides a high degree of freedom to the user in allocating the analysis work in an optimal way. This is particularly attractive for structural analysis departments in industry in order to emancipate themselves from the constraints that are often imposed on them by large centralized computer departments. There is also a very great potential for finite element analysis in smaller firms where in-house hardware for engineering analysis was cost prohibitive.

The generally expected big breakthrough in low-cost computer systems has not yet happened to the expected extent. One explanation refers to the fact that the field is prudently observing the further evolution of prices and technology. As more competitors are rapidly entering the market, some further reduction of prices can duly be expected. However, there is also an additional explanation that will be relevant for many years to come - a hugh education gap. For performing finite element analysis in an effective way, we need structural analysts who also possess considerable data processing skills. The notion of a black box analysis system, into which the user feeds a description of a structure together with supports and loads and after some computer runs gets a complete answer to his problem, is simply a misconception, even if we include the best of all conceivable pre- and postprocessing systems.

In most real life situations of finite element analysis the interesting part of the game starts just after the first results have been obtained. There is a good potential for obtaining an improved insight into the structure's behavior by repeating an analysis under varied conditions (new load cases; modified support conditions, geometry or material; or appending some dynamic or nonlinear analysis). As long as the finite element mesh is not changed considerably, a skilled analyst can add such analysis iterations at a cost which, apart from computer time, is small in relation to the cost of the first analysis. In this case he must be able to administer, access, and update his input data, intermediate data, and results inside his computer system in a highly professional way. This is also the reason why plenty of secondary and archival storage is required for effective work. In large computer centers the user can rely upon the support of experienced specialists; on his own minicomputer system he must act as data processing expert by himself. Just some experience in FORTRAN programming is certainly not sufficient.

At present there is an extreme shortage of structural analysts with a good background in data processing. Structural analysts who have always worked with tables, code books, and desktop calculators need intensive additional training in data processing in order to keep up with the changing technology. Consulting firms and education centers still have a big market for service. In the aerospace department of our university we have installed a curriculum where about 25 percent of the lectures and exercises for engineering students are devoted to data processing. The majority of the graduates have been soaked up by industry for work in finite element analysis, and the demand far surpasses the supply.

Supercomputers

The design goal of increasing central processing speed through large-scale parallelization led to the architectural concepts of array computers and pipeline processors in the early sixties (the ILLIAC IV and CDC-STAR computers are early examples of actual realizations). It has been known from the beginning that the utilization of these concepts for anything near their maximum processing speed requires major changes in software and algorithmic thinking. At first glance, finite element analysis requires enough numerical operations of a highly repetitive character to make parallel architectures worth an indepth investigation. However, it is well known that the majority of finite element applications are I/O bound on contemporary, fast, sequential machine architectures. Therefore, it is sensible to utilize even faster arithmetic processors only if the speed of data transmissions is increased accordingly.

Highly parallel machines that have become available more recently, such as the ICL DAP (which is integrated into central memory) [27], or the CRAY computers (which also offer a very high speed for scalar operations), have attracted considerable interest from the developers of large finite element software. For the ICL DAP we arrived at the conclusion that ASKA could be adapted with a relatively small effort just by reprogramming about six low level subroutines. This result is mainly due to the particular structure of the data modules in ASKA (hypermatrices [28, 19, 20]) and is, therefore, not necessarily valid for other software systems. On the CRAY computers large general purpose finite element software systems have already been installed with acceptable effort. For the nonlinear software system ADINA on CRAY1, time ratios with respect to CDC 7600 of three to six (unmodified program) and six to eleven (modified program for vector processing) have been reported [42]. This report estimates that with improved I/O capability a speed ratio exceeding twenty and a cost ratio of 1/7 relative to CDC 7600 will be possible. For the CRAY computers, with their high scalar processing speed and optimizing FORTRAN compilers, it is quite likely that utilization of only a fraction of the theoretical maximum speed will be considered satisfactory (avoiding the technical and financial risks of major software modifications). This was the case for the CDC 6600 (and 7600) computers, where maximum utilization of instruction stack and/or parallel processing units was frequently sacrificed in favor of retaining software compatibility with other architectures.

The high processing speed of supercomputers is worth detailed consideration. In contrast to some critical real time applications where higher processing speed is absolutely essential, in finite element analysis we are primarily interested in better overall turn-around time (i.e., the time between submitting the job and receiving the results). In a highly multiprocessing environment with a large number of users competing for the hardware resources (which is mandatory due to the high price of supercomputers) only a few privileged users can expect that the turn-around time will not be substantially longer than the accumulated processing time. At contemporary, heavily loaded, large computer centers a common complaint is that the larger finite element runs have a turn-around time that is orders of magnitude longer than the CPU time. This is different only for computer systems that are loaded with only a fraction of their full processing capacity.

This leads to the economic aspects. Supercomputers are only of interest for finite element analysis if, compared to other machines, they provide faster turn-around times at about the same cost level, or substantially lower processing costs at about the same turn-around time (or both). For the next five years we can safely assume that the accumulated finite element processing on low-cost machines will be substantially larger than the total of finite element processing on supercomputers.

Peripheral Equipment

With respect to direct access backing storage the situation is far from being satisfactory. This has been a problem since we have had electronic computers. Electromechanical storage devices (disk drives) have approached their technological limits with respect to recording density, access time, cost-effectiveness and, last but not least, reliability. Long-term backing storage (permanent disk files) is an important cost factor at present in finite element analysis, and its reliability causes major problems in work on large projects. Also, speeding up the data transmissions between backing storage and central memory could improve throughout and response times to its full extent on nearly any computer system that is presently used for finite element analysis. The advent of all-electronic storage devices with large capacity, high reliability, environment independence (temperature, moisture, dust), high speed, and good cost-effectiveness has been expected for several years, and it will have an even stronger impact on finite element analysis than contemporary low cost computers.

Add-on array/vector processors that can be attached to a computer as peripheral devices in order to speed up the numerical operations have been on the hardware market for several years. They are particularly attractive for minicomputers, provided that the accuracy of the floating point number representation is sufficient (i.e., a mantissa length of at least 32 bits or, even better, a double precision option that is compatible with the data format of the central processor). The necessary software modifications are analogous to those for the ICL DAP (see above).

Finally, it should be mentioned that we expect cheaper and more powerful graphic devices with comprehensive local intelligence (microprocessors, large local storage). This will improve engineering analysis productivity due to better pre- and postprocessing [29]. The present trend towards standardization in computer graphics will also reduce portability problems of software for pre- and postprocessing.

Software Tools

The prospects for further progress in basic software engineering tools [51, 52] (in particular, advanced programming languages and database management systems that are suited for CAD) are rather discouraging. We will have to be content if in the near future we can be sure that standard FORTRAN 77 is implemented properly on all computer systems of interest. Our present software tools are still mainly text editors, FORTRAN compilers, various loader software (binders, linkage editors, segment generators, overlay systems), command languages, and file systems. For very large software projects it is still worth the effort to invest some work in improving (or even replacing) some of these tools on a particular machine. This is a serious obstacle for the highly desirable shift to smaller, more intelligible and better manageable software packages.

Whether the new programming language Ada [53, 54] could really improve the quality and productivity of program development in the near future is still highly controversial [55, 56]. In the author's opinion the situation here is quite similar to the situation in the late sixties with regard to PL/1. At that time we decided not to replace FORTRAN by PL/1 for the development of finite element production software, and only from hindsight we can say that this decision has been correct. In the future we would certainly not abandon FORTRAN in favor of Ada unless Ada will be successfully implemented on all computer systems that are of interest for finite element analysis.

NONLINEAR AND OTHER SPECIAL PURPOSE SOFTWARE

Nonlinear Software

A program could be characterized as general purpose when it allows problems from a general domain to be solved without the necessity of modifying the source code due to particularities of a problem (in our case: topology, geometry, material, kinematic constraints, loads, time-dependence) [7]. As a consequence, no special particularities of the problem may be implicitly contained in the code. This is a crucial point in software for nonlinear finite element analysis. Rightly enough, for the two nonlinear software systems that have been prominent for many years, MARC and ANSYS, the developers offer comprehensive user support and consulting services. This is absolutely necessary because the user is dependent on detailed knowledge about theories, algorithms, and assumptions behind the program features. Considerable experience is necessary for the selection of models and algorithms, as well as for monitoring the iteration steps. There are also many problems where it is desirable to modify the program.

Software for nonlinear analysis cannot be developed by merely extrapolating successful design concepts of general purpose system for linear analysis [30]. This is the reason why the latter includes only such nonlinear analysis features for which their general software philosophy is well suited (e.g., elastoplastic analysis, linear buckling, some areas of large displacement analysis). For a general purpose system there is an inherent conflict of interests between the software developer, who wants to implement only well-established methods for solving "reasonably" nonlinear problems with a general field of application, and the researcher in nonlinear analysis, who is interested in handling the "most interesting nonlinear problems" not too rarely with a highly speculative haut gout: large rotations plus several hundred percent strain plus incompressible material plus instability, preferably all combined.

The best software engineering concepts available are just good enough in developing a useful product for nonlinear analysis. Unfortunately, just the opposite is the reality in many places. There are only a few institutions where experts in nonlinear analysis and software engineers cooperate closely. We all know the researcher who believes in all innocence that several thousand hours spent with the computer in FORTRAN-programming his algorithms and element models (in order to produce examples of highly academic interest) were sufficient qualification for turning out a useful product for the software market, taking care of the software engineering aspects with his left hand, while working on the nonlinear algorithms with his right hand. It is not too exaggerated to say that software engineering lacks due recognition in the nonlinear analysis quarters of academia.

The rapid expansion of linear finite element analysis in industry resulted in a growing request for solving nonlinear problems, also far outside the pioneering industries (aerospace, nuclear engineering and defense) that have big research budgets. There are many users (e.g., in the car industry, offshore technology, and soil mechanics) who are looking for software packages or who have even started their own software development. In many respects the situation resembles that of pre- and postprocessors: good programs are not necessarily bulky (10,000 to 40,000 FORTRAN statements can be sufficient), and good problem orientation as well as excellent user support are extremely important. We can, therefore, expect that in the future a larger number of flexible special purpose programs for highly nonlinear analysis will evolve, together with the experts that are capable of utilizing them effectively.

Automated Design

In order to affect the design, model definition and results of finite element analysis must be coupled to the data that are relevant to the various links in the design chain [13]. For the large general purpose systems this is considered to be an important task of pre- and postprocessing. Highly automated communication is necessary in order to be able to obtain structural analysis results in the early stages of product development where design modifications are still relatively cheap. Many in-house developments in industry are aimed at closing this communication gap. The lack of good general purpose database software for CAD is responsible for a large amount of unproductive parallel work.

Automated optimization of structures is still confined to the research environment (with a few exceptions, e.g., detail design of special parts). The necessary access to internal data and the iterative nature of optimization favors the utilization of relatively small finite element programs with simple data structures and limited problem size. Also, small minicomputer systems (in the price range of 10,000 to 50,000 dollars) that are operated off-line in the design office are quite attractive for that purpose.

Adaptive Mesh Refinement

There are two ways to refine a finite element mesh (and thus increase the number of degrees of freedom in the model). Either the number of elements in the mesh can be increased (reducing a size parameter h that describes the maximum element size), or more basis functions per element can be used (increasing the order p of the polynomial shape functions for displacement models). Thus there are two extremes for establishing convergence to the exact solution. In the h-convergence process the mesh size parameter h is reduced and the element order p is kept unchanged (thus utilizing more elements of the same order). In the p-convergence process the order of the elements p is increased without changing their arrangement in the mesh (thus keeping the mesh size parameter h unchanged). Both convergence processes have numerical and practical limitations: the h-convergence process eventually results in loss of significant digits as the condition number rapidly increases with decreasing h. The difficulties associated with increasing p are mainly increasing connectivity (bandwidth), coarser representation of geometry, and problems with the representation of boundary conditions, stresses, and displacements.

It is a very old experience (recently also supported by theoretical investigations) that p-convergence is considerably faster than h-convergence in most applications. However, there are also reasons for using lower order elements. Therefore, most general purpose systems offer both first- and second-order elements in their libraries (higher order elements are quite rare), and most experienced analysts avoid combining elements of different orders in the same mesh unless there are very strong reasons for doing so (see Chapter 3 for more detail).

The idea of integrating into software more or less automated procedures for mesh refinement is nearly as old as finite element analysis itself. However, it is critically dependent on the availability of economic and feasible criteria for the local discretization error. Progress in this area has to be considered as the most important short-term benefit of the on-going research in adaptive techniques. Effective indicators of the local discretization error are a highly desirable feature in finite element software systems, and software extensions for supporting an improved reanalysis are certainly conceivable.

On the other hand, a high degree of automatization of adaptive mesh refinement would affect a finite element software system in many critical parts, even up to the satellite processors. We can predict with little risk that automated mesh refinement will not be available as an integrated feature in the large general purpose software systems. At least the p-convergence method can be implemented conveniently in satellite processors [34, 35]. From a software point of view, it is a considerable advantage of the p-convergence method that the basic element mesh is not changed during the adaptation process. The general problem and data structures are thus not affected, and the evolving additional degrees of freedom can be easily processed in satellite software. This is due to the fact that the rigid body modes are already constrained in the initial solution. Therefore, the additional unknowns can be determined in a cheap and accurate way by iterative methods [34].

The p-convergence method also has the advantage that the coarseness of the finite element mesh will be limited mainly by the precision that is required for modeling the geometry and boundary conditions. This can result in considerable reduction of the data preparation effort (although not for all applications).

Postprocessing will be seriously affected due to the necessity of interpolating the final results. On the other hand, the h-convergence method will always affect the mesh generation. Reanalysis without changing the core software is certainly more expensive; however, postprocessing is possible with existing software.

Adaptive mesh refinement is most attractive in some special applications. Fracture mechanics is a good example [34]. From a software point of view fracture mechanics should be supported by satellite processors anyway (e.g., modification of length and direction of the crack, calculation of various integrals). It seems to be a good strategy to begin the investigation and development of software concepts for adaptive discretization techniques by developing appropriate special purpose programs.

Utilization of Microprocessors

Large scale integration in conjunction with mass fabrication yields microprocessors with excellent cost effectiveness. Processing speed and memory size are large enough that the utilization of microprocessors for finite element analysis has been under serious investigation since about 1975. There are two basic possibilities: to use a single microprocessor for rather limited problems, or to integrate in some way a very large number of microprocessors in order to obtain an extremely powerful finite element machine.

The first alternative is quite straightforward. The microprocessor is just the heart of a cheap microcomputer system that includes a keyboard with CRT display for the user/system communication, floppy disks and cassettes for secondary and archival storage. Several finite element software systems have already been developed for such a configuration (see [6, 31, 32, 45, 46] and Chapter 12 for more recent examples). The price for the hardware (including a CRT display, floppy disk storage and a mechanical printer) is presently in the range of 15,000 to 50,000 dollars. A prominent example is the WANG 220 series, which offers a sufficiently accurate data format (13 decimal digit mantissa) and a CPU speed of roughly 1,000 floating point operations per second. The software is generally coded in Basic. Software portability is extremely low since the special features of a particular microcomputer system have to be fully utilized. More comprehensive packages are organized as chains of program modules that can be executed in sequence; also, overlay techniques are used to a large extent.

The typical mode of operation is single user/interactive, thus providing a finite element desktop computer. Initially, the software packages were developed for (and often in) small civil engineering offices; however, there are other interesting areas of application, e.g., for analyzing crude models in the early design phase or for checking out more detailed computations. It can be expected that the successful packages will extend their chain of program modules further into all relevant areas that are typical for desktop computing. Rather than a finite element software system with pre- and postprocessing, we will then have a general library of analysis and design programs that includes a few finite element modules also.

The second alternative for utilizing microprocessors is aimed at very high computing power by organizing the work of a very large number of microprocessors within a single system. This is basically an array computer concept with relatively intelligent array elements. Present experimental array sizes are typically in the range of 16 and 256; however, if useful results are obtained, the arrays could be considerably larger. The fundamental problems of array computers, synchronization of the parallel processing, and organization of the data exchange between the array elements, require the development of new algorithms, and new program and data structures for finite element analysis.

One approach is to develop an array architecture where the communication between the microprocessors, as well as their synchronization, would accomodate, as far as possible, the particular requirements of finite element analysis [33]. The result is then a special purpose computer for finite element analysis. Many software engineering problems of finite element analysis are thus handed over to the computer architects. In technical discussions the author had the strong impression that the computer architects are now intimately concerned with the same problems which we had to solve on the software level, i.e., design decisions about structuring the element routines (closed form/numerical integration), assembling the higher level discretization matrices (connectivity problems), methods for solving the linear equations (direct or iterative), and data structures. Since, at least for linear analysis, we have been able to reduce the basic program and data structures to only a few, rather simple and consistent concepts [20], it can be expected that the computer architects will also arrive at a quite effective design.

Another approach is to begin with an existing architecture that is more of a general purpose nature [27]. Due to the larger market potential, it can be expected that the hardware is much cheaper than in the previous approach. However, the architectural constraints require considerable effort for the software design. Most likely, entirely new concepts for structuring both programs and data are required. The advent of microprocessor arrays has also stimulated new interest in iterative techniques for solving the load/deflection equations [36, 30].

EXAMPLES OF JOINT SOFTWARE DEVELOPMENT ACTIVITIES

We can certainly not venture to make a worldwide instantaneous record of all present projects for finite element software; simply to collect all relevant information would take so much time that the resulting picture would be obsolete. We restrict ourselves rather to presenting a few examples that could have some influence on the development of software for research work in Europe. There are a very large number of research projects in finite element analysis that are primarily supported by a variety of public funds and which continue to contribute to the software confusion. Each isolated project is not large enough to yield a proper software package that could be passed to users in industry in order to provide effective and rapid transfer of technology. As the primary emphasis (and funding) of the research work is concentrated upon analysis methods, the main goal of programming is just to obtain, within a minimum of time, the results of sample studies for publication. In no way does this mean that the amount of programming and computer time spent on those projects is small. The lack of flexible, well structured, basic software requires that existing programs be patched in an inefficient and error-prone way. In many countries millions of dollars are wasted every year in parallel and unproductive programming work that does not yield useful software for the desirable transfer of technology from research to applications.

The problem was recognized independently in several countries a long time ago and there have been several plans for improving the transfer of technology (e.g., the National Software Center in the United States). The most comprehensive effort to coordinate software development for finite element analysis in research institutions is the Club Modulef, which was established in 1975 in France [38]. At present, the Club Modulef has 72 members, the majority being research institutes and universities. To obtain the objectives of the Club Modulef, it is essential that among its members we find a heavy preponderance of applied mathematicians and numerical analysts (only a minority belong to engineering departments). About one quarter of the members are located outside France (Canada, Spain, Switzerland, Germany, Italy, Netherlands, United States, Mexico, Israel).

The Club Modulef

The Club Modulef is a nonprofit organization with its official headquarters at INRIA (Institut National de Recherche d'Informatique et d'Automatique, F 98150 Rocquen Court), and it is managed by a president (nominated by INRIA) and a controlling committee of twelve members. Each member has access to all computer programs in the library for his own scientific work and retains the full property rights of the codes which he makes available to the Club. The Club Modulef takes no responsibility for the distributed programs, including their documentation and maintenance. The legal construction of the Club makes commercial software distribution quite difficult since there is an inherent conflict between the principle of software sharing and the fact that every contributor retains the full property rights to his own programs. If a member wants to make the software available outside the Club, he needs the consent of all members that have property rights in the modules that are required in addition to his own programs.

In Modulef the notion of a program module is similar to that of a functional module in NASTRAN or of a processor in ASKA. There are standards for calling, programming, and insertion of modules [39]. An impressive variety of modules have already been implemented, including:

a) modules for mesh generation (comprehensive tools, in particular for two-dimensional continua)
b) equation solvers (skyline Cholesky, Crout and Gauss; wavefront; hypermatrix Cholesky)
c) eigenproblem solvers (inverse iteration with shift, inverse subspace iteration, Lanczos method, Householder tridiagonalization)
d) integrators (predictor-corrector, Runge-Kutta, multistep)
e) two-dimensional viscous incompressible fluid motion.

This brief list of major modules highlights the orientation of Modulef towards providing a research tool for numerical analysis. The concepts for the implementation of finite element models also differ specifically from those in general purpose software aimed at analysis in industry. The user can control the element formulation according to the variational approach, the interpolation functions, the metric, and the method of numerical integration. In concordance with this philosophy the element library comprises at present only elements for two- and three-dimensional continua (heat transfer and elasticity). For future development the following features have been announced: more mesh generators (in particular for three-dimensional continua), new element types (plates, shells, membranes), structural optimization, fluid mechanics, graphics, and substructure analysis.

Unfortunately, data management is somewhat underdeveloped. There are tools for dynamic storage allocation in central memory and for communication with secondary storage (sequential and paged direct files). Sixteen basic data structures are standardized and documented in detail [40]; the construction of additional data structure is also described [39]. However, the level of abstraction for handling the data appears to be insufficient. In particular, the overall control of data organization on a level above the individual data modules is missing. Therefore, too many details of structuring the data have to be handled explicitly in the program modules, down to pointer arrays for partitioned data. The data can be kept on a variety of external files; a notion of a uniform data base on long term storage seems to be completely lacking. This is not in favor of handling large complex problems, and implementation of substructure analysis will not be easy. Nevertheless, the Club Modulef appears to be quite a successful organization for coordinating the development of software in research institutions, and an impressive amount of work has already been done (Ref. [38] contains forty references).

Coordinated Software Activities in Sweden and Germany

A similar need has been realized in other countries. In Sweden a study group financed by STU (the Board for Technical Development) has been established in order to investigate possibilities of integrating the software development for finite element analysis. This group presently concentrates its attention on the various methods for data management [41]. This is certainly the core problem, and the approach to its solution will determine the feasibility of the whole project. Basically there are two extreme possibilities. The first approach is to couple relatively large programs similarly to the way that pre- and post-processors communicate with core programs. Internally the programs would retain their methods of data organization, and existing software packages could be included without major modifications. The second approach is to start with a data base concept that is tailored to the requirements of finite element analysis. Drawing from the experience with existing software, we are now in a much better position than ten years ago for developing the appropriate tools. Unfortunately, this would require reprogramming the whole software nearly from scratch, and this is presumably cost-prohibitive.

The same dilemma has been encountered in recent efforts towards coordination of the software development in Germany, originating in the "Schwerpunkt nichtlineare Berechnungen im konstruktiven Ingenieurbau," sponsored by DFG (Deutsche Forschungsgemeinschaft). The costs for developing a large, entirely new software system could certainly not be justified. However, the development of a relatively small package of software tools that can be used for checking out new nonlinear algorithms is presently being discussed. It has also been proposed to utilize one or more of the nonlinear software systems that are already in a highly advanced state of development (e.g., LARSTRAN 80 [26]) as a tool for research and education.

Software development in research environments could certainly be much better coordinated and more effective if there were standardized software tools for data base management of technical data implemented on all major computer systems. Since such a data base management system for efficient support of both interactive graphics and finite element analysis does not yet exist, we will have to wait for an organization which is willing to invest the necessary millions for its development.

REFERENCES

1 Pilkey, W., Saczalski, K., and Schaeffer, H., Structural Mechanics Computer Program, University Press of Virginia, Charlottesville, 1974.

2 Henrywood, R. K., "The Design, Development and Support of a Major Finite Element System," Computer Aided Design, Vol. 5, 1973, pp. 160-165.

3 Schrem, E., "Development and Maintenance of Large Finite Element Systems," in Pilkey, W., Saczalski, K., Schaeffer, H. (Eds.), Structural Mechanics Computer Programs, University Press of Virginia, Charlottesville, 1974, pp. 669-685.

4 Swanson, J. A., "Present Trends in Computerized Structural Analysis," Computers and Structures, Vol. 10, 1979, pp. 33-37.

5 Schaeffer, H. G., "A Review of the International Symposium on Structural Mechanics Software," Computers and Structures, Vol. 8, 1978, pp. 589-598.

6 Fredriksson, B., and Mackerle, J., "Overview and Evaluation of Some Versatile General Purpose Finite Element Computer Programs," in Robinson, J. (Ed.), Finite Element Methods in the Commercial Environment (Proceedings of the World Congress, October 1978, Bournemouth), Robinson and Associates, Dorset, pp. 389-419.

7 Sollogoub, P., Wahl, L., and Dreyer, F., "Main Computer System Programs, Presentation, Criteria for Selection," CNEXO/CTICM, 1978 (to be obtained from: CNEXO, B.P. 337, F-29273 Brest, or CTICM, 20 rue Jean Jaures, F-92807 Puteaux).

8 Taig, I. C., "Selection Criteria for Structural Analysis Programs," AGARD Report No. 670, January 1979, NATO-AGARD, Neuilly sur Seine, France, pp. 11-20.

9 Fenves, S. J., Perrone, N., Robinson, A. R., and Schnobrich, W. C., Numerical and Computer Methods in Structural Mechanics, Academic Press, New York, 1973.

10 Noor, A. K., and McComb, H. G., Trends in Computerized Structural Analysis and Synthesis (Proceedings of the Symposium, Oct. 30-Nov. 1, 1978, Washington, D.C.), Pergamon Press, Oxford, 1978.

11 Spooner, J. B., "A History of the Finite Element Method," in Robinson, J. (Ed.), World Congress on Finite Element Methods in Structural Mechanics (Oct. 12-17, 1975), Robinson and Associates, Verwood, 1975, pp. A1-A22.

12 Schrem, E., "Trends and Aspects of the Development of Large Finite Element Software Systems," Computers and Structures, Vol. 10, 1979, pp. 419-425.

13 MacNeal, R. H., "One Man's View of Trends in Finite Element Analysis," in Gloudeman, J. F., and Rosahoff, R. E. (Eds.), Computational Aspects of the Finite Element Method, Bundesanstalt fur Materialprufung, Berlin, 1979, pp. 1-19.

14 Noor, A. K., Kamel, H. A., and Fulton, R. E., "Substructuring Techniques - Status and Projections," Computers and Structures, Vol. 8, 1978, pp. 621-632.

15 Lopez, L. A., "FINITE: An Approach to Structural Mechanics Systems," International Journal for Numerical Methods in Engineering, Vol. 11, No. 5, 1977, pp. 851-866.

16 Dodds, R. H., Lopez, L. A., and Pecknold, D. A., "Numerical and Software Requirements for General Nonlinear Finite Element Analysis," University of Illinois, Urbana, 1978.

17 Bell, K., Hatlestad, B., Hansteen, O. E., and Araldsen, P. O., "NORSAM - A Programming System for the Finite Element Method," SINTEF, Trondheim, 1973.

18 Mo, O., Klem, H. F., Pahle, E., Harwiss, T., "Finite Element Programs Based on General Programming Systems," Computers and Structures, Vol. 8, 1978, pp. 703-715.

19 Schrem, E., "From Program Systems to Programming Systems for Finite Element Analysis," in Bathe, K. J., Oden, J. T., and Wunderlich, W. (Eds.), Formulations and Computational Algorithms in Finite Element Analysis (Proceedings of the U.S.-German Symposium, Aug. 9-13, 1976, Boston), MIT Press, 1977, pp. 163-190.

20 Schrem, E., "Programmbausteine und Datenstrukturen fur die Implementation der Methode der finiten Elemente," Dissertation, Universitat Stuttgart, 1978.

20a Soerensen, M., "A Case Study Based on TOPAS," in Robinson, J. (Ed.), Finite Element Methods in the Commercial Environment (Proceedings of the World Congress, October 1978, Bournemouth), Robinson and Associates, Dorset, 1978, pp. 1-6.

21 Andrew, L. V., "Rockwell International's Subcommittee for Computerized Structural Analysis," AGARD Report No. 670, January 1979, NATO-AGARD, Neuilly sur Seine, France, pp. 1-9.

22 Storaasli, O. O., "On the Role of Minicomputers in Structural Design," Computers and Structures, Vol. 7, 1977, pp. 117-123.

23 Swanson, J. A., "Use of Minicomputers for Large Scale Structural Analysis Programs," Computers and Structures, Vol. 7, 1977, pp. 291-294.

24 Storaasli, O. O., and Foster, E. P., "Cost Effective Use of Minicomputers to Solve Structural Problems," Proceedings of the AIAA/ASME Conference on Structures, Structural Dynamics and Materials, Bethesda, Maryland, April 3-5, 1978, Paper No. 78-484.

25 Schrem, E., "ASKA auf Minicomputern," in Pahl, P. J., Stein, E., and Wunderlich, W. (Eds.), Finite Elemente in der Baupraxis (Proceedings of the Conference, April 13-14-1978, Hannover), Wilhelm Ernst und Sohn, Berlin, 1978, pp. 338-343.

26 Hermann, P., Knudson, W., and Schneider, S., "Considerations for the Design of Programs for Nonlinear Finite Element Analysis," in Gloudeman, J. F., and Rosanoff, R. A. (Eds.), "Computational Aspects of the Finite Element Method," Bundesanstalt fur Materialprufung, Berlin, 1979, pp. 177-178.

27 Streiner, P., and Schrem, E., "Vielzweckprogramme fur die Methode der Finiten Elemente und Neuere Tendenzen der Rechnertechnologie," in Finite Element Congress (Proceedings of the Conference, Nov. 13-14, 1978, Baden-Baden), IKOSS, Stuttgart, 1978, pp. 67-76.

28 Schrem, E., "Computer Implementation of the Finite Element Procedure," in Fenves, S. J., Perrone, N., Robinson, A. R., and Schnobrich, W. C. (Eds.), Numerical and Computer Methods in Structural Mechanics, Academic Press, New York, 1978, pp. 79-121.

29 Romans, G., Iveson, F., and de Groot, H., "Graphic Systems and Their Effect on the Finite Element Method," in Robinson, J. (Ed.), Finite Element Methods in the Commercial Environment, Robinson and Associates, Dorset, 1978, pp. 518-530.

30 Schrem, E., "Structural Aspects of Software Systems for Nonlinear Finite Element Analysis," in Bergan, P. G., Larsen, P. K., Pettersson, H., Samuelsson, A., Soreide, T., and Wiberg, N.-E. (Eds), Finite Elements in Nonlinear Mechanics, TAPIR, Trondheim, 1978, pp. 621-645.

31 Backx, E., Rammant, J. P., and Schymkowitz, G., "Case Study on Desk Computers: Finite Element Analysis in Basic," Proceedings of the Second World Congress, Robinson and Associates, Dorset, 1978, pp. 670-680.

32 Backx, E., Rammant, J. P., and Schymkowitz, G., "Interactive Engineering Software for Desktop Computers," Finite Element Systems Seminar, June 6-7, 1979, Southampton.

33 Jordan, H. F., and Sawyer, P. L., "A Multi-Microprocess System for Finite Element Structural Analysis," Computers and Structures, Vol. 10, 1979, pp. 21-29.

34 Peano, A., Pasini, A., Riccioni, R., and Sardella, L., "Adaptive Approximation in Finite Element Structural Analysis," Computers and Structures, Vol. 10, 1979, pp. 333-342.

35 Szabo, B. A., "Adaptive Finite Element Software Systems Based on P-Convergence," in Gloudeman, J. F., and Rosanoff, R. A. (Eds.), Computational Aspects of the Finite Element Method, Bundesanstalt für Materialprüfung, Berlin, 1979, pp. 99-113.

36 Wilson, E. L., "Special Numerical and Computer Techniques for the Analysis of Finite Element Systems," in Bathe, K. J., Oden, J. T., and Wunderlich, W., (Eds.), Formulations and Algorithms in Finite Element Analysis, Massachusetts Institute of Technology, Boston, 1977, pp. 3-25.

37 Zhongyue, F., "An Outline of the Aeronautical Structural Analysis System HJFX-I," Aircraft Strength Research Institute, Shaaxi PRC, 1979.

38 Begis, D., and Perronnet, A., "Presentation du Club MODULEF," October 1979, IRIA Domaine de Voluceau, F-78150 Rocquencourt.

39 Perronnet, A., "Normes d'Appel, de Programmation, d'Insertion des Modules," October 1977, IRIA Domaine de Voluceau, F-78150 Rocquencourt.

40 Perronnet, A., "Description des Structures de Donnees," February 1979, IRIA Domaine de Voluceau, F-78150 Rocquencourt.

41 Fredriksson, B., Petersson, H., Tägnfors, H., Johansson, Th., Bengtsson, A., and Oppelstrup, J., "Samordnat Specifikationsprojekt Inom FEM-Omradet," STU-Project 79-3188, Lägesrapport 790901, ITM, Stockholm, 1979.

42 Oakes, W. R., and Browning, R. V., "Experiences Running ADINA on a CRAY-I," in K. J. Bathe (Ed.), Nonlinear Finite Element Analysis and ADINA, MIT Report 82 448/9, 1979, pp. 27-41.

43 Dodds, R. H., and Lopez, L. A., "A Generalized Software System for Nonlinear Analysis," in Adey, R. A. (Ed.), Engineering Software, Pentech Press, Plymouth, 1979, pp. 55-77.

44 Foster, E. P., and Storaasli, O. O., "Structural Analysis on a Minicomputer," in Adey, R. A. (Ed.), Engineering Software, Pentech Press, Plymouth, 1979, pp. 43-54.

45 Collington, D. J., and Adey, R. A., "An Engineering Problem Solving System for Small Computers," in Adey, R. A. (Ed.), Engineering Software, Pentech Press, Plymouth, 1979, pp. 78-93.

46 Backx, E., Rammant, J. P., and Schymkowitz, G., "Interactive Engineering Software for Desktop Computers," in Adey, R. A. (Ed.), Engineering Software, Pentech Press, Plymouth, 1979, pp. 161-179.

47 Schrem, E., "Finite Element Software in the Next Decade," Proceedings of the World Congress on Finite Element Methods in Structural Mechanics, Robinson and Associates, Verwood, 1975, pp. R.1-R.18.

48 Gallagher, R. H., "Computerized Structural Analysis and Design - The Next Twenty Years," Computers and Structures, Vol. 7, No. 4, 1977, p. 495.

49 Nagy, D. A., "Software Engineering for Finite Element Analysis," Journal of the Structural Division, ASCE, Vol. 104, No. ST8, August 1978, pp. 1287-1298.

50 Fredriksson, B., and Mackerle, J., Structural Mechanics Finite Element Computer Programs, Linkoping Institute of Technology, S-58183 Linkoping, Report LiTH-IKP-R-054, 1978.

51 Howden, W. E., "Contemporary Software Development Environments," ACM, Vol. 25, May 1982, pp. 318-329.

52 Wassermann, A. I., and Gutz, S., "The Future of Programming," ACM, Vol. 25, March 1982, pp. 196-206.

53 Ichbiah, J. D. (Ed.), Reference Manual for the Ada Programming Language, U.S. Dept. of Defense, Advanced Research Projects Agency, 1980.

54 Barnes, J. G. P., "An Overview of Ada," Software - Practice and Experience, Vol. 10, 1980, pp. 851-887.

55 Hoare, C. A. R., "The Emperor's Old Clothes," ACM, Vol. 24, February 1981, pp. 75-83.

56 Ledgard, M. F., and Singer, A., "Scaling Down Ada," ACM, Vol. 25, February 1982, pp. 121-125.

CHAPTER ELEVEN

APPLICATION OF INTERACTIVE GRAPHICS AND OTHER PROGRAMMING AIDS

I. Grieger
University of Stuttgart
West Germany

H. A. Kamel
University of Arizona
Tucson, Arizona

ABSTRACT

The subject of pre- and postprocessing of finite element data, sometimes called "auxiliary finite element techniques," has gained importance over the last several years. Preprocessors include model generation, model display and verification, model editing, and node and element renumbering. Postprocessing is concerned with representation of results. Computer graphics and interactive processing play a central role in the activities. Most present day auxiliary finite element software is not readily portable and is too dependent upon a particular display device or a specific analysis program.

INTRODUCTION

The intensive utilization of the finite element method led to the development of suitable pre- and postprocessors which save time in data preparation and representation of results. Since various hardware and several finite element codes are used, it is desirable that pre- and postprocessors be hardware-independent and appropriate for different finite element programs. Integrated interactive structural analysis seems to be the current trend [1]. In going beyond analysis to the associated automatic model generation and presentation of results, the process changes from that of "computer analysis" to "computer-aided analysis". An increase in the computer costs over what is necessary for the analysis itself is to be expected, but the resulting savings in labor and the faster response usually more than compensate for the additional expense.

The use of interactive systems to enhance the man-machine dialog has grown dramatically during the past years. Further increase in the use of display consoles is expected in the future. In addition to the development of appropriate hardware, improved programming techniques have been introduced. A system for man-machine communication consists of the user (who plays an important role and must remain in control), the computer system (hardware) and the program (software). Often, the hardware is given and the problem of successfully incorporating the user into the process can only be solved with an appropriate system design.

In this context one has to distinguish among several functions associated with what one may call "auxiliary finite element software". Preprocessors perform such tasks as geometry definition, geometry discretization (mesh generation), model display and verification, model editing, node and element renumbering as well as load and boundary condition definiton. Postprocessing is concerned with interpretation of results.

Many commercial organizations (mainly software houses and hardware manufacturers) are developing and marketing packages aimed at finite element model manipulation. Some of these aim at enhancing a specific analysis program. Others are linked to a specific hardware product designed to support popular finite element programs. The third group of programs is independent of both hardware and analysis programs. There are obvious advantages and disadvantages to each alternative.

Apart from the development of user-oriented pre- and postprocessor software, research efforts have been directed at some fundamental points associated with mesh generation and software engineering. Among the subjects addressed are algorithms for geometry definition, discretization of irregular shapes, and a new and promising subject, grid optimization.

The process of model generation is by no means divorced from that of computer-aided design and computer-aided manufacturing. It has long been recognized that an integration of the functions of design (synthesis) and analysis would represent an ideal working environment. Although this is indisputable in principle, its practical implementation is not straightforward by any means, and attempts to construct a formal link between a design database and analysis programs for complex objects have been typically costly and laborious. It is in the nature of complex systems that an increase in size brings with it a decrease in reliability and flexibility. We may still see some success in such integration attempts, but an acceptable solution will only be possible after significant advances are made in computer software design technology, and more effective use is made of available hardware.

INTERACTIVE GRAPHICS HARDWARE

Computer graphics hardware belongs to one of two main categories: interactive and passive. Interactive graphics devices are represented by the different types of cathode ray tubes and associated input equipment (e.g., light pen, digitizer). Passive graphics devices include mainly plotters and microfilm recorders, which have existed for many years and are required for many pre- and postprocessors.

The graphics display hardware [2] is of most interest here, and some assessment of their relative merit is in order. Three important types of interactive graphics devices can be distinguished:

1 Refresh vector displays,
2 (refresh) raster displays,
3 storage displays.

The refresh vector display (e.g., Adage, Evans & Sutherland, Vector General, Megatek) is the most sophisticated. It can have powerful hardware features such as graphical transformations, zooming, clipping, etc. The picture which is stored in the display buffer must be refreshed at a certain rate in order to produce a steady image. A disadvantage of a refresh vector display is that the amount of graphical information that can be drawn at any one time is limited by the size of the display buffer and the speed of the display processor. On the other hand, depending on the programming technique, any part of the picture can be changed without erasing the entire screen. For interactive work, the input of information from the display console to the computer is significant. An important device for the feedback from the user to the computer on a refresh display is the light pen, which is a light-sensitive graphical device. The light pen has two functions: picking and tracking. Picking may be used to select a graphics entity, to identify a displayed entity or to activate a light button for program control. Tracking may involve the placing of a tracking cross (or a similar light source) at any desired position on the display surface in order to allow the user to address the screen, to place a graphics entity, or to designate that position as an area of interest. This operation can also be performed on a data tablet with a stylus.

In addition to the analog input devices there also exist other advantageous devices such as the alphanumeric keyboard and function keys. The latter can be used to request a particular operation from the application program using illuminated keys. On the other hand, the alphanumeric keyboard provides a typewriter-like symbolic input to the applications program.

Television technology is the basis for raster display devices (e.g., Ramtek, Hewlett-Packard, Tektronix), which are also refreshed. The refreshing of the picture is done scan line by scan line from a memory buffer which contains an image of the raster picture. Most of the structure of the picture is lost when it is transferred to this buffer. The raster display is normally equipped with indirect graphical input devices, such as a joystick, knobs, tracking ball, rolling mouse, tablet, etc., to position a cursor on the display surface. The position of the input device can be read in hardware coordinates. Some raster displays can be addressed with a light pen. Also, the selective erasure of individual display elements is feasible.

The storage display (e.g., Tektronix) is a special form of a cathode ray tube which does not require refreshing. The picture is retained flicker-free until it is erased. The storage display is, like the raster screen, only equipped with indirect graphical devices. The function of the light pen is taken over by a graphics cursor. The amount of display is unlimited, and new information may be added at any time. The main disadvantage of storage tube displays, however, is the fact that selective erasure is not possible. The generation of the display is slow in comparison to the refresh displays. Therefore, the erasure of the screen should be kept down to a minimum for the convenience of the user. To introduce dynamic features to the display, the so-called "write through" capability is added to storage tubes. The capabilities of the work station influences directly the convenience and, therefore, the acceptability by the user [3].

For some work stations a piece of hardware for the input of data from drawings or sketches is important. The digitizer is a tablet of the size of a drawing board. Graphical information can be digitized directly from a drawing, placed on the tablet, and stored in the computer. Some digitizers can also be used as plotters and vice versa.

For the different types of display, various configurations of interactive station and computer are possible. A simple solution (which is realized in turnkey systems) is the connection of a cathode ray tube to a small computer (Fig. 1a). The display processor as well as the display buffer can be separate or in the memory of the small computer if a refresh display is used. The simulation of a display buffer for storage displays, where it is not necessarily needed, also has great advantages for interactive work.

If the display is based on a storage tube (or a raster tube where refreshing is done at the display terminal), there are no timing problems associated with picture-refreshing. Therefore, telephone lines can be used to transmit the picture (Fig. 1b).

The timeshared, large computer (Fig. 1c) contains a powerful central processor and a large core memory. It also contains large random-access auxiliary disk storage. Various types of activities may be serviced concurrently. Remote graphics consoles make use of their local computing power when possible. The central computer is only called upon when large-scale computation, or access to the central data bank is needed. At the same time, batch processing may be performed in the background. The timesharing of several consoles on a common computer has several advantages [4]:

1 The power of the large computer and the large memory facilities are available for the individual console.

2 Timesharing gives all consoles access to a common data bank, avoiding duplication of data and programs in individual smaller computers.

3 Timesharing can provide communication between consoles.

However, timesharing seems to become more difficult with graphics consoles because of the high demand placed by the display of large complex problems.

Due to the variety of hardware encountered in industry, the application software may operate in any one of the following configurations:

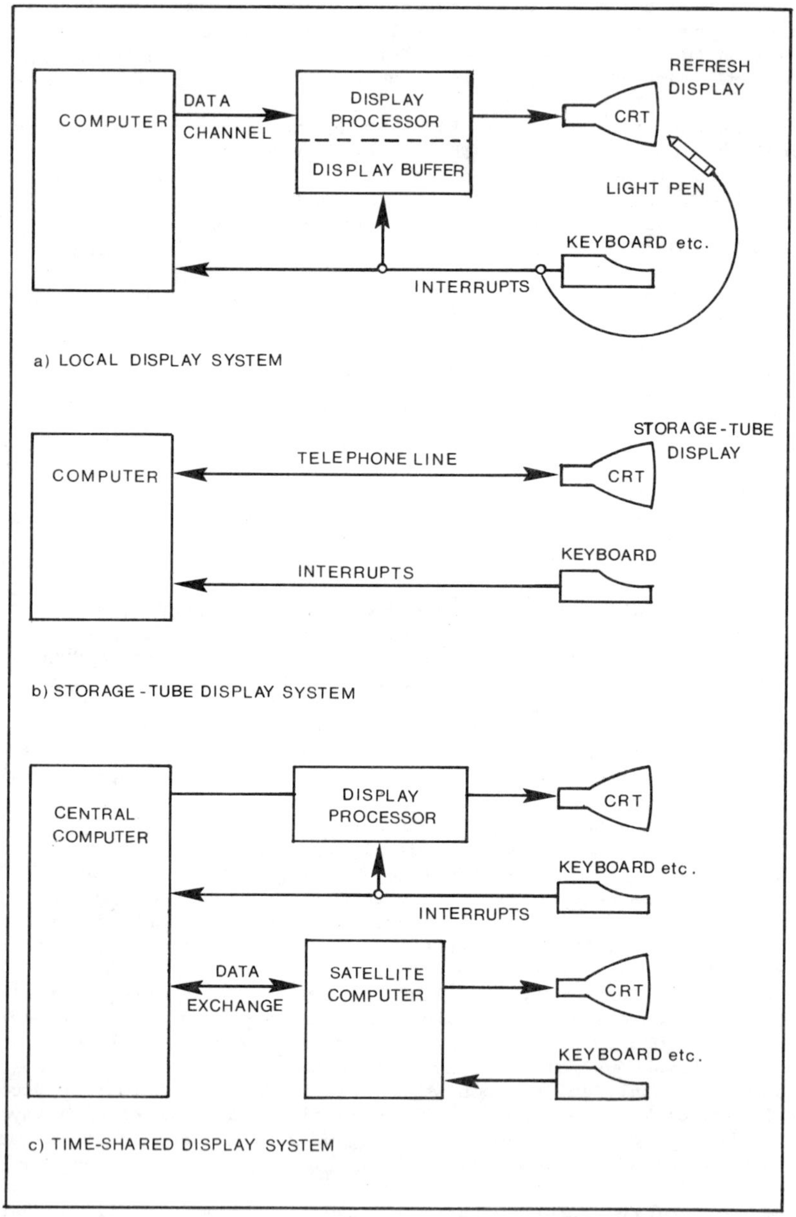

Fig. 1 Interactive Display Systems

1 Small computer with display,
2 Large computer with display,
3 Large computer with intelligent graphics terminal.

In the latter configuration, where a large computer is connected to a small computer with a graphics console, some operations are performed on the large computer and others are executed on the small one. Finite element pre- and postprocessing may be preferred on a stand-alone graphics system, with the data transferred to and from the main computer where the anaysis takes place.

INTEGRATED STRUCTURAL ANALYSIS

The procedural steps which are explained in this section are basic to setting up design criteria for general purpose pre- and postprocessors. The idealization of a given structure is always the first step in the analysis process. The actual structure is replaced by a collection of finite elements, and thus is replaced by an idealized or computational model. Following the conceptual idealization of the structure, the necessary input data (e.g., coordinates, geometric data, loading) must be prepared. The preparation of the input data for a complex structure is a time-consuming operation and will most likely contain errors. The error diagnostic system of a modern finite element program will automatically detect most of the data input errors before extensive computation has been carried out. However, some typical user errors (e.g., wrong nodal point coordinates, wrong element connections, overlapping elements) would not be detected in this manner. In these cases a graphical representation of the structure is invaluable.

Structural analysis, which is accomplished interactively in many cases, consists of three major parts:

1 Preprocessing (problem description, model generation, checking and modification),
2 Intermediate processing (program control over the various computation steps, evaluation of intermediate results),
3 Postprocessing (representation of results).

The concept of integrated structural analysis is shown in Fig. 2. A finite element program needs input data (nodal point coordinates, element connections, degrees of freedom, loads, geometric and elastic data, etc.). The results of the computation (displacements, stresses, vibration modes, plastic zones, crack propagation, etc.) are output on various devices. In the traditional analysis environment the input data are on punched cards, and the output is produced on a line printer. Today, plotters and microfilm output devices are heavily used in the structural analysis field. The input of data for computational purposes, as well as special output processing, involves the use of interactive graphics. A typical input device is the digitizing tablet. However, digitizing of large volumes of data is tedious, and methods have been developed for the semiautomatic or automatic digitizing and scanning of data. Alternatively, the relevant data are taken from a common geometric (design) data bank.

In the design of general purpose pre- and postprocessors for finite element programs incorporating graphics, the following points should be taken into account:

1 There exists several finite element programs, each with its own points of strength.
2 Finite element computations are performed on a large variety of computer and graphics hardware (refresh, storage, raster displays, plotters, etc.). Sometimes different hardware exist within the same organization.
3 Many of the pre- and postprocessing operations apply to different engineering disciplines.

It is advantageous, therefore, that pre- and postprocessors should be largely independent of hardware, finite element programs and engineering

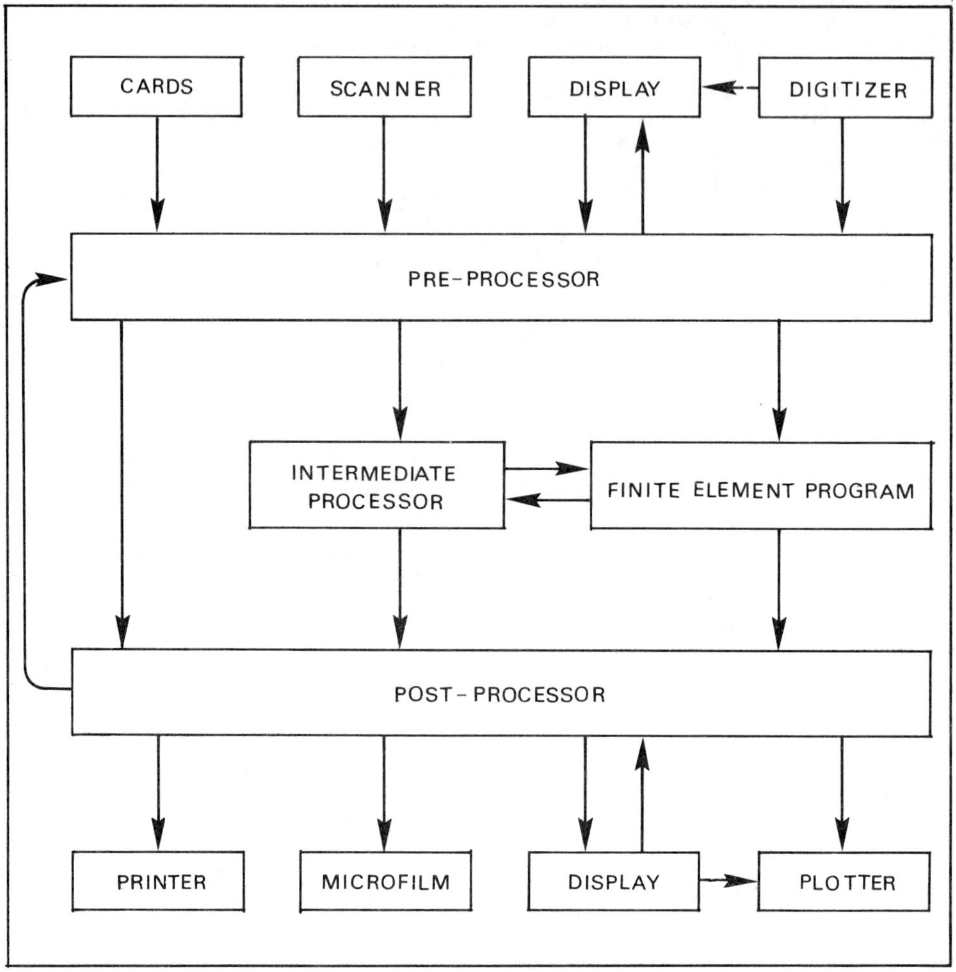

Fig. 2 Integrated Structural Analysis

disciplines. In spite of this, specialized programs in this field have their place. (Pre- and postprocessors are often application-dependent in order to produce efficient software solutions.) The programs should be modular and flexible so that extensions and alterations may be introduced without difficulties. Efficiency, software reliability and maintainability (see Chapter 10) are also important for the user acceptance of pre- and postprocessors.

All large finite element systems support pre- and postprocessing to some degree. Pre- and postprocessors are offered by software houses, hardware manufacturers and universities. The material compiled by Frederikson and Mackerle [5] represents an important source of information about the program. Some caution is necessary, however, in comparing the features of various programs (see also Chapter 10). Users' conferences organized by hardware manufacturers, as well as by large finite element system developers, are a source of information. Papers related to pre- and postprocessing are also presented at software and computer-aided design conferences and published in professional journals.

PREPROCESSING

Preprocessing comprises all activities associated with preparing, generating, checking, and altering the data before the main structural analysis is performed. Programs have been written (see [6]) to

1 generate nodal point coordinates,
2 generate element connectivities,
3 generate boundary conditions,
4 generate nodal and distributed loads,
5 generate geometric and elastic data,
6 check data for syntax and reasonableness,
7 display and plot data,
8 renumber nodal points to reduce the bandwidth,
9 prepare connectivity data for the coupling of substructures,
10 transform input data into a format suitable for the analysis program.

In preparation for a finite element analysis, the process of model geometry generation has two distinct stages. First a mathematical definition of the geometry is accomplished, and then the discretization process is carried out.

Geometry Definition

The definition of the geometry of a structure is the basis of all mesh generation programs (see Fig. 3). In creating the geometric model, mathematical methods for the representation of curves, surfaces, and bodies, typical of those employed in computer-aided design may be used. Some of the methods used in the description of two-dimensional domains (plane and curved surfaces) for analysis purposes are based on mathematics used in finite element computations. A typical example is to be found in isoparametric element formulation. Such methods are usually not as sophisticated as those used in surface design, producing discontinuties in slopes and curvatures at patch boundaries. They are nonetheless popular due to the familiarity of the analysts with their formulation, the associated ease of implementation, as well as their ability to describe discontinuous geometry. Although these methods are generally adequate, it has been found in certain applications, such as the analysis of arbitrary shells, that the results may be extremely sensitive to curvature, thus encouraging the use of the more sophisticated formulations for these purposes.

Curves

Plane and space curves may be defined in parametric form [7,8]. For curves of greater complexity a piecewise continuous parametric representation is necessary. The most popular one is the cubic curve [9] due to its ability to incorporate points of inflexion. Also the mathematical spline (in its simplest form) [10, 11] leads to a series of cubic curves joining at the points where the curves are continuous in position, slope and curvature. Of the many possibilities for parametric representation the Bezier [12] and B-spline [13,14] curves may be mentioned. The Bezier method of representation, originally developed for the French automobile industry, derives the parametric shape of a particular curve from a so-called control polygon connecting n + 1 vertices. The resulting parametric curve of order n passes through the two endpoints and is tangential to the polygon's first and last sides. The shape of the control polygon influences the shape of the curve. The control exerted by the polygon is global in the sense that change of the position of one of the points will produce a change of the shape of the curve overall. If relatively few points are used in the polygon, the control of the shape of the curve is good. If the Bezier curve is based on several segments, the problem of geometric continuity between the segments arises.

The B-spline approximation avoids many of these shortcomings. This approach is based on polynomial splines (basic splines) in which the Bezier formulation

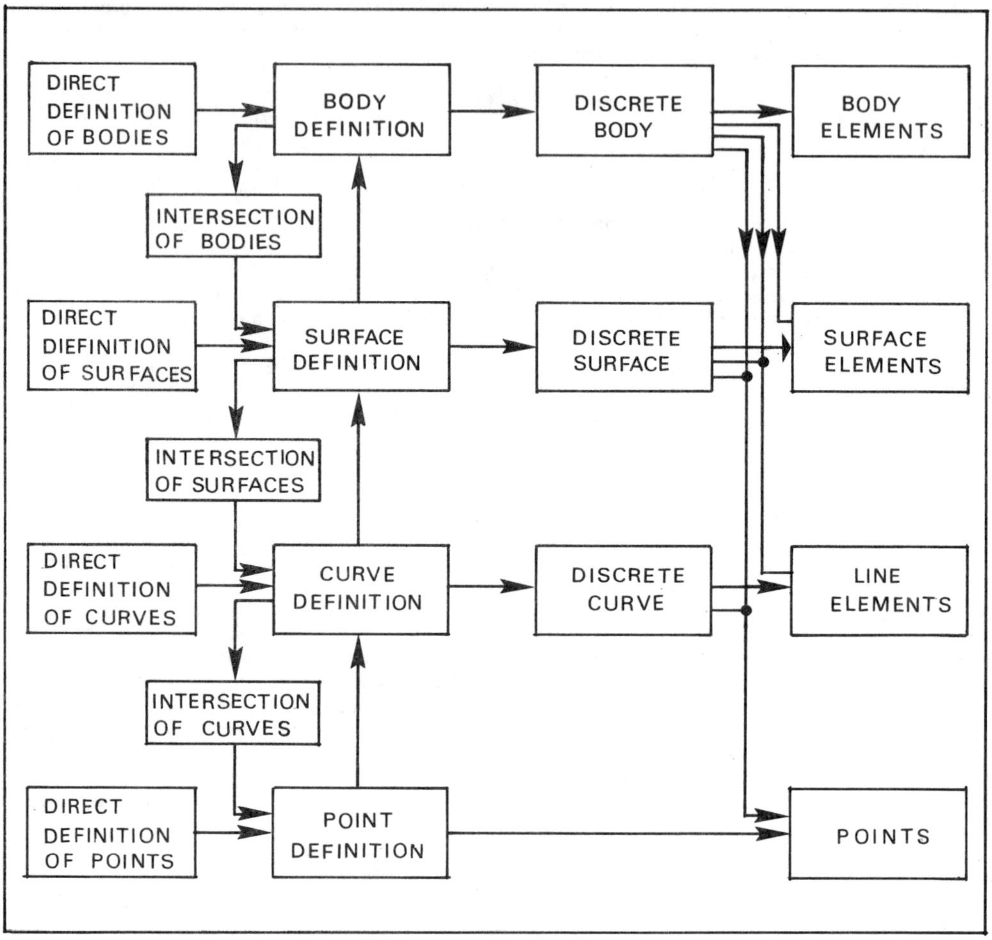

Fig. 3 Possible Paths in Model Generation

is incorporated as a subset. The B-spline curve is also based on a control polygon. The blending functions involve the fitting of a piecewise continuous curve and provides for continuity of geometric derivatives at segment boundaries through constraint conditions. It has local control, so that the effect of moving a point on the shape of the curve applies only to the immediate neighborhood of the point. It is possible to form closed or open curves, as in the case of the Bezier method, and introduce discontinuities in the derivatives. Many positive features of the B-spline curves (and surfaces) make their application attractive in computer graphics.

Surfaces

The representation of surfaces is an important feature in computer-aided geometric design of many engineering objects, such as aircraft, cars and ships. Among the various possibilities the most powerful are the nonanalytic surfaces. It can be stated that the techniques for curve generation may also be extended to surfaces. Parametric forms, as well as the approximation of a surface by patches, lead to a method of surface definition which can be carried out interactively. Three main surface definition techniques can be distinguised [15]: Cartesian product surfaces (e.g., bi-cubic surface [7,9], two-dimensional spline interpolation [16, 17], Bezier surfaces, B-spline surfaces and finite elements), lofting surfaces (the surface is defined by a set of, usually, planar curves [18], such as cross-sections of a fuselage or waterlines and transverse offsets of a ship), and the boolean summation of transfinite surfaces (e.g., Coons surfaces [19], Gordon's extended surfaces [20], which are interpolated by meshes of curves using spline blending functions and triangular surface patches [21]).

A number of publications address the question of curve and surface description for various applications. The automobile industry uses both Bezier surfaces and B-splines. Coons surfaces [22], splines [23], and B-splines [24] are applied in the definition of ship hull geometry. The problem of surface fairness is solved, for example in [24], in an elegant way by taking the curvature into account. A major research effort at Cornell University is described in [25]. Among the subjects discussed are methods for representation of three-dimensional surfaces using interactive graphics.

An example of the use of cubic splines as a basis for mathematical surface definition, followed by a finite element analysis, is given by Liu [26]. He describes an approach by which the smoothness of the surface generated for arbitrary curved shell analysis may be optimized using the unknown twist vectors at the patch corners as controlling parameters.

Bodies

The definition of three-dimensional solid objects is mainly used for computer-aided design in mechanical engineering. The term often used here is geometric modelling [27], which may use several forms of representation. The line model is well-suited for the generation of technical drawings. Further possibilities are the surface model and the volume model, which are easily perceived by the designer, who may visualize bodies where parts are added or subtracted. In this case, techniques of set theory can be applied. Generally, one would say that geometric operations can be performed on geometric objects. Interactive manipulation [28] is also important in mechanical engineering design.

Input of the Geometry

Techniques for the input of the geometry of a three-dimensional object into the computer often rely on the interactive use of digitizers and tablets. The digitizing of data, on- or off-line, is an activity which needs high user concentration. The error rate increases rapidly with elapsed time. It is important, therefore, that error recovery is possible. Again, automation of the process should result in minimization of the required manual digitization [29]. Future research may be directed at designing hardware to perform automatic digitizing and software to convert the information to the correct format required for the description, which may be performed interactively at the time of design, removing the need for drawings as a method of object definition.

There are several ways to display a solid. For complicated solids various pictorial views are required for a complete understanding of the structure. Orthogonal projections are well-established requirements in the field of engineering design. With this type of drawing the length, breadth and depth coordinates of a solid are fully represented by at least two views which are sufficient for digitization [30, 31, 32, 33, 34]. The main problem, however, is the assembly of a solid from various views [35]. An interesting development [36] is the use of several pens on the digitizing tablet. One pen can be placed in one view, and the other can be used for digitizing of data in the other view. The digitizing of key points in various views gives a three-dimensional transformation matrix. The digitizing of the subsequent data produces three-dimensional coordinates.

The digitizing of points gives insufficient information about the structure. Additional information is needed for the use of the digitized data in finite element preprocessors [37].

Finite Element Mesh Generation

Many papers exist which deal with mesh generation algorithms (see the survey in [38]). In this section we deal primarily with methods for the automatic subdivision of complex geometric configurations into elements and the associated computation of the position of intermediate grid points. The simplest and most widely solved problem is the two-dimensional one, in which a complex shape or an interconnected set of domain shapes is subdivided into triangular or quadrilateral subdomains. Next in degree of difficulty is the problem of definition and discretization of three-dimensional surfaces which may be interconnected. The additional problems arise from the need to determine a method for the definition of the location of the surface in space, as well as the fact that several surfaces may intersect along the same curve. At such intersections surface parameter continuity may be required, although not necessarily. Finally, we have the case of three-dimensional solid continua, where a body bounded by such surfaces may be subdivided into a number of tetrahedron, pentahedron or hexahedron elements.

The model creation involves both mathematical definition in continuous form and subsequent discretization into finite elements (subspaces). The procedure by which this may be accomplished is not unique and may take several forms, as is evident from Fig. 3. It is possible, for example, to generate continuous forms for both curves and surfaces and then discretize both independently. Since the curves form the surface boundaries, care must be taken that the discretization is compatible. Alternatively, one may proceed from a continuous curve directly to a discrete curve format and use this information to form the discrete surface (patch) without necessarily providing a continuous surface definition. It is also possible to define curves in discrete form directly by digitizing point by point and then proceed to generate discrete forms for both surfaces and solids.

Another approach evolves from disregarding the natural geometric hierarchy and proceeding directly to the definition of the surfaces in continuous form. Once the surfaces have been defined, their intersection is computed, thus defining their boundary curves as well as the form of the solids bounded by them. All of the above approaches have their advantages and disadvantages. A truly general purpose model generation program should allow all possible paths so that the user may choose whichever approach may best suit his particular problem.

Turning to mesh generation, the algorithms can be classified into different groups. One approach is based on topologically regular meshes, needing a parametric partition [39, 40, 35, 41, 42, 43, 44, 46, 47, 48, 49, 50, 51, 52]. In some methods the subdivision of a two-dimensional domain into triangular elements results in an irregular mesh [53, 39, 54, 55, 56, 57, 58]. The problem of mesh refinement [59, 60] is also important. However, the use of natural coordinates [61, 62, 63] is independent of the manner of mesh generation. Cook [64] develops and uses the concept of "natural coordinates" to generate surface and volume grids. Another effort based on the same concept is presented by Aral [65]. A process for checking solid models by means of computing and displaying the intersections of the elements of the model with a series of planes is described in [66].

A method of subdividing a two-dimensional area bounded by an arbitrary polygon into triangular elements is given by Bykat [60]. The method subdivides the area first into a number of convex subregions. This is followed by an automatic preconditioning of the boundaries by introducing additional boundary points to eliminate sudden changes in grid spacing. Automatic boundary refinement is applied at re-entrant corners. Finally, all convex regions are triangulated, producing well-shaped elements. A two-dimensional mesh generator with many interesting features is described by Gabrielson [67]. It is based on the definition of multi-connected four-sided regions (i, j grids) in which intermediate points are computed by linear interpolation. It accepts input alphanumerically via the terminal in the form of data cards, digitizer output or directly from a larger geometric database intended for computer-aided manufacturing.

Some authors present attempts at developing a language to be used as a means for input description. An early attempt was associated with the initiation of the ASKA program [68]. In a more recent example, the SAIL language [69], developed at Boeing Aircraft Co., is a FORTRAN-like structural input language which generates input data for several finite element programs. Silvester [70] describes the MAG-NET language, which is a tool for the description of finite element models. It allows geometric and topologic changes, unions of separate models, and addition and removal of model constituents. Input may be through a keyboard or graphics cursor. It is designed particularly for repetitive structures. A mesh generator based on B-spline curve representation [71] uses a command language for the generation of points, lines, circles and various other curve and surface types. It has the ability to calculate surface intersections.

Best results can be obtained with an interactive mesh generation program [72, 73, 74, 75, 76, 77, 78] because the user can control the mesh size on the screen. The mesh can be generated partly by the program and partly by the user in an interactive mode.

Other efforts deserve attention. An excellent example of a special purpose mesh generation program is one developed by Leick and Potvin [49]. An analysis program was written to handle tubular joints (which are prevalent in offshore tubular structures). The associated mesh generator produces a fine grid near stress concentration areas and a course grid far away from them. The grid characteristics are defined in terms of few parameters. Kalkani [79] describes a mesh generation program for highway excavation cuts. Line, triangular and quadrilateral elements are automatically generated by straight-line interpolation for the nodes and increments for the elements. Another example is an algorithm by Preiss [80], which checks topological consistency of plate and solid models. It is part of an in-house NANSAP preprocessor. In problems where model geometry changes due to chemical reactions or physical phase changes, such as models with ablating boundaries, the problem of automatic model generation is further complicated. Weeks and Cost [81] propose an algorithm for tracking such boundaries, in conjunction with an automatic mesh generator, and a finite element program for the calculation of transient thermal and stress analysis of such structures.

Renumbering of Nodes and Elements

In most programs a bandwidth or wavefront optimizer is necessary to reduce subsequent solution times [82, 83, 84, 85, 86]. A method of renumbering elements in order to achieve improved storage in preparation for a frontal solution, and other methods not requiring a stiffness assembly, is given by Bykat [87]. It presents a modification of the Cuthill-McKee algorithm [88] and requires a reasonable choice of the first element. Gray et al [89] describes two methods for automatic renumbering of nodes for water network analysis. The method for nodes can be extended to finite element programs and is aimed at the minimization of matrix fill during the solution process.

Mesh Optimization

Among the most interesting areas of current research in model generation is that of mesh optimization [90, 91]. Here the stress is on devising the optimum mesh configuration for a particular element type and an approximate number of degrees of freedom in order to obtain an optimum solution for the problem at hand. It is obvious that a clear definition of what constitutes an optimum solution is necessary. It will be found, for example, that high accuracy in a peak stress value, achieved by an optimized grid, may be associated with poor deflection results. It is also obvious that a grid may be optimum for one specific loading case but far from it for another.

A paper by Turcke and McNeice [92] introduces the node coordinates of the mesh as independent unknowns in the finite element variational formulation. The solution, which is based on a minimization of the potential energy of the system, provides both displacement values as well as new node coordinates. Certain constraints have to be imposed on the node relocation to ensure meaningful results.

Caroll [93] extends grid optimization to the area of vibrational mode computation. He shows that a different optimum grid is associated with each mode. Saad and Turcke [94] and Melosh and Killian [95] show the superiority of an optimized mesh over one obtained by uniform refinement. The introduction of additional freedoms and elements is allowed in [95], based on local solutions to study the effect of element subdivision. Denayer [50] extended some algorithms given in [39] for the generation of topologically uniform grids. The mapping process from a parent grid to the area under consideration is chosen so as to achieve certain optimal conditions which translate into a variational formulation lending itself to a finite element solution. Carey [96] presents a method for selective refinement of a finite element mesh near an area of interest. Lagrangian constraints are used to maintain continuity with the rest of the model. Results show good convergence in the solution of the Poisson equation with a singularity in two dimensions.

POSTPROCESSING

Postprocessing comprises all manipulation and display activities of the results after the structural analysis has been performed. Programs have been written (see [6]) to:

1 display and plot results (displacements, stresses, strains, bending moments, residual loads, reaction forces, etc.) in various presentations,
2 generate and display contour lines,
3 compute and display principal stresses,
4 display the deflected shape of the structure,
5 display vibration mode shapes,
6 generate time history displays of deflections and stresses,
7 display element stresses and/or print stress values adjacent to the elements on the display surface,
8 prepare plots and tables suitable for inclusion in reports summarizing the analysis,
9 superpose loading cases to produce results for various loading combinations,
10 extract maximum stress value and stress excesses,
11 select data for display,
12 extract data for use by subsequent processing programs,
13 convert output data into a format suitable for another analysis program.

This list should show only the variety of operations for which postprocesses are used. Many postprocessors are batch plotting programs. However, an interactive display program is more advantageous than a passive postprocessor. Although postprocessing is often directly related to preprocessing, special display techniques are often employed at this stage.

Contouring of stress and deflection results is a useful and popular postprocessing operation. Reference [97], for example, gives a FORTRAN program which admits several subregions, each divided into triangular or quadrilateral elements. The problem of contouring within higher-order element boundaries is mathematically intriguing. An initial effort has been conducted by Akin and Gray [98], in which they lay out the fundamental relationships and provide some numerical examples. A follow-up [99] utilizes a predictor-corrector method to trace such contours accurately. Similarly, Meek and Beer [100] describe a method for tracing deflections across higher-order elements. It is based on a process involving averaging nodal values, followed by element subdivision and local linearization. Results are given for triangular and quadrilateral elements.

Akin and Stoddart [101] present an algorithm for plotting intersections of isoparametric solids with an arbitrary plane and show the subsequent plots of stress or displacement contours on the resulting mesh. The plots are generated point by point in a random order, and they are suitable for graphics terminals or electrostatic plotters. Fray et al [66] describes a method for calculating the intersection of a plane with second-order isoparametric solid brick elements.

The use of color graphics [102] plays an emerging role in the display of results. A paper describing an algorithm for clipping and capping a solid polyhedron [103] is directly applicable to the display of three-dimensional solids. It produces an input file for the well-distributed hidden-line program, MOVIE.BYU [104]. A version of the program for sixteen-bit minicomputers, called MOVIE.ARIZONA, has also been developed. A two- and three-dimensional half-tone and color program for the output of finite element results is described by Murai and Tateishi [105]. It has some mesh generation capabilities, is capable of solving the hidden-line and -surface problems and contouring. Furthermore, it uses inexpensive hardware.

Reference [106] gives an example of the use of computer graphics as an integral part of a complex analysis. Refresh scope hardware and color graphics are used advantageously to help perform nonlinear analysis of frames.

PRE- AND POSTPROCESSING SOFTWARE

Auxiliary finite element programs may be developed for specific hardware or may be intended to be hardware-independent. Hardware-dependent packages are usually associated with turnkey systems including graphics. In the same manner, pre- and postprocessors may be tailored to a specific analysis program or may be intended for use by a number of different programs. There are advantages and disadvantages to system-dependent and system-independent packages. Whether the package is dependent on hardware or the analysis program or on both, it is usually well-maintained by the originators. Should the hardware or analysis program change, the auxiliary software is readily changed and tested. Furthermore, the pre- and postprocessor programs would cater well to the idiosyncrasies of the analysis program and would utilize special hardware features most effectively. On the other hand, the user's dependence on a single source hampers his freedom of action. Should a particular type of hardware be dropped by the manufacturer, or if it proves to be ineffective, the required changeover to another system is usually costly in both lost production time and manpower. Furthermore, if the auxiliary software is dependent on the analysis program, and the user has several in-house programs, the personnel training problem may become excessive. In the case of general purpose auxiliary software the training may be more demanding but need only be done once for all programs. A maximum flexibility of action is guaranteed. On the other hand, it is more time-consuming to maintain software that is independent of hardware and the analysis program. Any change in hardware or analysis program characteristics has to be carefully studied as to its effect on the pre- and postprocessors. The group performing the maintenance has to have continuous access to all hardware and software in question. This is only possible for extremely large organizations. It may be accomplished, however, through a well-organized user's group.

Turning to specific software reported in the literature, there is an early survey, mainly of preprocessors, by Napolitano et al [107]. It is perhaps appropriate here to start by mentioning those packages that support popular analysis software. First, auxiliary software specifically aimed at particular analysis programs will be surveyed. Following that, analysis-independent software will be considered.

Of all commercial programs, perhaps the one most used in practice is NASTRAN. An early survey of NASTRAN pre- and postprocessors is given in [108]. As mentioned earlier, it is important to preserve the mesh generation geometry and logic for later use in the input of loads and boundary conditions. A pioneering effort to that effect was conducted by Cook [109], who used spline representation of curves and surfaces for geometry definition. The resulting preprocessor was intended for the NASTRAN program. A general purpose postprocessor for NASTRAN which operates in both batch and timesharing environments is described in [110]. A modeling system is described in [111] which is based on a hierarchical representation of geometry and has parametric representation of curves, surfaces and volumes. An interactive pre- and postprocessing system is IGFES [112]. It is modular and uses storage tube graphics as well as plotters. It includes both two- and three-dimensional shell mesh generators and model editors. An interactive program for the creation of NASTRAN data has been developed mainly for the analysis of ship hulls [113].

One of the most popular programs in the civil engineering field is STRUDL. It has graphics pre- and postprocessing capabilities, as typified in [114].

DASA [115] is a utility package of subroutines to support the SESAM-69 and NORSAM systems. It allows the user to implement special and general purpose data generators using its subroutines as building blocks. It is based on the concept of a mesh, defined by a system of orthogonal surfaces, that may assume prismatic, cylindrical or spherical shapes. The generated model may be modified later to introduce local details. The system also allows automatic mesh refinement as well as load and boundary condition generation.

Moving on to program-independent auxiliary software, an early example is given by the work of Bousquet and Yates at Lockheed LMSC [116], the previewing and model-editing package operated on storage displays. A number of commercially available packages exist today, as well as others that are in the public domain. The UNISTRUC package [117] uses the so-called "drag method" to develop three-dimensional node and element arrangements from two-dimensional ones, and two-dimensional ones from one-dimensional strings. The FASTDRAW program [118, 119] has been developed by McDonnell-Douglas and serves as a preprocessor for STRUDL, NASTRAN and ANSYS. Another popular commercial program, developed by SDRC, is SUPERTAB [30, 120, 121, 122]. Tektronix has developed a software package [123] for use on its stand-alone intelligent graphics device. It has extensive interactive editing capabilities, and a new mesh generation module has been announced. A package called FEMALE [124] is intended as a general purpose program. However, it seems that the program is still in an early stage. The SUPERNET preprocessor [48] supports line, surface and solid elements and follows a geometric hierarchy. Interfaces are being written for analysis programs such as ASKA, NASTRAN, MARC and ANSYS. However, SUPERNET may be run in batch or interactively only on Computer Vision hardware. A postprocessor is also under development. An interactive three-dimensional shell mesh generator is described in [125]. It uses refresh displays, light pen, and keyboard. Initial input defining the outlines of surface patches is introduced via cards. The user may view the outlines and perform certain operations. Afterwards, the mesh generator may be invoked and results displayed and edited.

Several packages of pre- and postprocessing software have been developed in a university environment as a by-product of research efforts or out of necessity to facilitate access to available finite element software. The GIFTS system [73, 126] is one example. It has two- and three-dimensional model, load and boundary condition generation capabilities. It is designed to run in minimum core space, and at present its postprocessor handles all but solid models. Interfaces exist with the SAP4, STAGS, NASTRAN, ANSYS, and DAISY programs, and others are under development. Apart from pre- and postprocessing modules, GIFTS is also capable of static and dynamic analysis on a number of mainframes and minicomputers. The program is supported by a user group and is distributed by the University of Arizona. The INGA system [72], developed at the University of Stuttgart, is also based on a modular design, and from its beginning it was designed to be machine- and display-independent [127]. Currently the interactive system is installed on various types of large and small computers with different types of graphics hardware (refresh, raster and storage displays as well as plotters). The pre- and postprocessors are operational in conjunction with ASKA at many installations. However, other finite element programs (e.g., NASTRAN) are also supported at a few locations. The preprocessor FEMGEN [46], developed at the University of Lund in Sweden, is intended to support analysis programs such as ASAS, ASKA, NASTRAN, and STARDYNE, and uses storage tube terminals, plotters, and line printers. Straight lines and circular arcs may be defined in terms of geometric points or as the intersections of standard mathematical surfaces such as planes, cylinders, and cones. An example of a structural analysis preprocessor with an interface to a computer-aided design system is McDonnel-Douglas' CGSA [128], coupled to the comprehensive CADD computer-aided design system.

Some programs have an integrated pre- and postprocessing capability which may often be important in special purpose codes in which the processes of model generation and computation are interwoven. An interesting example is the TOTAL program reported by Beaubien [129]. It is a two-dimensional analysis program designed to simulate the failure mechanism in layered orthotropic composites.

It has a built-in pre- and postprocessor which helps keep track of the progress of cracks.

DESIGN OF INTERACTIVE SOFTWARE

Associated with interactive graphics software, special problems in design methodology, software reliability, portability and testing arise. Requirements for developing general pre- and postprocessing systems are formulated by Tischler and Bernier [130] and discussed by Herness and Tocher [6]. The concepts of a modular system in which the pre- and posprocessors interact with the analysis programs via a standard database is well represented by GIFTS [126] and INGA [131]. The design of interactive pre- and postprocessor systems is described in [132], which discusses procedures of program design, testing, overlaying, data handling and command language design. The problem of program portability is more complex than it is for standard batch analysis programs. The main body of the code should be programmed independently of the machine. Computer dependency will arise in the data handling and graphics areas [133]. The different graphics systems perform essentially the same operations, but often in too general a manner. The introduction of graphics standards should, therefore, further improve program portability. An early engineering attempt to produce hardware-independent graphics software is the FLING set of subroutines [134]. However, the situation will change when the American [135] and German [136] procedures for standardization of graphical data processing are successfully complete.

ACKNOWLEDGMENTS

The authors gratefully acknowledge the help of various members of the staff at both ISD and the University of Arizona. Particular thanks are due to Ms. Juanita Alvarez, who typed the final manuscript, and Ms. Devi Gunara, who kindly prepared the drawings.

REFERENCES

1 Grieger, I., "Integrated Interactive Structural Analysis with Finite Elements," Proceedings of CAD78 (3rd Int. Conf. on Computers in Engineering and Building Design), IPC Science and Technology Press, England, 1978, pp. 789-802.

2 Newman, W. M., and Sproull, R. F., Principles of Interactive Computer Graphics, 2nd ed., McGraw-Hill, New York, 1979.

3 Lillehagen, F. M., Riesenfeld, R. F., and Frogner, S., "New Dimensions in Man-Machine Communications," Computer Applications in the Automation of Shipyard Operation and Ship Design III, North-Holland Publishing Co., Amsterdam, 1979, pp. 351-358.

4 Prince, M. D., Interactive Graphics for Computer-Aided Design, Addison-Wesley Publishing Co., Reading, MA, USA, 1971.

5 Frederikson, B. and Mackerle, J., "Structural Mechanics: Pre- and Post-Processor Programs -- Surveys and Availability," Advanced Engineering Corporation (AEC), Box 3044, S-580 03, Linköping, Sweden, 1977.

6 Hernes, E. D., and Tocher, J. L., "Design of Pre- and Postprocessors," Structural Mechanics Computer Programs, University Press of Virginia, Charlottesville, 1974, pp. 887-898.

7 Forrest, A. R., "Curves and Surfaces for Computer-Aided Design, " Ph.D. Dissertation, University of Cambridge, England, 1968.

8 Rogers, D. F., and Adams, J. A., Mathematical Elements for Computer Graphics, McGraw-Hill Book Co., New York, 1976.

9 Peters, G. J., "Interactive Computer Graphics Application of the Parametric Bi-cubic Surface to Engineering Design Problems," Computer-Aided Geometric Design, Academic Press, New York, 1974, pp. 259-302.

10 Ahlberg, J. H., Nilson, E. N., and Walsh, J. L., The Theory of Splines and Their Applications, Academic Press, New York, 1967.

11 Greville, T. N. E., Theory and Applications of Spline Functions, Academic Press, New York, 1969.

12 Bezier, P., Numerical Control -- Mathematics and Applications, (translated by A. R. Forrest), John Wiley & Sons, London, 1972.

13 Riesenfeld, R. F., "Application of B-Spline Approximation to Geometric Problems in Computer-Aided Design," Ph.D. Dissertation, Syracuse University, 1973.

14 de Boor, C., A Practical Guide to Splines, Springer-Verlag, New York, 1978.

15 Forrest, A. R., "Mathematical Principles for Curve and Surface Representation," Curved Surface in Engineering, IPC Science and Technology Press, Guildford, England, 1972, pp. 5-13.

16 Birkhoff, G., "Smooth Surface Interpolation," Journal of Mathematics and Physics, Vol. 39, 1960, pp. 258-268.

17 de Boor, C., "Bicubic Spline Interpolation," Journal of Mathematics and Physics, Vol. 41, 1962, pp. 212-218.

18 Wu, S. C., Abel, J. F., and Greenberg, D. P., "An Interactive Computer Graphics Approach to Surface Representation," Communication of the ACM, Vol. 20, No. 10, 1977, pp.703-712

19 Coons, S. A., "Surfaces for Computer-Aided Design of Space Forms," MIT Project MAC, Report MAC-TR-41, 1967.

20 Gordon, W. J., "Blending Function Methods of Bivariate and Multivariate Interpolation and Approximation," SIAM Journal on Numerical Analysis, Vol. 8, No. 1, 1971, pp. 158-177.

21 Barnhill, R. E., Birkhoff, G., and Gordon, W. J., "Smooth Interpolation in Triangles," Journal of Approximation Theory, Vol. 8, No. 2, 1973, pp. 114-128.

22 MacCallum, K. J., "The Application of Computer Graphics to the Preliminary Design of Ship Hulls," Ph.D. Dissertation, Imperial College, London, 1970.

23 Theilheimer, F., and McKee, J. M., "The Role of Splines in Computer-Aided Ship Design," 1st Intern. Symp. on Computer-Aided Hull Surface Definition, SNAME, Annapolis, MD, 1977.

24 Munchmeyer, F. C., Schubert, C., and Nowacki, H., "Interactive Design of Fair Hull Surfaces Using B-splines," Computer Application in the Automation of Shipyard Operation and Ship Design III, North-Holland Publishing Co., Amsterdam, 1979, pp. 67-76.

25 Abel, J. F., Greenberger, D. P., McGuire, W., Gallagher, R. H., "Interactive Graphics for Finite Element Analysis," Proceedings of 7th Conf. on Electronic Computation, St. Louis, MO, Aug. 1979, (ASCE Publication).

26 Liu, D., "Finite Element Analysis of Arbitary Shells," Ph.D. Dissertation, University of Arizona, December 1978.

27 Baer, A., Eastman, C., and Henrion, M., "Geometric Modelling: A Survey," Computer-Aided Design, Vol. 11, No. 5, Sept. 1979, pp. 253-272.

28 Grieger, I., "Interactive Techniques for Mechanical Design and System Aspects," Proceedings on Computer-Aided Design in Mechanical Engineering, Cooperative libraria universitaria del politecnico (clup), Politecnico di Milano, 1976, pp. 215-229.

29 Kamel, H. A. and Navabi, Z., "Digitizing for Computer-Aided Finite Element Model Generation," ASCE Design Automation Conference, St. Louis, MO, July, 1979.

30 "SUPERTAB Interactive Finite Element Model Generation System," Structural Dynamics Research Corporation (SDRC), Cincinnati, OH, 1976.

31 White, P. R., and Garett, R. E., "A Generalized Interactive Three-Dimensional Input System," Proceedings of CAD 76 (2nd Int. Conf. on Computers in Engineering and Building Design), IPC Science and Technology Press, England, 1976, pp. 275-282.

32 Yi, C., Besant, C. B., and Jebb, A., "Three-Dimensional Digitizing Techniques for Computer-Aided Animation," Proceedings of CAD 76 (2nd Int. Conf. on Computers in Engineering and Building Design), IPC Science and Technology Press, England, 1976, pp. 292-295.

33 Thornton, R. W., "Interactive Modelling in Three Dimensions Through Two-Dimensional Windows," Proceedings of CAD 78 (3rd Int. Conf. on Computers in Engineering and Building Design), IPC Science and Technology Press, England, 1978, pp. 204-211.

34 Liardet, M., "PICAX -- Polyhedron Input to the Computer Using an Axonometric Drawing," Proceedings Int. Conf. Interactive Techniques in Computer-Aided Design (Bologna, Sept. 21-23, 1978), I.E.E.E., New York, 1978, pp. 344-355.

35 Sagawa, K., "Automatic Mesh Generation for Three-dimensional Structures," Theory and Practice in Finite Element Structural Analysis, University of Tokyo Press, 1973, pp. 687-703.

36 Sutherland, I. E., "Three-Dimensional Data Input by Tablet," Proceedings of the I.E.E.E., Vol. 62, No. 4, 1974, pp. 453-461.

37 Speth, J. F., "Strukturierung digitalisierter Daten," Dipl. -Ing. Thesis at the ISD, University of Stuttgart, 1977.

38 Buell, W. R., and Bush, B. A., "Mesh Generation -- A Survey," Transactions of the ASME, Series B, Journal of Engineering for Industry, Vol. 95, No. 1, 1973, pp. 332-338.

39 Kamel, H. A., and Eisenstein, H. K., "Automatic Mesh Generation in Two- and Three-dimensional Interconnected Domains," Proceedings IUTAM Symp. on High Speed Computing in Elastic Structures, Université de Liège, Belgium, Vol. 61, Tome 2, 1971, pp. 455-475.

40 Zienkiewicz, O. C., and Philips, D. V., "An Automatic Mesh Generation Scheme for Plane and Curved Surfaces by Isoparametric Coordinates," Int. Journal for Numerical Methods in Engineering, Vol. 3, No. 4, 1971, pp. 519-528.

41 Ohtmer, O., "Zur automatischen Generierung und Kondensierung großer Massenund Steifigkeitsmatrizen," Angewandte Informatik, 12/72, 1972, pp. 569-574.

42 Fujii, T., and Yuki, T., "Automatic Data Generation and Large Matrix Operation for Three-Dimensional Plate Structural Analysis," Theory and Practice in Finite Element Structural Analysis, University of Tokyo Press, 1973, pp. 671-686.

43 Neal, B. K., "A Finite Element Mesh Generation Program for Arbitrary Two- and Three-Dimensional Structures," Second International Conference on Structural Mechanics in Reactor Technology, M 4/5, Vol. 5, Berlin, 1973.

44 Yeung, S. F., and Hsu, M. B., "A Mesh Generation Method Based on Set Theory," Computers and Structures, Vol. 3, No. 5, 1973, pp. 1063-1077.

45 Yu, J. C., "Automatic Generation of Finite Element Mesh Within a Bandwidth and an Efficient Solution of the Bandmatrix," Theory and Practice in Finite Element Structural Analysis, University of Tokyo Press, 1973, pp. 651-670.

46 Johansson, T., "FEMGEN -- A General Finite Element Mesh Generator," User's Manual, Lund University Computing Centre, also in Finite Element Methods in the Commercial Environment, Vol. 2, Robinson and Associates, England, 1979, pp. 497-516.

47 Singh, S., "A Computer-Aided Finite Element Idealization and Mesh Generation System," Proceedings of CAD 76 (2nd Int. Conf. on Computers in Engineering and Building Design), IPC Science and Technology Press, England, 1976, pp. 213-218.

48 Buck, K. E., Bodisco, U. von, and Winkler, K., "SUPERNET -- Generierungsprogramm für finite Elemente," Benutzerhandbuch, BBC (Brown Boveri), Mannheim, 1976, Revision 1979.

49 Leick, R. D., and Potvin, A. B., "Automated Mesh Generation for Tubular Joint Stress Analysis," Computers and Structures, Vol. 7, No. 1, 1977, pp. 73-91.

50 Denayer, A., "Automatic Generation of Finite Element Meshes," Computers and Structures, Vol. 9, No. 4, 1978, pp. 359-364.

51 Haugerud, M. H., "Interactive 3D Mesh Generation by an Idealization and Mapping Technique," Proceedings of CAD 78 (3rd Int. Conf. on Computers in Engineering and Building Design), IPC Science and Technology Press, England, 1978, pp. 753-766.

52 de Castel, J. and Finifter, D., "Concise Description and Automatic Finite Element Modelling of Ship Structures with DEMAIN," Computer Application in the Automation of Shipyard Operation and Ship Design III, North-Holland Publishing Co., Amsterdam, 1979, pp. 277-286.

53 Frederick, C. O., Wong, Y. C., and Edge, F. W., "Two-dimensional Automatic Mesh Generation for Structural Analysis," Int. Journal for Numerical Methods in Engineering, Vol. 2, No. 1, 1970, pp. 133-144.

54 Suhara, J., and Fukuda, J., "Automatic Mesh Generation for Finite Element Analysis," Advances in Computational Methods in Structural Mechanics and Design, UAH Press, Huntsville, AL, 1972, pp. 607-624.

55 Saw, G. B. and Smith, R. G., "Automatic Nodal Triangulation for Finite Elements," Computer-Aided Design, Vol. 5, No. 1, 1973, pp. 33-35.
56 Cavendish, J. C., "Automatic Triangulation of Arbitrary Planar Domains for the Finite Element Method," Int. Journal for Numerical Methods in Engineering, Vol. 8, No. 4, 1974, pp. 679-696.
57 Tracy, F. T., "Graphical Pre- and Postprocessor for Two-Dimensional Finite Element Method," SIGGRAPH-ACM Report Computer Graphics, Vol. 11, No. 2, 1977, pp. 8-12.
58 Schools, A. J. G., Beukering, L. H. Th. M. v., Suiter, M. L. C., "Gebruikershandleiding voor de tweedimensionale Meshgenerator TRIQUAMESH," Technische Hogeschool Eindhoven, Afdeling der Werktingbouerkunde, Report WE 78-01, January, 1978.
59 Cavendish, J. C., "Local Mesh Refinement Using Blended Finite Elements," Journal of Computational Physics, Vol. 19, No. 2, 1975, pp. 211-228.
60 Bykat, A., "Automatic Generation of Triangular Grids: I -- Subdivision of a General Polygon into Convex Subregions. II -- Triangularisation of Convex Subregions," Int. Journal for Numerical Methods in Engineering, Vol. 10, No. 6, 1976, pp. 1329-1342.
61 Akyus, F. A., "Natural Coordinate Systems -- An Automatic Input Data Generation Scheme for a Finite Element Method," Nuclear Engineering and Design, Vol. 11, 1970, pp. 195-207.
62 Gordon, W. J. and Hall, C. A., "Construction of Curvilinear Coordinate System and Application to Mesh Generation," Int. Journal for Numerical Methods in Engineering, Vol. 7, No. 4, 1973, pp. 461-477.
63 Cook, W. A., "Body Oriented (Natural) Coordinates for Generating Three-Dimensional Meshes," Int. Journal for Numerical Methods in Engineering, Vol. 8, No. 1, 1974, pp. 27-43.
64 Cook, W. A., "INGEN: A General Purpose Mesh Generator for Finite Element Codes," Applications using ADINA, MIT Report, 82448-6, 1977, pp. 328-348.
65 Aral, K., "Data Generation for a 3D Finite Element System," ASME PVP Conference, Miami, 1974.
66 Fray, A. E., Hall, C. A., and Porsching, T. A., "An Application of Computer Graphics to Three-Dimensional Finite Element Analysis," Computers and Structures, Vol. 10, 1979, pp. 149-154.
67 Gabrielson, V. K., "Mesh Generation for Two-dimensional Regions Using a DVST Graphics Terminal," Sandia Laboratories, Report No. SAND76-8231, July 1976.
68 Argyris, J. H., Kamel, H. A., Sorensen, M., Schmid, G., and Pretsch, H., "ASKA: An Automatic System for Kinematic Analysis," Programmer's Manual, ISD Report No. 8, Stuttgart, Oct. 1965.
69 "The ASTRA System," Boeing Document D2-125179-8, May 1972.
70 Silvester, P.O., "The MAG-NET-78 Finite Element Model Description Language," U.S. - Japan Seminar on Int. Finite Element Analysis, Cornell University, August 1978.
71 Golden, M. E., "Geometric Structural Modelling: A Promising Basis for Finite Element Analysis," Computers and Structures, Vol. 10, 1979, pp. 347-350.
72 Grieger, I., "Interactive Graphical Pre- and Postprocessing for Finite Element Analysis with INGA," Proc. 6th Structural Analysis SIG Meeting Univac User Association/Europe, Speery Univac Int. Div., London, 1977, pp. 102-123.
73 Kamel, H. A., and McCabe, M. W., "GIFTS: Graphics-Oriented Interactive Finite Element TimeSharing System," Structural Mechanics Software Series, Vol. 1, University Press of Virginia, Charlottesville, 1977, pp. 145-226.
74 Wüstenberg, H., "Interaktive Generierung von zweidimensionalen Idealisierungen," Dipl.-Ing. Thesis at the ISD, University of Stuttgart, 1977.
75 Uerkvitz, M., "Interaktive Generierung dreidimensionaler idealisierungen," Dipl.-Ing. Thesis at the ISD, University of Stuttgart, 1978.
76 Grieger, I., "Geometry Elements in Computer-Aided Design," Computers and Structures, Vol. 8, No. 3/4, May 1978, pp. 371-381.
77 Haber, R., Shephard, M., Abel, J., Gallagher, R., and Greenberg, D., "A Generalized Graphic Preprocessor for Two-Dimensional Finite Element Analysis," SIGGRAPH-ACM Report Computer Graphics, Vol. 12, No. 3, 1978, pp. 323-329.
78 Gerhard, M. A. and Greenlaw, R. C., "SLIC -- An Interactive Mesh Generator for Finite Element and Finite Difference Application Programs," CAFEM 5 (5th Int. Seminar on Computational Aspects of the Finite Element Method),

BAM Seminar Preprint 10, Berlin, 1979, pp. 149-160.

79 Kalkani, E. C., "Mesh Generation Program for Highway Excavation Cuts," Int. Journal for Numerical Methods in Engineering, Vol. 8, No. 2, 1974, pp. 269-394.

80 Preiss, K., "Checking of the Topological Consistency of a Finite Element Mesh," International Report, SRI International, Poulter Laboratory, May 1978.

81 Weeks, G. E. and Cost, T. L., "An Algorithm for Automatically Tracking Ablating Boundaries," Int. Journal for Numerical Methods in Engineering, Vol. 14, 1970, pp. 441-449.

82 Grooms, H. R., "Algorithm for Matrix Bandwidth Reduction," Proceedings of the ASCE, Journal of the Struct. Division, Vol. 98, No. ST1, 1972, pp. 203-214.

83 Collins, R. J., "Bandwidth Reduction by Automatic Renumbering," Int. Journal for Numerical Methods in Engineering, Vol. 6, 1973, pp. 345-356.

84 Rodrigues, J. S., "Node Numbering Optimization in Structural Analysis," Proceedings of the ASCE, Journal of the Struct. Division, Vol. 101, No. ST2, 1975, pp. 361-376.

85 Akhras, G. and Dhatt, G., "An Automatic Node Relabelling Scheme for Minimizing a Matrix or Network Bandwidth," Int. Journal for Numerical Methods in Engineering, Vol. 10, 1976, pp. 787-797.

86 Gibbs, N. E., Poole, W. G. and Stockmeyer, P. K. "An Algorithm for Reducing Bandwidth and Profile of A Sparse Matrix," SIAM Journal of Numerical Analysis, Vol. 13, No. 2, April 1976, pp. 236-250.

87 Bykat, A., "A Note on an Element Ordering Scheme," Int. Journal for Numerical Methods in Engineering, Vol. 11, No. 1, 1977, pp. 194-198.

88 Cuthill, E. and McKee, T., "Reducing the Bandwidth of Sparse Symmetric Matrices," Proceedings of the 24th National Conf. of ACM, 1969, p. 69.

89 Gay, R. K. L., Chin, K. K., Chua, S. H., Chan, C. H., and Ho, S. Y., "Node Reordering Algorithm for Water Network Analysis," Int. Journal for Numerical Methods in Engineering, Vol. 12, 1978, pp. 1241-1259.

90 Shephard, M. S. and Gallagher, R. H. (Editors), Finite Element Grid Optimization, ASME Special Publication PVP-38, June 1979.

91 Shepard, M. S., "The Generation of Optimal Finite Element Meshes," Proceedings of the 7th Conf. on Electronic Computation, St. Louis, MO, Aug. 1979, (ASCE Publication).

92 Turcke, D. J. and McNeice, G. M., "Guidelines for Selecting Finite Element Grids Based on an Optimization Study," Computers and Structures, Vol. 4, 1974, pp. 499-519.

93 Caroll, W. E., "Inclusive Criteria for Optimum Grid Generation in the Discrete Analysis Technique," Computers and Structures, Vol. 6, 1976, pp. 333-337.

94 Saad, M. and Turcke, D. J., "A Preprocessing Technique for Improved Mesh Generation," Finite Element Methods in the Commercial Environment, Vol. 2, Robinson and Associates, England, 1979, pp. 465-484.

95 Melosh, R. J. and Killian, D. E., "Finite Element Analysis to Attain a Prospected Accuracy," Proc. 2nd National Conf. on Computing and Structures, 1976.

96 Carey, G. F., "A Mesh-Refinement Scheme to Finite Element Computations," Comp. Meth. in Appl. Mech. and Engineering, Vol. 7, No. 1, 1976, pp. 93-105.

97 Kalkani, E. C., "Computer Plotting of Stress Contours in Excavated Slopes," Int. Journal for Numerical Methods in Engineering, Vol. 10, 1976, pp. 1261-1280.

98 Akin, J. E. and Gray, W. H., "Contouring on Isoparametric Surfaces," Int. Journal for Numerical Methods in Engineering, Vol. 11, 1977, pp. 1893-1897.

99 Gray, W. H., and Akin, J. E., "An Improved Method for Contouring on Isoparametric Surfaces," Int. Journal for Numerical Methods in Engineering, Vol. 14, 1979, pp. 451-458.

100 Meek, J. L. and Beer, G., "Contour Plotting of Data Using Isoparametric Element Representation," Int. Journal for Numerical Methods in Engineering, Vol. 10, No. 4, 1976, pp. 954-957.

101 Akin, J. E. and Stoddart, W. C. T., "Plane Intersections and Contours for General Isoparametric Solids," Computers and Structures, Vol. 10, 1979, pp. 155-157.

102 Christiansen, H. N., "The Emerging Role of Color Graphics," Finite Element Methods in the Commercial Environment, Vol. 1, Robinson and Associates, England, 1979, pp. 103-112.

103 Stephenson, M. B., and Christiansen, H. N., "A Polyhedron Clipping and Capping Algorithm and Display System for Three-Dimensional Finite Element Models," SIGGRAPH-ACM Report, Computer Graphics, Vol. 9, No. 3, 1975.

104 Christiansen, H.N., and Stephenson, M. B., "MOVIE.BYU -- A Computer Graphics Software System," Journal of the Technical Councils of ASCE, April 1979.

105 Murai, S. and Tateishi, R., "A Study on Image Processing for Results Obtained for Finite Element Analysis," U.S. - Japan Seminar on Interdisciplinary Finite Set Analysis, Cornell University, August 1978.

106 Gruss, J. L., Mutryn, T. A. and McGuire, W., "Computer Graphics and Nonlinear Frame Analysis," Proceedings of the 7th Conf. on Electronic Computation, St. Louis, MO, Aug. 1979, (ASCE Publication).

107 Napolitano, G., Monti, R., and Murino, P., "Preprocessors for General Purpose Finite Element Programs," Structural Mechanics Computer Programs, University Press of Virginia, Charlottesville, VA, 1974, pp. 807-823.

108 Eversting, G.C., and McKee, J. M., "A Survey of Pre- and Postprocessors for NASTRAN," Structural Mechanics Computer Programs, University of Virginia, Charlottesville, VA, 1974, pp. 825-847.

109 Cook, W. L., "Automated Input Data Preparation for NASTRAN," GSC-11039, Goddard Space Flight Center, Greenbelt, MD, April 1969.

110 Raibstone, A. J. and Pipano, A., "RINA -- An Interactive System for the Rapid Interpretation of NASTRAN Results," Sixth NASTRAN Users' Colloquium, NASA Conf. Pub. 2018, Oct. 1977.

111 Stanten, E. L., "An Automated Data Generator for NASTRAN," Sixth NASTRAN Users' Colloquium, NASA Conf. Pub. 2018, Oct. 1977.

112 Lorensen, W. E., "Interactive Graphics Support for NASTRAN," Sixth NASTRAN Users' Colloquium, NASA Conf. Pub. 2018, Oct. 1977.

113 Armit, A. P. and Lemke, H. U., "ICON: The Interactive Creation of NASTRAN Data. A System Description," Computer-Aided Design, Vol. 7, No. 3, 1975, pp. 145-150.

114 Peacher, D. L. and Appleton, J. H., "Computer Design of Reinforced Concrete Structures," Proceedings of the 7th Conf. on Electronic Computation, St. Louis, MO, Aug. 1979, (ASCE Publication).

115 Pahle, E. and Flatlandsmo, K., "DASA Data for Structural Analysis General Description," Aker Group and Computers, Oslo, Norway, 1976.

116 Bousquet, R. D. and Yates, D. N., "A Low Cost Interactive Graphics System for Large-Scale Finite Element Analysis," Computers and Structures, Vol. 3, 1975, pp. 1321-1330.

117 Park, S. and Washom, C. J., "Drag Method as a Finite Element Mesh Generation Scheme," Computers and Structures, Vol. 10, 1979, pp. 343-346.

118 "FASTDRAW Interactive Graphics System," McDonnell-Douglas Automation Co., Document B1298083, 1973.

119 Nolan, L. E., "A Distributed Structural Design Graphics System," Proceedings of the 7th Conf. on Electronic Computation, St. Louis, MO, Aug. 1979, (ASCE Publication).

120 Korcese, J. "Stress Analysis on a Budget," Machine Design, March, 1979.

121 Jackson, R. and Olsofka, F., "Design Analysis of a Centrifugal Compressor Impeler," ASME Eastern Design Engineering Conference, Boston, MA, 1979.

122 Argus, G. D. and Maddux, K., "Lightweight Component Design via Computer-Aided Engineering," SAE Paper no. 790984, Oct. 1979.

123 Romans, G., Ineson, F., de Groot, H. "Graphic Systems and Their Effect on the Finite Element Method," Finite Element Methods in the Commercial Environment, Vol. 2, Robinson and Associates, England, 1979, pp. 518-530.

124 Shoppee, G. J. V., Jeanes, P. J., and Griffin, T. B., "A Finite Element Modeling and Analysis Language for Engineering the Program FEMALE," Advances Engineering Software, Vol. 1, No. 1, 1978, pp. 37-41.

125 Dwyer, T. J., Hasegawa, T., and Lynn, K. R., "General Purpose Structural Graphics System (GPSGS)," ASME, PVP Conference, Miami, June 1974.

126 Kamel, H. A. and McCabe, M. W., "Geometry and Function Definition for Discrete Analysis and its Relationship to the Design Database," Proc. Int. Symp. on Computer-Aided Hull Definition (SCAHD77), Annapolis, MD, Sept. 1977.

127 Grieger, I., "Uber den Einsatz von Bildschirmgeraten bei der Berechnung von Tragerken," Dr.-Ing. Dissertation, University of Stuttgart, 1972.

128 Norman, W. A., "Computer-Aided Structural Design Applied to Production Aircraft," MacAir Report 77017, NATO 46th Structural Material and Panel Meeting, Voss, Norway, Sept. 1977.

129 Beaubien, L. A., "TOTAL: Interactive Graphics System for the Two-Dimensional Analysis of Linear Elastic Solids," Structural Mechanics Software Series, Vol. 1, University Press of Virginia, Charlottesville, 1977, pp. 275-346.

130 Tischler, V. A. and Bernier, L. J. D., "Consideration for Developing a General Finite Element Pre- and Postprocessing System," Structural Mechanics Computer Programs, University Press of Virginia, Charlottesville, 1974, pp. 849-863.

131 Grieger, I., "INGA -- Interactive Graphic Analysis," User's Reference Manual, ISD Report No. 156, 2nd Ed., ISD, University of Stuttgart, 1979.

132 Kamel, H. A., "Design and Implementation of Interactive Engineering Software," U.S. - Japan Seminar on Interdisciplinary Finite Element Analysis, Cornell University, August 1978.

133 Grieger, I. and Wagemann, G., "Maschinen- und Geräteunabhangigkeiteine moderne Forderung," Graphische Datenverarbeit. 79, Schriftenreihe Nr. 4 der Österreichischen Computer Gesellschaft, Wien, 1979, pp. 103-117.

134 Batdorf, W. J. and Kapur, S. S., "FLING -- A FORTRAN Language for Interactive Graphics," Numerical and Computer Methods in Structural Mechanics, Academic Press, New York, 1973, pp. 513-542.

135 "Status Report of Graphics Standard Planning Committee (GSPC)," SIGGRAPH-ACM Report, Computer Graphics, Vol. 13, No. 3, 1979.

136 Deutsches Institut fur Normung e.v., Norm-Entwurf DIN ISO 7942, Informations verarbeitung, Graphisches Kernsystem (GKS), Funktionale Beschreibung, Beuth Verlag, Berlin, 1982; see also ISO/DIS 7942, Information Processing, Graphical Kernel System (GKS), Functional Description, Version 7.0, ISO/TC 97/SC 5 N690.

CHAPTER TWELVE

PARTIAL LIST OF MAJOR FINITE ELEMENT PROGRAMS AND DESCRIPTION OF SOME OF THEIR CAPABILITIES

B. Fredriksson and J. Mackerle
Linköping Institute of Technology
Department of Mechanical Engineering
Division of Solid Mechanics
Linköping, Sweden

ABSTRACT

In this chapter we describe a few of the hundreds or thousands of finite element programs available today. The computer software described is divided into programs for teaching and research, programs for desktop and minicomputers, and general purpose programs for midi- and maxi-computers. We also discuss to some extent available literature about how to find information about a specific computer program or how to find a computer program for your needs. Information is presented also about organizations that compile information about finite element software.

INTRODUCTION

The very rapid development of computer hardware capabilities has implied an equally rapid development of computer software. The finite element method has probably been and is still one of the fields in which computer software is developing the most rapidly. The applicability of the finite element method is essentially limited by the computer hardware capabilities. The wide range of computers available today may, from a finite element point of view, be divided as in Fig. 1. Until a few years ago programs for FEM have essentially been running on what we call maxi-computers such as CDC, Univac, or IBM. Today many FEM-programs are running on so-called midi- or mini-computers such as PRIME, VAX, DEC, NORD, etc. Today the capability of desktop computers such as HP-9845 or Tektronix 4051 is high enough to make it possible to run finite element programs with applications to practical problems. The boundaries between the different types of computers as presented in Fig. 1 are still moving and will probably do so even in the future. We will, for instance, probably soon have desktop computers with FORTRAN. The micro-computer technology will have a great influence on computer software for FEM in the future.

In this chapter we will present programs and some of their capabilities for the whole range of computers as given by Fig. 1.

GUIDELINES FOR SOFTWARE SELECTION, IMPLEMENTATION AND PROGRAM EVALUATION

The potential user of a FEM program is essentially faced with three main problems. The first is how to find information about existing programs. When

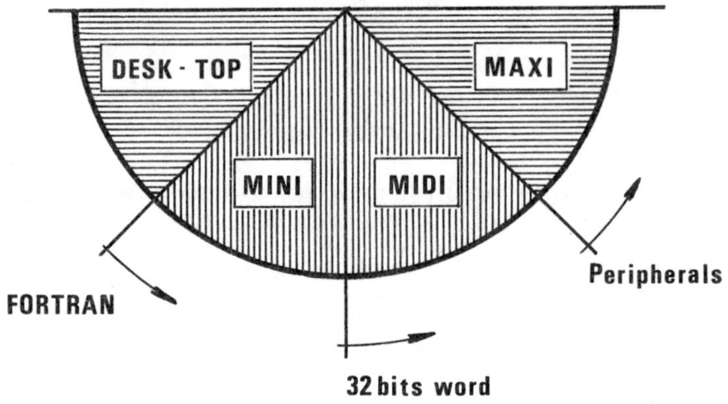

Fig. 1 A possible division of computers

he knows about the sources of information available he is next faced with the problem of how to sort out the programs that are of interest to him. When a number of programs out of hundreds or thousands are selected the third problem is to sort out the best one for his needs.

To solve the first problem we refer to the section, "How to Find Literature About Existing Structural Mechanics Software," and, "Software Dissemination Practices and Information Organizations," of this chapter.

The second problem was how to sort out programs of interest. The documentation available is mostly not suited for rational search. To read through descriptive surveys for hundreds of programs is very hard. Searching program catalogues [A-11 - A-14][1] which summarize the program capabilities in a tabular form is much easier. It is easy to look through a catalogue and find out the capabilities of a program but it is still hard to memorize and systematically evaluate programs. It seems rational to leave this job to the computer. The tabular information in a catalogue could easily be stored in a database. The search in this database could be done by the computer in a way similar to that used when, for instance, searching for scientific papers through the information systems available at libraries. For more information about such systems see, for instance, Refs. (1,2).

When the potential user of a FEM program is searching using information sources mentioned above he will surely end up with a number of programs. To sort out the best one is very difficult. The user has to define the most essential features and then thoroughly evaluate the programs both theoretically and practically by usage. One should also be open to the alternative that the best answer could be not one but perhaps two programs.

The reader may ask: Is it really worth all this trouble to try to find a program that fulfills my requirements? My requirements are rather specific and I will probably not find a program that fulfills all of them. Is it not better for me to develop my own program? In our opinion, the answer to this question is definitely no. First of all there are so many programs, good programs, available today that he will surely find some program that is rather close to his needs. Secondly, there are programs available that are very rationally programmed, making it possible for the user to add his own routines and in that way fulfill all requirements. The user should be aware of the fact that developing a finite element computer program requires a lot of manpower. Many programs are available free of charge; other programs could be purchased. The price of the commercially available programs seems at first sight to be rather high. However, if you compare this to the cost of developing your own program it is very cheap. You will then also get a program developed by experts on programming and finite elements. From there on you can start to develop your own routines for your

---

[1]Refers to Appendix citations

specific needs. Besides that, you then have caught up with technology - you have won time. You can start your own development from a higher level.

What is said above is valid for the case in which the user is in a design office that aims to use FEM as an analysis tool for its own needs. If the user is, for instance, a consultancy company that also wants to market the program as a product, the aspects of developing programs will be different.

SUMMARY OF MAJOR FINITE ELEMENT PROGRAMS

Programs for Use in Teaching the Finite Element Method

The teaching of fundamentals of the finite element method or their research application requires application of computer programs. The structural analysis method used in large general-purpose programs can be subdivided into a series of simple operations which are under the control of the user. These well-defined operations can be:

- Mathematical description of the model, input data
- Generation of element matrices
- Assembly of element matrices into structural matrix
- Solution of the resulting linear equations
- Calculations of node and element displacements, stresses, etc.
- Presentation of results

A set of modular programs or blocks of routines already thoroughly tested, built a kernel of the educational or research codes presented in this section. A student/researcher connects these routines or completes them with self-written routines into a tailor-made program, a general-purpose or a special-purpose finite element program. A user of this executable program does not have to know anything about programming. He has to describe the model only in accordance with the input requirements.

Descriptions of some general programming systems follow. The abstract of programs CAL, MODEL, MINIFEM is presented.

For pure "problem solving" applications in an educational environment it is very important that the programs used are easy to use. This makes the interactive or conversational input-mode programs attractive. In addition, it is important that the error diagnostics for the program are good. For this "problem solving" purpose there are many of the established general-purpose programs that may be used, perhaps with some modifications. The general-purpose programs, in addition, have the advantage that realistic applications could be studied.

In a more research-oriented use of the FEM as, for instance, in diploma works or doctor students applications, it is important that it is easy to incorporate self-written routines. Even here some of the general-purpose programs are suitable. For this to be rational it requires, in our opinion, that the program has a database architecture and a data management system. There are some such programs available. See, for instance, ASKA, FINITE, NASTRAN, or SPAR.

Below we describe three programs developed mainly for educational/research purposes.

Program name: CAL (3,4)

Prof. E. L. Wilson, Dept. of Civil Engineering, University of California, Berkeley, CA 94720, USA

Program summary. CAL is a matrix interpretive language and small capacity structural analysis program (up to 100 DOF). It contains over 40 subroutines which can be used within CAL or can be used in the development of other programs. Operations exist for both static and dynamic analyses. Dynamic analysis can be performed by either the step-by-step or mode superposition method. In order to simulate the behavior of structural algorithms which involve iterations, multilevel looping operations can be used. The present version has three different elements: three-dimensional truss; three-dimensional beam; and three nine-noded isoparametric finite elements. CAL is written in standard FORTRAN IV utilizing dynamic storage allocation. It is designed to be used by students in structural analysis courses. No attempt has been made to extend the capacity of the program to use low speed storage effectively. In its present form it is being used at several universities.

Machine version available. CDC 6400, IBM 370. The program can also be used on minicomputers (16 bit words) with a minimum of modification. It can be run in either batch or timesharing mode.

Program name: MODEL (5,7)

Prof. J. E. Akin, Department of Mechanical Engineering, Rice University, Houston, Texas 77251, USA

Program summary. MODEL, Modular Finite Element Program, has been developed as an educational tool and a basic research code. The various operations of the finite element method have been separated into several parts. This allows the user to set up one programming concept at a time. It is also possible to develop a series of blocks that stand alone or can be combined to fulfill various tasks of the special purpose application. The complete code contains over 150 modular subroutines. For a given application the analyst must supply those subroutines that involve problem dependent calculations. These are usually constructed from the available modules. All other operations such as generalized input of topology, properties, boundary conditions, printing of results, etc., are executed by the existing modules. The basic code is designed for steady-state banded symmetric formulations and utilizes an in-core solution algorithm. Subroutines are also available for the direct time integration of transient and dynamic applications. MODEL is written in standard FORTRAN IV. One-dimensional and 3-8 node two-dimensional isoparametric finite elements are available. The program is used at a number of universities and industrial companies.

Development criteria in connection with MODEL design. Conserve storage space, reduce run time, and minimize the programming effort required to solve a new type of problem.

Machine version available. IBM 360, CDC 7600, CDC 6600, DEC 10.

Program name: MINIFEM (8)

Prof. R. L. Taylor, Department of Civil Engineering, University of California, Berkeley, CA 94720, USA

Program summary. The program can be utilized to solve one-, two- and three-dimensional problems which may be linear or nonlinear, steady-state or transient. The program is separated into two basic parts: data input module and preprocessor, and solution and output modules. Each of the modules can be very complex. The program is written in FORTRAN IV and is listed in Ref. (8). In order to build a program which can solve many types of problems a macro-programming language is introduced. This language is associated with a set of compact subprograms, each designed to compute one or a few basic steps necessary in a finite element solution process. For simplicity, all equations are retained in core. Therefore, the program capacity is limited by the computer used. The program is written to serve as a research and educational tool. The various modules can be added or changed as desired.

Programs for Desk-Top and Mini-Computers

Until recently, finite element programs have been installed almost exclusively in mini-, midi-, and maxi-computers. For using the capabilities that most of the programs include, it is necessary to assemble different hardware units such as printers, plotters, and graphical devices. For some desk-top computers, all of these features are built together, forming a degree of integration that is very attractive for the practicing engineer. This makes the FEM much more "available." In addition to these attractive hardware features, many of the existing programs are in a conversational mode so that they are very easy to use. The capacity of the desk-top computers are such that most of the programs available are special-purpose programs rather than general-purpose programs.

Finite element programs for desk-top computers are now only in BASIC, but FORTRAN programs should also be available in the near future. The programs surveyed here are only in BASIC.

Program name: SPACEFRAME

Developed and supported by Technische Datenverarbeitung, Dipl. Ing. Heinz Pircher, A-8010 Graz, Luthergasse 4., Austria. Also supported by Teknisk Data A/S, Boks 86, Bryn N-Oslo 6, Norway and Advanced Engineering Consultants AB, Box 3044, S-580 03 Linköping, Sweden.

General information. User's and theoretical manual available. The program is implemented on Hewlett-Packard 9830, 9831, 9835, 9845, IBM 5110, IBM Sl, and Olivetti P6060.

Program capability. Linear statics, second-order theory and eigenfrequency analysis for spaceframes and trusses. 450 elements and 500 nodal points. Unlimited loading cases (sequential processing). Capacity may depend on machine configuration. A number of different load types are available: point loads, line loads, temperature change, self-weight, prescribed displacements, centrifugal mass forces, load series for influence lines. The output is element displacements, element internal forces and element stresses on extreme fibers. The graphics output are axonometric representation of: undeformed structure, element numbers, nodal point numbers, deformed structure, internal forces and vibration modes.

Solution methods. Matrix displacement method; Gauss elimination; geometric stiffness with iterative modifications.

Element library. Beam/truss element with two nodal points; eccentric connections; constant section and up to six degrees of freedom per nodal point. Elastic spring support/link elements with up to six components.

Notable items. Input in conversational mode; extensive load combinations; profile data input via tables; steel dimensioning; concrete dimensioning; parts of the structure may be analyzed without change of input data; results from different construction stages may be superimposed. Program modules for prestressed bridges, cable geometry, computation of prestress-forces, design checks for allowable load, ultimate load and maximum tensile stresses. Geometrically nonlinear and stability analyses are possible.

Program name: AXISHELL

Developed and supported by Technische Datenverarbeitung, Dipl. Ing. Heinz Pircher, A-8010 Graz, Luthergasse 4, Austria. Also supported by Teknisk Data A/S, Boks 86, Bryn N-Oslo 6, Norway, and Advanced Engineering Consultants AB, Box 3044, S-580 03 Linköping, Sweden.

General information. User's and theoretical manual available. The program is implemented on Data-General MICRO-NOVA and Hewlett-Packard 9845S.

Program capability. Linear statics with Fourier series expansion in circumferential direction. 250 elements, 250 nodal points, and 20 Fourier terms. Unlimited loading cases (sequential processing). Capacity may be limited by the machine configuration. The following load types are included: constant load over an angle symmetric or antisymmetric, distributed surface loads, temperature change, point load, dead weight, distributed load in defined direction and inertia forces. All loads except inertia forces may be expanded in Fourier series. The output are for each loading case and each Fourier term and on selected angles, element displacements, and element internal forces in element centers. The graphics output is an axisymmetric representation of: three-dimensional undeformed structures, element and nodal point numbers, deformed structures, and internal forces.

Solution methods. Matrix displacement method, Gauss elimination with Fourier series expansion.

Element library. Conical axisymmetric thin shell element with two nodal points and up to four degrees of freedom per node - unsymmetric loads through Fourier series expansion. Elastic spring and link element with up to four components.

Notable items. Input in conversational mode. Extensive load combinations: dead, live, live with sign change, load exclusion, load exclusion with sign change. Results for any angle may be obtained.

Program name: FEMBAS

Developed and supported by Advanced Engineering Consultants AB, Box 3044, S-580 03 Linköping, Sweden.

General information. User's manual available. The program is implemented on Hewlett-Packard 9845 and Tektronix 405112.

Program capability. Linear statics analysis of two- and three-dimensional trusses, two-dimensional frames, plane stress and plane strain problems, axisymmetric shells and solid problems could be analyzed. The program is modularly designed and it is possible to include any element with three degrees of freedom per node. Different types of elements could be included on user's request. A number of fixed load types for trusses and beams are included. Line loads and surface load types are included. The output is displacements and stresses for user specified nodes and elements. Graphics output is structure geometry, node and element numbers and deformed structure.

Solution method. Matrix displacement method, Gauss elimination with skyline band method.

Element library. Linear truss element, cubic beam element. Isoparametric bilinear plane stress and strain element. Bilinear axisymmetric element.

Notable items. Input in conversational mode. Modularity implies that the analysis and reanalysis is directed by the user. Easy to modify loads and/or structure or boundary condition and perform reanalysis. Easy to include user specified elements on request.

Program name: FESDEC

Developed by Engineering Computer Services, Ltd., Piccadilly, Tamworth, Staffs B78 2ER, England. Sales and technical support in the United States and Canada is provided by H. G. Engineering, Ltd., 260 Lesmill Rd., Don Mills, Ontario, Canada M3B 2T5.

General information. FESDEC stands for a Finite Element System for Desktop Computers. The program is written in extended BASIC and uses the modular design principle. Program modules can communicate with each other by modifying the data base; no data is passed from one module to another in common storage areas. FESDEC is implemented on the Hewlett-Packard 9845. The program has been designed to operate about 60 K bytes. Problem size is limited only by the amount of the secondard storage available.

Program capability. The program can handle linear elastic static and dynamic analysis of two- and three-dimensional structures. Two-dimensional mesh generation and an ability to do the mesh plotting is included in the system. The results of an analysis may be viewed as deflected shape plots and two-dimensional stress vector and contour diagrams.

Element library. Isoparametric membranes, shells and solid elements.

Notable items. Local coordinate system may be skewed at a node. Linear constraints may be applied for any user.

A lot of programs are available on mini-computers. For details, the reader is referred to catalogues [A-11 - A-13]. The reader is also referred to the section "Summary of Major Finite Element Programs" of this section. Many of the programs presented there are also available on mini- and/or midi-computers. In this section we will describe some FEM programs that are not classified as general purpose but rather as special purpose programs for mini-computers.

Program name: SPACEFRAME

This is the FORTRAN version of the desktop BASIC program described earlier. Development and support are the same.

General information. User's and theoretical manuals are available. The program is implemented on Data General NOVA, Data General ECLIPSE, Interdata 8132, Hewlett-Packard 3000, NORD 10S, UNIVAC 90/30, SIEMENS 4004, IBM S1, PRIME.

Program capability. In addition to the desktop program this program can perform linear response analysis and critical rotations. Depending on computer configuration, 2000 elements and 1000 nodal points could be analyzed. Output and graphical output is the same as for the desktop program.

Solution methods. In addition to the desktop program, the determinant search and modal superposition methods are used.

Element library. Beam/truss elements with two nodal points, eccentric connections, constant section and up to six DOF per nodal point, flange element, bend element, elastic spring/link elements with up to six components.

Notable items. Same as for the desktop version.

Program name: MISES 3

Developed and supported by Technische Datenverarbeitung, Dipl. Ing. Heinz Pircher, A-8010 Graz, Luthergasse 4, Austria. Also supported by Teknisk Data A/S, Boks 86, Bryn N-Oslo 6, Norway and Advanced Engineering Consultants AB, Box 3044, S-580 03 Linköping, Sweden.

General information. User's and theoretical manuals are available. The program is implemented on Data General NOVA, Data General ECLIPSE, Hewlett-Packard 3000, Interdata 8/32, UNIVAC 90/30, PRIME.

Program capability. Linear statics and nonlinear material behavior analysis. Two-dimensional plane stress/strain problems, three-dimensional and axisymmetric solid problems and three-dimensional trusses could be analyzed. Nodal point loads, distributed surface loads, mass forces, temperature loads and surface loads from primary stress state are included. Primary output is element oriented, nodal point displacements, element Gauss-point stresses, plastic zones. Secondary results are nodal point oriented, stresses (linearly extrapolated from Gauss-points) or stresses computed via element shape functions. Von Mises or Tresca equivalent stresses, principal stresses and directions. Graphics output are axonometric representation of undeformed structure, element and nodal point numbers, deformed structure, isostress lines, stresses as vectors, and plastic zones. Seven hundred elements, 1500-10000 nodal points (secondary result limited when nodal points greater than 1500 for 16-bit machines). Five hundred is maximum bandwidth. Capacity depends on machine configuration.

Solution method. Gauss elimination, initial strain. Material laws, von Mises and Drucker-Prager.

Element library. Two-dimensional eight-node biquadratic isoparametric element. Isoparametric parabolic three-dimensional element with curved edges. Isoparametric parabolic axisymmetric element with curved edges. Two/three-dimensional rod linear element.

Notable items. Special functions for excavation, temperature loads automatically from MISHEAT3 (described below). Isostress lines may be obtained in a section within a three-dimensional element. Elements may be disconnected, coordinate input in several user-defined systems. Input coordinates may be Cartesian, cylindrical or spherical. Automatic mesh generation through use of "super-elements". Layered material possible in visco-plastic analysis.

Program name: MISHEAT3

Developed and supported by Technische Datenverarbeitung, Dipl. Ing. Heinz Pircher, A-8010 Graz, Luthergasse 4, Austria. Also supported by Teknisk Data A/S, Boks 86, Bryn N-Oslo 6, Norway and Advanced Engineering Consultants AB, Box 3044, S-580 03 Linköping, Sweden.

General information. User's and theoretical manuals are available. Program implemented on Data General NOVA and ECLIPSE, Hewlett-Packard 3000, Interdata 8/32 PRIME.

Program capability. This is a program for two-, three-dimensional, and axisymmetric stationary and instationary temperature, magnetic flow potential problems. Element and nodal point capacity as for MISES3. The following boundary conditions could be used: convection, conduction, radiation, prescribed field values and supplied or removed heat on boundaries. The primary output are element oriented, temperature and temperature gradients. Secondary results are nodal point oriented, temperature and temperature gradients. Graphics output are axonometric representation of structure, element and node numbers, isotherm lines, temperature gradients as vectors.

Solution methods. Gauss elimination, Galerkin for time steps.

Element library. Parabolic elements with curved edges for two-, three-dimensional and axisymmetric elements.

Notable items. Same element as MISES3; temperatures may be transported automatically. Isotherms may be obtained in a section within a three-dimensional element, coordinate input in several user-defined systems. Input coordinates may be Cartesian, cylindrical, or spherical. Automatic mesh generation through use of "super-elements".

Program name: SHELL

Developed and supported by Technische Datenverarbeitung, Dipl. Ing. Heinz Pircher, A-8010 Graz, Luthergasse 4, Austria. Also supported by Teknisk Data A/S, Boks 86, Brun N-Oslo 6, Norway and Advanced Engineering Consultants AB, Box 3044, S-580 03 Linköping, Sweden.

General information. User's and theoretical manuals are available. The program is implemented on Data General NOVA and ECLIPSE, Hewlett-Packard 3000 and Interdata 8/32, PRIME.

Program capability. Linear statics and dynamics analysis of general shells. Reduction to plate and/or membrane problems. Loads may be global/local, constant/variable line load and surface load, point loads, self weight, centrifugal mass forces, influence surfaces, prescribed deflections and load by function. The number of elements may be 400-600 and the number of nodal points may be 1200-2000. Maximum front width is 308. Capacity depends on computer configuration. The output is element displacements at nodal points and eccentric points, element stresses, element forces, principal stresses, principal forces and spring element forces. The graphics output is axisymmetric representation of undeformed structure, element and nodal point numbers, eccentric connections, upper/lower/middle surface of element, thickness vector, deformed structure, stresses/forces as vectors and influence surfaces as isolevel lines.

Solution methods. Gauss elimination with frontal solution technique, reduced integration. Determinant search technique.

Notable items. Load combination max/min, dead/live loads. Thickness vector may be specified off-normal to element mid-surface.

Program name: GIFTS 4 (32-37)

Prof. H. A. Kamel, Aerospace and Mechanical Engineering Department, University of Arizona, Tucson, Arizona 85721, USA

General information. GIFTS is a graphically-oriented structural analysis package developed and used in an educational environment. The system is designed to fit in a relatively small core area and, therefore, it is specifically suited to time sharing and mini-computer systems. Development started about five years ago. GIFTS 4 has been supported by the Office of Naval Research and the United States Coast Guard. It is in the public domain and may be obtained for a nominal charge from the University of Arizona in the form of the source code on magnetic tape and the user's, theoretical and systems manuals. At present the GIFTS package is installed on DG ECLIPSE, PDP, DEC, PRIME, CDC 6000 series and IBM 370 series of computers. Support and user's group exists. User's workshop and courses are held.

Program capability. GIFTS 4 is not a single program but a collection of modules present in a program library. Analysis capabilities include static solution package, natural vibration package, transient response package and constrained substructuring package. Linear elastic material.

Pre- and postprocessor capabilities. GIFTS pre- and postprocessor part may be used together with GIFTS analysis routines or with other finite element programs. All data generated by the system are stored in a number of files. In order to interface the system to a particular program, it is only necessary to write two simple linking programs to pass data back and forth between two sets of program files. Pre- and postprocessor capabilities are as follows. Automatic model generation and interactive model editor. Display of model outlines or detailed element plots. Choice of absolute viewing direction or incremental rotations. Generation and display of load and boundary conditions. A plot of the deformed model. User may change the display scale, or create loading cases by linearly combining a number of loading cases. A bandwidth optimization routine is included, although the programs are not bandwidth limited. Module for reduction of analysis results.

Element library. Elements are classified into three categories. In the first one the elements may be generated and displayed in unstressed and in stressed form. GIFTS can compute their mass distribution, stiffness matrix, equivalent nodal loads and stresses. Represented elements: rod, beam, membrane and plate bending elements. Elements within the second category can be generated and displayed only. Elements in the last category can be stored only.

Solution methods.
Equation solver - Matrix partitioning, Cholesky decomposition procedure
Eigenvalue and dynamic analysis - Subspace iteration method; the Houbolt method (third order backward difference scheme).

Notable items. Substructuring and constrained substructuring capabilities. The program may also be used to extract practically any subset of information from the database and print them in an organized manner. HELP command.

Program name: PREFEM (22)

Developed and supported by Advanced Engineering Corporation, Landalagången 6, S-411 30 Göteborg, Sweden.

General information. User's manual available. The program is implemented on IBM 360, 370, 3033 and UNIVAC 1100.

Program capability. The program is tailored for bending analysis of rectangular elastic plates. An incorporated preprocessor reduces the manual effort for preparing input data to an absolute minimum. The program is also equipped with a postprocessor which presents the computed results on lucid tableaux, printer diagrams and plotter diagrams.

Plates of variable stiffness, plates with holes, with distributed loads, line loads and point loads, with rigid and elastic supports and with supports subject to settlements are easily analyzed.

Solution method. Mixed method, Gaussian elimination.

Element library. Mixed rectangular plate bending elements with four corner deflections and four edge moments as unknown quantities.

Notable items. Fixed or free format input. The program is very simple to use.

Program name: SERFEM (23)

Developed and supported by Advanced Engineering Corporation, Landalagången 6, S-411 30 Göteborg, Sweden.

General information. User's manual available. The program is implemented on IBM 360, 370, 3033 and UNIVAC 1100.

Program capability. The program is tailored for in-plane analysis of rectangular elastic plates. An incorporated preprocessor reduces the manual effort for preparing input data to an absolute minimum. The program is also equipped with a postprocessor which presents the computed results on lucid tableaux, printer diagrams and plotter diagrams.

Plates of variable stiffness, plates with holes, with distributed loads, line loads and point loads, with rigid and elastic supports and with supports subject to settlements are easily analyzed.

Solution method. Displacement method, Gaussian elimination.

Element library. Rectangular plane stress elements with eight degrees of freedom (incompatible bending modes normally included).

Notable items. Fixed or free format input. The program is very simple to use.

General Purpose Finite Element Programs

In this survey it is, of course, impossible to present all the existing programs. Considerable effort is spent on the further development of widely used general purpose program systems and the new programs being developed. Thousands of finite element programs are in use all over the world. The chances of newly developed general purpose programs succeeding in the competitive market are probably very small. Instead of replacing the established software systems by completely new ones, it appears to be more practical and economic to build upon the old systems when new features are developed. Readers interested in the development trends and aspects of large general purpose finite element systems are referred to (9-23).

Most of the surveyed programs are well known and widely used. We shall also concentrate our attention on some of the relatively new and less known programs. Programs are presented in a descriptive and tabular form. Two categories may be distinguished. In the first category the main development effort has been done on the performance of linear static/dynamic calculations. The second represents the programs specially designed for nonlinear analysis.

Descriptive survey

This section gives a descriptive survey of general information, program capabilities, pre- and postprocessor capabilities, solution methods used, element library review and notable items. A quick reference for the program capabilities is given in Tables 1 to 4. The following programs are surveyed: ADINA, ANSYS, ASAS, ASKA, BERSAFE, MARC, MISA, MSC/NASTRAN, NEPSAP, PAFEC, SAMCEF, SAP and SESAM 69.

Program name: ADINA (24-27)

Prof. K. J. Bathe, Department of Mechanical Engineering, Massachusetts Institute of Technology, Cambridge, MA 02139, USA

General information. ADINA stands for Automatic Dynamic Incremental Nonlinear Analysis. The code was developed on experiences obtained from codes SAP IV and NONSAP. Development started in 1974. The program is fully operational but new routines are continuously developed. Research and development efforts are financed by a user's group of ADINA. Members of the user's group pay a yearly contribution and in return obtain the source code of the program and all new developments as long as they are members of the group. The source code is transmitted with sample data cases and their solutions. ADINA is a proprietary code. It is implemented on CDC 6400/6600/7600, IBM 360/370 and UNIVAC 1108/1110. Documentation consists of the program description, sample analyses and user's manual.

User's conferences and courses are being held each year.

Program capability. ADINA is a general purpose linear and nonlinear static and dynamic three-dimensional finite element analysis program. ADINAT has been employed for the solution of heat transfer and analogous field problems. The nonlinearities may be due to large displacements, large strains, and nonlinear material behavior. The material description available is: linear elastic, nonlinear elastic, thermoelastic, elastic-plastic, and thermo-elastic-plastic and creep for one-dimensional elements. For the two-dimensional elements: isotropic linear elastic, orthotropic linear elastic, isotropic thermo-elastic, curve description model, concrete model, elastic-plastic material, thermo-elastic-plastic-creep and Mooney-Rivlin material. Three-dimensional elements: isotropic and orthotropic linear elastic, isotropic thermo-elastic, curve description model, concrete model, elastic-plastic material and thermo-elastic-plastic creep. The program can be used to restart at preselected time steps. Vibration and dynamic analysis includes computation of eigenvalues and eigenmodes, and dynamic response. Dynamic spectral analysis is not possible. Stability and analysis includes: nonlinear collapse, dynamic and postbuckling.

Pre- and postprocessor capabilities. ADINA and ADINAT programs do not include any pre- or postprocessors. These are available through the user's group. MIT does not plan to develop other pre- and postprocessors.

Some pre- and postprocessing programs used in connection with ADINA are a series of programs developed at Civil Engineering Laboratory, Port Hueneme (28), FEMGEN mesh generator (29-30), INGEN (31), GIFTS (32-37).

Element library. General truss, beam, two- and three-dimensional isoparametric (or subparametric) elements are available. Depending on the element type, four different analysis procedures are available: linear elastic analysis, materially nonlinear only analysis, total Lagrangian formulation, updated Lagrangian formulation.

Solution methods.

Equation solver	- Compacted out-of-core solver
Eigenvalues	- Determinant search, subspace iteration is being incorporated
Dynamic response	- Implicit time integration (Newmark or Wilson) or explicit time integration (central difference method)
Nonlinear problems	- Incremental solution, Newton-Raphson method

Notable items. ADINA offers a very large range of applications, but some important features are missing. Substructuring is not possible but is currently under development. Specified displacement boundary conditions as an option is also under development. It is possible and easy to incorporate ones own element types. An effective usage of the program requires intensive training.

Program name: ANSYS (38-42)

Swanson Analysis Systems, Inc., P.O. Box 65, Houston, PA 15342, USA

General information. The program has been used commercially since 1970. It is widely available in the United States through many computer utility networks and also outside the USA. The program can be used on a computer time sharing basis or on an in-house royalty basis. The documentation consists of user's manual, examples manual, verification manual, theoretical manual and introductory manual. Programmer's manual is not scheduled for release to the general user community. Training seminars are available through Swanson Analysis Systems consulting service and through CDC centers. ANSYS can be run in batch, time-sharing and fully interactive graphic processing. It is implemented on CDC, IBM, UNIVAC, CRAY, AMDAHL, PRIME (mini), MODCOMP (mini) and VAX (mini) machines.

Program capability. The program capabilities include structural and heat transfer analyses. The structural analyses can handle static and dynamic linear and nonlinear analysis. Heat transfer includes steady-state and transient analysis, conduction, convection and radiation. Coupled thermal-fluid flow capability, coupled thermal-electric capability and wave motion analysis are also included.

Pre- and postprocessor capability. PREP 5 and PREP 7 are mesh generators. PREP 6 is transient boundary condition generator. Two-, three-dimensional and intersecting shell mesh generators are available. Data sets for transient dynamic analysis may be generated. Element reordering routines for wave front minimization. Geometry plotting is available for all elements in the ANSYS library, including isometric and perspective views. Plotting of stresses, displacements and temperatures are possible. The program permits variables calculated from a solution run and stored on a data file to be included in a number of mathematical operations (addition, subtraction, multiplication, etc.).

Element library. Finite elements available in the library number more than forty for static and dynamic analyses, thirteen for heat transfer analyses, three for thermal-fluid analyses, three for thermal-electric analyses, and two for wave motion analyses. All element types are represented. Special structural elements include masses, springs, dampers, sliding interfaces, gap interfaces and cables. Arbitrary stiffness, matrix elements are also available.

Solution methods.

Equation solver	- Wave front method
Condensation	- Guyan's reduction
Eigenvalues	- Jacobi eigenvalue extraction
Dynamic response	- Modal superposition; Harmonic response; Implicit quadratical integration
Nonlinear problems	- Incremental method

Notable items. New features added to the program are announced to the user on the printout. Effective data checking and error messages tell the user of difficulties which the program has encountered in his data. Solution time and core size estimates are also given. Restart capability. Other notable program options: seismic loading, spectrum analysis, linear multipoint constraint equations, both primary and secondary creep, large deflection in dynamic analysis, etc.

Program name: ASAS (43-47)

Atkins Research and Development, Woodcote Grove, Ashley Road, Epsom, Surrey KT18 5BW, England

General information. Development started in 1970. The program system consists of a number of programs, e.g., ASAS G - general purpose finite element program; ASAS HEAT - a general purpose heat conduction program; ASAS RESPONSE - general purpose dynamic response program. The documentation consists of user's manual, programmer's manual, theoretical manual, and comparative sample problems manual. Program system is installed on IBM, CDC, UNIVAC, AMDAHL, HONEYWELL, DEC, PRIME and XEROX computers. User's conferences are held each year. Atkins Computing runs two day "Introduction to ASAS" courses regularly.

Program capability. The program can solve linear elastostatic isotropic and anisotropic problems. Eigenvalue, linear response and spectral analysis of dynamic systems can be handled. Possibility for steady-state heat transfer problems. Transient heat transfer problems can be analyzed in a separate program. Special purpose programs for offshore engineering applications.

Pre- and postprocessor capabilities. Application dependent and independent programs are available. MESH3 and MESH4 may be used to generate two-dimensional meshes with control over mesh size and growth pattern, and automatic nodal matching between adjacent regions. MESHMOD provides an interactive facility for editing and amending these meshes at a Tektronix terminal. ASDIS is an interactive viewing program which operates in timesharing or batch mode with a storage tube or hardcopy plotter, respectively. It can handle any viewing angle, has zoom facilities, provides automatic scaling, etc. ASBAND - bandwidth optimization; ASASLOCO - load factoring and combination; FATJACK - dynamic fatigue analysis of offshore jackets. A system called ENGRAVE is under development. It will provide geometry generation, mesh generation, selection, editing, viewing and output modules. It will supersede the generation, selection, editing, viewing and output modules. It will supersede the ASDIS program and provide considerably enhanced facilities based on a common databasing system.

Element library. Element library contains the elements based on displacement and force equilibrium formulation. All element types are represented. Special purpose elements are represented by membrane crack tip elements and warped shear panels. A family of stress-hybrid membrane elements is under development.

Solution methods.

Equation solver	- Wave front method in-core; partitioned Cholesky out-of-core
Condensation	- Guyan's reduction
Eigenvalues	- Superspace iteration, Jacobi, Householder, QL, Householder Sturm sequence
Dynamic response	- Newmark β-method

Notable items. Automatic handling of self-weight and centrifugal forces; rigorous data checks and cross checks; the system is economical for any size problem with automatic selection of frontal or three-partition out-of-core solution, and unlimited load cases in one run; stress checks against allowed stress levels; constrained relation possibilities; no possibility for initial stress and strain calculations.

Program name: ASKA (48-68)

Statik und Dynamik Forschungsgesellschart GmbH, Postfach 80 1044, 7 Stuttgart 80, West Germany

General information. ASKA stands for Automatic System for Kinematic Analyses. The development started about 1965. The range of organizations that maintain an ASKA installation comprises large corporations (in-house use), data centers (use on service basis) and universities (research). The program consists of the following parts: ASKA I, ASKA II, ASKA III-1, ASKA III-2, ASKA-HS, ASKA-CS, ASKA-FM and ASKA-HEAT. There exists a comprehensive program documentation contained in thirteen volumes and includes theoretical manuals, user's reference manuals, training manuals, etc. ASKA is implemented on IBM, ICL, UNIVAC, CDC, Honeywell, Burroughs, VAX and PRIME computers. A user's conference is held every year.

Program capability. The program can handle linear elastic isotropic and anisotropic structures. Structures with nonlinear material properties, elastic-plastic materials and creep may be analyzed. For elastic-plastic material the von Mises yield criterion with associated Prandtl-Reuss flow rule is adopted. Isotropic, kinematic and mixed hardening are included. Additionally, a Drucker-Prager generalization of the linear and the parabolic Mohr-Coulomb laws with non-associated flow rule may be adopted. Dynamic capabilities include eigenvalue analysis, linear response and spectral analysis. A multilevel substructuring technique is incorporated. The program has several so-called rigid formats for limited range of applications. For problems that cannot be solved by means of the rigid format, the user writes his own steering program to perform the appropriate analysis steps (so called APC program). This program is a series of calls to ASKA processors that perform the solution steps required.

Pre- and postprocessor capabilities. FEMGEN (29,30) finite element mesh generator is used as a preprocessor program. The program may be used either in batch or interactively from a timesharing terminal. It is directed by a command language which is easy to learn. FEMGEN automatically generates topology and coordinates, the intersection points and space curves are easily obtained. Extensive plotting facilities are available for checking and viewing. The structure may be saved on a database for later reloading, changing or further development. FEPS, Finite Element Plotting System, is used as a postprocessor program.

Element library. Flange, beam, membrane, plate, shell, axisymmetric and solid elements are included in ASKA element library. The material properties can be isotropic or anisotropic. Element types can be combined to model various types of load paths. The system design philosophy allows quite simple incorporation of new element types. Extensive library of beam elements. They differ in the shape of the cross-section (solid, thin-walled closed, thin-walled open, including torsion bending effects) and in the placement of their nodes (e.g., eccentric connection).

Solution methods.

Equation solver	- Partitioned Gauss-elimination
Condensation	- Guyan's reduction
Eigenvalues	- Simultaneous vector iteration; Householder, Jacobi
Dynamic response	- Modal superposition with the option of analytical integration of harmonic linear and delta function; Numerical integration of user specified functions; Direct integration
Nonlinear problems	- Initial strain/stress method

Notable items. A large number of options are available. A comprehensive set of data checks (more than 600 different error messages). Restart facility. Analysis of axisymmetric structure with nonaxisymmetric loads is possible. General hypermatrix operations. User access to internal data makes it possible to apply ones own defined subroutines, which then can be used in the APC program to perform special analysis. The approach of integrated evolution is followed in the concept of ASKA 80 (12) presently under development. The introduction of a net type allows further differentiation without the need to break the software into a large number of incompatible derivatives.

Program name: BERSAFE (70-84)

Central Electricity Generating Board, Research and Development Department, Berkeley Nuclear Laboratories, Berkeley, Gloucestershire GL3 9PB, England

General information. Development started in 1967 at the Berkeley Nuclear Laboratories. The program consists of BERSAFE, BERDYNE, FLHE and a large number of pre- and postprocessor programs. The system was initially designed for power plant problems, but its versatility has permitted its application to a large number of other analysis problems outside the power industry. BERSAFE and its associated programs are fully available also to users outside the CEGB. The system may be used on client's own computer under a licensing agreement, or alternatively at the CEGB Computing Bureau. Documentation consists of manuals to all modules and theoretical reports for some of the modules. The system is implemented on IBM, UNIVAC and ICL computers. A user's group exists.

Program capability. BERSAFE can perform linear and nonlinear isotropic and anisotropic elasto-plastic analysis of arbitrary structures subjected to pressures, point loads, body forces, rotational forces and temperature distributions. BERDYNE can handle the linear elastic behavior of arbitrary two- or three-dimensional structures subjected to free, forced undamped or forced damped vibrations. The FLHE program is designed to perform the calculation of steady-state or transient temperatures in arbitrary structures subject to thermal loading. The nonlinear materials version of the BERSAFE system includes isotropic and kinematic hardening. Plasticity and creep may also be performed with thermal transient loading. Routines for special rock behavior properties are also included. The program may also be used for electromagnetic potential calculations.

Pre- and postprocessor capabilities. BERMESH, BERGEN, BERCYL, etc., are the programs for mesh generation of two- and three-dimensional structures. DATAGEN is the program for mesh and other input data modifications. POINTA is an interactive graphics pre- and postprocessing system. It consists of generating, editing and plotting parts. Facilities are also provided for allocating and checking loads and constraints. PLOT 3 program, a module of POINTA system, can display the important analysis results. Interactive display of output variables such as stresses and temperatures is also available. The postprocessing programs include BERPLOT (plotting of meshes and analysis results), ELOPPER (comprehensive output program for results from an elastic analysis), etc.

Element Library. About fifty different element types are available in the element library. They are categorized under plane stress, plane strain, axisymmetric, three-dimensional beams and shells. These can be further classified into two groups: simple and complex. Geometry and loading data may be specified in Cartesian, polar or cylindrical coordinates, irrespective of element type used. A decoupling feature included in the program enables any number of DOF at any node to be independent between different elements meeting at that node (useful e.g., for crack problems or shear slip problems). Singular elements are also included in the BERSAFE system. They are used around the crack tip so that the radial (from tip) displacement varies as $\sqrt{r}$, whereas circumferentially the variation is a standard polynomial form. Mainly for elastic, can be used for nonlinear cases (when the displacement variation is unknown).

Solution methods.

Equation solver	- Frontal solution method
Eigenvalues	- Sturm sequence
Dynamic response	- Direct time integration
Nonlinear problems	- Initial stress method; initial strain method; tangential stiffness method.

Notable items. The program is particularly effective for crack analysis, where it has been applied extensively (85-90). Special techniques for fracture mechanics is included in the system. User specified stiffness. Automatic bandwidth optimizer. Substructuring technique is presently also available.

Program name: MARC (91-98)

MARC Analysis Corporation, 260 Sheridan Avenue, Palo Alto, CA 94306, USA

General information. The program is based on research work carried out by Dr. P. V. Marcal and his colleagues. In 1969 MARC Analysis Company was formed to develop the current MARC system. The program has since been widely used via CDC computer centers, University Computing Company, etc. MARC Analysis arranges one week courses at intervals of about two months to introduce new users to the MARC system of programs. New features added to the program are announced in MARC Corporation's Quarterly Newsletter.

The program documentation includes User Information Manual, Program Input Manual and Demonstration Problems Manual. Program is implemented on IBM, CDC, UNIVAC and PRIME computers.

Program capability. The program is capable of dealing with both linear and nonlinear static and dynamic analyses. It is built of three different libraries: element, material and structural. The material library contains 35 different models. Examples of material models are generalized Maxwell Mooney large-strain elasticity, hypoelasticity, von Mises and Mohr-Coulomb plasticity, temperature and strain rate dependent yield stress, von Mises type of creep, pure volumetric (swelling) and pure deviatoric creep, anisotropic behavior for elasticity-plasticity-creep, viscoplasticity, low tension and cracking, etc.

The structural library contains procedures for linear static nonlinear static, linear dynamic, modal and proportional damping, and lumped masses for dynamic analysis, large displacement, buckling, elastic-plastic buckling, creep buckling, transient and steady-state heat transfer, etc. Nonlinear geometric or material behaviors may be included in dynamic analysis.

Pre- and postprocessor capabilities. MARC has 2- and 3-dimensional mesh generators, bandwidth optimization. Plane or perspective plotting of a mesh is provided. The 3D program permits perspective display of solid 3D structures with hidden lines removed. Postprocessor plotting facilities. They include plotting isotherms, isostress and isostrain components and deformed geometry. For 3D solid elements, plots are displayed as perspective plots of user selected sections.

Element library. All general element types are represented. More than sixty different elements are available. Some special element types include: special pipe bend element, 1D truss/gap element in space, 1D gap and friction link in space, generalized plane strain element, axisymmetric torsional element, linear and nonlinear spring, concentrated masses, etc.

Solution methods.

Equation solver	- Gaussian elimination
Eigenvalues	- Inverse power sweep
Dynamic response	- Modal superposition; Duhamel exact integration, Implicit Newmark's β-method; Explicit central difference method, Houbolt operator; Step-by-step using tangent stiffness
Nonlinear problems	- Tangent stiffness; Initial strain.

Notable items. MARC is probably the most advanced program for nonlinear and complex analysis existing today. It is mainly developed for analyses of nonlinear problems. The program contains many notable items including: tying degrees of freedom; joining shell and solid - fine and coarse mesh; user supplied constraints; the program checks the mesh quality from an energy point of view; all nonlinear material behavior may be combined with geometric nonlinear behavior; great versatility of problem description exists in the program as a result of the "User Subroutines" in which a program user describes a very general problem by means of a short subroutine; a restart feature permits restart at an increment of a problem whether it is nonlinear or a series of elastic analyses on the same structure, etc. Substructuring is not yet included in the program.

Program name: MISA (99-102)

Mitsui Engineering Shipbuilding Company, Ltd., Technical Research and Development Headquarters, 6-4, Tsukiji 5-Chome, Shuo-Ku, Tokyo, Japan

General information. MISA stands for the MItsui Structural Analysis Program. Development started in 1971. The program has been in practical use since 1974. The program system is designed to have high performance pre- and postprocessors, thus special efforts have been applied for the saving of manpower and computer time. MISA is applicable to a large scale structural analysis with minimum and automatic I/O data preparation. Functions of the program can be optioned depending on the kind of calculation. The program is implemented on IBM computers. A large amount of documentation has been prepared, particularly for the user's convenience.

Program capability. MISA is limited to linear stress analysis and steady-state heat conduction analysis followed by thermal stress analysis of structures. Capabilities for extension to dynamic and nonlinear problems. The program structure consists of an executive module, three pre- and postprocessing modules, and six analysis modules. Each module consists of several submodules. A dynamic serial structure has the function of bringing the modules needed during execution from the program library into the main storage. Multilevel substructuring is available. For the identical substructures within the structure, the time for data preparation and matrix calculation can be efficiently reduced by use of the COPY option. This option can be used for all levels of the structure, independent of substructure boundary conditions. The DOF of joints for a combined structure can be determined automatically. The hierarchy of the structure can be determined automatically.

Pre- and postprocessor capabilities. Preprocessor parts have the following capabilities: generation of structure, load and restraint condition, using super-elements as units of input; checking of data at an early stage; nodes renumbering to reduce the bandwidth; graphic display of the structure, load and boundary conditions. Input generator can generate one-three dimensional meshes with arbitrary subdivisions including cylindrical, spherical, and conical surfaces. Postprocessor has the possibility of plots of contour lines or intensity levels of stress components, principal stresses and equivalent stresses; plotting of displacements or deformations; printout of the results suitable for formal reports; combination of the results for load conditions. Further extension of pre- and postprocessing capabilities is under development. Usage of the interactive modes, including free format feature and graphic CRT are being investigated for the MISA system. Data generation is the most highly developed feature of MISA compared with other general purpose programs.

Element library. The library contains 27 different elements for stress analysis and 16 elements for heat conduction analysis. All element types are represented. Displacement and Pian's hybrid formulation.

Solution methods.
Equation solver - Wave front method; LDU decomposition.

Notable items. MISA is a user-oriented program with main emphasis on the user's convenience. Restart function and constrained relations option are available. Nonsymmetric loads on an axisymmetric structure can be treated.

Program name: MSC/NASTRAN (103-121)

The MacNeal-Schwendler Corporation, 815 West Colorado Blvd., Los Angeles, CA 90041, USA

General information. Development started in 1966 and was sponsored by NASA. Today there are three versions of NASTRAN. The official version is distributed by NASA through COSMIC. One version is distributed by Sperry Univac. The version described here is the MSC/NASTRAN. This is the version maintained and continuously developed by MacNeal-Schwendler Corporation. MSC/NASTRAN documentation consists of user's manual, theoretical manual, application manual, basic training manual, analyst's guide and programmer's manual. The program is marketed and serviced from MSC's offices in Los Angeles, Munich and Tokyo. User's conferences are held each year in the United States and Europe. NASTRAN educational courses are available. NASTRAN is implemented on CDC, CYBER, IBM, AMDAHL, FACØM, ITEL, UNIVAC, DEC, VAX computers.

Program capability. MSC/NASTRAN is a self-contained system and cannot be described as a suite of small programs. It is a large-scale general-purpose computer program that can solve linear static and dynamic as well as material (introduced in Fall 1979) and geometric nonlinear problems. Heat transfer, aero-elasticity, acoustics, electromagnetism and other field problems can also be run in batch, timesharing or fully interactive graphic mode. NASTRAN has a number of so-called rigid formats which are prepackaged programs for static, dynamic and buckling analysis. For problems that cannot be solved by these rigid formats the user may write his own program performing the appropriate computational steps. The user writes a so-called Direct Matrix Abstraction Program (DMAP).

Pre- and postprocessor capabilities. Interactive graphics capabilities for input data are under development. MSGMESH generates finite element models of structures from analysis-supplied descriptions of one-, two- and three-dimensional regions and associated interconnection specifications. NASPLOT reads the plot file and generates correctly formatted input files for virtually any type of pen plotter. TEK- provides for a TEKTRONIX plotting capability in an interactive mode. There exists a number of pre- and postprocessors developed by users. For their review see Refs. (122-127). BANDIT-matrix bandwidth reduction.

Element library. A large number of elements are available. All types are represented. New developed elements are being continuously incorporated, e.g., higher-order plate, membrane and shell elements. Special purpose elements: shear panel and out-of-plane membrane, singular plastic element, rigid elements, elements for field problems, thermo-fluid element, scalar elements, general elements described by influence coefficients, etc.

Solution methods.

Equation solver	- Partitioned LDL^t decomposition for symmetric matrices; LDU^t decomposition for nonsymmetric matrices;
Condensation	- Guyan's reduction
Eigenvalues	- Determinant method; Inverse power with shifts; Givens and QR-method
Dynamic response	- Modal superposition; Numerical integration of uncoupled systems; Direct integration by Newmark β-method
Nonlinear problems	- Incremental method (tangent stiffness)

Notable items. MSC/NASTRAN is a very powerful program that enables the experienced user to analyze a great variety of problems. A large number of options are available. General matrix operations. Multipoint constraint. Rigid body motion. Multilevel substructuring. Restart capability.

Program name: NEPSAP (128-130)

Dr. S. Nagarajan, Lockheed Missiles and Space Company, Inc., P.O. Box 504, Sunnyvale, CA 94088, USA

General information. NEPSAP stands for Nonlinear Elastic-Plastic Structural Analysis Program. The program was developed at Lockheed to handle a wide range of nonlinear problems. It is offered for public use (binary or binary and source codes) for the first year license fee and the annual license renewal. NEPSAP is operational on the UNIVAC, CDC and CYBER computer systems. Training and documentation are available.

Program capability. The NEPSAP is a modular program in its structure. It is a general-purpose, three-dimensional nonlinear code capable of large displacements, thermo-elastic-plastic and creep analysis of arbitrary structures. The size of structural models analyzed is limited only by the available core size. Analytical capabilities also include: linear multiload analysis, nonlinear buckling, bifurcation buckling and vibration analysis, linear and nonlinear transient dynamic analysis, steady-state as well as nonlinear transient thermal stress analysis. Available material behavior: linear thermoelasticity, thermoplasticity, isotropic hardening with linear or piecewise linear strain hardening or kinematic hardening with linear strain hardening, orthotropic elasticity and composite materials, isotropic incompressible elastic material as well as incompressible thermo-elastic-plastic materials, creep behavior using the Odquist-Norton stationary creep power law with time-hardening and temperature-dependent material creep properties, etc.

Pre- and postprocessor capabilities. Input data can be generated by a flexible preprocessor program. Topology, boundary conditions and other data needed for the analysis are prepared and saved on a tape or mass storage data base. Free-field input of data using keywords. Bandwidth optimization. Error checking of data. Extensive printout control options. Minimum/maximum stress tables for each element group. Complete graphic package for model debugging and verification as well as display of results.

Element library. Wide range of different element types is available. Special purpose elements such as elements for incompressible materials, plate and shell elements with anisotropic multilayered construction, nonlinear straight and curved pipe elements, gap and contact elements.

Solution methods.

Equation solver	- Variable band skyline matrix solver
Dynamic analysis	- Newmark, Houbolt, Park or any user-defined refractoring intervals and variable time steps
Nonlinear problems	- Modified (tangent) stiffness approach with user-specified load and temperature increments

Notable items. Multi-point constraint conditions. Sliding boundaries, skewed coordinates and DOF. Multi-global coordinate systems, cylindrical and spherical coordinates. Restart and analysis data save options. Sophisticated database to administer data files to enable a very flexible modular structuring of the program especially useful for interactive applications.

Program name: PAFEC (131-132)

PAFEC, Ltd., Thane Road, Lenton Industrial Estate West, Nottingham NG7 2TG, England

General information. Development started in 1965 at Nottingham University. In 1976 the PAFEC Group at the University became too large to exist within an academic framework. An independent private limited company was formed to exploit PAFEC and to continue its development. The PAFEC is a suite of programs, built in a modular form. Program code is designed to be easy to modify and inhouse users are encouraged to do this to solve any special problem. Source program available at standard price. Program can also be rented by arrangement. The last program version PAFEC75 is documented in theory, results, easidata, get started, data preparation and system manuals. Program runs on IBM, CDC, UNIVAC, Xerox Sigma, Honeywell, Burroughs, DEC, PRIME, ICL and GE computer systems. User's group exists. Courses on the FEM and the PAFEC run twice a year at Nottingham or at other sites upon request.

Program capability. The PAFEC can handle static and dynamic analysis of linear elastic isotropic and anisotropic structures. Some limited large displacement analyses can be performed. A heat transfer part is included in the program. Available material behavior includes nonlinear elastic materials, temperature-dependent properties, elasto-plasticity and creep. A dynamic analysis part can handle eigenvalues and eigenmodes and dynamic response. Dynamic spectral analysis is not yet available. Eigenvalue stability analysis and dynamic stability analysis is included in the program.

Pre- and postprocessor capabilities. PIGS is an interactive graphics suite. It is used for checking and correcting input data on a graphics console. A user can communicate with PIGS via a cursor or the keyboard. The program is ideally suited to any of the Tektronix range of equipment fitted with a cross-hair cursor. There are eight 2D and eight 3D PAF BLOCKS developed for mesh generation. Graphical facilities include IN.DRAW and OUT.DRAW modules. IN.DRAW module produces drawing of the structure before any deformation takes place. OUT.DRAW module shows the analysis results-displacements or stresses in a structure.

Element library. There are about fifty different element types in the element library; both displacement and hybrid elements are included. Force element will be made available. All membrane elements have an axisymmetric capability. There are also thermal elements 2D and 3D plus boundary layer elements.

Solution methods.

Equation solver	- Gaussian elimination: In-core and out-of-core Cholesky decomposition; Frontal solution method
Condensation	- Dynamic condensation by an automatic method for choosing masters
Eigenvalues	- Householder tridiangonalization and QL method
Dynamic response	- Newmark β-method with variable β
Nonlinear problems	- Incremental method.

Notable items. Calculation is divided into ten phases, restarts being possible at the end of any phase. Multilevel substructuring technique is included. More than 200 error messages are available. Certain axisymmetric elements have a capability for responding to a load which is not axisymmetric by superposition of circumferential harmonics.

Program name: SAMCEF (133-145)

University of Liege, LTAS, Rue de val Benoit, 75, 4000 Liege, Belgium.

General information. Program development started in 1967. The program system consists of ASEF, OPTIM, DESSIN, DYNAM, SAMNL, REPOYN, POSTPRO, STABIL, and POSTFAC. Program is offered for the standard price or for the yearly license fee. Documentation consists of a user's manual, a theoretical manual and comparative sample problem solution. SAMCEF is implemented on IBM, CDC, UNIVAC and SIEMENS computers. User's group exists.

Program capability. The program can handle linear and nonlinear static problems. The material could be isotropic, anisotropic, temperature-dependent, nonlinear elastic or elastic-plastic. The part of the program for the geometric nonlinearities includes large displacements. A large strain assumption is under development. Heat transfer part is included in the SAMCEF. Dynamic analysis part can handle eigenvalues and eigenmodes, dynamic response and dynamic spectral analysis. Stability analysis is limited to the eigenvalue computation. The program can handle structural optimization problems (weight optimization).

Pre- and postprocessor capabilities. Mesh generators for two- and three-dimensional structures are available. Preprocessing part consists of a few steps. Input data from the mesh generator or hand prepared data are checked in data analyzer for the geometry and element compatibility. Options for improvement of computational efficiency have been developed: automatic choice of local axes, elimination of singularities, fixations, etc. Plotting facilities of input and output modes are available. These provide verification of the input model and present output results. Special options such as zooming, rotations, and automatic extraction of external contours are available. Static deflections and modal shapes, isolines, principal stresses, transient responses, etc., can be plotted.

Element library. The SAMCEF system offers a fairly comprehensive finite element library. About 100 different element types are available. Most of them are displacement (or temperature) elements, but also equilibrium (or heat flux) and hybrid elements are included in the library. All element types are represented. Some special-purpose elements include: local stiffness element, shell stiffner, special convection elements, tying elements, and fluid elements.

Solution methods.

Equation solver	- Frontal solution method
Condensation	- Iron's - Guyan's reduction
Eigenvalues	- Simultaneous iteration
Dynamic response	- Modal superposition and Newmark β-method
Nonlinear problems	- Incremental, Newton-Raphson

Notable items. The SAMCEF system is a highly modular organized system. It seems to be a very general program system which includes a large number of capabilities. The communication files are organized in such a way that the information contained in them are easy to access for nonstandard applications. Fluid-solid interaction studies are possible. It is also possible to include initial stresses and strains. The system handles incompressibility and has a multilevel superelement facility.

Program name: SAP V (146-152)

SAP User's Group, Dept. of Civil Engineering, University of Southern California, University Park, Los Angeles, CA 90007, USA

General information. SAP V is the additional modification of the SAP IV developed by Prof. E. L. Wilson at the University of California, Berkeley. Network availability: United Computing Systems (USC); University Computing Company (UCC); and TYMSHARE. The program also can be purchased for the standard price which includes the tape, manual and program updating for a one-year period. User's group exists. A yearly user's conference is held. The SAP program is well known and, therefore, the description as follows is brief.

Program capability. SAP V is a general three-dimensional, linear, static and dynamic finite element program. Dynamic analysis part can handle: eigenvalue and eigenvector solution, forced dynamic response by mode superposition, frequency response analysis using mode superposition, response spectrum analysis. Buckling analysis is possible. Heat transfer analysis is not included.

Pre- and postprocessor capabilities. A pre- and postprocessor graphics subroutine which activates a Calcomp or SC 4020 plotter was added to the SAP V version. Plotting of the undeformed and deformed structure and the vibration mode shapes of a structure are possible. Several pre- and postprocessor programs developed by users are also available.

Element library. The element library of SAP V consists of eight different element types both for a static or dynamic analysis. 3D truss element, beam element, plane stress element, plane strain and axisymmetric element, 3D solid element, plate and shell element, boundary element and pipe element are represented. To these a general finite element and a geometric stiffness matrix for plate and beam elements were added.

Solution methods.

Equation solver	-	Gauss elimination
Eigenvalues and dynamic analysis	-	Mode superposition, determinant search method, subspace iteration solution, direct step-by-step integration

Notable items. Bandwidth minimization subroutine. Substructuring is not available.

Program name: SESAM-69 (153-168)

A. S. Computas, Postboks 310, 1322 Høvik, Norway

General information. Development started in 1968. SESAM-69 is a modular system containing a number of programs which could be used as autonomous programs or to be integrated in the general multilevel superelement program. A. S. Computas submits the program modules for rent or sale. Program documentation is extensive; each modular program has its own user's manual. Theoretical manuals are also available. Program system is implemented on UNIVAC, IBM, CDC, and GE computer systems. User's group was established in 1977.

Program capability. SESAM-69 can handle elastic, static and dynamic analysis; elasto-plastic analysis; analysis of crack propagation, linear or nonlinear; steady-state or transient heat transfer analysis. Dynamic analysis is available for computation of eigenvalues and eigenmodes, and dynamic response. Dynamic spectral analysis is not included in the program. Stability analysis: postbuckling and nonlinear collapse. Structures in dynamic analysis may be fully or partially submerged in an ideal fluid. Modular programs included in the system are: piping system analysis, thin shell analysis, thick and thin shell analysis, analysis of solids, general superelement program, three-dimensional frame analysis, two- and three-dimensional membrane analysis, general postprocessing and plotting program, elasto-plastic membrane analysis, crack analysis program, elasto-plastic analysis of solids, loading program, stationary nonlinear temperature fields and analysis of heat conduction in solids. Calculation of three-dimensional acoustic fields.

Pre- and postprocessor capabilities. A three-dimensional interactive graphics preprocessor has been developed featuring material properties and element generation, geometry description, specification of boundary conditions, assembly of superelements, and specification of loads. Generation of all element types available in SESAM-69 is possible. Representation of the true geometry is quickly obtained by deforming the easily generated regular mesh. Data generators for using in batch mode are also available. Output of results may be obtained in either Cartesian or cylindrical coordinates. In analysis where superelement technique is used, the output of results may refer to coordinate system which is different from superelement to superelement. Extensive plotting package is available.

Element library. Each direct analysis program contains elements for analyzing one particular type of structure. In the superelement program all available element types may be combined together. Element library contains all element types (with exception of plate elements), displacement formulation. In addition, springs, masses and constraint equations may be specified. Elements for linear/nonlinear fracture mechanics analysis are available. A number of elements for piping analysis.

Solution methods.

Equation solver	- Crout triangularization of submatrices, Gaussian elimination
Condensation	- Guyan's reduction, modal synthesis technique
Eigenvalues	- Householder's tridiagonalization, simultaneous iteration
Dynamic response	- Modal superposition, numerical integration of uncoupled systems
Nonlinear problems	- Incremental Euler-Cauchy method, true and modified Newton-Raphson for iterative solutions

Notable items. The program system seems to be a powerful program for the large structural mechanics analyses. To the authors' knowledge this was the first program which utilized the multilevel substructuring technique. The program has special links to other postprocessor programs such as stress check, fatigue check, dynamic wave load, stochastic analysis, etc. Save and restart facilities.

General purpose finite element computer programs presented previously in this section may be classified as the "classical-designed" programs. Different finite element system configurations are represented in Fig. 2, namely, the classical system with sequential file, a more flexible system with random file management, and software virtual machines. General purpose program systems should have a long lifetime in order to amortize their large development and maintenance costs. Entry of new elements, capabilities and thus insertion of new routines should be done easily. Therefore, for the development of a general purpose finite element program system incorporation of an effective data management system and program structure is one of the main tasks. Among the programs presented previously, the ASKA and NASTRAN systems are general purpose systems with a well

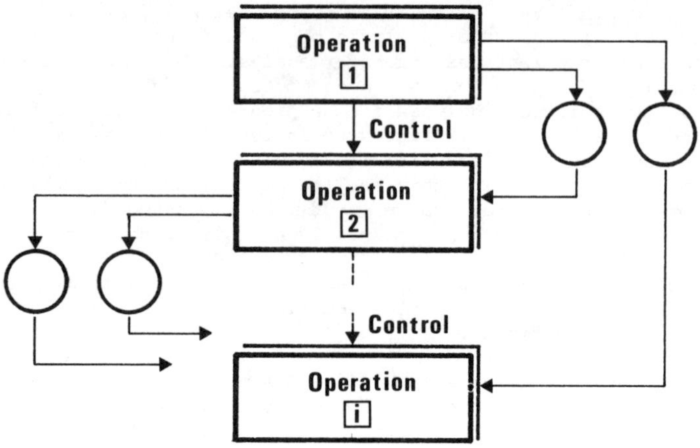

System with sequential files

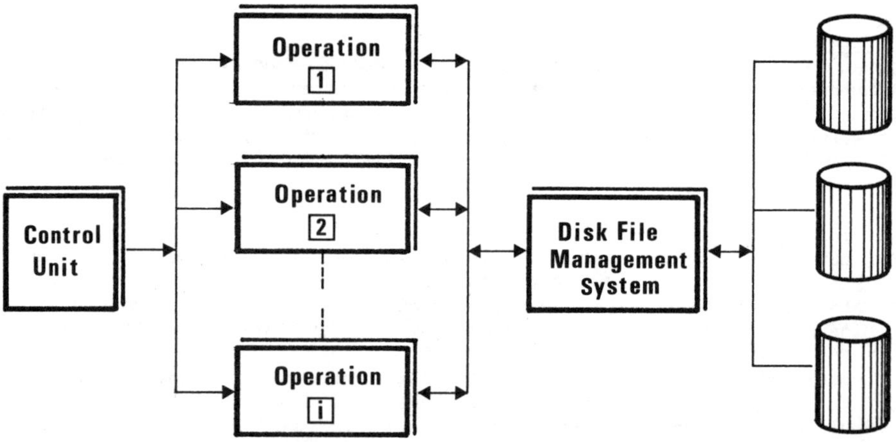

System with random files

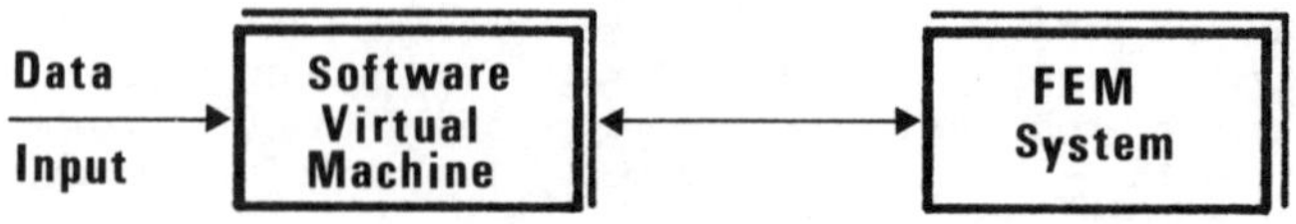

System with virtual machine

Fig 2

defined database and data management systems. These programs are thus well suited for inclusion of user routines and also for data communication. The development in the area of database-coupling philosophy for finite element computer programs are presently intensive.

To give an example of the modern software design technology trend, two more programs will be described; namely, the programs FINITE and SPAR:

Program name: FINITE (169-175)

Civil Engineering Department, Attn. Dr. L. A. Lopez or Dr. D. Rehak, University of Illinois, Urbana, IL 61801, USA

General information. The FINITE system is an example of software virtual machine, a general purpose structural mechanics system designed with emphasis on structural modeling. FE system operates through POLO virtual machine. The POLO system was developed by combining a hierarchically structured software virtual memory with a database management system. FINITE has been developed to satisfy three types of users groups; practicing civil engineers, civil engineering researchers, and software engineers. The system operates in both the interactive and batch modes. User's communication with the system is via a problem oriented language. New subroutines may be inserted easily. Linkages between these subroutines and the system are established via POLO commands.

Program features. Hypermatrix solution scheme. Generalized structural modeling. Multilevel substructuring combined with static condensation. Various forms of linear constraints may be applied. Extensive element library, combination of different element types is possible. New developed element types such as hybrid elements, transitional elements, nonsymmetric elements, etc., can easily be incorporated into the system. Mesh and load generators are available. Substructure may be repeatedly used with or without its associated loads.

Program name: SPAR (176-181)

Engineering Information Systems, Inc., Attn. Dr. W. D. Whetstone, 5120 West Campbell Avenue, Suite 240, San Jose, CA 95130, USA

General information. SPAR (Structural Performance Analysis and Redesign) system is a collection of modules called processors that perform the analysis of large structural systems. All processors may be divided into one of the five groups: geometry, elements, statics, dynamics, and thermal. The main part of the SPAR system is the unified database. Communication between the individual processors is possible through this database only. Results of each processor are stored in the unified database. Described design concept has many advantages, such as automatic inclusion of restart, possibility for multiple analyses through the parallel database access, etc. The large problem size capability is due to use of sparse hypermatrix storage, secondary storage and dynamic core allocation.

Program features. Thermal, stress, vibration and buckling analysis may be handled. Free-field data input. Matrix algebra operations. Multiple coordinate systems. Mesh generators are available. Interactive graphics utilities. The SPAR code runs on CDC CYBER 173. The program has also been implemented on the PRIME 400 minicomputer.

Table 1 Analysis Capabilities

STATIC ANALYSIS

		ADINA	ANSYS	ASAS	ASKA	BERSAFE	MARC	MISA	MSC/NASTRAN	NEPSAP	PAFEC	SAMCEF	SAP V	SESAM · 69
RANGE OF APPLICATION	Linear elastostatics	●	●	●	●	●	●	●	●	●	●	●	●	●
	Non-linear statics	●	●		●	●	●		●	●	●	●		●
	Linear dynamics	●	●	●	●	●	●		●	●	●	●	●	●
	Non-linear dynamics	●	●				●			●				
	Heat transfer	●	●	●	●	●	●	●	●	●	●	●		●
THEORY ASSUMPT	Small displacements	●	●	●	●	●	●	●	●	●	●	●	●	●
	Small strains	●	●	●	●	●	●	●	●	●	●	●	●	●
	Large displacements	●	●			●	●		●	●	●	●		●
	Large strains	●					●							
MATERIAL PROPERTIES	Isotropic	●	●	●	●	●	●	●	●	●	●	●	●	●
	Anisotropic	●	●	●	●	●	●	●	●	●	●	●	●	●
	Linear elastic	●	●	●	●	●	●	●	●	●	●	●	●	●
	Non-linear elastic	●			●	●	●				●	●		●
	Temperature dependent	●	●		●	●	●		●	●	●	●	●	●
	Elasto-perfectly plastic	●	●		●	●	●			●	●	●		●
	Elasto-strain hardening	●	●		●	●	●			●	●	●		●
	Viscoelastic		●				●							●
	Creep	●	●		●	●	●			●	●			●
ACCEPTABLE LOADING	Static	●	●	●	●	●	●	●	●	●	●	●	●	●
	Function of time	●	●		●	●	●		●	●	●	●	●	●
	Deformation-dependent		●		●	●	●		●		●		●	●
	Others	●	●		●		●							
	General variation	●	●	●	●	●	●	●	●	●	●	●	●	●
	Axisymmetric var. only													
	Point loads	●	●	●	●	●	●	●	●	●	●	●	●	●
	Line loads	●	●	●	●	●	●	●	●	●	●	●	●	●
	Surface loads	●	●	●	●	●	●	●	●	●	●	●	●	●
	Volume loads	●	●	●	●	●	●	●	●	●	●	●	●	●
	Suppr./prescribed displ.	●	●	●	●	●	●	●	●	●	●	●	●	●
	Initial strains/stresses	●	●		●	●	●	●			●	●	●	●
	Thermal	●	●	●	●	●	●	●	●	●	●	●	●	●
	Centrifugal		●	●		●	●	●	●	●	●	●		●
	Others													●

Table 2 Analysis Capabilities (Cont'd)

		ADINA	ANSYS	ASAS	ASKA	BERSAFE	MARC	MISA	MSC/NASTRAN	NEPSAP	PAFEC	SAMCEF	SAP V	SESAM - 69
DYNAMIC ANALYSIS														
RANGE OF APPLIC.	Eigenvalues, eigenmodes	●	●	●	●	●	●		●	●	●	●	●	●
	Dynamic response	●	●	●	●	●	●		●	●	●	●	●	●
	Dynamic spectral anal.		●	●	●	●	●		●			●	●	●
ACTIONS	Prescr. time depen. forces	●	●	●	●	●	●		●	●	●	●	●	●
	Prescr. displacements	●	●		●	●	●		●	●	●	●	●	●
	Prescr. velocities		●		●	●	●		●		●	●	●	
	Prescr. accelerations		●	●	●	●	●		●		●	●	●	
MASS	Kinematic consistent	●	●	●	●	●	●		●		●	●		●
	Lumped	●	●	●	●	●	●		●		●	●	●	●
STABILITY ANALYSIS														
RANGE OF APPLICAT.	Eigenvalue		●		●		●		●	●	●	●	●	
	Non-linear collapse	●	●				●		●	●				●
	Dynamic	●	●				●				●			
	Postbuckling	●	●				●							●
OTHER CAPABILITIES														
	Constrained relations		●	●	●	●	●	●	●	●		●	●	●
	Substructuring		●	●	●	●		●	●		●	●		●
	Same substr. can be inserted repeated.		●	●	●			●	●			●		●
	No restriction on the no. of substruct.		●	●	●			●	●		●			●
	Automatic renumbering of nodes, elem.		●			●	●	●	●	●	●		●	
	Structural optimization algorithm											●		
	Own element types easy to incorpor.	●		●	●	●			●		●	●		●
	Local system of axes		●	●	●	●	●	●	●	●	●	●	●	●
	No. of load cases not limit. (same run)	●	●	●	●		●		●	●				●
	Modificat. without compl. re-calculat.		●		●	●	●	●	●					●
	Restart capability		●	●	●	●	●	●	●	●	●	●		●
	Free-field input		●	●	●	●	●		●	●	●			

Table 3 Pre- and Postprocessor Capabilities

		ADINA	ANSYS	ASAS	ASKA	BERSAFE	MARC	MISA	MSC/NASTRAN	NEPSAP	PAFEC	SAMCEF	SAP V	SESAM - 69
PRE PROCESSOR														
INPUT DATA CHECKING AND GENER.	Graphical, passive		●	●	●	●	●	●	●	●	●	●	●	●
	Graphical, interactive		●	●	●	●	●				●			●
	Generator for 2-D mesh		●	●	●	●	●	●	●	●	●	●	●	●
	Generator for 3-D mesh		●	●	●	●	●	●	●	●	●	●	●	●
	Loading generator		●		●	●	●	●	●		●			●
	Boundary conditions		●		●	●	●	●	●	●	●		●	●
	Material properties table										●	●		●
PLOTS AND CRT DISPL.	Complete structure		●	●	●	●	●	●	●	●	●	●	●	●
	Part of structure		●	●	●	●	●	●	●	●	●	●	●	●
	"Blow up" option		●	●	●	●	●	●	●	●	●	●		●
	Ability to model rotation		●	●	●	●		●			●	●	●	●
	Hidden-line capability		●				●							
	Orthographic views		●	●	●	●	●	●	●	●	●	●	●	●
	Perspective views		●		●	●	●	●	●	●		●		●
IMPROVEMENT OF COMPUT. EFFICIEN.			●			●	●	●	●	●	●	●	●	
POSTPROCESSOR														
PLOT ROUTINES	Contour plots		●		●	●	●	●	●	●	●	●		●
	Undeformed/defor. geometry		●	●	●	●	●	●	●	●	●	●	●	●
	Isocurves		●		●	●	●	●		●	●	●		●
	Natural vibrat. mode shapes		●	●	●	●	●		●	●	●	●	●	●
	Time history generation		●		●	●	●			●	●	●		●
	Extract values exceedances		●		●	●				●				

Table 4 Element library

	Element type	ADINA	ANSYS	ASAS	ASKA	BERSAFE	MARC	MISA	MSC/NASTRAN	NEPSAP	PAFEC	SAMCEF	SAP V	SESAM - 69
Structural displacement elements	Truss members	●	●	●	●	●	●	●	●	●		●	●	●
	Beam	●	●	●	●	●	●	●	●	●	●	●	●	●
	Membrane	●	●	●	●	●	●	●	●	●	●	●	●	●
	Plate		●	●	●	●	●	●	●	●	●	●	●	●
	Shell, axisymmet.	●	●		●		●	●	●	●		●		
	Shell, general		●	●	●	●	●	●	●	●	●	●	●	●
	Solid, axisymmet.	●	●	●	●	●	●	●	●	●	●	●	●	●
	Solid	●	●	●	●	●	●	●	●	●	●	●	●	●
	Crack - tip		●	●	●	●	●							●
	Pipe		●		●	●	●			●			●	●
	Shear - panel			●	●				●					
	Isoparametric	●	●	●	●	●	●	●	●	●	●	●	●	●
Struct. equilibrium elem.				●								●		
Heat conduction elem.		●	●		●	●	●	●	●	●	●	●		●
Fluid - solid interaction			●		●		●		●			●		●
Thermal - fluid			●											
Thermal - electric			●											
Wave motion			●				●		●					

HOW TO FIND LITERATURE ABOUT EXISTING STRUCTURAL MECHANICS SOFTWARE

The first and most difficult problem that the user of a finite element computer program is faced with is how to find information about existing programs. How do I find the best one for my needs?

To answer the questions we present below some of the sources of reviews of available structural mechanics computer programs.

Structural Mechanics Computer Programs: Surveys, Assessments and Availability (1)

Edited by W. D. Pilkey, K. Saczalski and H. G. Schaeffer.

Abstract: The book contains reviews of structural mechanics computer programs in civil engineering, mechanical engineering, nuclear engineering, applied mechanics, aerospace engineering, and marine engineering. Programs are presented by summary of their capabilities, details of availability and source for more detailed information. Included chapters also deal with subjects as programs for building analysis and design, bridge design, structural members, stability, nonlinear analysis, structural optimization, fracture mechanics, piping systems, plastic analysis, shock wave propagation, transient analysis, etc.

The second part of the book contains papers discussing pre- and postprocessors, computer graphics and future trends in software developments.
Availability: University Press of Virginia, Box 3608, University Station, Charlottesville, VA 22903, USA.

Structural Mechanics Software Series (182)

Edited by N. Perrone and W. Pilkey
Abstract: The objective of this series of books is to provide access for the technical community to structural analysis and design computer programs. The first three volumes are available. Each volume contains sufficient documentation of several of the programs available on nationwide commercial computer networks that can be accessed by remote terminal devices connected via phone lines. Another role of this series is to inform the reader, through reviews, what is new in software in different branches of engineering.

Vol. 1 - Presented programs: BOSOR4, GIFTS, preprocessor for SAP, TOTAL, BEAM, BEAMSTRESS, SHAFT. Review articles: Computer-aided building design, bridge design, floor analysis, crash simulation.

Vol. 2 - Presented programs: SAP V, UCIN, WHAMS, DISK, TWIST, GRILL, TABS 77. Review articles: Finite element programs for pressure vessels, European finite element programs, cantilever retaining wall design, bridge rating systems.

Vol. 3 - SAP6, BOSOR5, GIFTS/SAP interface. Review articles: nonlinear analysis programs, programs for multipoint boundary value problems, rotor dynamics programs, fracture mechanics programs and mixed methods analysis.

Books available from University Press of Virginia, Box 3608, University Station, Charlottesville, VA 22903, USA.

Structural Mechanics Program Catalogues [A-11 - A-14]

Compiled by B. Fredriksson and J. Mackerle
The following publications catalogue programs of interest to people seeking finite element software.

Structural Mechanics: Finite Element Computer Programs - Surveys and Availability - This book presents a compact summary of more than 600 programs developed in the United States, Japan and Europe, which are presented in tabular form. A short abstract is given for each program. Programs for desktop and minicomputers are included. The addresses of program developers and approximately 2,000 references to papers describing programs and their applications are given.

Structural Mechanics: Pre- and Postprocessor Programs - Surveys and Availability - Compact summaries of about 260 programs are presented in tabular form. Programs and their applications are described by 360 references and papers.

Finite Element Review - Approximately 250 finite elements are presented in tabular form. All element groups and formulations are presented. There are over a thousand references on developed elements and their applications.

Stress Analysis Programs for Fracture Mechanics - Approximately 80 programs are summarized. The addresses of program developers and over 600 references are given.

Books available from AEC - Advanced Engineering Company, Box 3044, S-580 03 Linköping, Sweden.

Program Bibliography with Abstracts (183-184)

Published by NTIS, National Technical Information Service.

Computer programs in structural analysis - design problems are cited. Detailed analyses of structural problems - applied and theoretical - including stress analysis, vibration problems, shear stress analysis, deformation analysis and others. This bibliography is regularly updated.

Available from NTIS, U.S. Department of Commerce, Springfield, VA 22161, USA.

Journals with Activities in Engineering Software Information

NEAS (Newsletter of Engineering Analysis Software). The periodical dedicated to the dissemination of structural mechanics software information encompassing the areas of civil, mechanical and aerospace engineering design and analysis. Published monthly. Available from Frank Maga and Associates, P.O. Box 2435, Sepulveda, CA 91343, USA.

AES (Advances in Engineering Software). The aims of this journal are to provide accurate and up-to-date information on engineering software, and to act as a link between the originators of software and the engineering community. Published quarterly by CML Publications, 125 High Street, Southampton SO1 OAA, England.

SOFTWARE DISSEMINATION PRACTICES AND INFORMATION ORGANIZATIONS

The purpose of these organizations could be defined as an effort to establish a center for the effective application of the computer and software in practice of a specific field of engineering. Some of the main objectives of these organizations should be named.

- Keep the members of the organization informed about the state-of-the-art of computational structural mechanics and current development trends, and eventually coordinate the development
- Program selection and evaluation
- Maintain limited program library and distribute the programs
- Serve as a distribution source for the program revisions
- Cooperate in software coordination activities
- User experience activities, continued evaluation and feedback based on actual use of a program
- Information exchange, user training and education.

Short reviews of engineering software organizations and user groups in the United States and Europe are presented in Table 5. The addresses of these organizations are given in Appendix I. For more detailed information about these groups, see Ref. (185).

A. BOOKS AND MONOGRAPHS

11 Fredriksson, B. and Mackerle, J., "Structural Mechanics: Finite Element Computer Programs - Surveys and Availability," AEC - Advanced Engineering Corporation, Box 3044, S-580 03 Linköping, Sweden, 1980.

12 Fredriksson, B. and Mackerle, J., "Structural Mechanics: Pre- and Postprocessor Programs - Surveys and Availability," AEC - Advanced Engineering Corporation, Box 3044, S-580 03 Linköping, Sweden, 1977.

13 Fredriksson, B. and Mackerle, J., "Finite Element Review," Report AEC-L-003, AEC - Advanced Engineering Corporation, Box 3044, S-580 03 Linköping, Sweden, 1978.

14 Fredriksson, B. and Mackerle, J., "Stress Analysis Programs for Fracture Mechanics," AEC - Advanced Engineering Corporation, Box 3044, S-580 03 Linköping, Sweden, 1979.

Table 5 Software Centers and Information Organizations

	Government User Group	University User Group	Indep. Profess. User Gr.	Hardware User Group	Program Development	Program Distribution	Program Evaluation	Information Services	Education	User Experience Exchan.	Note
AEC; Sweden			●		●	●	●	●	●		Program catalogues
Argonne Code Center	●				●	●	●	●	●		ERDA Prog. Summary
ASIAC	●					●		●			Air Force newsletter
APEC			●		●	●	●	●	●	●	Building design
CACT; France	●				●	●	●	●	●	●	Civil engng, bulletin
CEPA			●		●	●		●	●	●	Civil engng
CIAD; Netherlands			●		●	●	●	●	●	●	Civil engng
COMMON				●		●		●	●		IBM computers
COSMIC	●					●	●	●	●	●	Comp. Progr. Abstract
DECUS				●		●		●	●	●	Digital Equipment
EUROCOPI; Italy	●					●		●			Program catalogues
FACTS	●				●	●	●	●	●		Construction engng
HEEP	●							●	●		Highway engng
HUG				●	●			●	●		Honeywell computer
ICES			●		●	●		●	●	●	ICES Journal
IITRI			●			●	●	●	●	●	Newsletter
NCC; England	●							●	●	●	Information center
NISEE		●				●		●	●		Earthquake engng
SHARE				●	●	●		●	●	●	IBM computers
STORE	●				●	●		●	●	●	Newsletter
SWAP				●	●	●		●	●		WANG computers
VIM				●	●	●		●	●	●	Control Data comp.

REFERENCES

1 Pilkey, W., Saczalski, K., and Schaeffer, H., Structural Mechanics Computer Programs-Surveys, Assessments and Availability, University Press of Virginia, Charlottesville, Virginia, 1974.

2 Fredriksson, B., and Mackerle, J., "Overview and Evaluation of Some Versatile General Purpose Finite Element Computer Programs," Second World Congress on Finite Element Methods, Bournemouth, England, October 1978, pp. 390-419.

3 Wilson, E. L., "CAL- Computer Analysis Language for the Static and Dynamic Analysis of Structural Systems," University of California, Berkeley, Dept. of Civil Engineering, Rep. No. UCSESM 77-2, Jan. 1977.

4 Wilson, E. L., "CAL - A Computer Analysis Language for Teaching Structural Analysis," Computers & Structures, Vol. 10, 1979, pp. 127-132.

5 Akin, J. E., and Stoddart, W. C. T., "Computer Programs for Implementing the Finite Element Method," Rep. ESM 75-1, Dept. of Engineering Science and Mechanics, University of Tennessee, 1975, 202 pp.

6 Akin, J. E., "A General Purpose Educational and Research Code: MODEL," Proceed. of the Symp. on Applicat. of Computer Methods in Engineering, Los Angeles, California, August 1977, pp. 1209-1216.

7 Akin, J. E., "Typical Applications of the MODEL Code," Rep. ESM 75-2, Dept. of Engineering Science and Mechanics, University of Tennessee, 1975, 125 pp.

8 Taylor, R. L., "Computer Procedures for Finite Element Analysis," in The Finite Element Method,by O. C. Zienkiewicz, McGraw-Hill Book Co. Ltd., 1977, pp. 677-757.

9 Schrem, E., "The Assessment of Large-Scale Software System for Finite Element Structural Analysis," Finite Element Congress, IKOSS, Baden-Baden, Nov. 1974.

10 Schrem, E., "Development and Maintenance of Large Finite Element Systems," in Pilkey, W., Saczalski, K., Schaeffer, H., (Eds), Structural Mechanics Computer Programs, University Press of Virginia, Charlottesville, 1974, pp. 669-685.

11 Schrem, E., "From Program Systems to Programming Systems for Finite Element Analysis," in Bathe, K. J., Oden, J. T., Wunderlich, W.,(Eds), Formulations and Algorithms in Finite Element Analysis, MIT, Cambridge, 1976, pp. 163-190.

12 Schrem, E., "Trends and Aspects of the Development of Large Finite Element Software Systems," Computers & Structures, Vol. 10, 1979, pp. 419-425.

13 Schrem, E., "Finite Element Software in the Next Decade," World Congress on Finite Element Methods in Structural Mechanics, Bournemouth, October 1975.

14 Schrem, E., "Functional Software Design and Its Graphical Representation," Computers & Structures, Vol. 8, No. 3/4, 1978, pp. 491-502.

15 Schrem, E., and Streiner, P., "General Purpose FE Programs and New Tendencies in Computer Technology," Int. Finite Element Congress, Baden-Baden, West Germany, November 1978.

16 Betess, J. A., "A Data Structure for Finite Element Analysis," Int. J. Num. Meth. Engng., Vol. 11, No. 12, 1977, pp. 1799-1800.

17 Dunham, R. S., Becker, E. B., and Guerra, F. M., "Organization and Functional Purpose of Finite Element Computer Programs," ASME Pressure Vessel and Piping - Materials - Nuclear Conf., Miami, June 1974.

18 Felippa, C. A., "Database Management in Scientific Computing - 1. General Description," Computers and Structures, Vol. 10, Nos. 1/2, April 1979, pp. 53-61.

19 Fenves, S. J., "Future Directions of Structural Engineering Applications," Computers and Structures, Vol. 10, 1979, pp. 3-6.

20 Hansteen, H. B., Miller, R. E., and Wahlström, S. O., "Systems for Large Engineering Problem Solutions," Proc. Int. Symp. on Large Engng. Syst., University of Manitoba, Winnipeg, Canada, August 1976, pp. 19-37.

21 Swanson, J. A., "Present Trends in Computerized Structural Analysis," Computers and Structures, Vol. 10, 1979, pp. 33-37.

22 Bäcklund, J., and Petersson, H., "PREFEM - A Computer Program for Bending Analysis of Rectangular Slabs by the Finite Element Method,"(in Swedish), Chalmers University of Technology, Department of Structural Mechanics, Publ. 72:3, Göteborg 1972.

23 Petersson, H., and Bäcklund, J., "SERFEM - A Computer Program for In-Plane Analysis of Plates by the Finite Element Method," Chalmers University of Technology, Division of Building Construction, Publication 74:1, Göteborg 1974.

24 Bathe, K. J., "ADINA - A Finite Element Program for Automatic Dynamic Incremental Nonlinear Analysis," Acoustics and Vibration Laboratory, Mechanical Engng. Dept., Rep. 82448-1, MIT, Cambridge, September 1975; Revised May 1977.

25 Bathe, K. J., "Static and Dynamic Geometric and Material Nonlinear Analysis Using ADINA," Acoustics and Vibration Laboratory, Mechanical Engng. Dept., Rep. 82448-2, MIT, Cambridge, May 1976; Revised May 1977.

26 Bathe, K. J., "ADINAT - A Finite Element Program for Automatic Dynamic Incremental Nonlinear Analysis of Temperatures," Acoustics and Vibration Laboratory, Mechanical Engng. Dept., Rep. 82448-5, MIT, Cambridge, May 1977.

27 Bathe, K. J., "Some Recent Developments in Computational Capabilities for Nonlinear Finite Element Analysis," 4th Int. Conf. on Struct. Mech. in Reactor Technol., San Francisco, August 1977.

28 Crawford, J. E., "Pre- and Postprocessors for General Purpose 3-Dimensional Finite Element Programs," Proc. of the ADINA Conf., MIT, Cambridge, Mass., August 1977, pp. 295-311.

29 Johansson, T., "FEMGEN - A General Finite Element Mesh Generator," Proc. of the ADINA Conf., MIT, Cambridge, Mass., August 1977, pp. 312-327.

30 Johansson, T., "FEMGEN - A General Finite Element Mesh Generator," Proc. 2nd World Congress on Finite Element Methods, Bournemouth, October 1978, pp. 498--516.

31 Cook, W. A., "INGEN: A General Purpose Mesh Generator for Finite Element Codes," Proc. of the ADINA Conf., MIT, Cambridge, Mass., August 1977, pp. 328-348.

32 Kamel, H. A., and McCabe, M. W., "A Graphics Interactive Finite Element Time Package," Office of Naval Research Report, Contr. Number N 00014-67-A-0209 0016, 1973.

33 Kamel, H. A., and McCabe, M. W., "The GIFTS System," Int. Symposium on Struct. Mechanics Software, University of Maryland, College Park, Maryland, 1974.

34 Kamel, H. A., and McCabe, M. W., "Applications of GIFTS III to Structural Engineering Problems," University of Arizona, Technical Report No. 1, April 1976.

35 Kamel, H. A., and McCabe, M. W., "GIFTS IV Documentation, User's Manual and Systems Manual," University of Arizona, May 1976.

36 Kamel, H. A., "Interactive Computer Graphics as a Tool in Teaching Structural Analysis," J. Struct. Div., ASCE, Vol. 104, August 1978, pp. 1299-1314.

37 Kamel, H. A., "GIFTS 4 Modelling Guide," University of Arizona, Tucson, Arizona, 1977.

38 "ANSYS, User's Manual," Swanson Analysis Systems, Inc., updated July 1979.

39 "ANSYS, Examples Manual," Swanson Analysis Systems, Inc., April 1978; updated July 1979.

40 "ANSYS, Verification Manual, " Swanson Analysis Systems, Inc., June 1976; updated April 1979.

41 "ANSYS, Theoretical Manual," Swanson Analysis Systems, Inc., November 1977.

42 "ANSYS, Introduction Manual," Swanson Analysis Systems, Inc.; updated March 1979.

43 "ASAS User Manual," Atkins Research and Development, Ashley Road, Epsom, Surrey, United Kingdom, November 1976.

44 Robinson, J., and Spooner, J. B., "ASAS - A Commercial Finite Element System with Displacement and Force Continuity Options," IKOSS Finite Element Congress, Baden-Baden, West Germany, November 1973.

45 Spooner, J. B., "The Development of a Major Finite-Element System," IKOSS Finite Element Congress, Baden-Baden, West Germany, November 1973.

46 Spooner, J. B., "ASAS - Progress Towards Engineering Generality," IKOSS Finite Element Congress, Baden-Baden, West Germany, November 1975.

47 Henrywood, R. K., and Sheffield, J. D., "ASAS - A General Purpose Finite Element Analysis System," Computer Aided Design, Vol. 8, No 1, January 1976, pp. 2-8.

48 Argyris, J. H., "ASKA - User's Reference Manual," ISD Report No. 73, 1971, University of Stuttgart, West Germany.

49 Brönlund, O. E., and Buhlmeier, J., "DYNAN - User's Reference Manual," ISD Report No. 97, 1971, University of Stuttgart, West Germany.

50 "ASKA III-1, Material Non-Linearities, User's Reference Manual," ASKA UM 207, 1972, Stuttgart, West Germany.

51 "ASKA III-2, Linear Buckling, User's Reference Manual," ASKA UM 209, 1973, Stuttgart, West Germany.

52 "ASKA Part II - Linear Dynamic Analysis, User's Reference Manual," ASKA UM 211, 1974, Stuttgart, West Germany.

53 Schrem, E., and Roy, J. R., "Introduction to ASKA I," ASKA UM 201, Reprint 1975, Stuttgart, West Germany.

54 "ASKA Part II - Linear Dynamic Analysis, Lecture Notes and Example Problems. Training Manual," ASKA UM 212, 1974, Stuttgart, West Germany.

55 Balmer, H., and Doltsinis, J. S., "ASKA Part III-1, Material Non-Linearities. Lecture Notes with Example Problems," ISD Report 132, 1972, University of Stuttgart, West Germany.

56 Nagy, D., "ASKA Part III-2, Linear Buckling, Lecture Notes and User's Guide; Training Manual," ASKA UM 210, 1974, Stuttgart, West Germany.

57 Argyris, J. H., "ASKA - Automatic System for Kinematic Analysis," Nuclear Engineer. and Design, Vol. 10, 1969, pp. 441-455.

58 Argyris, J. H., Brönlund, O. E., and Sorensen, M., "Computer Aided Structural Analysis. The Machine-Independent System ASKA," Nord. Data-70 Conference, Aug. 1970, Copenhagen, Denmark.

59 Bergmann, H. W., "ASKA - A Large-Scale Software System for Finite Element Analysis," Advances in Matrix Methods of Struct. Anal. and Design, University of Alabama Press, Huntsville, 1970.

60 Meijers, P., "Review of the ASKA Program," Numerical and Computer Meth. in Struct. Mech., Academic Press, New York, 1973, pp. 123-149.

61 Balmer, H. A., and Doltsinis, J. S., "Extensions to the Elastoplastic Part of ASKA-Material Laws, Bending Elements," ISD Rep. No. 204, Stuttgart, 1977.

62 Parisch, H., and Skinner, R., "ASKA - HS - Axisymmetric Continua with Arbitrary Loads," ASKA UM 224, ISD, Stuttgart, 1978.

63 Knapp, H., "ASKA - CS - A Special Package for Cyclic Symmetric Structures under General Loads," in ASKA Extensions, E. Schrem (ed.), ISD Rep. 239, Stuttgart, 1978.

64 Balmer, H. A., Doltsinis, J. S., and Koenig, M., "Elasto-Plastic and Creep Analysis with the ASKA Program System," Comput. Meth. in Applied Mechanics and Engineer., Vol. 3, 1974, pp. 87-104.

65 Argyris, J. H., and Schrem, E., "ASKA, Software Engineering for the Seventies in Structural Analysis," Second Int. Conf. on Struct. Mech. in Reactor Technol., Sept. 1973, Berlin, Paper M 1/4.

66 Brönlund, O. E., and Straub, K., "A Brief Description of DYNAN A (ASKA IIA) and DYNAN B (ASKA IIB)," ISD Report No. 139, University of Stuttgart, West Germany, 1973.

67 Just, W., and Kinder, A., "ASKA-T, A Special Package for Steady State and Transient Temperature Fields," Proc. ASKA User's Meet., 1978, pp. 79-87.

68 König, M., et al, "Buckling Analysis with the ASKA Program System," Comp. Meth. Appl. Mech. Engng., Vol. 16, 1978, pp. 185-212.

69 Doltsinis, J. S. et al, "ASKA-FM," ASKA UM 226, Stuttgart, West Germany, 1979.

70 Hellen, T. K., "BERSAFE (Phase 1): A Computer System for Stress Analysis, Part 1: User's Guide," RD/B/N 1761, CEGB Report, Berkeley Nuclear Lab., Berkeley, United Kingdom

71 Hellen, T. K., "BERSAFE (Phase 1): A Computer System for Stress Analysis, Part 2: Advice and Sample Problems," RD/B/N 1813, CEGB Report, Berkeley Nuclear Lab., Berkeley, United Kingdom.

72 Hellen, T. K., "A User's Guide to BERSAFE Phase II, " RD/B/M 2508, CEGB Report, Berkeley Nuclear Lab., Berkeley, United Kingdom.

73 Hellen, T. K., and Protheroe, S. J., "The BERSAFE Finite Element System," Computer Aided Design, Vol. 6, No. 1, 1974, pp. 15-24.

74 Reynen, J., "A Substructure Version of BERSAFE," Finite Element Workshop Meeting, University of Stuttgart, West Germany, Sept. 1973.

75 Hellen, T. K., "The Application of the BERSAFE Finite Element System to Nuclear Design Problems," First Internat. Confer. on Struct. Mech. in Reactor Technol., Sept. 1971, Berlin, Paper M6/1.

76 Fullard, K., "FLHE - A Finite Element Program for the Calculation of Temperatures in Arbitrary Structures; Part I: User's Guide, Part II: Theory," RD/B/N 1849, 202, CEGB Reports, Berkeley Nuclear Lab., Berkeley, United Kingdom.

77 Fullard, K., "FLHE Phase II: An Extended Version of the Finite Element Heat Conduction Program, Part I - User's Guide," RD/B/N 2865, CEGB Report, Berkeley Nuclear Lab., Berkeley, United Kingdom.

78 Fullard, K., "FLHE: A Finite Element Program for the Calculation of Temperatures in Arbitrary Structures," First Internat. Confer. on Struct. Mech. in Reactor Technol., Sept. 1971, Berlin.

79 Fullard, K., "Thermal Transient Analyses Involving Large Temperature Gradients, Solved by Means of FLHE," RD/B/N 3831, 1976, CEGB Report, Berkeley Nuclear Lab., Berkeley, United Kingdom.

80 Heilen, T. K., and Harper, P. G., " A User's Guide to BERSAFE Phase III Level 1 for Plasticity and Creep Analysis," RD/B/N 3597, 1976, CEGB Report, Berkeley Nuclear Lab., Berkeley, United Kingdom.

81 Harper, P. G., "Automatic Timestep Control for Creep in BERSAFE Phase III," RD/B/N 3797, 1976, CEGB Report, Berkeley Nuclear Lab., Berkeley, United Kingdom.

82 Hellen, T. K., and Harper, P. G., "BERSAFE Phase III: Plasticity and Creep Analysis Mathematical Theory," RD/B/N 3765, 1976, Berkeley Nuclear Lab., Berkeley, United Kingdom.

83 Leech, A., "BERDYNE (Phase 1) - A Computer System for Dynamic Analysis of Structures," MS/C/P295, CEGB Report, CEGB Computing Centre, United Kingdom.

84 Leech, A., and Spires, R. W., "A User's Guide to BERDYNE, Phase 2," CS/C/P 496, 1977, CEGB Report, CEGB Computing Centre, United Kingdom.

85 Hellen, T. K., and Jerram, K., "Finite Element Techniques in Fracture Mechanics," Int. Conf. on Welding Research Related to Power Plant, Southampton, Sept. 1972.

86 Hellen, T. K., "The Finite Element Calculation of Stress Intensity Factors Using Energy Techniques," Second Conf. on Structural Mechanics in Reactor Technology, Paper G 5/3, Berlin, Sept. 1973.

87 Hellen, T. K., "The Use of the J—Integral for Nonlinear Fracture Mechanics," CEGB Report RD/B/N 3770, 1976.

88 Hellen, T. K., and Blackburn, W. S., "Calculation of Stress Intensity Factors in Two- and Three-Dimensions Using Finite Elements," Comput. Frac. Mech., Nat. Congr. on Pressure Vessels and Piping, San Francisco, Calif., Jun. 23-27, 1975, ASME, New York, pp. 103-120.

89 Hellen, T. K., "On Special Isoparametric Elements for Linear Elastic Fracture Mechanics," Int. J. for Numer. Meth. in Engng., 11, 1977, pp. 200-205.

90 Hellen, T. K., and Blackburn, W. S., "The Use of a Path Independent Integral in Nonlinear Fracture Mechanics," Fourth Conf. on Struct. Mech. in Reactor Technol., San Francisco, Aug. 1977.

91 "MARC-CDC, Nonlinear Finite Element Analysis Program, User Information Manual," Vol I, Publication No. 17309500, Control Data Co., Minneapolis, Minn.

92 "MARC-CDC, Program Input Manual," Vol II, Publication No. 17311600, Control Data Co., Minneapolis, Minn.

93 "MARC-CDC, Demonstration Problems Manual," Vol III, Publication No. 17311700, Control Data Co., Minneapolis, Minn.

94 "MARC Course Notes," Vol.IV; published by MARC Analysis Company.

95 "MARC Background Papers," Vol.V; published by MARC Analysis Company.

96 Ayres, D. J., "Elastic-Plastic and Creep Analysis Via the MARC Finite Element Computer Program," Numerical and Computer Methods in Structural Mechanics, ed.by S. J. Fenves, Academic Press, New York, 1973, pp. 247 - 263.

97 Fine, D. S., "An Evaluation of the MARC Program," Chevrolet Engng., Analysis Rep., March 1974.

98 Marcal, P. V., "Nonlinear Analysis with a General-Purpose Program in a Commercial Environment," Second World Congress on Finite Element Methods, Bournemouth, England, October 1978, pp. 563 576.

99 Tanaka, N. et al, "The Mitsui Structural Analysis Program System (MISA) by the Finite Element Method," Japan Shipbuilding and Marine Engng., Vol. 10, No. 2, 1976, pp. 5-22.

100 Iwaki, T. et al, "MISA - A General Purpose FEM Program," Computers and Structures, Vol. 10, 1979, pp. 311-322.

101 Ishii, T., and Ito, M., "The Role of Executive Functions in Large Scale F.E.M. Programs," Fifth Nat. Symp. on the Finite Element Methods, Tokyo, Japan, June 1977.

102 Nishihara, S., and Nomura, D., "Automated Data Processing for Multi-Level Substructure Methods," Fifth Nat. Symp. on the Finite Element Methods, Tokyo, Japan, June 1977.

103 "MSC/NASTRAN Basic Training Manual," MacNeal-Schwendler Company, Los Angeles, California, USA, Rep. MSR-46, July 1977.

104 "MSC/NASTRAN - Demonstration Problem Manual," MacNeal-Schwendler Company, Los Angeles, California, USA, November 1978.

105 "MSC/NASTRAN - User's Manual," MacNeal-Schwendler Company, Los Angeles, California, USA, Rep. MSR-39, February 1978.

106 "MSC/NASTRAN - Application Manual," MacNeal-Schwendler Co., Rep. MSR-32, 1979.

107 "MSC/NASTRAN - Programmer's Manual," MacNeal-Schwendler Co., Rep. MSR-50, Sept. 1976.

108 "MSC/NASTRAN MSGMESH - Analysis Guide," MacNeal-Schwendler Co., Rep. MSR-48A, April 1978.

109 "MSC/NASTRAN - Aeroelastic Supplement," MacNeal-Schwendler Co., 1979.

110 Rogers, J. L., "Guide to a Condensed Form of NASTRAN," NASA-Rp-1019, L-11900, Hampton, VA, Sept. 1978, p. 297.

111 Jones, R. F., "Some Time and Cost Comparisons Using NASTRAN and other Finite Element Computer Programs," The Third NAVY-NASTRAN Colloquium, Washington, D.C., March 1972.

112 Lee, H. P., "NASTRAN Thermal Analyzer, Vol. I: The NASTRAN Thermal Analyzer Manual," NASA-Goddard Space Flight Center, X-322-76-16, December 1975.

113 Nagy, L. I., "Evaluation of NASTRAN From the User's Point of View," JSAE Symposium of Analysis and Design of Automobile Body Structures, Tokyo, November 13, 1973.

114 MacNeal, R. H., and McCormick, C. W., "The NASTRAN Computer Program for Structural Analysis," Computers and Structures, Vol. 1, 1971, pp. 389-412

115 MacNeal, R. H., "Some Organizational Aspects of NASTRAN," Nuclear Eng. and Design, Vol. 29, 1974, pp. 254-265.

116 MacNeal, R. H., Harder, R. L., and Mason, J. B., "NASTRAN Cyclic Symmetry Capability," NASTRAN User's Experiences, NASA TM-X-2893, 1973, pp 395-422.

117 Eames-Jones, J., "A NASTRAN Compatible Finite Element Program for a Mini-Computer," NASTRAN User's Conference, Munich, April 1977.

118 Tocher, J. L., and Herness, E. D., "A Critical View of NASTRAN," Numerical and Computer Methods in Structural Mechanics, Fenves, S. J., (Ed.) Academic Press, New York, 1973, pp. 151-174.

119 Wall, S. E., "The Management of Large Problems with NASTRAN," NASTRAN User's Conf., West Germany, April 1975.

120 Wills, C. M. R., and Roe, D., "NASTRAN - A Finite Element Program for Structural Analysis," Computer Aided Design, pp. 172-175, July 1972.

121 Schaeffer, H. G., "MSC/NASTRAN - Static and Normal Modes Analysis," Schaeffer Analysis, Inc., 1979.

122 Everstine, G. C., and McKee, J. M., "A Survey of Pre- and Postprocessors for NASTRAN," in W. Pilkey, et al, Structural Mechanics Computer Programs, University Press of Virginia, Charlottesville, 1974, pp. 825-847.

123 Lorensen, W. E., "Interactive Graphics Support for NASTRAN," Sixth NASTRAN User's Colloquium, NASA Conf. Public. 2018, October 1977, pp. 305-325.

124 Raibstein, A. I., and Pipano, A., "RINA - An Interactive System for the Rapid Interpretation of NASTRAN Results," Sixth NASTRAN User's Colloquium, NASA Conf. Public. 2018, October 1977, pp. 341-355.

125 Stanton, E. L., "An Automated Data Generator for NASTRAN," Sixth NASTRAN User's Colloquium, NASA Conf. Public. 2018, October 1977, pp. 419-434.

126 Newton, P., and Sodha, R., "An Efficient Postprocessing Environment for MSC/NASTRAN or Other Analysis Systems," NASTRAN User's Conf., Munich, May 1979.

127 Brunner, M., "Interactive Handling of NASTRAN," NASTRAN User's Conf., Munich, May 1979.
128 Sharifi, P., "User's Manual for NEPSAP," Lockheed Missiles and Space Co. Rep., Sunnyvale, Ca., April 1974; and revisions.
129 Sharifi, P., and Yates, D., "Nonlinear Finite Element Method and Its Application to Large-Scale Structural Problems," World Congress on Finite Element Methods and Structural Mechanics, Bournemouth, England, Oct. 1975.
130 Sharifi, P., and Yates, D., "Nonlinear Thermo-Elastic-Plastic and Creep Analysis by the Finite Element Method," AIAA J., Vol. 13, Sept. 1974, pp. 1210-1215.
131 Henshell, R. D., "PAFEC 70 - User's Manual," Nottingham University, Mechanical Engineer. Dept., 1972, Nottingham, United Kingdom, 1972.
132 Henshell, R. D., "PAFEC 75 Theory, Results,", "PAFEC 75 Easidata," "PAFEC 75 Get Started," "PAFEC 75 Data Preparation,","PAFEC 75 Systems," PAFEC, Ltd., Nottingham, United Kingdom.
133 De Veubeke, B. F., Sander, G., and Beckers, P., "Dual Analysis by Finite Elements - Linear and Nonlinear Applications. Part I: Linear Applications. Part II: Nonlinear Theories - Nonlinear Shell Theory. Part III: Appendix," Rep. SA-22, University of Liege, Belgium.
134 Kabiala, A. P., and De Veubeke, B. F., "Stability Analysis by Finite Elements," Rep. SA-16, University of Liege, Belgium.
135 Fleury, C., and De Veubeke, B. F., "Structural Optimization," Rep. SA-34, University of Liege, Belgium.
136 Fleury, C., and Geradin, M., "Optimality Criteria and Mathematical Programming in Structural Weight Optimization," Rep. SA-39, University of Liege, Belgium.
137 Sander, G., "Applications de la Méthode des Eléments Finis à la Flexion des Plaques," Rep. SF-4, University of Liege, Belgium.
138 Nyssen, C., "La Méthode de Newton-Raphson Appliquée à la Résolution des Problémes Elasto-Plastiques par Eléments Finis," Rep. SF-42, University of Liege, Belgium.
139 Geradin, M., "Computational Efficiency of Equilibrium Models in Eigenvalue Analysis," Rep. VA-1, University of Liege, Belgium.
140 Geradin, M., "Error Bounds for Eigenvalue Analysis by Elimination of Variables," Rep. VA-2, University of Liege, Belgium.
141 De Veubeke, B. F., Geradin, M., and Huck, A., "Structural Dynamics," Rep. VA-11, University of Liege, Belgium.
142 Geradin, M., "Analyze Dynamique Duale par la Méthode des Eléments Finis," Rep. UF-13, University of Liege, Belgium.
143 Geradin, M., "Les Grandes Méthodes Numériques de l'Analyze Dynamique des Structures," Rep. UF-29, University of Liege, Belgium.
144 Huck, A., "Méthodes Numériques en Résponse Dynamique Avec Amortissement Structural," Rep. UV-30, University of Liege, Belgium.
145 Sander, G., "Récents Progrés dans l'Analyse des Structures par la Méthode des Eléments Finis," Third Testing Symposium, Frascati, Italy, March 1974.
146 Wilson, E. L., et al, "SAP - A Structural Analysis Program for Linear Systems," Nuclear Engng. and Design, Vol. 25, 1973, pp. 257-274.
147 Spencer, R. B., and Howard, G. E., "Implementation of SAP IV on a Mini-computer Disc Operating System," Fourth Inter. Conf. on Struct. Mech. in Reactor Technol., San Francisco, Paper G 7/8, Aug. 1977.
148 Goodzeit, C. L., "Applications of SAP to Structural Design Using Pre- and Postprocessors," Brookhaven Nat. Lab., Rep. CONF-760627-1, Upton, N.Y., 1976.
149 Miura, H., and Imam, H., "SAP V: A General Three-Dimensional Linear, Static, and Dynamic Finite Element Structural Analysis Program," in W. Pilkey, et al, (Eds.), Structural Mechanics Software Series, Vol. II, Univ. Press of Virginia, Charlottesville, 1978, pp. 15-130.
150 Bathe, K. J., et al, "SAP IV: A Structural Analysis Program for Static and Dynamic Response of Linear Systems," Rep. No. EERC 73-11, College of Engineering, Univ. of California, Berkeley, June 1973.
151 Norton, R. L., Ed., "SAP IV Sample Problems," Rep., Dept. of Civil Engn., Univ. of Southern California, August 1974.

152 Wilson, E. L., "SOLID SAP - A Static Analysis Program for 3-D Solid Structures," UC-SESM 71-19, Dept. of Civil Engng., Univ. of California, Berkeley, Dec. 1972.

153 Araldsen, P. O., and Egeland, O., "General Description of SESAM-69," Sem. on the Practical Application of the Finite Element Method, University of Norway, Trondheim, Norway, January 1971.

154 "SESAM-69, Super Element Structural Analysis Program Modules, General Description," Computas A/S, Det Norske Veritas, Norway, December 1976.

155 Engja, H., Gudbrandsen, G., Bjerkås, E., and Bjørnstad, H., "Finite Element Program for Piping System Analysis (SESAM-69)," User's Manual NV-323, Det Norske Veritas, Oslo, Norway, 1972.

156 Kråkeland, B., Johansson, P. I., Pahle, E., Blaker, B., and Klem, H. F., "Thin Shell Analysis, (SESAM-69)," User's Manual NV-331, Det Norske Veritas, Oslo, Norway, 1974.

157 Wergeland, J. H., "Thick/Thin Shell Analysis (SESAM-69)," User's Manual NV-332, Det Norske Veritas, Oslo, Norway, 1974.

158 Aasen, E., Kråkeland, B., Pahle, E., Blaker, B., and Klem, H. F., "Analysis of Solids (SESAM-69)," User's Manual NV-333, Det Norske Veritas, Oslo, Norway, 1974.

159 Sandsmark, N., and Egeland, O., "Plastic and Viscoelastic Stress Analysis of Solids of Revolution (SESAM-69)," User's Manual NV-334, Det Norske Veritas, Oslo, Norway, 1972.

160 Kråkeland, B., Johansson, P. I., Pahle, E., Blaker, B., and Klem, H. F., "General Superelement Program (SESAM-69)," User's Manual NV-336, Det Norske Veritas, Oslo, Norway, 1974.

161 Bjørnstad, H., "3-Dimensional Frame Analysis, (SESAM-69)," User's Manual NV-337, Det Norske Veritas, Oslo, Norway, 1973.

162 Kråkeland, B., Wergeland, J. H., Pahle, E., Blaker, B., and Klem, H. F., "Membrane Analysis, (SESAM-69)," User's Manual NV-339, Det Norske Veritas, Oslo, Norway, 1974.

163 Sandsmark, N., "Stationary Nonlinear Analysis of Temperature Fields, (SESAM-69)," User's Manual, NV-610, Det Norske Veritas, Oslo, Norway, 1973.

164 Egeland, O., "General Load Program, (SESAM-69)," User's Manual NV-423, Det Norske Veritas, Oslo, Norway, 1972.

165 Egeland, O., and Araldsen, P. O., "SESAM-69, A General Purpose Finite Element Method Program," Computers and Structures, Vol. 4, January 1974, pp. 41-68.

166 Mo, O., "Elasto-Plastic Analysis," General Description of NV 342 and NV 349, Det Norske Veritas, Oslo, Norway, 1976.

167 Wergeland, J. H., et al, "Practical Finite Element Application and Finite Element Program Development - Ten Years of Experience as General Purpose Finite Element Program Supporters," 2nd World Congress on Finite Element Method, Bournemouth, England, Oct. 1978, pp. 171-187.

168 Mo, O., Klem, H. F., Pahle, E., and Harwiss, T., "Finite Element Programs Based on General Programming Systems," Computers and Structures, Vol. 8, 1978, pp. 703-715.

169 Lopez, L. A., "FINITE - An Approach to Structural Mechanics Systems," Int. J. for Numer. Meth. in Engng., Vol. 11, No. 5, 1977, pp. 851-866.

170 Lopez, L. A., "POLO - Problem Oriented Language Organizer," Comp. and Struct., Vol. 2, 1972, pp. 555-572.

171 Lopez, L. A., "POLO Programmer's Guide", Civil Eng. System Lab., Univ. Of Illinois at Urbana, Urbana, Ill., 1973.

172 Lopez, L. A., "FILES - Automated Engin. Data Management System," J. Struct. Div., ASCE, Vol. 101, 1975, pp. 661-676.

173 Lopez, L. A., "FINITE - A POLO II Subsystem for Structural Mechanics," Civil Engng. Systems. Lab., Univ. of Illinois at Urbana, Urbana, Ill., 1975.

174 Dodds, R. H., et al, "Numerical and Software Requirements for General Nonlinear Finite Element Analysis," Illinois Univ. at Urbana-Champaign, Dept. of Civil Engng., Rep. UILU-ENG-78-2020, Sept. 1978.

175 Dodds, R. H., Lopez, L. A., "A Generalized Software System for Nonlinear Analysis," in Engineering Software, ed. by R. A. Adey, Pentech Press, London, 1979, pp. 55-77.

176 Whetstone, W. D., "SPAR Structural Analysis System Reference Manual, Program Execution," NASA CR-145098, 1976; Revision Feb. 1977.

177 Whetstone, W. D., "SPAR Structural Analysis System Reference Manual," NASA CR-158970, 1978.

178 Jones, C. E., et al, "SPAR Structural Analysis System Reference Manual, Demonstration Problems," NASA CR-145098-3, Feb. 1977.

179 Whetstone, W. D., "EISI/SPAR Reference Manual," Engng. Inform. Syst., Inc., San Jose, Calif., Aug. 1976.

180 Giles, G. L., and Haftka, R. T., "SPAR Data Handling Utilities," NASA TM-78701, 1978.

181 Foster, E. P., and Storaasli, O. O., "Structural Analysis on a Minicomputer," in Engineering Software, ed. by R. A. Adey, Pentech Press, London, 1979, pp. 43-54.

182 Perrone, N., and Pilkey, W., Structural Mechanics Software Series, University Press of Virginia, Charlottesville, Virginia, Vol. I - 1977; Vol. II - 1978; and Vol. III - 1979.

183 Grooms, D. W., ed., Structural Mechanics Software, Vol. 2, May 1975-May 1977, NTIS/PS-77/0525, NTIS, Springfield, VA 22161, June 1977.

184 Carrigan, B., ed., Structural Mechanics Software, Vol. 2, July 1977-June 1979, NTIS/PS-79/0706, NTIS, Springfield, VA 22161, July 1979.

185 Moone, E. C. E., "Software Coordination Efforts," Computers and Structures, Vol. 6, 1976, pp. 489-496.

186 Sollogoub, P., et al, "Main Computer Systems Programs, Presentation, Criteria for Selection," CNEXO/CTICM, Brest/Puteaux, France, 1978.

187 Backx, E., et al, "Case Study on Desk Computer: Finite Element Analysis in BASIC," Proc. Second World Congress, Robinson and Assoc., Dorset, 1978, pp. 670-680.

188 Backx, E., et al, "Interactive Engineering Software for Desktop Computers," in R. A. Adey, ed., Engineering Software, Pentech Press, Plymouth, 1979, pp. 78-93.

189 Collington, D. J., and Adey, R. A., "An Engineering Problem Solving System for Small Computers," in R. A. Adey, ed., Engineering Software, Pentech Press, Plymouth, 1979, pp. 78-93.

APPENDIX I

ADDRESSES OF THE SOFTWARE AND INFORMATION ORGANIZATIONS

1 AEC, Advanced Engineering Corporation, Box 3044, S-580 03 Linköping, Sweden

2 Argonne Code Center, Mrs. Margaret Butler, Argonne National Labs., Argonne, Illinois 60439, USA.

3 ASIAC, Aerospace Structures Information and Analysis Center, AFDL-FBR, Wright-Patterson AFB, Dayton, Ohio 45433, USA

4 APEC, Automated Procedures for Engineering Consultants, Mrs. Doris J. Wallace, Executive Secretary, Automatic Procedures for Engineering Consultants, Grant-Deneau Tower, Suite M-15, Fourth and Lodlow Streets, Dayton, Ohio 45402, USA

5 CACT, Centre d'Assistance au Calcul Technique, Professor S. Bernaert, Vice Director, CACT, 9, rue la Perouse, 74784 Paris, Cedex 16, France

6 CEPA, Civil Engineering Program Applications, Mr. Joseph Rodgers, Executive Secretary, CEPA, P.O. Box 1532, Rockville, Maryland 20850, USA

7 CIAD of Holland, Mr. J. C. Le Clercq, Director of CIAD, P.O. Box 74, Zoetermeer, Netherlands

8 COMMON, Mr. Robert G. Bostrom, Administrative Director, COMMON, 435 N. Michigan Avenue, Chicago, Illinois 60611, USA

9 COSMIC, Computer Software Management and Information Center, Miss Maragaret Park, Manager, Information Service, 112 Barrow Hall, University of Georgia, Athens, GA 30502, USA

10 DECUS, Digital Equipment Corporation Users Society, Mrs. Angela J. Cossette, Executive Secretary, DECUS, Digital Equipment Corporation, Maynard, Mass., USA

11 EUROCOPI, European Computer Program Institute, 21020 Centro Euroatom di Ispra, Varese, Italy

12 FACTS, Federal Agencies Computer Time-Sharing System, Mr. Henry A. Borger, Program Manager, Federal Construction Council, Building Research Advisory Board, 2101 Constitution Avenue, N.W., Washington, D. C. 20018, USA

13 HEEP, Highway Engineering Exchange Program, Mr. John Bridwell, Director, Division of Technical Computing, Kentucky Department of Transportation, Frankford, KY 40601, USA

14 HUG, Honeywell Users Group, Mr. Wallace Juntunen, Honeywell Administration Service, 2701 4th Avenue South, Minneapolis, Minnesota 55408, USA

15 ICES Users Group, Inc., Frederick E. Hajjar, Executive Director, ICES Users Group, Inc., P. O. Box 8243, Cranston, Rhode Island 02910, USA

16 IITRI, IIT Research Institute Structural Mechanics Computer Library, Mr. R. L. Chiapetta, Senior Research Engineer, IIT Research Institute, 10 West 35th Street, Chicago, Illinois 60616, USA

17 NCC, The National Computing Centre Ltd, Oxford Road, Manchester M1 7ED, England

18 NISEE , National Information Service for Earthquake Engineering, Dr. Ken Wong, NISEE/Computer Applications, 729 Davis Hall, University of California, Berkeley, California 94720, USA

19 SHARE, Inc. SHARE Program Library Agency, Triangle Universities Computation Center, P. O. Box 12076, Research Triangle Park, N. C. 27709, USA

20 STORE, Structures Oriented Exchange, Dr. Nicholas Perrone, Office of Naval Research, Code 439, 800 North Quincy Street, Arlington, Virginia 22217, USA

21 SWAP, Society for Wang Applications and Programs, Mr. Jason R. Taylor, Executive Director, SWAP, 836 North Street, Tewksburg, Massachusetts 01876, USA

22 VIM, Users Group for CDC 6000 Series Machines, Mr. A. L. Siegel, Computer Center, Battelle Memorial Institute, 505 King Avenue, Columbus, Ohio 43201, USA

CHAPTER THIRTEEN

FINITE ELEMENTS IN THE TIME DOMAIN

O. C. Zienkiewicz
University College of Swansea
United Kingdom

ABSTRACT

The use of finite elements in space and time domains is demonstrated as a particular case of "weighted residual" formulations. In problems of constant spatial boundaries, these techniques are equivalent to the use of finite elements in time on the semi-discretized equations of such form as

$$[C]\{\dot{a}\} + [K]\{a\} + \{f\} = 0$$

and

$$[M]\{\ddot{a}\} + [C]\{\dot{a}\} + [K]\{a\} + \{f\} = 0$$

Various two and three step schemes are developed by the "finite element in time" process, and it is shown that in addition to several well known "finite difference" expressions, new formulations with special merits appear.

In convective problems where the K matrix is nonsymmetric, alternative formulation becomes feasible to eliminate instabilities associated with convective terms. It is shown that in such problems, the use of full space-time finite elements may be desirable.

INTRODUCTION

The finite element method may be, most generally, considered as a process of approximation to continuum problems by a series of undetermined parameters ($\{a\}$ or $\{a_i\}$) and prescribed trial (shape) functions ($[N]$ or $[N_i]$).[1] The continuum problem is generally defined in a domain Ω of independent variables with its associated boundaries Γ. In the early days, the problem domain was generally associated only with the space coordinates (x, y, z), and if the time "coordinate" entered the formulation, a semi-discretization followed in which the parameters remained time variable. This resulted in a system of ordinary differential equations for the parameters $\{\underset{\sim}{a}\}$ which was solved either analytically or by the use of a finite difference discretization. Clearly, however, the use of the

[1] $[N]$ and $\{a\}$ are used in this chapter for matrices and vectors, respectively. $[N_i]$ or $\{a_i\}$ denote component submatrices or vectors, though often such quantities may be scalars.

finite element discretization in the time domain was an obvious extension, and this has been introduced as a practical possibility by Oden [1], Argyris and Sharpf [2], Fried [3], Zienkiewicz [4,5] and others.

Two distinct classes of finite elements in the time domain exist:

In the first, the finite element process is applied to the ordinary differential equation resulting from the semi-discretization process.

In the second, direct finite element shape functions are defined in the space-time domain.

Unless the problem space boundary is changing with time, the combined space-time domain is "prismatic", and the expansions used for the combined shape functions can be written in a product form as

$$[N(\underset{\sim}{x},t)] = [\bar{N}(\underset{\sim}{x})]\hat{N}(t) \tag{1}$$

If this is the case, both processes of discretization can be made identical, and hence it is always desirable to proceed from the partially discretized forms. Indeed, the large part of this paper will be concerned with such a two stage process starting from ordinary matrix differential equations of the form

$$[C]\{\dot{a}\} + [K]\{a\} + \{f\} = 0 \tag{2}$$

or

$$[M]\{\ddot{a}\} + [C]\{\dot{a}\} + [K]\{a\} + \{f\} = 0 \tag{3}$$

The first of these arises from such problems as heat transfer, seepage, etc. by a semi-discretization of the relevant partial differential equations. The second typifies the dynamic behavior of solids. In all of the above it is not essential to even use the finite element discretization in the space variables. Other legitimate approximations can be introduced, or indeed Eqs. (2) or (3) may themselves model a physically discrete situation.

On infrequent occasions, such as for instance those which may arise in dealing with the thermal behavior of ablating structures, the space boundary surface may change with time, and the use of "nonprismatic" space-time elements may be advantageous. Indeed a similar situation is encountered in a formulation of convective diffusion heat flow problems which utilizes the characteristic directions. We shall discuss this in a general context in a later section of this chapter. A particularly interesting application of this kind was recently introduced by Finn and Varoglu [6,7].

In what follows we shall invariably use a weighted residual or Galerkin form of discretization. This allows us to obtain as a special case the more usual forms of finite element approximation which result from the stationarity of a specified functional. Other, more interesting approximations will differ from such special cases when the weighting functions are not the same as the shape functions. Here we shall rediscover many standard recurrence formulae, alternatively derived. Indeed the process of applying finite elements in the time domain appears to encompass all alternative methods of time discretization and, in addition, presents many new and interesting possibilities.

The notation and theoretical basis will follow the author's text [8], but some, more mathematical proofs may be found in other sources, such as, for instance, the excellent treatise by Strang and Fix [9].

THE WEIGHTED RESIDUAL PROCESS

Continuum problems are generally defined by a differential equation (or a set of such equations) which must be satisfied in the problem domain Ω of independent variables (such as x, y, t, etc.). In addition, certain conditions need to be satisfied on the boundary of the domain

$$\partial\Omega \equiv \Gamma \tag{4}$$

Denoting the independent variable (or variables) as $\{\phi\}$, we can symbolically write the problem as a requirement that

$$\{A(\{\phi\})\} = 0 \quad \text{in } \Omega \tag{5a}$$

$$\{B(\{\phi\})\} = 0 \quad \text{on } \Gamma \tag{5b}$$

where {A} and {B} are suitable operators.

In the finite element method the unknown function is expanded as an approximation

$$\{\phi\} \approx \{\hat{\phi}\} = \sum_{i=1}^{n} [N_i]\{a_i\} \equiv [N]\{a\} \tag{6}$$

where

$$[N_i] = [N_i(x,y,z,t, \text{ etc.})] \tag{7}$$

are prescribed shape-functions, and $\{a_i\}$ is a set of independent parameters.

Because in general it will be impossible to satisfy Eq. (5) exactly by the appropriate expansion, we shall satisfy it approximately by writing

$$\Omega[W_j]^T\{A(\hat{\phi})\}d\Omega + \Gamma[\bar{W}_j]^T\{B(\hat{\phi})\}d\Gamma = 0 \tag{8}$$

where W_j, $\bar{W}_j$ are again a set of arbitrary test (or weighting) functions.

As the number of parameters {a} grows and as the number of arbitrary weighting functions becomes larger, $\{\hat{\phi}\} \to \{\phi\}$, and the approximation improves.[2]

On substitution of expansion (6), Eq. (8) yields a set of simultaneous algebraic equations in $\{a_i\}$ (i = 1 to n) which when solved gives an approximation to $\{\phi\}$. If the operators {A}, {B} are linear, then this equation can be written in the equivalent matrix form as

$$[H]\{a\} = -\{f\} \to \{a\} = -[H]^{-1}\{f\} \tag{9}$$

If in expansion (6) we allow $\{a_i\}$ to remain a function of one independent variable, say

$$\{a_i\} = \{a_i(t)\} \tag{10}$$

and we use a shape function given in terms of the other variables, say

$$[N_i] = [N_i(x,y, \ldots)] \tag{11}$$

then assuming weighting functions to be similarly defined,

$$[W_j] = [W_j(x,y, \ldots)] \tag{12}$$

the approximate relation will result in a <u>semi-discretized</u> form, given typically by a set of equations such as (2) or (3).

As an example, consider for instance the transient heat equation

$$A(T) = -\frac{\partial}{\partial x}\left(k\frac{\partial T}{\partial x}\right) - \frac{\partial}{\partial y}\left(k\frac{\partial T}{\partial y}\right) + C\frac{\partial T}{\partial t} + Q = 0 \quad \text{in } \Omega \tag{13}$$

with $B(T) \equiv \phi = 0$ on the space boundary Γ at all values of time. (This 'boundary condition' is also valid here for all values of x,y at t=0.)

The problem domain is illustrated in Fig. 1. This domain is 'open' since the problem is of interest for all $t \geq 0$. In practice we could limit our solution to a certain range and divide the resulting domain into elements (or otherwise discretize) to write

$$T \approx \hat{T} = \Sigma N_i(x,y,t)a_i \tag{14}$$

with N_i and a_i components being simple scalars.

---

[2]Certain conditions have to be satisfied by the shape and weighting functions for this to be strictly true. Such conditions are discussed in detail elsewhere [8,9].

Writing the weighted form as[3]

$$\int_{\Omega} W_j \left(-\frac{\partial}{\partial x} k \frac{\partial \hat{T}}{\partial x} - \frac{\partial}{\partial y} k \frac{\partial \hat{T}}{\partial y} + C \frac{\partial \hat{T}}{\partial t} + Q\right) dx\,dy\,dt + \int_{\Gamma} \bar{W}_j \,\phi\, d\Gamma = 0 \tag{15}$$

we can drop the second term by choosing $\bar{W}_j = W_j = 0$ on all boundary points j and enforcing the boundary condition.

An integration by parts (or use of Green's theorem) allows us to write

$$\int_{\Omega} \left(\frac{\partial W_j}{\partial x} k \frac{\partial \hat{T}}{\partial x} + \frac{\partial W_j}{\partial y} k \frac{\partial \hat{T}}{\partial y} + W_j C \frac{\partial \hat{T}}{\partial t} + W_j Q\right) dx\,dy\,dt = 0 \tag{16}$$

$$j = 1 - n$$

On substitution of expansion (14) we have now a set of algebraic equations in the form

$$[H]\{a\} + \{f\} = 0 \tag{17}$$

where

$$H_{ji} = \int_{\Omega} \left(\frac{\partial W_j}{\partial x} k \frac{\partial N_i}{\partial x} + \frac{\partial W_j}{\partial y} k \frac{\partial N_i}{\partial x} + W_j C \frac{\partial N_i}{\partial t}\right) dx\,dy\,dt$$

$$f_j = \int_{\Omega} W_j Q \; dx\,dy\,dt \tag{18}$$

It is immediately apparent that: a) if a large time domain is considered, the size of the problem can become excessively large; and b) the algebraic equation system is, in general, nonsymmetric even if the Galerkin/Bubnov type of weighting is used, i.e.

$$W_j \equiv N_j \tag{19}$$

This symmetry arises from the presence of the last term of the expansion defining H_{ji}.

To reduce the size of the problem, it is obviously possible to reduce the time of the domain to the length of one time step Δt and to establish a recurrence relation between known values of T_o (or T_n) at $t=t_o$ (or $t=t_n$) and those at $t_1=t_o + \Delta t$ or $(t=t_{n+1})$.

Clearly there is little advantage in using an irregular distribution of space-time elements, and in general we shall write

$$N_j(x,y,t) = \bar{\bar{N}}_k(x,y)\bar{N}_\ell(t) \tag{20}$$

with a similar expansion used for the weighting function W_j (each space-time point is now characterized by k and ℓ).

An alternative procedure is to apply a semi-discretization and to write in place of Eq. (14)

$$T \approx \hat{T} = \Sigma\, N_i(x,y)\; a_i(t) \tag{21}$$

where the parameters a_i define the temperature field at a fixed point of space but at varying times. With $\bar{\bar{\Omega}}$ now representing the x,y section of the domain we have in place of Eq. (17) a set of ordinary differential equations

$$[C]\frac{d}{dt}\{a\} + [K]\{a\} + \{f\} = 0$$

$$[C]\{\dot{a}\} + [K]\{a\} + \{f\} = 0 \tag{22}$$

---

[3]Note that $\int_{\Omega} (\;)\, dx\,dy\,dt \equiv \iiint (\;)\, dx\,dy\,dt$

where

$$C_{ji} = \int_{\bar{\bar{\Omega}}} \bar{\bar{W}}_j \, C \, \bar{\bar{N}}_i \, dx\,dy$$

$$K_{ji} = \int_{\bar{\bar{\Omega}}} \left(\frac{\partial \bar{\bar{W}}_j}{\partial x} k \frac{\partial \bar{\bar{N}}_i}{\partial x} + \frac{\partial \bar{\bar{W}}_j}{\partial y} k \frac{\partial \bar{\bar{N}}_i}{\partial y}\right) dx\,dy \tag{23}$$

$$f_j = \int_{\bar{\bar{\Omega}}} \bar{\bar{W}}_j \, Q \, dx\,dy$$

All of the above matrices, as well as the parameter set, can be a function of t, and in general, the coefficients k and C may vary with time or exhibit nonlinear characteristics depending on the parameters themselves.

If now, to Eq. (22) we apply a trial function expansion in time, i.e., $\{a\} = \Sigma\, N_\ell(t)\{\dot{a}\}_\ell$ where $\{a\}_\ell$ is the set of parameters defined at a time instant 1, then again a set of approximate algebraic equations will be obtained. The reader can verify that this final approximation will be precisely the same as that given by Eq. (17) providing that the product shape functions of Eq. (20) are used. For this reason in what follows, we shall assume as a starting point the semi-discretized form given by Eqs. (2) and (3). Various approximations and resulting recurrence relationships will now be discussed.

SIMPLE TWO POINT RECURRENCE RELATIONSHIPS FOR FIRST ORDER EQUATIONS (HEAT CONDUCTION PROBLEMS, ETC.)

Weighted Residual Approach

We shall now consider the first order Eq. (2) and show how a simple kind of recurrence scheme can be devised.

Proceeding in the usual manner of discretization, with time as the independent variable, we can write

$$\{\underset{\sim}{a}\} \approx \{\hat{a}\} = \Sigma\, N_\ell \,\{a\}_\ell \tag{24}$$

where $\{a\}_\ell$ stands for a nodal set of $\{a\}$ at a time ℓ. The shape functions $N_\ell(t)$ are taken to be the same for each component of a vector $\{a\}$, and therefore, N_ℓ is a scalar.

The lowest order of polynomial necessary for the shape function N_ℓ is that of first order because only first order derivatives are involved in Eq. (2).

Consider now a typical time 'element' of length Δt with $\{a\}_\ell$ taking on nodal values $\{a_n\}$ and $\{a_{n+1}\}$ as shown in Fig. 2. The interpolation (shape) functions and their first time derivatives can be written in terms of local variables as

$$\begin{aligned} &0 \le \xi \le 1 && \xi = t/\Delta t \\ &N_n = 1 - \xi && \dot{N}_n = -1/\Delta t \\ &N_{n+1} = \xi && \dot{N}_n = 1/\Delta t \end{aligned} \tag{25}$$

A typical weighted residual equation can now be written assuming that the full domain of investigation corresponds with that of one element;

$$\begin{aligned} \int_o^1 W_j\big([C](\{a\}_n \dot{N}_n + \{a\}_{n+1}\dot{N}_{n+1}) \\ + [K](\{a\}_n N_n + \{a\}_{n+1} N_{n+1}) + \{f\}\big)d\xi = 0 \qquad j = 1 \end{aligned} \tag{26}$$

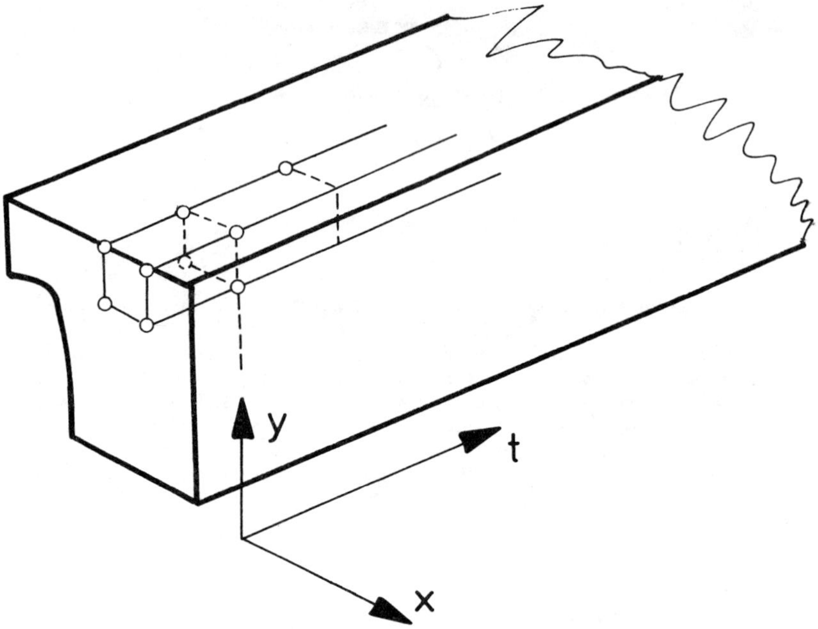

Fig. 1 A 'prismatic' space-time region

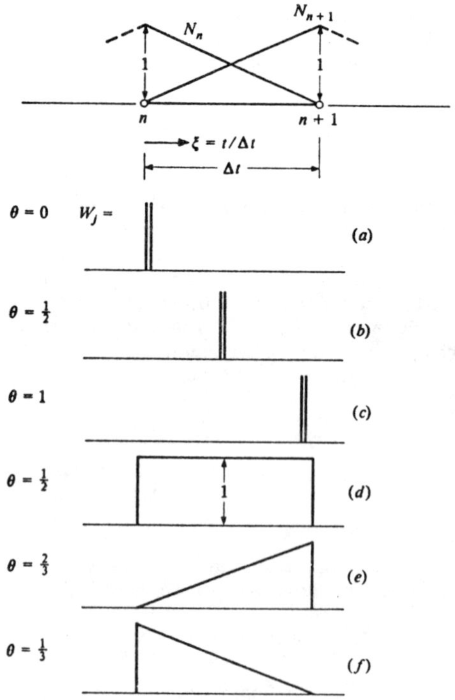

Fig. 2 Shape functions and weight functions for two point recurrence formulae

Since the problem is an initial value one, one of the parameter sets $\{a_n\}$ is assumed known, and the equation will serve to determine $\{a_{n+1}\}$ approximately. Immediately on inserting Eq. (25) a recurrence relation can be written as

$$\left([K] \int_0^1 W_j \xi d\xi + [C] \int_0^1 W_j d\xi/\Delta t\right)\{a\}_{n+1}$$

$$+ \left([K] \int_0^1 W_j (1-\xi) d\xi - [C] \int_0^1 W_j d\xi/\Delta t\right)\{a\}_n \tag{27}$$

$$+ \int_0^1 W_j \{f\} d\xi = 0$$

in which various weighting functions can be inserted. In the above, matrices [K] and [C] have been assumed to be independent of t. Quite generally, expression (27) can be rewritten for any weighting function as

$$([C]/\Delta t + [K]\theta)\{a\}_{n+1} + (-[C]/\Delta t + [K](1-\theta))\{a_n\} + \{\bar{f}\} = 0 \tag{28}$$

$$\theta = \int_0^1 W\xi \, d\xi / \int_0^1 W \, d\xi \tag{a}$$

$$\bar{f} = \int_0^1 W\{f\} d\xi / \int_0^1 W \, d\xi \tag{b}$$

From the above, $\{a_{n+1}\}$ can be found by a simple solution of equations since $\{a_n\}$ and $\{\bar{f}\}$ are known.

It is logical and convenient to assume that the same interpolation is applied to the function $\{f\}$ as that used for the unknown vector $\{a\}$. If this interpolation is adopted, we find that

$$\{\bar{f}\} = \{f\}_{n+1}\theta + \{f\}_n(1-\theta) \tag{29}$$

If the function varies smoothly in time, such an interpolation is acceptable but on occasion may be misleading. In such cases, it is simple to evaluate the expression (28b) exactly. This allows 'impulse' and other discontinuous inputs to be used.

At this stage, we observe that if $\theta=0$ and [C] is a diagonal (lumped)[4] matrix, the solution for $\{a_{n+1}\}$ is trivial, and each individual component can be computed directly from its precursors. Such schemes are known as explicit whilst those in which $\theta \neq 0$, requiring the solution of a nondiagonal system of equations, are known as implicit. We shall see later that this computational convenience is accompanied by a serious drawback which requires the use of Δt not exceeding a certain magnitude.

The reader will recognize in Eq. (28) a well known series of finite difference formulae with a modification of using a weighted loading term $\{\bar{f}\}$. In Fig. 2 we show a series of weighting functions and the resulting values of θ. The first three, (a) to (c), represent point collocation weighting applied to n, n + 1/2, and n + 1, respectively, and give the well known forward difference (Euler), mid-difference (Crank-Nicholson), and backward difference formulae.

The schemes shown in Fig. 2(e) and (f) represent Galerkin type processes. The scheme (e) was first suggested by the author and is equivalent to the normal use of the Galerkin procedure with the weighting corresponding to the unknown function, and this scheme has been shown to lead to considerable computational advantages [10].

[4] If finite element discretization is in fact used in the space domain, we find, in general, that such matrices as [C] are not diagonal unlike those arising in finite difference discretization. There are several possible methods for diagonalizing such matrices without loss of accuracy. A survey of literature and description of several such processes is given in Ref. [8], pages 535-539.

An alternate approach to deriving a time marching scheme of the above type is possible. Here we shall write Eq. (2) as a set of equations

$$[C]\{\nu\} + [K]\{a\} + \{f\} = 0$$
$$\{\nu\} - \{\dot{a}\} = 0 \tag{30}$$

Assuming now a linear interpolation of the type given in Eq. (24) and Eq. (25) for both variables $\{\nu\}$ and $\{a\}$ and weighting the individual equations by independent functions $\bar{W}$ and W, respectively, we have, on performing operations identified to those which gave Eq. (28),

$$[C](\{\nu\}_{n+1}\bar{\theta} + \{\nu\}_n(1-\bar{\theta})) +$$
$$[K](\{a\}_{n+1}\bar{\theta} + \{a\}_n(1-\bar{\theta})) + \{f\}_{n+1}\bar{\theta} + \{f\}_n(1-\bar{\theta}) = 0 \tag{31}$$
$$\{\nu\}_{n+1}\theta + \{\nu\}_n(1-\theta)\} - (\{a\}_{n+1} - \{a\}_n)/\Delta t = 0$$

In the above we have implicitly assumed that $\{f\}$ varies according to a linear interpolation as in Eq. (29).

If now we take starting values $\{\nu\}_n$ and $\{a\}_n$ such that they satisfy the first of Eq. (30), we observe that $\bar{\theta}$ does not enter the formulation and we can now write simply

$$[C]\{\nu\}_{n+1} + [K]\{a\}_{n+1} + \{f\}_{n+1} = 0 \tag{32}$$

and

$$\{\nu\}_{n+1}\theta + \{\nu\}_n(1-\theta) - (\{a\}_{n+1} - \{a\}_n)/\Delta t = 0$$

On elimination of $\{\nu\}_{n+1}$ above yields the recurrence algorithm

$$\{\nu\}_{n+1} = \frac{1}{\theta\Delta t}(\{a\}_{n+1} - \{\hat{a}\}_{n+1}) \tag{33a}$$

where we define

$$\{\hat{a}\}_{n+1} = \{a\}_n + \Delta t(1-\theta)\{\nu\}_n \tag{33b}$$

and

$$([C]/\Delta t + [K]\theta)\{a\}_{n+1} = -\theta\{f\}_{n+1} + [C]\{\hat{a}\}_{n+1}/\Delta t \tag{33c}$$

In the above we first compute $\{\hat{a}\}_{n+1}$ from Eq. (33b) involving only simple component operations and follow by determining $\{a\}_{n+1}$ from Eq. (33c). This requires only multiplication by the matrix [C] to determine the right hand side. Since this matrix is often diagonal, some operations are saved as compared with the algorithm given in Eq. (28). The calculation is completed by determining $\{\nu\}_{n+1}$ from Eq. (33c).

The reader can verify that $\{\nu\}_n$ is eliminated by using the condition

$$[C]\{\nu\}_n + [K]\{a\}_n + \{f\}_n = 0 \tag{34}$$

identity with the previous recurrence scheme of Eq. (28) is obtained.

In the foregoing we have assumed the domain of the approximation to correspond to a time Δt and have established a recurrence relation between two successive values of $\{a_{n+1}\}$ and $\{a_n\}$. The computation can obviously proceed in a step-by-step manner using a sequence of such domains. It is, however, possible to apply the procedure to the whole domain of time simultaneously, assuming this domain to be divided into a finite number of elements. Using, for instance, the linear expansions of Eq. (25) but integrating over the whole domain, we note that unless the weight functions are confined to a single element, several sets of $\{a_i\}$ will be included simultaneously in a typical equation. For instance, if the Galerkin procedure is used and we assume that

$$W_j = N_j$$

then, if the whole domain is included, three successive values are involved in a typical equation, as shown in Fig. 3. For a constant time interval Δt the following expression is obtained, which can be verified by the reader

$$([C]/2\Delta t + [K]/6)\{a\}_{n+1} + (2[K]/3)\{a\}_n + (-[C]/2\Delta t + [K]/6)\{a\}_{n-1} + \{\bar{f}\} = 0$$

$$\{\bar{f}\} = \{f\}_{n+1}/6 + 2\{f\}_n/3 + \{f\}_{n-1}/6 \tag{35}$$

Providing two initial values are known, such a formula can be used in a recurrent manner for evaluating $\{a\}_{n+1}$ from $\{a\}_n$ and $\{a\}_{n-1}$. We shall discuss in some detail such expressions in general in the section on multipoint recurrence schemes.

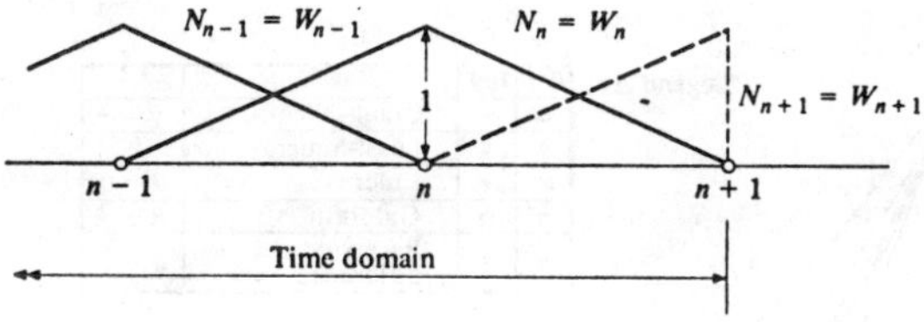

Fig. 3 A Galerkin scheme with linear shape functions applied to whole time domain

Variational Approaches

As the alternative to the weighted residual approach it is often possible to obtain a variational functional whose stationarity corresponds to the correct differential equations discussed in the time domain. For instance, in the second order dynamic equation Hamilton's principle [11] could provide a starting basis. Gurtin [12,13] establishes some other useful principles for both first and second order equations. Such variational functionals have been used by Wilson and Nickell [14], Fried [2,15], and Argyris [3,15]. However, it is well known that such variational principles are equivalent to the use of Galerkin procedures and will yield no new alternative numerical schemes. Zienkiewicz and Parekh [4] have used, for the first time, the finite element in time based on weighted residual forms.

One alternative which is not embedded explicitly in standard variational forms is that of using the least square procedure. In this procedure we write a functional minimizing the square of the error. In the context of one element representing the whole domain and of a linear interpolation function of Eq. (25) we thus minimize

$$\Pi = \int_0^1 ([C](\{a\}_n\dot{N}_n + \{a\}_{n+1}\dot{N}_{n+1}) + [K](\{a\}_n N_n + \{a_{n+1}\}N_{n+1}) + \{f\}^T)([C](\ldots.))d\xi \tag{36}$$

with respect to the variable $\{a_{n+1}\}$. The reader can verify that the final recurrence scheme now obtained is

$$\begin{aligned}&\{[C]^T[C]/\Delta t + ([K]^T[C] + [C]^T[K])/2 + [K]^T[K]\Delta t/3\}\{a\}_{n+1}\\&+ \{-[C]^T[C]/\Delta t - [K]^T[C] - [C]^T[K]/2 + [K]^T[K]\Delta t/6\}\{a\}_n\\&+ [K]^T \int_0^1 \{f\}\xi d\xi/\Delta t^2 + [C]^T \int_0^1 \{f\}d\xi/\Delta t = 0\end{aligned} \tag{37}$$

The above scheme obviously involves more computation but results in symmetric equations even if matrices [K] and [C] are not symmetric. Some experiments with such a scheme are given by Zienkiewicz and Lewis [16] and have been used successfully by others [17]. To compare the performance of various schemes outlined in this section, we shall consider a simple single variable equation with

$$K = C = 1; \quad f = 0$$

for an initial value of $a_0 = 1$. In Fig. 4 we show results obtained using $\Delta t = 0.5$ and $\Delta t = 0.9$ for various schemes. The least square process shows by far the greatest accuracy, but with associated larger computational cost. Here in the same example the central difference schemes give 'second best' results, and these schemes have been used most frequently in practical applications. As we see later, however, they often lead to oscillatory solutions which are troublesome, and, for that reason the backward difference scheme ($\theta = 1$) or 'Galerkin' scheme with $\theta = 2/3$ is often preferred.

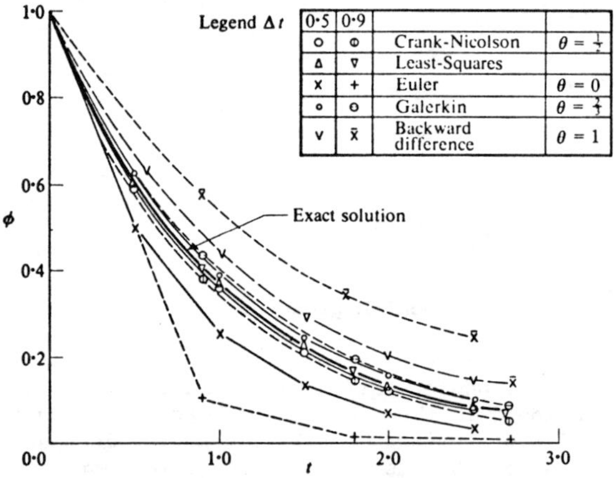

Fig. 4 Comparison of various time-stepping schemes on an initial value problem

In Fig. 5 results for larger time steps, t = 1.5 and 2.5, are shown for the same problem. Here an interesting phenomenon occurs. The forward integration gives either oscillatory or divergent results while the other schemes still retain an acceptable accuracy. The behavior shown here is that of instability, which we shall discuss in the next section.

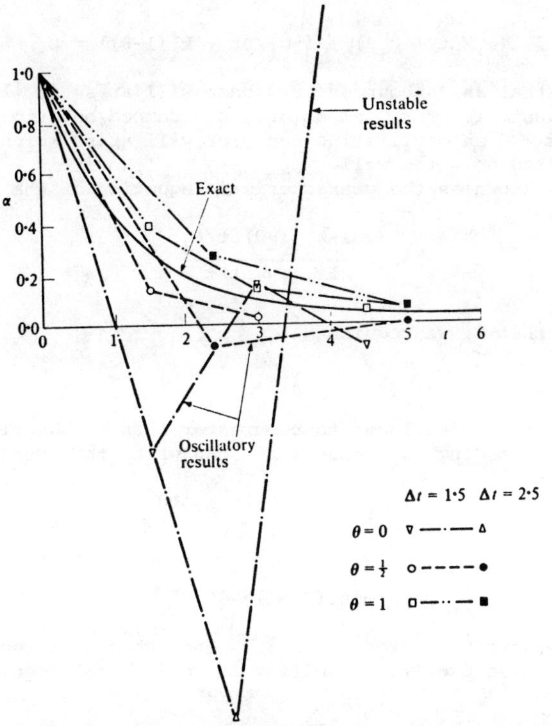

Fig. 5 Demonstration of instability in problems of Fig. 4

Oscillation and Instability for Two-Point Recurrence Schemes

As we have remarked in the introduction, for stability considerations it will be convenient to consider the system of decoupled equations in terms of the modal participation variables y_i, i.e., to deal with a set of independent scalar equations of the form (38) for the first order equation

$$c_i \dot{y}_i + k_i y_i + f_i = 0 \tag{38}$$

Clearly as any response can be written as a sum of such modes, we shall be able to synthesize the total response for a multi-degree-of-freedom system with eigenvectors $\{\bar{a}\}_i$ as

$$\{a\} = [\{\bar{a}\}_1, \{\bar{a}\}_2, \ldots] \begin{Bmatrix} y_1 \\ y_2 \\ \vdots \end{Bmatrix} \tag{39}$$

The recurrence relations written previously are obviously applicable here, and we shall consider the general recurrence relation of the form (28). For free response, i.e., with the forcing term set to zero, we can write this recurrence as

$$(c_i/\Delta t + k_i\theta)(y_i)_{n+1} + (-c_i/\Delta t + k_i(1-\theta))(y_i)_n = 0 \tag{40}$$

or writing

$$(y_i)_{n+1} = \lambda(y_i)_n \tag{41}$$

we have

$$\lambda(c_i/\Delta t + k_i\theta) + (-c_i/\Delta t + k_i(1-\theta)) = 0 \tag{42}$$

Immediately we see that an 'unbounded' response will arise if $|\lambda|>1$ and the solution will become unstable, for real solutions a damped behavior being generally noted. Further, if $\lambda<0$ an oscillating behavior will arise which clearly does not represent the required solution well.

Equation (42), known as the characteristic equation of the recurrence scheme, gives

$$\lambda = \frac{1-k_i(1-\theta)\Delta t/c_i}{1+k_i\,\theta\,\Delta t/c_i} \tag{43}$$

We see immediately that if we require

$$|\lambda|<1$$

the right-hand side of Eq. (43) has to be greater than -1. Noting that $k_i/c_i=\omega_i$, the eigenvalue corresponding to a mode i, we can write this requirement as

$$1-\omega_i\Delta t(1-\theta)>-1-\omega_i\Delta t\theta$$

or

$$\omega_i\Delta t(2\theta-1)>-2 \tag{44}$$

This condition is always satisfied for $\theta\geq 1/2$, and schemes of such kind are unconditionally stable. When $0<\theta<1/2$, stability is conditional requiring

$$\omega_i\Delta t < \frac{2}{1-2\theta} \tag{45}$$

This, in the example of Fig. 5, gives the limit of the time step as $\omega_i\Delta t\leq 2$ when the forward difference scheme ($\theta=0$) is used, and the violation of this condition has resulted in the divergent numbers shown.

The study of the characteristic value λ gives us, however, more information. In Fig. 6 we show how λ varies with some of the time-stepping schemes discussed. We note that, for most of these, λ becomes negative with a large time step, and in fact, the backward difference scheme with $\theta=1$ is the only one not showing this property. This means that for any $\theta<1$ oscillatory results can be obtained. Although mathematically it can be shown that the error for the mid-difference scheme with $\theta=1/2$ is of a higher order, this scheme can give less accurate results than the backward scheme for larger time steps, as shown in Fig. 5.

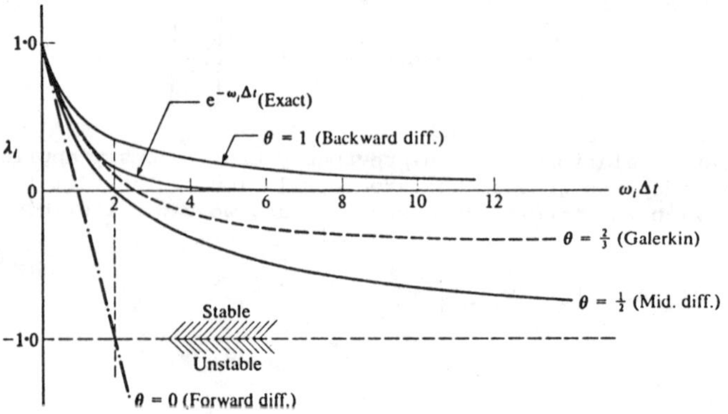

Fig. 6 Variation of λ with $\omega_i\Delta t$ for various recurrence schemes

The time response of a multi-degree-of-freedom system is a combination of all modal responses. Fortunately, the major part of the response corresponds generally to the modes with low eigenvalues ω_i. When an unconditionally stable scheme is used for a multi-degree-of-freedom system, we will usually utilize time steps much in excess of those corresponding to good accuracy for higher frequencies ω_i, and with the value of λ for the unconditionally stable schemes having a negative value, oscillations may not damp out as they should in practice. This is particularly noticeable with the Crank-Nicholson $\theta=1/2$ scheme, and numerical devices have to be used to eliminate such spurious oscillations [17,18]. All such devices consist in essence of averaging successive time steps of computation, and we should note that the most severe input starting such oscillations occurs at abrupt changes of the forcing term. Such abrupt changes should therefore be avoided, or particular care should be taken to deal with them. We shall discuss this matter in the next section.

An alternative procedure which helps to iron out the oscillation is the use of $\theta>1/2$. In this context a useful compromise has been found in the Galerkin scheme with $\theta=2/3$; this scheme has been shown to be very useful in practice with almost all oscillation and errors avoided.[5] In Table I [10] we show the results of a one-dimensional finite element problem where a bar at uniform initial temperature is subjected suddenly to zero temperatures applied at its ends. Here ten linear elements are used in the space dimension with L=1. The oscillatory errors occurring with $\theta=1/2$ are much reduced for $\theta=2/3$. The time step used here is much longer than that corresponding to the lowest eigen period, and the main cause of the oscillation is the abrupt discontinuity in temperature.

TABLE I

Percentage Errors for Finite Elements in Time ($\theta=2/3$) and Crank-Nicholson ($\theta=1/2$) Scheme; $\Delta t=0.01$

t	x=0·1		x=0·2		x=0·3		x=0·4		x=0·5	
	$\theta=\frac{2}{3}$	$\theta=\frac{1}{2}$	$\theta=\frac{2}{3}$	$\theta=\frac{1}{2}$	$\theta=\frac{2}{3}$	$\theta=\frac{1}{2}$	$\theta=\frac{2}{3}$	$\theta=\frac{1}{2}$	$\theta=\frac{2}{3}$	$\theta=\frac{1}{2}$
0·01	10·8	28·2	1·6	3·2	0·5	0·7	0·6	0·1	0·5	0·2
0·02	0·5	3·5	2·1	9·5	0·1	0·0	0·5	0·7	0·7	0·4
0·03	1·3	9·9	0·5	0·7	0·8	3·1	0·5	0·2	0·5	0·6
0·05	0·5	4·5	0·4	0·2	0·5	2·3	0·4	0·8	0·5	1·0
0·10	0·1	1·4	0·1	2·0	0·1	1·5	0·1	1·9	0·1	1·6
0·15	0·3	2·2	0·3	2·1	0·3	2·2	0·3	2·1	0·3	2·2
0·20	0·6	2·6	0·6	2·6	0·6	2·6	0·6	2·6	0·6	2·6
0·30	1·4	3·5	1·4	3·5	1·4	3·5	1·4	3·5	1·4	3·5

Conductivity = specific heat = 1

Conditionally stable schemes, and in particular, the explicit scheme, with $0\leq\theta<1/2$, will always result in instability as long as the time interval used in the calculation exceeds that specified by the highest eigenvalue of the system. This is a serious limitation on the use of explicit time schemes; nevertheless the computational time saving with no matrix inversion (or repeated solution) being required compensates often for the need of using many small time steps.

The estimation of the critical time step for conditionally stable schemes apparently requires the solution of the eigenvalue problem for the whole system. This is not so. The bound on the highest eigenvalue can be simply obtained by the consideration of an individual element. This is established by an important theorem proposed by Irons [20] which proves that the highest system eigenvalue

[5] Lambert [19] suggests, by different reasoning, $\theta=0.878 \approx 7/8$ as optimal.

must always be less than the highest eigenvalue of the individual elements. This theorem allows a very easy estimation of critical time steps to be made which will err on the safe side.[6]

We have not discussed the stability conditions for either the three-point scheme given by Eq. (30) or the recurrence relation obtained from the least square approximation given by Eq. (32), and we leave these as exercises for the reader to perform.

Accuracy and Initial Conditions

We have stated that in the first order problems discussed here the recurrence starts from some specified initial conditions. However, as in the problem of a rapid change of boundary condition discussed previously, such initial conditions may cause an abrupt discontinuity to appear at the start, and an alternative formulation is physically preferable. In this we start the whole problem from a solution which represents the system at rest, i.e., in which a = const., and the change of the initial conditions or of any suddenly applied forcing terms can then be considered as a disturbance on this steady system. The initial conditions, therefore, correspond to those of the steady state and are given for all times prior to a certain instant.

If we consider as an example the simple initial value problem on which we have based Figs. 4 and 5, then the problem can be restated as that requiring a solution of an equation

$$\dot{a} + a + f(t) = 0 \tag{46}$$

which is valid in the whole time domain, and where

$$f(t) = -1 \qquad (t<0) \qquad a = 1$$

$$f(t) = 0 \qquad (t\geq 0)$$

The resulting discontinuity in the new forcing term is shown in Fig. 7(i). Clearly such a discontinuity should be 'smoothed', and this can be done in many ways; such as, for instance, placing an interval which straddles the discontinuity as shown. In the same figure we show the numerical results obtained when such smoothing was applied for the very large time interval $\Delta t=2.5$. The reader will note that the smoothed solution does not show the violent oscillations previously noted and is more physically acceptable.

The process of starting from known steady solutions for $t<0$ and smoothing out any discontinuities will simplify the computation for multi-step schemes because it implies the knowledge of all the vectors $\{a\}$ at times prior to the initial instant. We have now shown that this simplification does, in fact, lead to more realistic answers, and we shall invariably apply it both in first and second order equations.[7]

In Fig. 7(ii) we show the use of such smoothing in a multi-degree-of-freedom system. A step rise in temperature is applied to one end of a bar at $t=0$. The suppression of oscillation and the general improvement in accuracy is noteworthy. Similar problems have been studied by Bettencourt et al [21] using multistep processes, and in all cases the improvement in performance has been remarkable.

---

[6] It is of importance to observe here that for the first order problems of the type of Eq. (2) the element eigenvalues increase as h^2 (h=element size). This means a very rapid decrease of stable Δt with mesh subdivision, and explicit schemes are therefore seldom used for such problems. This is not the case with dynamic problems when element eigenvalues are proportioned to h only.

[7] The smoothing of the discontinuities is in fact a natural consequence of the finite element formulation in the time domain and does not appear naturally in finite difference recurrence formulae.

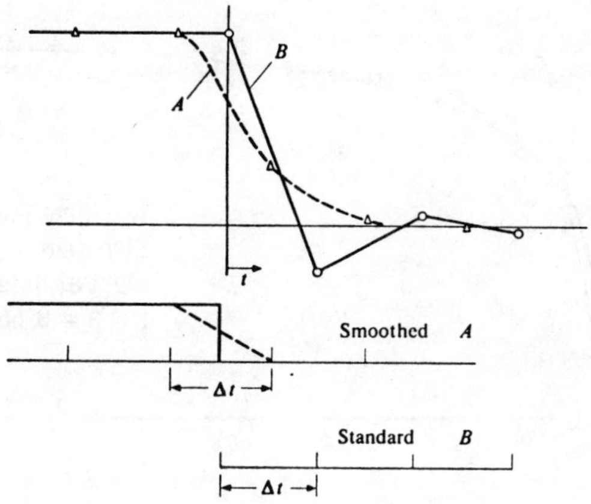

Fig. 7(i) Initial conditions interpreted as step change on steady state. Effect of smoothing discontinuity: θ=1/2, Δt=2·5

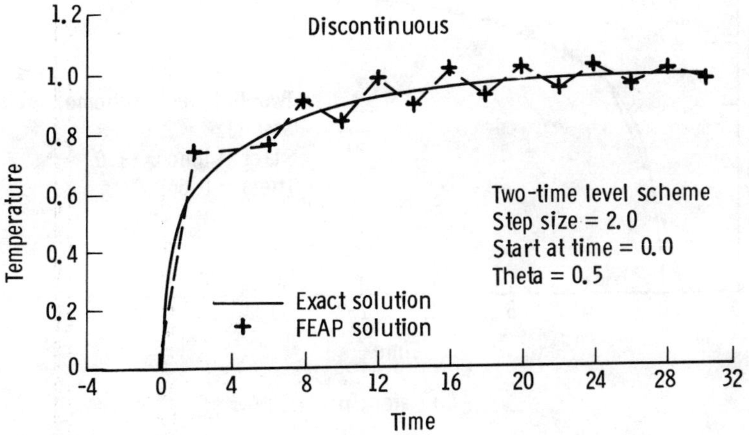

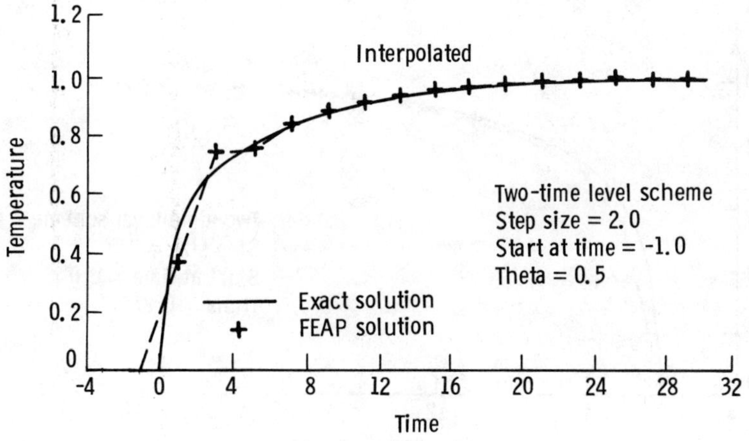

(a) Crank-Nicholson

Fig. 7(ii)

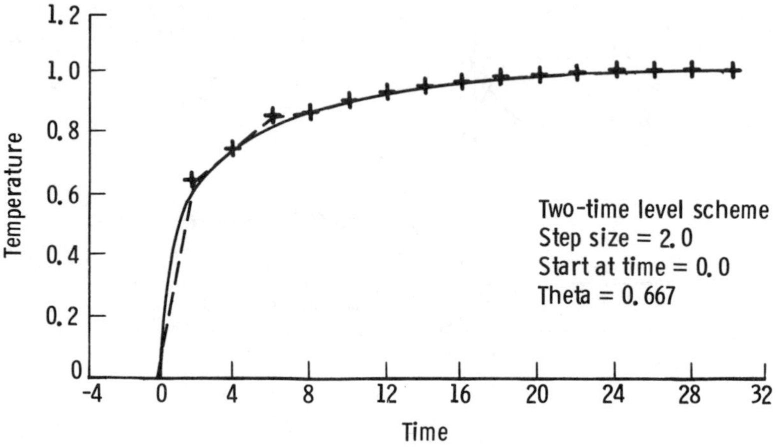

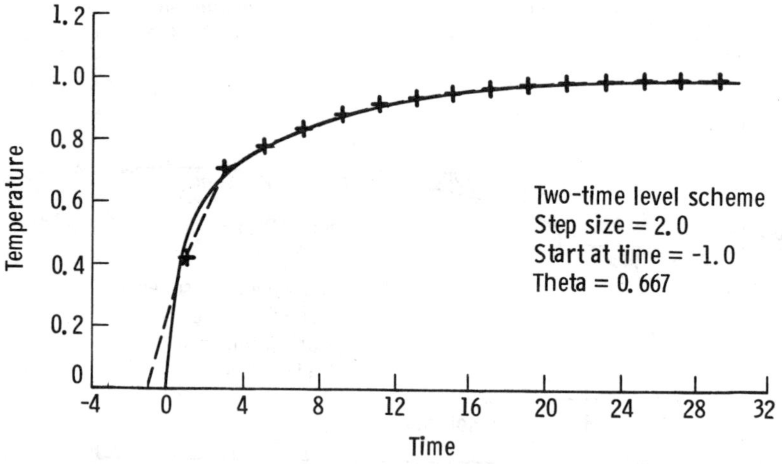

(b) Galerkin

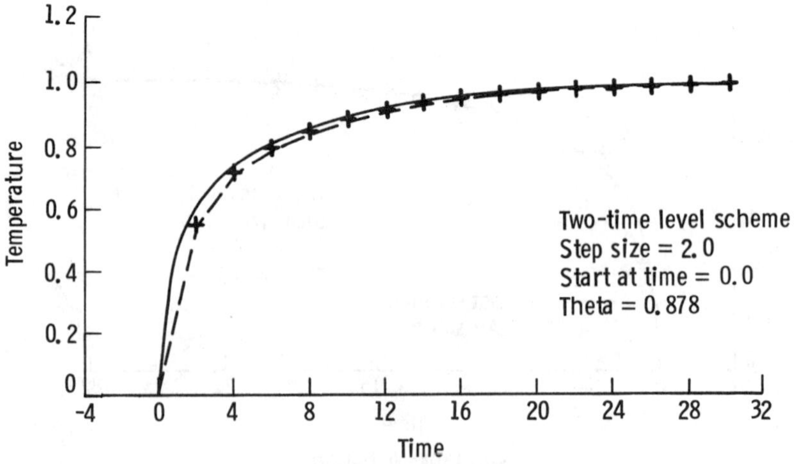

Fig. 7(ii) - Continued

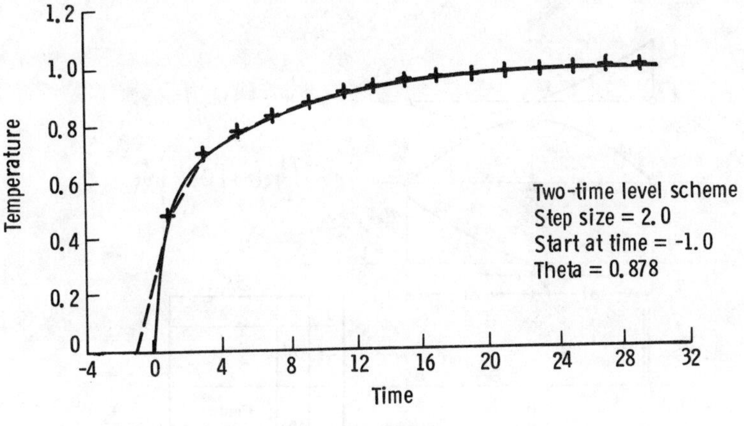

(c) Liniger

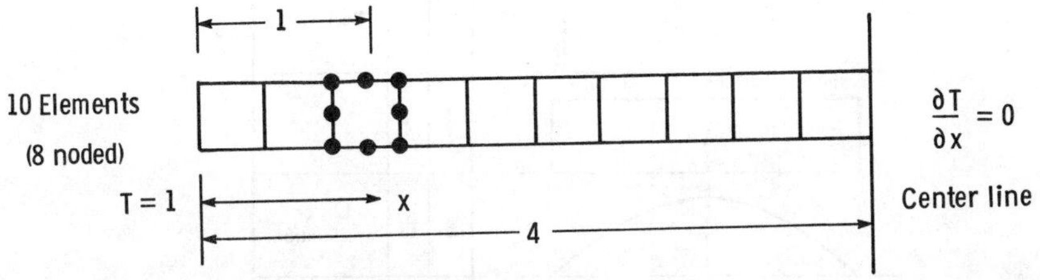

Fig. 7(ii) Transient heating of a bar. Comparison of discontinuous and interpolation (smoothed) initial conditions for two level schemes

THREE-POINT RECURRENCE SCHEMES FOR SECOND ORDER EQUATIONS

The Weighted Residual Algorithm

The procedures of the previous section can be applied directly to the second order Eq. (3), but the shape functions $N_i(t)$ have now to be at least of second order (parabolic) in t because a second order derivative has to be represented. We need now, thus, a minimum of three sets of $\{a\}_i$ to describe approximately the variation of this function. Once again we can write

$$\{a\} \approx \{\hat{a}\} \equiv \Sigma\, N_i\{a\}_i \qquad (47)$$

letting i=n, n+1, n-1.

The shape functions normalize to an interval $2\Delta t$, i.e., with $-1<\xi<1$, they are the standard parabolic ones shown in Fig. 8 and can be written as

$$\xi = t/\Delta t$$

$$N_{n+1} = \xi(1+\xi)/2$$

$$N_n = (1-\xi)(1+\xi) \qquad (48)$$

$$N_{n-1} = -\xi(1-\xi)/2$$

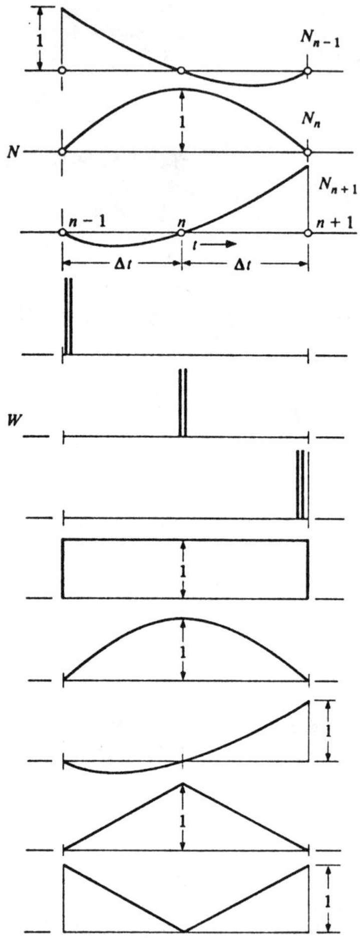

$$\gamma = \int_{-1}^{1} W(\xi + \tfrac{1}{2})\,d\xi \Big/ \int_{-1}^{1} W\,d\xi$$

$$\beta = \tfrac{1}{2}\int_{-1}^{1} W\xi(1 + \xi)\,d\xi \Big/ \int_{-1}^{1} W\,d\xi$$

γ	β	
$-\frac{1}{2}$	0	
$\frac{1}{2}$	0	Central explicit
$\frac{3}{2}$	1	Backward
$\frac{1}{2}$	$\frac{1}{6}$	
$\frac{1}{2}$	$\frac{1}{10}$	Linear acceleration
$\frac{3}{2}$	$\frac{4}{5}$	Galerkin
$\frac{1}{2}$	$\frac{1}{12}$	Fox Goodwin
$\frac{1}{2}$	$\frac{1}{4}$	Average acceleration

Fig. 8 Shape and weight functions for three point recurrence formulae

The time derivatives of these functions are given as

$$\dot{N}_{n+1} = (\frac{1}{2} + \xi)/\Delta t \qquad \ddot{N}_{n+1} = 1/\Delta t^2$$

$$\dot{N}_n = -2\xi/\Delta t \qquad \ddot{N}_n = -2/\Delta t^2 \tag{49}$$

$$\dot{N}_{n-1} = (-\frac{1}{2} + \xi)/\Delta t \qquad \ddot{N}_{n-1} = 1/\Delta t^2$$

We shall now use as a 'domain' of time the period of the size of the element $2\Delta t$ and assume that $\{a\}_n$ and $\{a\}_{n-1}$ are prescribed, thus leaving $\{a\}_{n+1}$ to be determined. The assumption of two known values in fact corresponds precisely to the requirement that two sets of initial conditions be known in order to solve the equation system. Thus we write a single weighted residual equation of the form

$$\int_{-1}^{1} W_j\{[M](\{a\}_{n-1}\ddot{N}_{n-1} + \{a\}_n\ddot{N}_n + \{a\}_{n-1}\ddot{N}_{n-1}) + [C](\{a\}_{n+1}\dot{N}_{n+1}$$

$$+ \{a\}_n\dot{N}_n + \{a\}_{n-1}\dot{N}_{n-1}) + [K](\{a\}_{n+1}N_{n+1} + \{a\}_n N_n + \{a\}_{n-1}N_{n-1}) + \{f\} = 0 \qquad (50)$$

$$j = 1$$

In an analysis similar to that used in deriving Eq. (28) we find that the above can be written as

$$([M] + \gamma\Delta t[C] + \beta\Delta t^1[K])\{a\}_{n+1}$$

$$+ (-2[M] + (1-2\gamma)\Delta t[C] + (\tfrac{1}{2} - 2\beta + \gamma)\Delta t^2[K])\{a\}_n \qquad (51)$$

$$+ ([M] - (1-\gamma)[C] + (\tfrac{1}{2} + \beta - \gamma)\Delta t^2[K])\{a\}_{n-1} + \{\bar{f}\}\Delta t^1 = 0$$

in which[8]

$$\gamma \equiv \int_{-1}^{1} W_j(\xi + \tfrac{1}{2})d\xi \Big/ \int_{-1}^{1} W_j d\xi$$

$$\beta = \int_{-1}^{1} W_j \tfrac{1}{2}\xi(1+\xi)d\xi \Big/ \int_{-1}^{1} W_j d\xi \qquad (52)$$

$$\{\bar{f}\} = \int_{-1}^{1} W_j\{f\}d\xi \Big/ \int_{-1}^{1} W_j d\xi$$

If the same interpolation is used for f as implied for a, then

$$\{\bar{f}\} = \{f\}_{n+1}\beta + \{f\}_n(\tfrac{1}{2} - 2\beta + \gamma) + \{f\}_{n-1}(\tfrac{1}{2} + \beta - \gamma) \qquad (53)$$

Expression (51) is in fact a general algorithm corresponding to that derived by Newmark [22] in a completely different manner and is one of the best known recurrence relationships (albeit not usually stated explicitly in the above form).

Once again various forms of weighting functions can be used ranging from point collocation to Galerkin forms. In Fig. 8 we show the values of β and γ corresponding to a series of such weightings. Newmark recommends that $\gamma=1/2$ be generally taken. This corresponds to symmetric weighting functions of all forms. Again, if $\beta=0$ and the matrices [M] and [C] are diagonal (lumped), then no inversion is necessary to determine $\{a\}_{n+1}$, and the scheme is explicit. One such scheme with $\gamma=1/2$ corresponds to the central difference formula which is extremely economical. However, just as we found in first order equations, we shall find that stability here is conditional and the time interval Δt has to be suitably limited. Such schemes have proved extremely efficient for many linear and non-linear problems in practice and are discussed in Refs. [23-26].

As we have already remarked, two starting values $\{a\}_n$ and $\{a\}_{n+1}$ are necessary to commence calculation. Frequently these are specified by the initial displacements and the initial velocity. This is inconvenient, and as was true with linear systems, it is always an easy matter to translate the problem to that of an initially steady system to which a perturbation is applied. Alternatively, various starting schemes have to be used to predict two successive values of the vector $\{a_i\}$.

---

[8] β and γ correspond to precisely the same symbols introduced by Newmark.

Stability of Three-Point Recurrence Schemes [27-31]

The stability of the schemes developed in the previous section can now be investigated using the procedures identical to those described in the section on oscillation and instability for two point recurrence schemes. First we note that the response can be studied by a series of uncoupled equations of the general form

$$m_i \ddot{y}_i + c_i \dot{y}_i + k_i y_i + f_i = 0 \tag{54}$$

In general to achieve such uncoupling, it is necessary to consider complex natural frequencies, but if the [C] matrix is of a suitable form, the mode decomposition can be accomplished using real eigenvalues of the free vibration

$$\omega_i^2 = k_i/m_i \tag{55}$$

It is mainly with this situation that we shall be concerned, although the arguments given below are quite general.

Once again we shall study the free response in which $f_i=0$ and assume a solution in the form of

$$\begin{aligned} (y_i)_{n+1} &= \lambda (y_i)_n \\ (y_i)_n &= \lambda (y_i)_{n-1} \end{aligned} \tag{56}$$

Substituting the above into the general recurrence relation (51) (now written for the single-degree-of-freedom system of Eq. (49), we have a characteristic equation

$$\begin{aligned} &\lambda^2[m_i + \gamma\Delta t c_i + \beta\Delta t^2 k_i] + \lambda[-2m_i + (1-2\gamma)\Delta t c_i + (\tfrac{1}{2} - 2\beta + \gamma)k_i] \\ &+ [m_i - (1-\gamma)\Delta t c_i + (\tfrac{1}{2} + \beta - \gamma)k_i] = 0 \end{aligned} \tag{57}$$

The roots of this equation can be found and will indicate the behavior of the numerical solution and, in particular, show whether this grows in an unbounded manner which obviously is a physically unacceptable situation. One difference from the solutions discussed in the section on oscillation and instability for two point recurrence schemes is apparent. The roots of the quadratic will generally be complex; this indeed would be expected from the fact that the solution corresponds to one of a damped oscillation. However, we shall still require that the absolute value (modulus) of the complex root satisfies

$$|\lambda| \leq 1 \tag{58}$$

for the oscillation to remain bounded.

The general case of a damped oscillation can be studied in detail by the reader, and here we shall consider answers only for the undamped case, i.e., putting the damping matrix $c_i=0$. We know that for such cases the true solution must be of the form given below

$$y_i = \bar{y}_i \, e^{i\omega t} \tag{59}$$

thus establishing the exact value of λ which is

$$\bar{\lambda} = \frac{(y_i)_{n+1}}{(y_i)_n} = \frac{e^{i\omega(t+\Delta t)}}{e^{i\omega t}} = e^{i\omega\Delta t} \tag{60}$$

This has an absolute value

$$|\bar{\lambda}| = 1 \tag{61}$$

thus indicating an undamped persisting oscillation.

Any numerical scheme which produces $|\lambda|<1$ will give a stable but artifically damped solution. Considering now the solution of the characteristic equation, Eq. (59), in which

$$c_i = 0$$

$$p_i \equiv \frac{k_i}{m_i}\Delta t^2 = \omega_i^2 \Delta t^2$$

we have

$$\lambda^2(1+\beta p_i) + \lambda[-2 + (\tfrac{1}{2} - 2\beta + \gamma)p_i] + [1 + (\tfrac{1}{2} + \beta - \gamma)p_i] = 0 \tag{62}$$

Writing

$$g = \frac{(\frac{1}{2}+\gamma)p_i}{1+\beta p_i} \qquad h = \frac{(\frac{1}{2}-\gamma)p_i}{1+\beta p_i}$$

we can obtain the roots of Eq. (57) as

$$\lambda_{1,2} = \frac{(2-g) \pm \sqrt{(2-g)^2 - 4(1+h)}}{2} \tag{63}$$

These roots will be complex if the quantity under the square root is negative, i.e., if

$$4(1+h) > (2-y)^2$$

or

$$p_i[4\beta - (\tfrac{1}{2}+\gamma)^2] > -4 \tag{64}$$

The modulus of λ is then

$$|\lambda| = \sqrt{1+h} \qquad \leq 1$$

which imposes the requirement

$$-1 < h = \frac{(\frac{1}{2}-\gamma)p_i}{1+\beta p_i} < 0 \tag{65}$$

Summarizing the results of Eqs. (64) and (65), we require therefore that

$$\beta \geq \frac{1}{4}(\tfrac{1}{2}+\gamma)^2$$

$$\gamma \geq \frac{1}{2} \tag{66}$$

$$\frac{1}{2}+\gamma+\beta \geq 0$$

to achieve stability, i.e., for the stability to be unconditional for all values of p_i.

If the above conditions are not satisfied, stability can still be achieved providing

$$p_i < p_{crit}$$

$$\Delta t < \Delta t_{crit}$$

where the critical value can be again found from Eq. (64).

Only two of the schemes shown in Fig. 8 are unconditionally stable ($\gamma=3/2$, $\beta=1$ and $\gamma=1/2$, $\beta=1/4$), and for all the others the stability is conditional. As remarked by Newmark, all schemes for which

$$\gamma = 1/2, \quad \beta \geq 1/4$$

are unconditionally stable and indeed show no artifical damping, i.e., $|\lambda|=1$. For conditionally stable schemes, such as the central difference expression, a simple calculation from Eq. (64) shows that with $\gamma=1/2$, $\beta=0$ we require for stability

$$p_i < 4$$

or

$$\omega_i \Delta t < 2$$

Putting $\omega_i=2\pi/T_i$, where T_i is the period, we can write the stability condition as

$$\Delta t \leq \frac{1}{\pi} T_i \tag{67}$$

An alternative but popular scheme with

$$\gamma = 1/2, \quad \beta = 1/6$$

requires for stability

$$\Delta t \leq \frac{\sqrt{3}}{\pi} T_i \tag{68}$$

as can easily be verified by the reader.

All schemes with $\gamma > 1/2$ show an appreciable numerical damping leading to inaccuracy of results. In Fig. 9 we show a plot of $|\lambda|$ against $\Delta t/T_i$ for various such schemes, showing how large this damping can be for larger values of Δt.

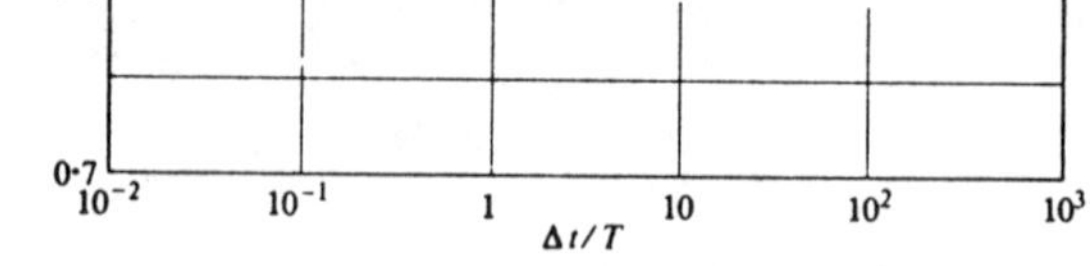

Fig. 9 Three level (Newmark) expression.
'spectral' radius, $|\lambda|$ versus $\Delta t/T$

In practice some degree of numerical damping is desirable because invariably the Δt used in unconditionally stable schemes will be much larger than that corresponding to the highest frequencies of the system which cannot be reproduced exactly and only lead to numerical noise. Ideally, therefore, we will seek schemes which have $|\lambda|=1$ for $\Delta t/T<1$ and show as much damping as possible when $\Delta t/T>1$.

One way of obtaining such performance is to include, deliberately, a damping matrix of a form

$$[C]_a = \varepsilon[K]\Delta t \tag{69}$$

Obviously, as $\Delta t \to 0$, this damping will disappear, and when $\Delta t \to \infty$, it will have a large value.

Such artificial 'adjustment' of numerical performance is of some interest and was used by Grant [32] to adjust the performance of an explicit $\gamma = \beta = 0$ Newmark scheme. A more sophisticated use is developed by Hilber et al. [33].

In addition to numerical damping, the value of $\underline{\lambda}$ obtained from the characteristic Eq. (57) will, by comparison with the exact λ of Eq. (59), give information on the relative period error.

Results are shown in Fig. 10 for the various schemes of second order.

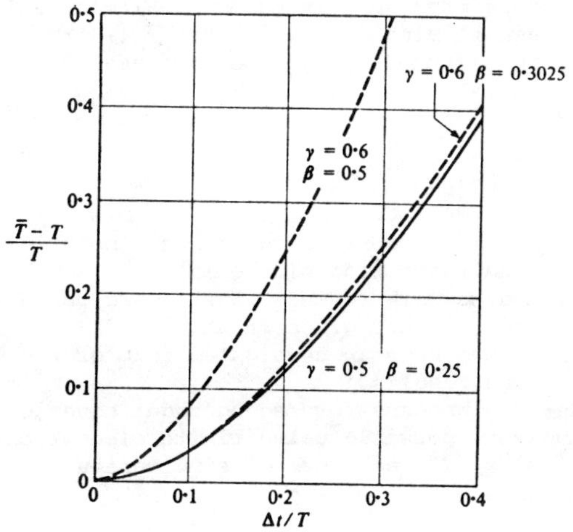

Fig. 10 Three level (Newmark) expression.
Relative period error versus $\Delta t/T$.

The Newmark Algorithm and Alternative

In conventional usage the Newmark algorithm is employed as a 'two point' formula. In this the three values of displacement, velocity, and acceleration $\{a\}_n$, $\{\dot{a}\}_n$ and $\{\ddot{a}\}_n$ at the start of the interval are used to compute $\{a\}_{n+1}$, $\{\dot{a}\}_{n+1}$ and $\{a\}_{n+1}$. The equations are written as follows

$$[M]\{\ddot{a}\}_{n+1} + [C]\{\dot{a}\}_{n+1} + [K]\{a\}_{n+1} + \{f\}_{n+1} = 0 \tag{70a}$$

(the equation of motion at $t=t_{n+1}$). Further, we approximate the integration as

$$\{a\}_{n+1} = \{\hat{a}\}_{n+1} + \beta\,\Delta t^2\{\ddot{a}\}_{n+1} \tag{70b}$$

$$\{\dot{a}\}_{n+1} = \{\hat{\dot{a}}\}_{n+1} + \gamma\,\Delta t\{\ddot{a}\}_{n+1} \tag{70c}$$

In the above

$$\{\hat{a}\}_{n+1} = \{a\}_n + \Delta t\{\dot{a}\}_n + (\tfrac{1}{2} - \beta)\Delta t^2\{\ddot{a}\}_n$$

$$\{\hat{\dot{a}}\}_{n+1} = \{\dot{a}\}_n + (1-\gamma)\Delta t\{\ddot{a}\}_n$$

are simply quantities grouping the initial variables. The logic behind the above expressions need not concern us here, but the reader can verify that if we write a similar recurrence between steps n-1 and n and supplement the six relations by a seventh, i.e., the equation of motion at n-1, it is possible to eliminate all velocities and accelerations and thus retrieve the three point expression of Eq. (51).

The two point formula has, however, some computational advantages. In the first place it is easy to vary the time interval Δt. In the second place the computation can be so organized as to avoid matrix multiplication of the non-diagonal matrix $[K]$ and thus to save storage and computation operations. Such multiplication always arises in the case of expression (51) as can be seen by noting that the solution for $\{a\}_{n+1}$ involves writing

$$\{a\}_{n+1} = \{[M] + \gamma\Delta t[C] + \beta\Delta t^2[K]\}^{-1}\{(\quad)\{a_n + (\quad)\{a\}_{n-1} - \bar{f}\Delta t^2\} \tag{71}$$

where bracketed terms involve $[K]$ and are given in Eq. (51).

The computational procedures in solving Eq. (65) most efficiently use $\{a\}_{n+1}$ as the primary variable and eliminate $\{\dot{a}\}_{n+1}$ and $\{\ddot{a}\}_{n+1}$ from (70a) by using the simple vector relationships (70b and 70c). We now have

$$\begin{aligned}\{a\}_{n+1} = \{[M] + \gamma\Delta t[C] + \beta\Delta t^2[K]\}^{-1}\{([C]\gamma\Delta t + [M])\{\hat{a}\}_{n+1} \\ - [C]\beta\Delta t^2\{\hat{\dot{a}}\}_{n+1} - \{f\}_{n+1}\beta\Delta t^2\}\end{aligned} \tag{72}$$

Now, although the identical matrix occurs in the solution of both equations, no $[K]$ multiplication in the right hand side exists.

On the debit side, the Newmark formula in standard usage is not self-starting because acceleration is not given in the initial condition and has to be computed from Eq. (2) and thus uses an unweighted form of the load vector which on occasion gives misleading results.[9]

To derive a single-step process for second order equations which avoid the above difficulty is, however, possible using finite element concepts. A simple alternative is to express Eq. (3) as a set of simultaneous first order equations by introducing velocity as a variable, e.g.,

$$\begin{aligned}[M]\{\dot{V}\} + [C]\{V\} + [K]\{a\} + \{f\} = 0 \\ \{V\} - \{\dot{a}\} = 0\end{aligned} \tag{73}$$

Now procedures identical to those used in the section on weighted residual approach can again be employed interpolating linearly both variables $\{V\}$ and $\{a\}$ and noting that two independent weighting functions W^a and W^b can now be used for each of the equations given above. We shall now have (as in writing Eq. (27))

$$\begin{aligned}[M](\{V\}_{n+1} - \{V\}_n) + [C]\Delta t[\theta\{V\}_{n+1} + (1-\theta)\{V\}_n] \\ + [K]\Delta t[\theta\{a\}_{n+1} + (1-\theta)\{a\}_n] + \{\bar{f}\}\Delta t = 0\end{aligned} \tag{74a}$$

and

$$\Delta t[\alpha\{V\}_{n+1} + (1-\alpha)\{V\}_n] - (\{a\}_{n+1} - \{a\}_n) = 0 \tag{74b}$$

In the above

---

[9] By not self starting we mean in the present context that an additional solution of Eq. (70a) has to be performed for n=0 before the standard computation is commenced. This should not be necessary since $\{a\}_o$ and $\{\dot{a}\}_o$ constitute the required starting conditions.

$$\theta = \int_0^1 W_\xi^a d\xi / \int_0^1 W^a d\xi \tag{75a}$$

$$\alpha = \int_0^1 W^b \xi d\xi / \int_0^1 W^b d\xi \tag{75b}$$

$$\{\bar{f}\} = \int_0^1 W^a \{f\} d\xi / \int_0^1 W^a d\xi \tag{75c}$$

In the above expression, just as in Eq. (52), $\{\bar{f}\}$ can be related to the weighted impulse of external forces.

Equations (74a) and (74b) allow a single step process to be used, and starting from initial values of $\{a\}_n$ and $\{V\}_n$, only values of $\{a\}_{n+1}$ and $\{V\}_{n+1}$ can be found. The same computational advantages as the Newmark algorithm offers can be preserved if we use

$$\{\hat{a}\}_{n+1} \equiv \theta\{a\}_{n+1} + (1-\theta)\{a\}_n \tag{76}$$

as the primary variable.

On eliminating $\{V\}_{n+1}$ from Eq. (74a) using (74b) with the introduction of the new variable we have

$$\begin{aligned} \{\hat{a}\}_{n+1} = \{[M] + \theta\Delta t[C] + \alpha\theta\Delta t^2[K]\}^{-1}\{[M](\{a\}_n + \theta(1-\alpha)\Delta t\{V\}_n) \\ + [C](\{a\}_n + (\theta-\alpha)\Delta t\{V\}_n)\theta\Delta t - \{\bar{f}\}\alpha\theta\Delta t^2\} \end{aligned} \tag{77}$$

Once $\{\hat{a}\}_{n+1}$ is evaluated, $\{a\}_n$ and $\{\dot{a}\}_{n+1}$ are available from simple vector operations which follow from Eqs. (76) and (74b).

We note that the matrix defining the simultaneous equations is identical, once again, to the Newmark equations providing

$$\begin{aligned} \alpha\theta &= \beta \\ \alpha + \theta &= \gamma + \frac{1}{2} \end{aligned} \tag{78}$$

Indeed the stability of the scheme can be shown to be identical to that of the Newmark scheme if the above identity is preserved. Full discussion of the scheme is given elsewhere [34], but the reader will note that it is not possible to obtain real values of α and θ for all combinations of β and γ. For unconditional stability we thus must have

$$\alpha = \beta \geq \frac{1}{2} \tag{79}$$

(with $\alpha = \beta = \frac{1}{2}$ we retrieve $\gamma = \frac{1}{2}$ $\beta = \frac{1}{4}$ as in the Newmark algorithm). For conditional stability

$$\alpha + \theta \geq 1 \tag{80}$$

and the limiting time step is given by

$$\omega_i \Delta t < 2/|\alpha - \theta| \tag{81}$$

This scheme is conveniently adaptable to explicit computation taking

$$\theta = 0 \qquad \alpha = 1$$

As is readily seen from Eq. (72), this does not require the diagonality of the [C] matrix. A similar scheme but derived by alternative methods has been suggested recently [35].

It appears that for many practical applications the single step scheme suggested by the use of time finite element processes has considerable advantages as compared with the more conventional algorithms.

Some Other Two Point Algorithms

It is, of course, possible to devise other two point algorithms by the use of different interpolations. For instance, if we do not assume independent interpolations of {a} and {á} but instead redefine the 'nodal' parameters as

$$\begin{Bmatrix} a \\ \dot{a} \end{Bmatrix} = \begin{Bmatrix} a \\ v \end{Bmatrix} \tag{82}$$

we can use a cubic interpolation and write in the interval of time[10]

$$\begin{aligned}\{a(t)\} \approx \{\hat{a}(t)\} &= \sum_{i=n}^{n+1} [H_i(t), H_i'(t)] \begin{Bmatrix} \{a\}_i \\ \{v\}_i \end{Bmatrix} \\ &= \sum [\bar{H}]\{b\}_i \end{aligned} \tag{83}$$

where H and H′ are Hermitian, cubic, interpolation functions illustrated in Fig. 11. Now a weighted residual form for the unknown $\{b\}_{n+1}$ can be written from Eq. (3).

$$\int_0^{\Delta t} [\bar{W}]^T([M]\{\ddot{\hat{a}}\} + [C]\{\dot{\hat{a}}\} + [K]\{\hat{a}\} + \{\hat{f}\})\, dt = 0 \tag{84}$$

in which $[\bar{W}]$ is defined similarly to $[\bar{H}]$.

The resulting equation system can be written as

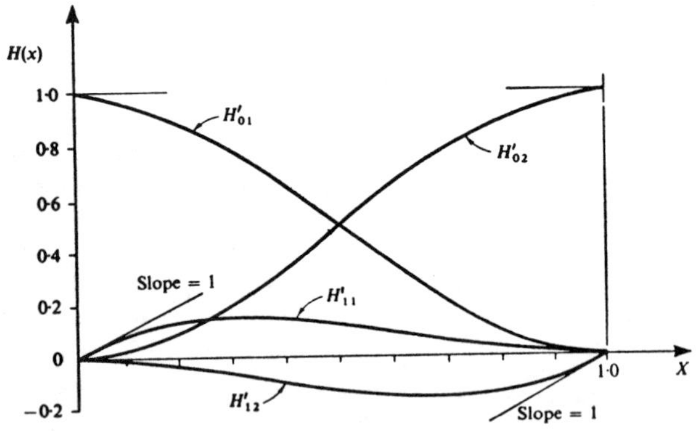

Fig. 11 Cubic interpolation functions in time

The resulting equation system can be written as

$$[A]\{b\}_{n+1} = -[C]\{b\}_n - \{q\} \tag{85a}$$

in which

---

[10]We implicitly assume that $[H_i, H_i'] \equiv [H_i[I], H_i'[I]]$ to preserve rules of matrix algebra and multiplication.

$$[A] \equiv \int_{o}^{\Delta t} [\bar{W}]([M][\ddot{\bar{H}}]_{n+1} + [C][\dot{\bar{H}}]_{n+1} + [K][\bar{H}]_{n+1})dt \tag{85b}$$

$$[C] = -\int_{o}^{\Delta b} [\bar{W}]^T([M][\ddot{H}]_n + [C][\dot{\bar{H}}]_n + [K][\bar{H}]_n)dt \tag{85c}$$

$$\{q\} = \int_{o}^{\Delta t} [\bar{W}]^T\{f\}dt \tag{85d}$$

Two matters are immediately apparent: firstly, because no part of it is diagonal, the matrix [A] is twice the size of the equation system requiring solution in the previous algorithm; and secondly, the matrix is only partly symmetric even if we use the Galerkin-Bubnov type of weighting, i.e., if we make

$$[\bar{W}] \equiv [\bar{H}]_{n+1} \tag{86}$$

If the damping term is omitted, we can, however, regain the symmetry of the first term involving the matrix [M] using an integration by parts. We can now write

$$\int_{o}^{\Delta t} [\bar{W}]^t_{n+1}[M][\ddot{\bar{H}}]_{n+1}\, dt \equiv$$

$$= -\int_{o}^{\Delta t} [\dot{\bar{H}}]^T_{n+1}[M][\dot{\bar{H}}]_{n+1}\, dt + \Big|_{o}^{\Delta t} [\bar{H}]_{n+1}[M][\dot{\bar{H}}]_{n+1} \tag{87}$$

The last term becomes identically zero due to the structure of $[\bar{H}]_{n+1}$, and symmetry is achieved. This artifice is identical to using as a starting point the Hamiltonian variational principle which is applicable in a system without damping. Such a procedure was introduced in Refs. [2] and [3] to derive the above algorithm. In Ref. [5], however, the weighted form of this algorithm is also presented.

This algorithm and indeed its most recent extended version is discussed by Argyris, et al [36], but has, for computational reasons, not gained popularity.

MULTIPOINT RECURRENCE SCHEMES

General

The procedures for deriving recurrence schemes by the weighting process can be extended to domains of $n\Delta t$ using higher order interpolation and indeed to the whole domain using a set of elements as we have shown in the section on weighted residual approach when formula (35) was derived. In this section we shall consider domains of three points for the first order equation (presuming the determination of $\{a_{n+1}\}$ from known values of $\{a_n\}$ and $\{a_{n-1}\}$ in which parabolic interpolation is used, and we shall consider four-point recurrence schemes for the second order equation (determine $\{a_{n+1}\}$ from $\{a_n\}$, $\{a_{n-1}\}$, and $\{a_{n-2}\}$) in which a cubic shape function determines the variation over the time domain.

Three-Point Schemes-First Order Equation

The first set of expressions is, in fact, already given by the derivation of the section entitled Three-Point Recurrence Schemes for Second-Order Equations. Indeed, if we put the second order term M=0, Eq. (51) will immediately result in

$$(\gamma[C] + \beta\Delta t[K])\{a\}_{n+1} + ((1-2\gamma)[C] + (\frac{1}{2} - 2\beta + \gamma)[K]\{a\}_n$$
$$+ (-(1-\gamma)[C] + (\frac{1}{2} + \beta - \gamma)[K])\{a\}_{n-1} + \{\bar{f}\} = 0 \qquad (88)$$

in which $\{\bar{f}\}$ is given by the previous interpolation expression (53) with β and γ having the same meaning as before. $\gamma = 1/2$ and $\beta = 1/3$ give an algorithm due to Lees [37] much used in practice for nonlinear problems [38]. $\gamma = 1/2$ and $\beta = 1/6$ result from the subdomain collocation (uniform $W_i = 1$) of Fig. 8. (This incidentally corresponds exactly to the recurrence formula (35) derived by considering linear interpolation over the whole time domain.) Once again the stability can be investigated as in the section on Stability of Three-Point Recurrence Schemes. Dahlquist [39] discusses the problem and establishes the following conditions for unconditional stability

$$\gamma \geq \frac{1}{2} \qquad \beta \geq \frac{1}{2}\gamma \qquad (89)$$

In Ref. [40] several optimal values of parameters are given.

Conditional stability can once again be achieved in certain circumstances. However, it is interesting to note that the central difference scheme with $\gamma = 1/2$ and $\beta = 0$ is now unconditionally unstable and cannot be used for any time interval.

Four-Point Schemes for Second and First Order Equations

Here the extension of the weighting procedure is obvious and can be done as an exercise by the reader. Using the time domain of $3\Delta t$, as shown in Fig. 12, and normalizing the coordinate as $\xi = 2t/3\Delta t$, the standard cubic shape functions can be used to obtain the expansion of

$$\{a\} \approx \{\hat{a}\} = \sum_{i=n-2}^{n+1} N_i\{a\}_i \qquad (90)$$

and a weighted residual form obtained. The reader is now invited to derive the explicit general form now given in terms of three independent parameters α, β, and γ, by using the previous established procedures.

This form is given as:

$$\{[M](\gamma-1) + (\frac{1}{2}\beta - \gamma + \frac{1}{3})[C]\Delta t + (\frac{1}{6}\alpha - \frac{1}{2}\beta + \frac{1}{3}\gamma)[K]\Delta t^2\}\{a\}_{n+1}$$
$$+ \{[M](-3\gamma + 4) + (-\frac{3}{2}\beta + 4\gamma - \frac{3}{2})[C]\Delta t + (-\frac{1}{2}\alpha + 2\beta - \frac{3}{2}\gamma)[K]\Delta t^2\}\{a\}_n$$
$$+ \{[M](3\gamma-5) + (\frac{3}{2}\beta - 5\gamma + 3)[C]\Delta t + (\frac{1}{2}\alpha - \frac{5}{2}\beta + 3\gamma)[K]\Delta t^2\}\{a\}_{n-1}$$
$$+ \{[M](-\gamma + 2) + (-\frac{1}{2}\beta + 2\gamma - \frac{11}{6})[C]\Delta t + (-\frac{1}{6}\alpha + \beta - \frac{11}{6}\gamma + 1)[K]\Delta t^2\}\{a\}_{n-2} \qquad (91)$$
$$+ \Delta t^2(\frac{1}{6}\alpha - \frac{1}{2}\beta + \frac{1}{3}\gamma)\{f\}_{n+1} + (-\frac{1}{2}\alpha + 2\beta - \frac{3}{2}\gamma)\{f\}_n\Delta t^2$$
$$+ (\frac{1}{2}\alpha - \frac{5}{2}\beta + 3\gamma)\{f\}_{n-1}\Delta t^2 + (-\frac{1}{6}\alpha + \beta - \frac{11}{6}\gamma + 1)\{f\}_{n-1}\Delta t^2 = 0$$

The general expression given here was derived by the author [40], and its general stability properties are discussed in detail by Wood [41]. Just as is the case in the previous three-point generalized Newmark expression given by Eq. (51), some of the permutations of the three constants result in already known and widely used expressions.

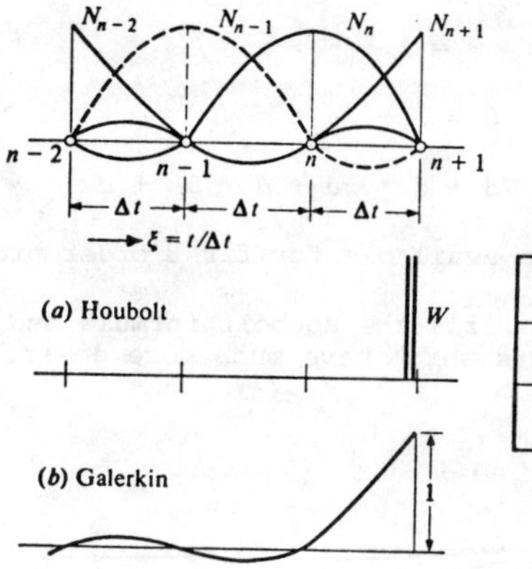

α	β	γ
30	9	3
$\frac{702}{35}$	$\frac{36}{5}$	$\frac{13}{5}$

$$\alpha = \int_0^3 W\xi^3 d\xi \Big/ \int_0^3 W d\xi$$

$$\beta = \int_0^3 W\xi^2 d\xi \Big/ \int_0^3 W d\xi$$

$$\gamma = \int_0^3 W\xi d\xi \Big/ \int_0^3 W d\xi$$

Fig. 12 A general four-point recurrence scheme using cubic shape functions. Houbolt (a) and Galerkin (b) as two special cases weighting

With $\alpha = 30$, $\beta = 9$ and $\lambda = 3$, the Houbolt [42] formula is recognized. This is unconditionally stable and has characteristics shown in Figs. 13 and 14 which the reader can compare with Figs. 9 and 10 for the Newmark schemes.

With

$$\alpha = 2 + 4\theta + 3\theta^2 + \theta^3$$

$$\beta = \frac{4}{3} + 2\theta + \theta^2 \tag{92}$$

$$\gamma = 1 + \theta$$

the so-called Wilson-θ procedure [27, 43] is obtained. This procedure was introduced to obtain improved high frequency mode elimination. $\theta = 1 \cdot 4$ to $2 \cdot 0$ have frequently been used here, and it can be shown that for unconditional stability $\theta > 1 \cdot 366$ is required [41]. It is of interest to remark that $\theta = 1$ reduces the four-point algorithm in the undamped case to that of Newmark ($\gamma = 1/2$; $\beta = 1/6$).

The algorithms proposed by Hilber et al [33] once again can be identified with the general four-level schemes with the introduction of artificial (negative or positive) damping of expression (69).

Clearly the general expression (85) possesses many other possibilities not yet fully tested in practice. For suitable choices of α, β, and γ, explicit expressions can be derived.

The general stability conditions for the undamped equations are not as simple as with the three-point expression and can be summarized as a requirement that for unconditional stability [41]

$$a > o \; ; \quad b > o \; ; \quad 3ab > c > o \tag{93a}$$

where a, b and c are related to α, β, and γ by

$$\gamma = 1 \cdot 5 + a$$

$$\beta = 3 + 3a + b \tag{93b}$$

$$\alpha = 6 \cdot 75 + 8 \cdot 5a + 4 \cdot 5b + c$$

The general form is now also available for first order problems simply by putting [M] = 0 [44].

The above formulation generalizes the Houbolt formula and can be programmed to allow many interesting variants which have much more desirable characteristics than the original.

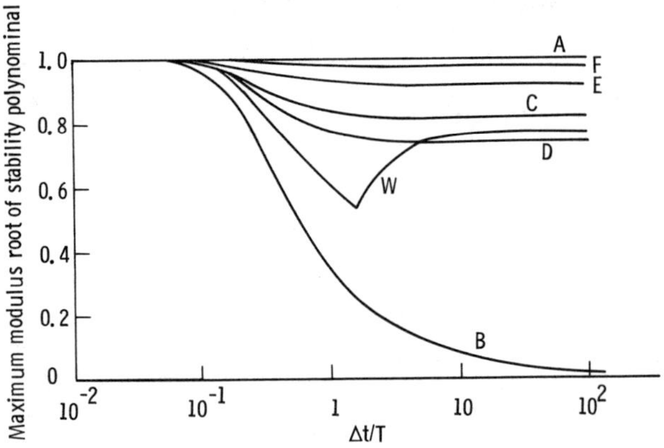

Curve label	a	b	c
A	1	0	0
B	1·5	1·5	0·75
C	5	1	0·1
D	1·5	0·5	0·25
E	1·5	0·15	0·1
F	50	1	1
W	0·9	0·393	0·0555

A) Zero damping, min. period elongation. B) Houbolt
W) Wilson ($\theta = 1.4$)

Fig. 13 Maximum modulus root of stability polynomial against

Although a large number of new and existing algorithms have here been derived using the finite element process in the time domain, many others exist and doubtlessly are valuable in practice. Park [45] assesses and reviews a series of currently used algorithms.

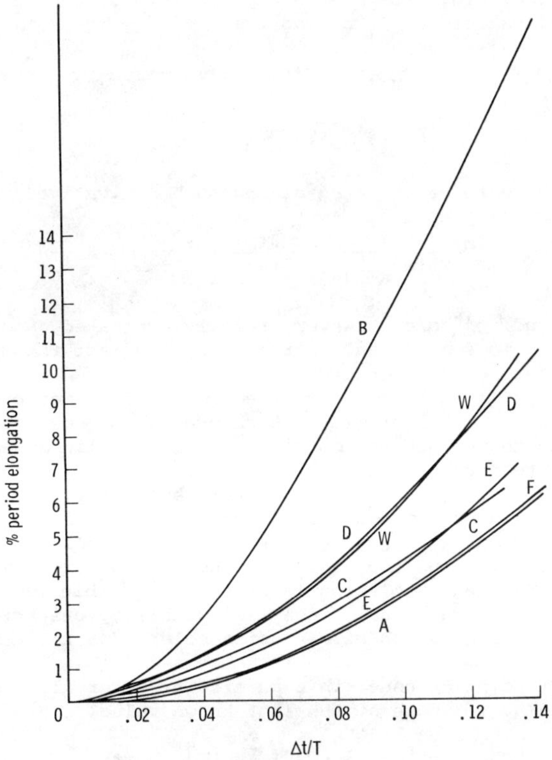

Fig. 14 Variation of percentage period elongation with Δt/T.

NONLINEAR TIME STEPPING SCHEMES

The major application of time marching procedures is to nonlinear problems, where one or more of the matrices [M], [C], [K] or {f} depend on the unknown vector {a}. Here the alternatives of analytical solution present in linear situations do not exist. Clearly the weighted residual expressions, such as given by Eqs. (26) and (50) for first and second order systems, respectively, remain valid, but their simplified, integrated forms (28) and (51) do not. Indeed, the full integration can only be carried out numerically, and, in general, iteration within each time step appears to be needed. Further, at each time step a different set of equations will require solution, thus making procedures costly.

In practice, with such nonlinear problems point collocation procedures have often been used (finite differences) avoiding the difficulties of integration in the time domain which become trivial. This loses some of the accuracy of the computation, and other alternatives exist. We can, for instance, turning our attention to Eq. (26) and assuming [C] and [K] to be variable with {a}, apply the interpolation expression, $\dot{N}$ and N, respectively, to the product vectors

$$\{q\} = [C]\{a\} \qquad \{p\} = [K]\{a\} \tag{94}$$

Now in place of Eq. (28) we shall have

$$(\{q\}_{n+1}/\Delta t + \{p\}_{n+1}\theta) + (-\{q\}_n/\Delta t + \{p\}_n\,(1-\theta)) + \{\bar{f}\} = 0 \tag{95}$$

An iterative process, e.g., the Newton-Raphson method, can be used to solve the above set of equations for $\{a\}_{n+1}$ noting that

$$\begin{aligned} \{q\}_{n+1} &= \{q(\{a\}_{n+1})\} \\ \{p\}_{n+1} &= \{p(\{a\}_{n+1})\} \end{aligned} \tag{96}$$

Tangent matrices have to be computed giving such derivatives as

$$\frac{\partial\{q\}}{\partial\{a\}_{n+1}} \quad ; \quad \frac{\partial\{p\}}{\partial\{a\}_{n+1}} \tag{97}$$

The vectors $\{q\}_n$ and $\{p\}_n$ are, however, readily evaluated, and errors in incomplete iteration are to some extent corrected by a direct recomputation of these vectors at the start of each interval.

The procedure can in this manner be applied to second order problems; for instance, starting with Eqs. (50) or (74). Such processes once again appear to be more consistent than the pointwise imposition of the nonlinear equation in conventional finite difference (or Newmark) schemes.

Iteration within a time interval can, however, be costly, and an alternative exists in making a cruder approximation to the variable matrices. Here mean values of the appropriate matrices $[M]$, $[\bar{C}]$ or $[K]$ are established by extrapolation from previous steps, and the linear expressions previously derived are used in the interval. Such extrapolation leads to more stable solutions [46-48] because within each interval the usual linearized stability criteria are obtained and further instability which may sometimes arise solely due to iteration is avoided.

A very simple extrapolation uses, in a particular interval, the values of the matrices corresponding to those at the last known value, i.e.,

$$[M]_{n+1} = [M]_n \; ; \; [C]_{n+1} = [C]_n \text{ , etc.} \tag{98}$$

and for first order problems and of the two- or three-point formulae previously developed can be used directly.

Culham and Varga [46] use such a scheme for the solution of a first order equation with a variable $[K]$ and combine it with a backward difference ($\theta = 1$) numerical scheme. Their results show a better accuracy than that obtainable with other schemes where iteration has been used.

In an explicit scheme with lumped matrices the use of approximation (98) is natural. Now the term

$$[K]_n\{a\}_n = \{p\}_n \tag{99}$$

is evaluated as a vector such as may be caused, for instance, by a nonlinear material or by the geometrical behavior of a structure, and the matrix $[K]$, in fact, is not explicitly formed. Such schemes appear extremely useful in many structural short-period investigations [23-25] and although the time interval is still subject to questions of stability, the simplicity of computation makes the scheme very commendable.

Another use of the assumption (98) is in the three-point schemes applied to first order equations in which all the matrices are subject to nonlinearity. This has been demonstrated as an effective procedure by Comini et al [38] for a heat conduction problem in which conductivity, specific heat, and heat generation all depend on temperature.

Indeed, at this point, we see a possible advantage of using the three-point formulation of the Newmark algorithm given by Eq. (51) rather than its conventional alternative, Eq. (70). In the former $[K]_n$ (etc.) correspond to mid-interval values rather than initial values, and thus the error in linearization is less severe. The stability of nonlinear schemes is generally (but not always) assured by satisfying linear stability criteria. For a full study of stability problems the reader should consult Refs. [49] to [51].

COMBINED IMPLICIT AND EXPLICIT PROCESSES

General

The computational advantages of explicit time stepping schemes are counterbalanced by the very small size of time step necessary when some elements exhibit high eigenvalues. In some problems, typified by that illustrated in Fig. 15, we may be faced with the situation in which a part I of a region is such that explicit processes with a reasonable time step size could be used and a part II in which stiffness or size of element is such that for the same time step an implicit process is necessary. It is, in such cases, possible to use simultaneously both algorithms and take advantage of the partial diagonalization of the matrices in the explicit region I. The procedures were first introduced by Belytschko and Mullen [52-54] and given an alternative form by Hughes [55,56] and Park et al [57-59]. Here we show that such a mixed formulation arises naturally with the weighted, finite-element-in-time, process. We shall illustrate the process on the first order problem of Eq. (2) for which we have developed the two-point formula of Eq. (28). The extension to other algorithms and to second order problems will follow identical lines and need not be discussed in detail.

Two possible approaches exist to the problem, i.e., nodal or element algorithm separations. In the first, the starting point is the semi-discretized set of ordinary differential equations. In the second, the separation is carried out at element levels. The first procedure results in an algorithm similar to those of Belytschko and Parks. The second is basically the process suggested by Hughes.

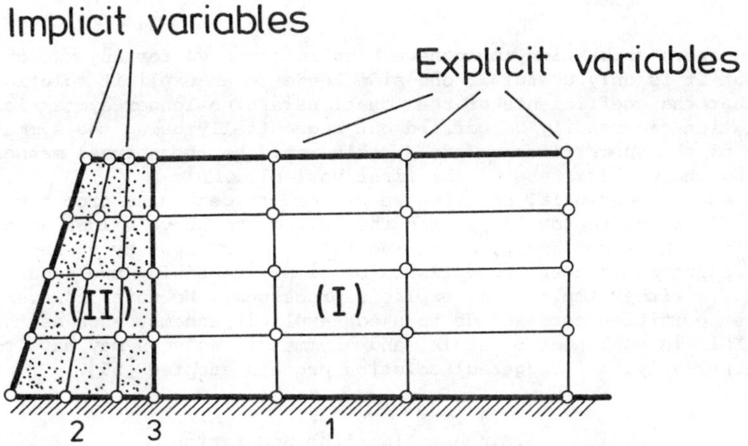

Fig. 15 A typical problem for which a mix of implicit and explicit processes is desirable.

Nodal Algorithm Separation

We shall start here with the semi-discretized form of Eq. (2), i.e.

$$[C]\{\dot{a}\} + [K]\{a\} + \{f\} = 0 \qquad (100)$$

in which [C] is assumed to be diagonal.

In the expansion following Eq. (24), we partition the vector $\{a\}_i$ into components $\{a\}_i^I$ and $\{a\}_i^{II}$ associated with explicit and implicit regions, respectively. We now have

$$\{\underset{\sim}{a}\} \approx \{\hat{a}\} = \sum_{i=n-1}^{n+1} [N_i^I, N_i^{II}] \begin{Bmatrix} \{a\}_i^I \\ \{a\}_i^{II} \end{Bmatrix} \qquad (101)$$

In the present case, we assume that $N_i^I = N_i^{II}$ and follow the forms given by Eq. (25), but obviously we could take different shape functions for each expansion.[11]

In weighted form analogous to that of Eq. (26) we now have

$$\int_0^{\Delta t} [W_i^I, W_i^{II}]^T \{[C](\{\hat{a}\}_n \dot{N}_n + \{\hat{a}\}_{n+1}\dot{N}_{n+1}) + [K](\{\hat{a}\}_n N_n + \{\hat{a}\}_{n+1} N_{n+1}) + \{f\}\} dt = 0 \tag{102}$$

The weighting functions W_i^I and W_i^{II} can now be so chosen as to make the algorithm explicit for the vector of unknown $\{a\}_i^I$ and implicit for $\{a\}_i^{II}$. Omitting algebraic detail, using the definitions of Eq. (101), and taking $\theta = 0$ for nodes in region I and $\theta = \bar{\theta}$ for nodes in region II, we can write Eq. (28) in a partitioned form as

$$\begin{bmatrix} [C]^{II}/\Delta t, & 0 \\ [K]^{II,I}\bar{\theta}, & [C]^{II,II}/\Delta t \\ & + [K^{II,II}]\bar{\theta} \end{bmatrix} \begin{Bmatrix} \{a\}^I \\ \{a\}^{II} \end{Bmatrix}_{n+1} + \begin{bmatrix} -[C]^{II}/\Delta t + [K]^{II}, & [K]^{I,II} \\ [K]^{II,II}(1-\bar{\theta}), & -[C]^{II,II}/\Delta t \\ & + [K]^{II,II}(1-\bar{\theta}) \end{bmatrix} \begin{Bmatrix} \{a\}^I \\ \{a\}^{II} \end{Bmatrix}_n + \begin{Bmatrix} \{\bar{f}\}^I \\ \{\bar{f}\}^{II} \end{Bmatrix} = 0 \tag{103}$$

The above separation could have been implemented for any two or more values of $\bar{\theta}$, but it is only useful if one side leads to an explicit solution. We observe that the coefficients of the equations are no longer symmetric. However, the solution can readily be carried out sequentially using the symmetric properties of the submatrices. Indeed, this would be the natural manner of utilizing the explicitness of the first variable.

In such a sequential solution we proceed to determine from the known values of $\{a\}_n$ first the vector $\{a\}_{n+1}^I$ and then using the above values as boundary conditions for the second part, determine $\{a\}_{n+1}^{II}$. As shown by Parks [59] this type of solution is best accomplished by simply combining two separate programs written for either implicit or explicit processes. We note, however, that if the first partition corresponds to a non-explicit scheme, such as that given by $\theta \neq 0$, this is no longer possible, and asymmetric solvers may have to be used, or alternatively, a 'staggered' solution process adopted [55].

Element Algorithm Separation

In this process we start from the fact that the semi-discretization was carried out, generally, by a spatial finite element process and that the semi-discrete system of Eq. (100) is obtained by an element assembly of the standard form defined below:

$$[c_{ij}] = \sum_{e=1}^{n} [c_{ij}]^e, \text{ etc.} \tag{104}$$

where e denotes the element contributions and the summation is carried out over all elements.

Now we shall consider two regions of elements I and II in the example of Fig. 15 and apply the same algorithm as before (i.e., $\theta = 0$ and $\theta = \bar{\theta}$) to the elements of each region.

---

[11] It is possible, if different shape functions are used, that a spatial discontinuity will be involved in the time space domain, but this need not concern us at this stage where discrete equations are being solved.

Partitioning the vector $\{a\}_i^{II}$ into three parts, the first corresponding to nodes in region I, the third in region III and the second of the interface, we can write the equivalent to Eq. (28) as

$$\begin{bmatrix} [C]^{11}/\Delta t, & 0, & 0 \\ 0, & [C]^{22}/\Delta t + [A], & [K]^{23}\bar{\theta} \\ 0, & [K]^{32}\bar{\theta}, & [C]^{33}/\Delta t + [K]^{33}\bar{\theta} \end{bmatrix} \begin{Bmatrix} \{a\}^1 \\ \{a\}^2 \\ \{a\}^3 \end{Bmatrix}_{n+1} +$$

$$\begin{bmatrix} -[C]^1/\Delta t + [K]^{11}, & [K]^{12}, & 0 \\ [K]^{21}, & -[C]^{22}/\Delta t + [B], & [K]^{23}(1-\bar{\theta}) \\ 0, & [K]^{32}(1-\bar{\theta}), & -[C]^{33}/\Delta t + [K]^{33}(1-\bar{\theta}) \end{bmatrix} \begin{Bmatrix} \{a\}^1 \\ \{a\}^2 \\ \{a\}^3 \end{Bmatrix}_{n} + \quad (105)$$

$$\begin{Bmatrix} \{\bar{f}\}^1 \\ \{\bar{f}\}^2 \\ \{\bar{f}\}^3 \end{Bmatrix} = 0$$

In the above

$$[A] = \sum_e^{II} [K]_e^{22}\,\bar{\theta}$$

$$[B] = \sum_e^{I} [K]_e^{22} + \sum_e^{II} [K]_e^{22}\,(1-\bar{\theta})$$

and the summations marked I and II refer to the appropriate element regions.

The resulting equations are still explicit in variables $\{a\}^1$ and, in addition, have a symmetry property thus allowing a simple symmetric program to be used throughout.

Which of the alternatives presented is superior depends on the usage and the problem presented. It is clear that either can be adopted to any of the algorithms discussed in this chapter and that, indeed, both forms spring directly from the finite-element-in-time concept.

Stability of the implicit-explicit processes has been studied extensively. Hughes and Liu [55] study the 'element' procedures while Park [59] gives a complete study of a variety of cases. It appears simply that in the mixed forms satisfaction of stability criteria within each separate domain automatically ensures stability of the whole scheme. This result is one which 'heuristically' we could anticipate.

CONVECTIVE/DIFFUSION PROBLEMS. PROBLEMS WITH CHANGING BOUNDARIES.

Convective/Diffusive Heat Transport Equation

In the discretization of Eqs. (2) and (3) we have implicitly assumed that the matrices occurring there are positive definite and, therefore, have real eigenvalues. If this is not the case, the conclusions concerning the stability of various algorithms are not valid, and it is possible for instability to occur. A typical problem of this class arises in a semi-discretized form of the convective/diffusive (heat) transport equation.

$$c \frac{\partial T}{\partial t} + U \frac{\partial T}{\partial x} + V \frac{\partial T}{\partial y} - \frac{\partial}{\partial x} (k \frac{\partial T}{\partial x}) + \frac{\partial}{\partial y} (k \frac{\partial T}{\partial y}) + Q = 0 \tag{106}$$

In the above, U(x,y,t) and V(x,y)t are known transport velocities. Here in contrast to Eq. (13), the addition of the second and third terms results in an asymmetric semi-discretized form even if Galerkin/Petrov methods are used. Now following exactly the same process as led to the semi-discretized form of Eq. (22) we have

$$\begin{gathered} [C]\{\dot{a}\} + [K]\{a\} + \{f\} = 0 \\ T \approx \hat{T} = \Sigma \bar{\bar{N}}_i (x,y)\; a_i(t) \end{gathered} \tag{107}$$

$$C_{ji} = \int_\Omega \bar{\bar{W}}_j \; c \; \bar{\bar{N}}_i \; dxdy$$

$$K_{ji} = \int_\Omega \{\frac{\partial \bar{\bar{W}}_j}{\partial x} k \frac{\partial \bar{\bar{N}}_i}{\partial x} + \frac{\partial \bar{\bar{W}}_j}{\partial y} k \frac{\partial \bar{\bar{N}}_i}{\partial y} + \bar{\bar{W}}_j U \frac{\partial \bar{\bar{N}}_i}{\partial x} + \bar{\bar{W}}_j V \frac{\partial \bar{\bar{N}}_i}{\partial y}\} dxdy \tag{108}$$

$$f_j = \int_\Omega \bar{\bar{W}}_j \; Q \; dxdy$$

It can be shown that even with the spatial discretization in which $\bar{\bar{W}}_j = \bar{\bar{N}}_j$ we can obtain unstable (oscillatory) results. To overcome the difficulty in such problems, special forms of weighting functions can be used [60 to 65]. The use of such so-called upwind weighting techniques has recently been extended to transient situations. With such spatial discretization, although the matrices [K] of Eq. (107) are still nonsymmetric, stable computation with some of the algorithms previously discussed are still possible, and the time discretization follows the path already described. Fuller discussion of this problem will be found in Refs. [66 to 69].

In this article we pursue a different line of attack which leads to a class of formulation with a standard diffusion (conduction) governing equation but with changing spatial boundaries.

Let us consider a coordinate change to be applied to Eq. (106). The new coordinates x', y', and t' are related to x, y and t by the requirement

$$\begin{gathered} dx' = dx - \frac{U}{c} dt \\ dy' = dy - \frac{V}{c} dt \\ dt' = dt \end{gathered} \tag{109}$$

Noting that

$$\frac{\partial x'}{\partial x} = \frac{\partial y'}{\partial y} = \frac{\partial t'}{\partial t} = 1 \; ; \quad \frac{\partial x'}{\partial t} = \frac{U}{c} \; ; \quad \frac{\partial y'}{\partial c} = \frac{V}{c} \quad \frac{\partial x'}{\partial y} = \frac{\partial y'}{\partial x} = \frac{\partial t'}{\partial x} = \frac{\partial t'}{\partial y} = 0$$

we can, by rules of partial differentiation, observe that

$$\begin{gathered} \frac{\partial T}{\partial t} = U \frac{\partial T}{\partial x'} + V \frac{\partial T}{\partial y'} + \frac{\partial T}{\partial t'} \\ \frac{\partial T}{\partial x} = \frac{\partial T}{\partial x'} \; ; \quad \frac{\partial T}{\partial y} = \frac{\partial T}{\partial y'} \end{gathered} \tag{110}$$

Equation (106) transforms simply in the above set of coordinates to the standard heat conduction form of Eq. (13), i.e.

$$\frac{\partial T}{\partial t'} - \frac{\partial}{\partial x'}\left(\frac{k}{c}\frac{\partial T}{\partial x'}\right) - \frac{\partial}{\partial y'}\left(\frac{k}{c}\frac{\partial T}{\partial y'}\right) + \frac{Q}{c} = 0 \tag{111}$$

The discretized form of this equation with standard Galerkin weighting has been fully discussed in the previous section of the chapter.

Further, since the coordinates x', y' and t' can be determined exactly or by numerical integration from relationships (104), it appears that the convective diffusion problem has been entirely reduced to the standard forms already known. However, a difficulty arises in that the boundary conditions of the form

$$\left.\begin{aligned} \phi &= \bar{\phi} \\ k\frac{\partial \phi}{\partial n} &= q \end{aligned}\right\} \text{ on } \Gamma(x,y) \tag{112}$$

are given generally on the true space domain whose shape does not change with time. Now, by virtue of relationships (104), the shape of the domain in the x' and y' coordinates changes. To illustrate the problem, consider a simple physical one-dimensional case governed by the equation:

$$\frac{\partial T}{\partial t} + \frac{u}{c}\frac{\partial T}{\partial x} + \frac{k}{c}\frac{\partial^2 T}{\partial x^2} + \frac{Q}{c} = 0 \tag{113}$$

with

$$\begin{aligned} T &= T_o \qquad x = o \\ & \qquad\qquad\qquad\qquad t \geq 0 \\ T &= T_L \qquad a = L \end{aligned} \tag{114}$$

In the above, c, u and k are taken as constants for the sake of simplicity. Now the equation in transformed coordinates becomes simply

$$\frac{\partial T}{\partial t'} + \frac{k}{c}\frac{\partial^2 T}{\partial x'^2} + Q = 0 \tag{115}$$

Figure 16a illustrates the time-space domain of the original problem, and the lines of constant x' which, in fact, represent 'characteristics of the propagation' part. In Fig. 16b the domain of the problem in the transformed coordinates is shown indicating the change of boundaries with time.

In Figs. 17a and 17b the same situation is illustrated for two-dimensional problems showing the distortion of the space time domain for a problem in which the velocities were not constant.

We note now that the simplification achieved by coordinate transformation is accompanied by an increase of difficulty due to the changes of spatial discretization.

Before proceeding further we note the behavior of the solution for the limiting case when $k = 0$. Now, in the <u>transformed</u> coordinate we have simply

$$\frac{\partial T}{\partial t'} + \frac{Q}{c} = 0 \rightarrow T = -\int_o^t \frac{Q}{c}\,dt \tag{116}$$

and T can be integrated exactly along the characteristic direction (x' = constant) providing initial conditions are known. Indeed, we note that in the absence of heat generation the temperature remains constant along the characteristic and in such a case the application of the boundary conditions on the line where characteristics leave the physical region is physically incorrect. With the above remarks in mind, we note that two possible ways of proceeding are possible.

In the first, limiting our attention to a time domain $t - t + \Delta t$, we choose $x = x'$ in the one-dimensional problem in Fig. 16 to apply at some point within the interval, e.g., at time $t + 1/2\,\Delta t$ as illustrated in Fig. 18 for both sets of coordinates. The approximate region is also shown there. In the domain $x' - t$ we now solve Eq. (115) by standard means (semi-discretizing and using, for instance, the algorithm of Eq. (28)), and a new set of temperatures at time $t + \Delta t$ is available to start the next step. As the new values are given, however, at the coodinates x' which can be evaluated, we change the spatial mesh at the next step and interpolate to new mesh positions. Now the new interval is again defined taking $x - t$, $x' = x$, at a time $t + 2\Delta t$ and the procedure is repeated.

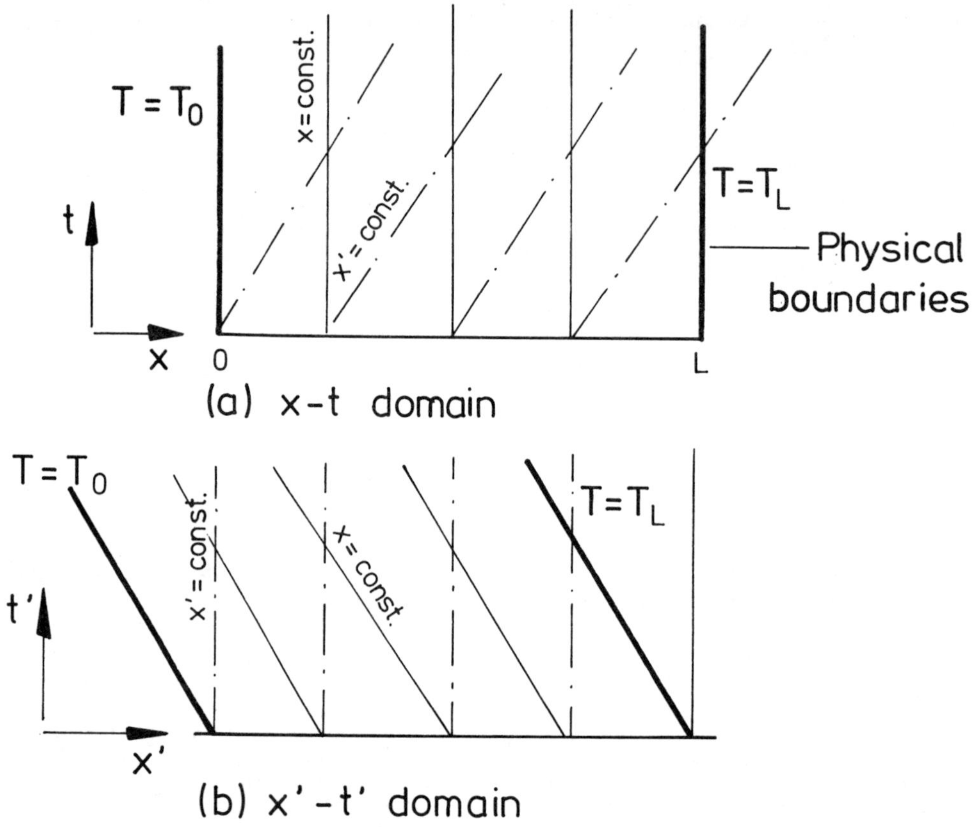

Fig. 16 Convective diffusive problem in one space dimension (a) original and (b) transformed coordination.

The method turns out to be identical to that suggested by Connor and Brebbia [70, 71] and derived by them physically. Basically, they note that the convection and conduction solutions can be used consecutively.

a) If we assume the velocities to be zero in the time interval Δt, a straightforward solution can be applied on the original mesh.

b) Turning off, as it were, the conduction, we now are concerned with the pure convection problem, and the new coordinates at which the results of a) are applicable are simply obtained by updating these to new positions given by $U/c\ \Delta t$. In practical computation to avoid changes of mesh at each time step, the temperatures are interpolated to the original mesh positions.

The second procedure is more precise. Here note is taken of the irregularity of the solution domain by using a full space-time element formulation. Such space-time elements can be drawn either in the original or transformed space domains of Figs. 16 and 17, and various forms of solution technique applied. Due to the presence of the first derivative, the matrices in Eq. (111) will no longer be symmetric but will approximate symmetry if the directions follow the characteristics. This process applied in the original domain was first used by

Finn and Varoglu [6, 7] and has achieved success in both one and two-dimensional solutions.

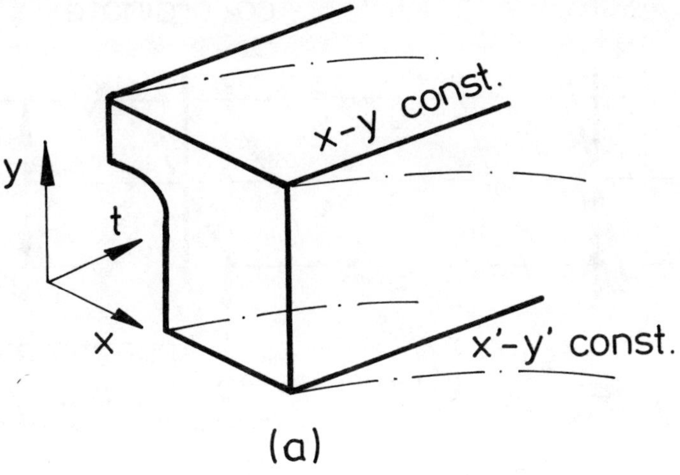

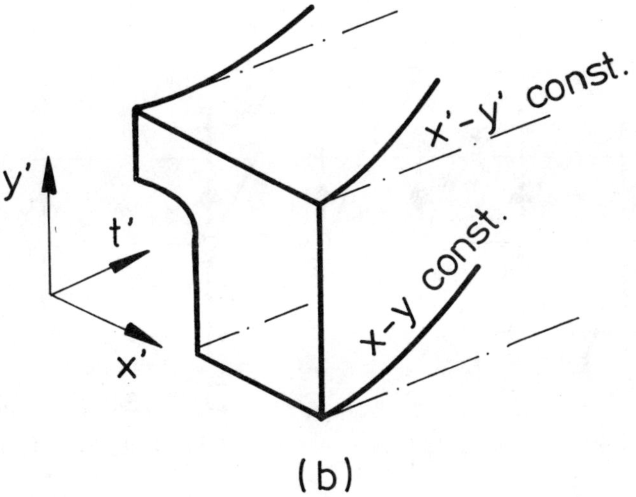

Fig. 17 Convective-diffusive problem in two space dimensions (a) original and (b) transformed domain.

General Problems with Changing Boundaries

In the previous section we have indicated the possibility of dealing with changing boundaries by various approximations. Some boundary change problems occur in another context; e.g., in ablating bodies where the surface is subject to combustion. Again, various solution possibilities are present following the details of the previous section.

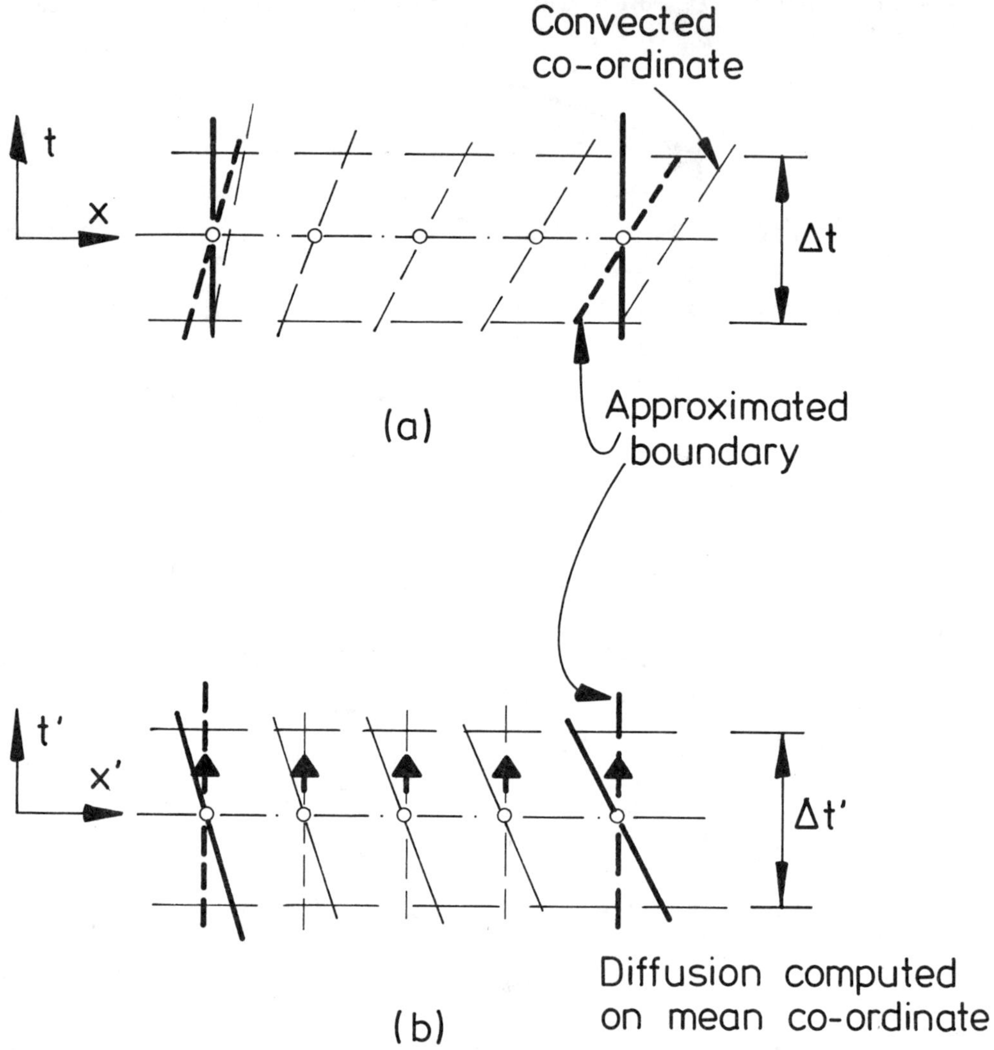

Fig. 18 An approximate treatment of changing boundaries in convective-diffusive domain (a) original and (b) transformed co-ordinate.

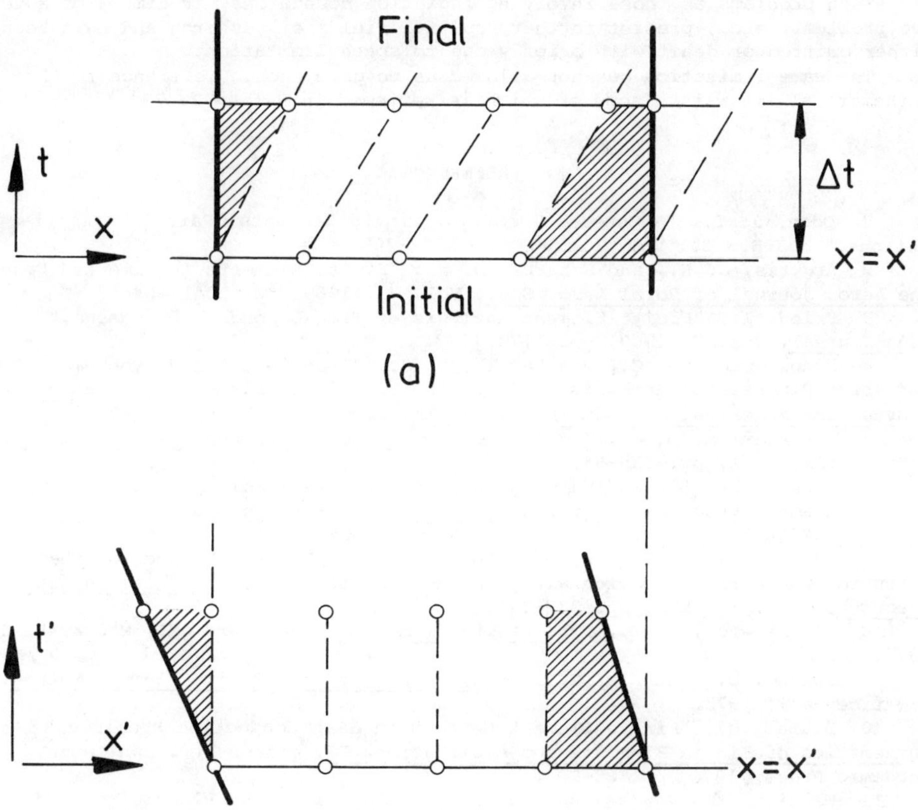

Fig. 19 Irregular time-space elements (mainly) oriented along characteristics (a) original and (b) transformed domains. (Reinterpolation to original mesh allows $x=x^1$ to be imposed at end of each step.)

CONCLUDING REMARKS

This survey has indicated the powerful possibilities given by the use of the finite element method (or of a more general form of weighted residual trial function approximation) in the time domain. Not only have all the conventional widely used time stepping algorithms been reproduced, but some alternatives have been derived. In addition, we feel that the use of finite elements in time gives a different perspective to the understanding and solution of the time domain problems even if the algorithms turn out to be identical.

The finite element viz-a-viz the finite difference operations in time has the advantage of being able to take into account efficiently the mean 'forces' in a dynamic or thermal problem and by suitably averaging impulsive actions which can now be accurately modeled.

Such problems as those involving radiation boundaries, treatment of advective problems, etc., present further fruitful fields of research and have been either omitted or dealt with briefly due to space limitation.

The same limitation has not allowed us to give enough reference to the mathematical literature some of which is reviewed in Ref. [72, 73].

REFERENCES

1 Oden, J. T., "A General Theory of Finite Elements, Part II - Applications," I.J.N.M.E., Vol. 1, 1969, pp. 247-259.

2 Argyris, J. H., and Scharpf, D. W., "Finite Elements in Time and Space," The Aero. Journal of Royal Aero. Soc., Vol. 73, 1969, pp. 1041-1044.

3 Fried, I., "Finite Element Analysis of Time Dependent Phenomena," AIAA Journal, Vol. 7, 1969, pp. 1170-1173.

4 Zienkiewicz, O. C., and Parekh, C. J., "Transient Field Problems - Two and Three Dimensional Analysis by Isoparametric Finite Elements," International Journal for Numerical Methods in Engineering, Vol. 2, 1970, pp. 61-71.

5 Zienkiewicz, O. C., The Finite Element Method in Engineering Science, McGraw-Hill, 1971, pp. 335-339.

6 Finn, W. D. L., and Varoḡlu, E., "An Efficient Solution for Heat Transport Problems," Proceedings of Conference on Numerical Methods in Thermal Problems, Edited by R. W. Lewis and K. Morgan, University of Swansea, 1979.

7 Varoḡlu, E., and Finn, N. D. L., "A Finite Element Method for the Diffusion-Convection Equation with Constant Coefficients," Advances in Water Resources, Vol. 1, 1973, pp. 337-341.

8 Zienkiewicz, O. C., The Finite Element Method, 3rd ed., McGraw-Hill, 1977.

9 Strang, C., and Fix, G. I., An Analysis of the Finite Element Method, Prentice Hall, 1973.

10 Zlamal, M., "Finite Element Methods in Heat Conduction Problems," Mathematics of Finite Elements and Applications II, edited by J. Whiteman, Academic Press, 1976, pp. 85-104.

11 Washizu, K., Variational Methods in Elasticity and Plasticity, 2nd ed., Pergamon Press, 1968.

12 Gurtin, M., "Variational Principles for Linear Elastodynamics," Arch. Rat. Mech. Anal., Vol. 16, 1964, pp. 34-50.

13 Gurtin, M., Variational Principles for Linear Elastodynamics and Plasticity, 2nd ed., Pergamon Press, 1975.

14 Wilson, E. L., and Nickell, R. E., "Application of the Finite Element Method to Heat Conduction Analysis," Nuclear Engineering and Design, Vol. 4, 1966, pp. 276-286.

15 Argyris, J. H., and Scharpf, D. W., "Finite Elements in Time and Space," Nuclear Engineering Design, Vol. 10, 1969, pp. 456-469.

16 Zienkiewicz, O. C., and Lewis, R. H., "An Analysis of Various Time Stepping Schemes for Initial Value Problems," International Journal of Earthquake Engineering Structural Dynamics," Vol. 1, 1973, pp. 407-408.

17 Wood, W. L., and Lewis, R. W., "A Comparison of Time Marching Schemes for the Transient Heat Conduction Equation," International Journal for Numerical Methods in Engineering, Vol. 9, 1975, pp. 679-689.

18 Jones, D. G., and Henshell, R. D., Oscillations in Transient Thermal Calculations (to be published).

19 Lambert, J. D., Computational Methods in Ordinary Differential Equations, Wiley, 1973.

19b Richtmyer, R. D., and Morton, K. W., Difference Methods for Initial Value Problems, Wiley Interscience, 1967.

20 Irons, B. M., "Applications of a Theorem on Eigenvalues to Finite Element Problems," CR/132/70, 1970, Department of Civil Engineering, University of Wales, Swansea.

21 Bettencourt, J. M., Zienkiewicz, O. C., and Cantin, G., "Consistent Use of Finite Elements in Time and the Performance of Various Recurrence Schemes for the Heat Diffusion Equation," International Journal for Numerical Methods in Engineering, Vol. 17, No. 6, June 1981, pp. 931-938.

22 Newmark, N. M., "Method of Computation for Structural Dynamics," Journal of Engineering Mechanics Div., ASCE, Vol. 85, EM3, 1959, pp. 67-94.

23 Belytschko, T., Chapetta, R. L., and Bartel, H. D., "Efficient Large Scale Nonlinear Transient Analysis by Finite Elements," International Journal for Numerical Methods in Engineering, Vol. 10, 1976, pp. 579-596.

24 Shantaram, D., Owen, D. R. J., and Zienkiewicz, O. C., "Dynamic Transient Behavior of Two and Three-Dimensional Structures Including Plasticity, Large Deformation and Fluid Interaction," International Journal of Earthquake Engineering Structural Dynamics, Vol. 4, 1976, pp. 561-578.

25 Krieg, R. D., and Key, S. W., "Transient Shock Response by Numerical Time Integration," International Journal for Numerical Methods in Engineering, Vol. 7, 1973, pp. 273-286.

26 Fu, C. C., "On the Stability of Explicit Methods for Numerical Integration of the Equations of Matrices in Finite Element Methods," International Journal for Numerical Methods in Engineering, Vol. 4, 1972, pp. 95-107.

27 Bathe, K. J., and Wilson, E. L., "Stability and Accuracy Analysis of Direct Integration Methods," Earthquake Engineering Structural Dynamics, Vol. 1, 1973, pp. 283-291.

28 Nickell, R. E., "On the Stability of Approximation Operators in Problems of Structural Dynamics," International Journal of Solids and Structures, Vol. 7, 1971, pp. 301-319.

29 Dunham, R. S. et al., "Integration Operators for Transient Structural Response," Computers and Structures, Vol. 2, 1972, pp. 1-15.

30 Goudreau, G. L., and Taylor, R. L., "Evaluation of Numerical Integration Methods in Elastodynamics," Computer Methods in Applied Mechanics and Engineering, Vol. 2, 1972, pp. 69-97.

31 Fox, L., and Goodwin, E. T., "Some New Methods for the Numerical Integration of Ordinary Differential Equations," Proc. Camb. Phil. Soc., Vol. 49, 1949, pp. 373-388.

32 Grant, J. E., "Response Computation Using Taylor Series," Proc. American Society of Civil Engineers, Vol. 97, EM2, 1971, pp. 295-303.

33a Hilber, H. M., Hughes, T. J. R., and Taylor, R. L., "Improved Numerical Dissipation for Time Integration Algorithms in Structural Mechanics," International Journal of Earthquake Engineering Structural Dynamics, Vol. 5, 1977, pp. 283-292.

33b Hilber, H. M., and Hughes, T. J. R., "Collocation, Dissipation and 'Overshoot' for Time Integration Schemes in Structural Dynamics," International Journal of Earthquake Engineering Structural Dynamics, Vol. 6, 1978, pp. 99-117.

34 Zienkiewicz, O. C., Wood, W. L., and Taylor, R. L., "An Alternative Single Step Algorithm for Dynamic Problems," International Journal of Earthquake Engineering Structural Dynamics, Vol. 8, 1980, pp. 31-40.

35 Collings, A. G., and Tee, C. J., "Generalized: Euler Numerical Integration Schemes for New Solution of Problems in Structural Dynamics," Proc. Sixth Australesian Conference on the Mechanics of Structures and Materials, Christchurch, New Zealand, 1977.

36a Argyris, J. H., and Dunne, P. R., Some Contributions to Nonlinear Solid Mechanics (Part II), International Symposium on Computing Methods in Applied Science and Engineering, Lecture Notes in Computer Science, Vol. 10, Springer-Verlag, 1979.

36b Argyris, J. H., and Chan, A. S. L., "Application of Finite Elements in Space and Time," Ingenieur Archiv, Vol. 41, 1972, pp. 235-257.

37 Lees, M., "A Linear Three Level Difference Scheme for Quasilinear Parabolic Equations," Mathematics of Computations, Vol. 20, 1966, pp. 516-622.

38 Comini, G., Del Guidice, S., Lewis, E. H., and Zienkiewicz, O. C., "Finite Element Solution of Nonlinear Heat Conduction Problems with Special Reference to Phase Change," International Journal for Numerical Methods in Engineering, Vol. 8, 1974, pp. 613-624.

39 Dahlquist, G., "A Special Stability Problem for Linear Multistep Method," B.I.T., Vol. 3, 1963, pp. 27-43.

40 Zienkiewicz, O. C., "A New Look at the Newmark, Houbolt and Other Time Stepping Schemes. A Weighted Residual Approach," International Journal of Earthquake Engineering Structural Dynamics, Vol. 5, 1977, pp. 413-418.

41a Wood, W. L., "On the Zienkiewicz Four Time Level Scheme for the Numerical Integration of Vibration Problems," International Journal for Numerical Methods in Engineering, Vol. 11, 1977, pp. 1519-1528.

41b Wood, W. L., "On the Zienkiewicz Three and Four Time Level Schemes Applied to the Numerical Integration of Parabolic Equations," International Journal for Numerical Methods in Engineering, Vol. 12, 1978, pp. 1717-1726.

42 Houbolt, J. C., "A Recurrence Matrix Solution for the Dynamic Response of Elastic Aircraft," Journal of Aero. Sci., Vol. 17, 1950, pp. 540-550.

43 Farhoomand, I., "Nonlinear Dynamic Stress Analysis of Two Dimensional Solids," Ph.D. Dissertation, 1970, University of California, Berkeley.

44 Cryer, C. H., "A New Class of Highly Stable Methods: A_o-Stable Methods," B.I.T., Vol. 13, 1973, pp. 153-159.

45 Park, K. C., "Evaluating Time Integration Methods for Nonlinear Dynamics in Finite Element Analysis of Transient, Nonlinear Structural Behavior," Applied Mechanics Symposia Series, ASME 1975.

46 Culham, W. E., and Varga, R. S., "Numerical Methods for Time Dependent Nonlinear Boundary Value Problems," J. Soc. Petrol. Eng., Dec. 1971, pp. 374-387.

47 Boggs, P. T., "The Solution of Nonlinear Systems of Equations by A-Stable Integration Techniques," SIAM Journal, Vol. 8, 1975, pp. 767-785.

48 Stricklin, J. A. et al., "Nonlinear Dynamic Analysis of Shells of Revolution by Matrix Displacement Methods," Proc. Conference on Structural Dynamics, ASME, Denver, Colorado, 1971.

49 Hughes, T. J. R., Caughey, T. K., and Liu, W. K., "Finite Element Methods for Nonlinear Elastodynamics Which Conserve Energy," Journal of Applied Mechanics, Vol. 45, No. 2, 1978, pp. 366-370.

50 Haug, E., Nguyen, Q. S., and de Rouvray, A. L., "An Improved Energy Conserving Implicit Time Integration Algorithm for Nonlinear Dynamic Structural Analysis," Transactions of the Fourth SMIRT Conference, San Francisco, California, August 1977.

51 Hughes, T. J. R., Pister, K. S., and Taylor, R. E., "Implicit-Explicit Finite Elements in Nonlinear Transient Anslysis," Computer Methods in Applied Mechanics and Engineering, Vols. 17/18, 1979, pp. 159-182.

52 Belytschko, T., and Mullen, R., "Mesh Partitions of Explicit-Implicit Time Integration," Formulations and Computational Algorithms in Finite Element Analysis, edited by J. K. Bathe et al., M.I.T. Press, 1977.

53 Belytschko, T., and Mullen, R., "Stability of Explicit-Implicit Mesh Partitions in Time Integration," International Journal for Numerical Methods in Engineering, Vol. 12, 1978, pp. 1575-1586.

54 Belytschko, T., Yen, H. J., and Mullen, R., "Mixed Methods for Time Integration," Proc. International Conference on Finite Elements in Nonlinear Mechanics (FENOMECH 78), September 1978, University of Stuttgart, West Germany.

55 Hughes, T. J. R., and Liu, W. K., "Implicit-Explicit Finite Elements in Transient Analysis: Stability Theory," Journal of Applied Mechanics, Vol. 45, 1978, pp. 371-374.

56 Hughes, T. J. R., and Liu, W. K., "Implicit-Explicit Finite Elements in Transient Analysis: Implementation and Numerical Examples," Journal of Applied Mechanics, Vol. 45, 1978, pp. 375-378.

57 Park, K. C., Felippa, C. A., and Deruntz, H. A., "Stabilization of Staggered Solution Procedures for Fluid-Structure Interaction Analysis," in Computational Methods for Fluid-Structure Interaction Problems, edited by T. Belytschko and T. L. Geers, ASME Applied Mechanics Symposia Series, Vol. 26, 1977, pp. 94-124.

58 Felippa, C. A., and Park, K. C., "Computational Aspects of Time Integration Procedures in Structural Dynamics," Journal of Applied Mechanics, Vol. 45, 1978, pp. 595-602.

59 Park, K. C., "Partitioned Transient Analysis Procedures for Coupled Field Problems: Stability Analysis," Journal of Applied Mechanics, Vol. 47, No. 2, June 1980, pp. 370-376.

60 Christie, I., Griffiths, D. F., Mitchell, A. R., and Zienkiewicz, O. C., "Finite Element Methods for Second Order Differential Equations with Significant First Derivatives," International Journal for Numerical Methods in Engineering, Vol. 10, 1976, pp. 1389-1396.

61 Heinrich, J. C., Huyakorn, P. S., Zienkiewicz, O. C., and Mitchell, A. R., "An 'Upwind' Finite Element Scheme for Two-Dimensional Convective-Transport Equation," International Journal for Numerical Methods in Engineering, Vol. 11, 1977, pp. 131-143.

62 Heinrich, J. C., and Zienkiewicz, O. C., "Quadratic Finite Element Schemes for Two-Dimensional Convective Transport Problems," International Journal for Numerical Methods in Engineering, Vol. 11, 1977, pp. 1831-1844.

63 Tabata, M., "A Finite Element Approximation Corresponding to the Upwind Finite Differencing," Memoirs of Numerical Mathematics, No. 4, 1977, pp. 47-63.

64 Tabata, M., "Uniform Convergence of the Upwind Finite Element Approximation for Semilinear Parabolic Problems," Journal Math. Kyoto Univ., Vol. 18, 1978, pp. 327-351.

65 Hughes, T. J. R., "A Simple Scheme for Developing 'Upwind' Finite Elements," International Journal for Numerical Methods in Engineering, Vol. 12, 1978, pp. 1359-1365.

66 Donea, J., Giuliana, S., and Laval, H., "Explicit Finite Element Solutions to Transient Convective-Conductive Heat Transfer Problems," Proceedings of the International Conference on Numerical Methods in Laminar and Turbulent Flow, Swansea, Wales, July 1978, John Wiley and Sons, New York, pp. 527-537.

67 Griffiths, D. F., "Towards Time Stepping Algorithms for Convective Diffusion," Proceedings of the Conference on the Numerical Analysis of Singular Perturbation Problems, Catholic University, Nijmegen, Holland, May 1978, Academic Press, London, 1979, pp. 199-216.

68 Mitchell, A. R., and Griffiths, D. F., "Semi-Discrete Galerkin Methods for Time Dependent Conduction Convection Problems," Proceedings of the Third Conference on the Mathematics of Finite Elements and Applications, Brunel, April 1978, Academic Press, 1979.

69 Morton, K. W., and Parrott, A. K., "Generalized Galerkin Methods for First Order Hyperbolic Equations," Journal of Computational Physics, Vol. 36, No. 2, 1980, pp. 249-270.

70 Connor, I. J., and Brebbia, C. A., Finite Element Techniques for Fluid Flow, Newness-Butterworth, London, 1976, pp. 33-42 and pp. 268-277.

71 Adey, R., and Brebbia, C. A., "Finite Element Solution for Effluent Dispersion," in Numerical Methods in Fluid Dynamics, edited by C. A. Brebbia and J. J. Connors, Pentech Press, London, 1974, pp. 325-354.

72 Cecchi, M. Morandi, "Error Continuation for Finite Element Solutions of Heat Transfer Problems in the Square Time Domain," in Mathematics of Finite Applications, Chapter 16, edited by C. J. Whiteman, Academic Press, 1976, pp. 203-207.

73 Alducin, V., and Oden, J. T., "Qualitative Analysis of Galerkin Approximation of a Class of Nonlinear Convection-Diffusion Problems," TICOM Report 78.8, University of Texas, Austin, 1978.

CHAPTER FOURTEEN

GLOBAL-LOCAL FINITE ELEMENT METHODS

S. B. Dong
Mechanics and Structures Department
School of Engineering and Applied Science
University of California
Los Angeles, California

ABSTRACT

Global-Local Finite Element Analysis refers to a numerical analysis technique that simultaneously utilizes conventional finite element modeling with classical Rayleigh-Ritz approximations. This technique enjoys the advantage of better modeling capabilities with substantially fewer degrees of freedom. The rudiments of this method are summarized herein. To date, the advantage of this approach has been clearly demonstrated in two elasto-static problem areas: fracture mechanics and problems involving a far field. A survey of the contributions to the literature in these two areas is given. Also, examples of other applications are cited.

INTRODUCTION

Approximate analysis within the realm of variational methods[1] may be conveniently divided into two main types: (classical) Ritz-Galerkin methods and finite element methods. Chronologically, the Ritz method (1), which appeared in 1909, preceded finite elements. And even before Ritz, similar ideas were successfully employed by Lord Rayleigh (2). For purposes of contrast, we will employ the term global variational methods interchangeable with Ritz-Galerkin methods. Finite elements did not emerge until the advent of large scale digital computers. This method is now universally acknowledged as one of the most powerful analysis tool available to engineers and applied scientists.

In global variational methods, the domain of the governing equation is treated as a whole, and the approximate solution is constructed from a sequence of linearly independent functions satisfying the geometric boundary conditions. Convergence is obtained by increasing the order of the approximation sequence. The domain in the finite element method, on the other hand, is subdivided into small regions, and within each of these regions elementary functions (typically, low order polynomials over each element) are used to describe its behavior.

---

[1] Approximate analysis is also referred to as the "direct method of the calculus of variation." See Courant and Hilbert (3), for example.

Continuity across element boundaries is enforced in terms of appropriate generalized coordinates. It has been shown that if certain completeness criteria are met by the approximation functions, convergence is assured by mesh refinements in which the element sizes are decreased.

For simply-shaped domains, global variational methods can yield excellent results with rapid convergence. However, realistic engineering problems typically involve domains of complicated geometry and inhomogeneous materials. Analysis of these problems by global variational methods is usually intractable because of difficulties in formulating a suitable sequence of approximation functions that meet the relevant boundary conditions and contain the mathematical essence describing the physical behavior. By means of finite elements, such complexities pose no exceptional difficulties. However, finite element methods are not without limitations. Problems containing singularities (cracked tip, etc.) can lead to serious discretization shortcomings. In the limit when the element size becomes infinitesimally small, the finite element analysis cannot mathematically converge to the true behavior because of the nature of the approximation polynomials. Also, problems with infinite or semi-infinite domains require truncation of the finite element model together with the need for artificial boundary conditions to preclude rigid body motions. While these approaches may be acceptable in some instances, there are attendant issues related to accuracy (convergence) and to computational effort as a consequence of an expanded discretization effort. On the other hand, global variational methods, whenever applicable, involve far less computation for achieving a comparable level of accuracy.

It is natural to consider the merger of these two types of approximate analysis techniques in order to capitalize on the merits of both. Mote (4) in 1971 demonstrated the feasibility of this approach with beam and plate vibration examples. We will follow Mote and refer to techniques utilizing the combined approximation fields as Global-Local Finite Element Methods (GLFEM). The descriptor local obviously refers to contemporary finite elements. In this chapter, we will discuss its general details, explore some of the modeling strategies and provide a survey of the progress to date.

In the following section, some examples are provided for motivation of GLFEM applications. Next, the basic equations of the technique are summarized and the principal global-local configurations are shown. A discussion is given of the interelement global-local continuity requirements. In the context of GLFEM, we will call attention to a closely akin method called the global element method (5) and note the salient difference which lies in interelement continuity considerations. Then, we will summarize the contributions to the technical literature wherein any GLFEM variant is employed. Here, mention will be made of problems not only in structural mechanics but also in other fields. In our discussion, we may allude to some closely akin methods relating to special and singular elements and boundary integral equation techniques. These topics are covered in Chapters 4 and 16 and any overlap here is restricted to that within the context of GLFEM.

EXAMPLES ILLUSTRATING GLOBAL-LOCAL FINITE ELEMENTS

To illustrate applications of GLFEM, three examples where this method enjoys advantages are given here.

Rectangular Plate

Consider the natural vibrations of a simply-supported rectangular, isotropic plate with thickness h and lateral dimensions a, b (see Fig. 1a). Denote its mass density by ρ and Young's modulus and Poisson's ratio by E and ν, respectively. Hamilton's principle for this plate has the form:

$$\delta \int_{t_1}^{t_2} L\, dt = 0 \tag{1}$$

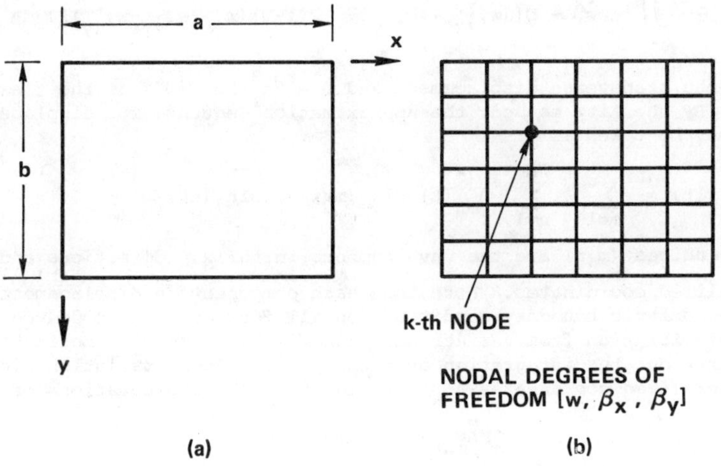

FIG. 1 Rectangular Plate of Thickness , Four Edges Simply-Supported.

(a) Global Region
(b) Finite Element Discretization

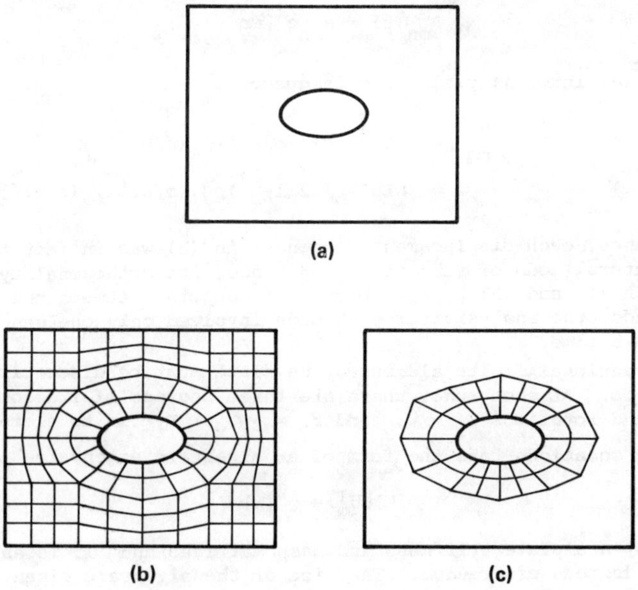

FIG. 2 Rectangular Plate of Thickness h with Hole, Four Edges Simply-Supported

(a) Diagram of Plate
(b) Finite Element Discretization
(c) Global-Local Finite Element Model

where the functional L is

$$L = \frac{1}{2} \iint_A \{\rho h \dot{w}^2 - D[(w_{,xx} + w_{,yy})^2 - 2(1-\nu)(w_{,xx}w_{,yy} - w_{,xy}^2)]\}\, dA \qquad (2)^2$$

with w as the transverse displacement and $D = Eh^3/12(1-\nu^2)$ as the flexural rigidity. By the Ritz method, the approximation sequence for displacement w(x,y,t) may be taken as

$$w(x,y,t) = \sum_{m=1}^{M} \sum_{n=1}^{N} A_{mn}(t) \sin(m\pi x/a) \sin(n\pi y/b) \qquad (3)$$

where the indices (m,n) are the wave numbers in the x,y directions and A_{mn}'s are the generalized coordinates. Note that each component in displacement form (3) meets the geometric boundary conditions on all four edges. To deduce the frequencies of vibration from variational principle (1), first substitute (3) into (2) and carry out the integration over the plate. Then, variation with respect to the generalized coordinates A_{mn}'s yield the following equations of motion:

$$M\ddot{A}_{mn} + K(m,n)A_{mn} = 0 \qquad (4)$$

where

$$M = \rho hab$$

$$K(m,n) = D\pi^4 ab[(m/a)^2 + (n/b)^2]^2 \qquad (5)$$

For simple harmonic motion

$$A_{mn}(t) = a_{mn}e^{i\omega_{mn}t} \qquad (6)$$

Substituting (6) into (4) yields the frequencies:

$$\omega_{mn}^2 = (D\pi^4/\rho h)[(m/a)^2 + (n/b)^2]^2$$

$$= \left(Eh^2\pi^4 / 12(1-\nu^2)\rho\right)[(m/a)^2 + (n/b)^2]^2 \qquad (7)$$

In this instance, each displacement component in (3) was in fact the exact solution for a natural mode of vibration, and hence, its orthogonality property was in evidence in (4) and (5) by the absence of coupling between the various components. Hence, the analysis for each mode involved only one generalized coordinate A_{mn} at a time.

By conventional finite elements, the plate must be discretized as exemplified in Fig. 1b. At each node, there are three degrees of freedom, i.e., displacement w and rotations $\beta_x = w_{,y}$ and $\beta_y = -w_{,x}$. By finite element methodology, the governing equations take the form of an algebraic eigenvalue problem.

$$[K]\{U\} = \omega^2[M]\{U\} \qquad (8)$$

where [K], [M] are plate stiffness and mass matrices and {U} is an ordered array of the nodal degrees of freedom. The size of the algebraic eigenvalue problem (8) is related to the finite element discretization process, which depends on the required accuracy of the modes to be investigated.

---

[2]Throughout this chapter, commas followed by subscripts indicate partial differentiation with respect to spatial variables and a dot denotes time differentiation.

In this example, it is obvious that the global variational method is far more convenient. There is only one equation to be evaluated for each unknown frequency.

Suppose this plate is modified slightly by the presence of a hole as shown in Fig. 2a. If this hole is small, then the frequencies should be nearly those for a plate without a hole. However, it would be a formidable task for the global variational method in selecting an approximation sequence that satisfies free edge boundary conditions around the hole in addition to those on the exterior edges. This problem can be routinely treated by finite elements. A schematic diagram of the discretization is shown in Fig. 2b. It is obvious that a substantive computational effort is needed. For a hole which is not large, the results should not differ from those for a holeless plate. Nevertheless, computation is required to quantify the frequencies.

GLFEM is ideally suited for this situation. Establish a finite element mesh around the hole as shown in Fig. 2c. The finite element degrees of freedom are intended to model the physical behavior around the hole. For the remainder of the plate, global approximation sequence (3) can be used. Continuity of displacements and rotations at the interface between the two regions must be enforced. More details on this important aspect of GLFEM will be discussed later. The number of degrees of freedom in this instance consists of the limited number of finite element coordinates and a sufficient number of terms in (3). This total should be substantially fewer than the finite element discretization shown in Fig. 2b. Moreover, there is little or no sacrifice in the modeling capability of combined approximation technique.

Soil-Structure Interaction

Consider the vertical loading of a circular concrete footing of radius a in smooth contact with a soil medium that extends over a semi-finite domain. This problem is illustrated in Fig. 3a, where the adopted coordinate system and notation are shown. By conventional finite elements, the footing and some portion of the soil must be discretized. A typical finite element mesh is shown in Fig. 3b. It is necessary in the solution procedure to impose some fixity condition to preclude rigid body motions and, customarily, zero displacements at the finite element boundary S_1 are taken. Accordingly, a relatively large finite element model must be adopted in order to minimize this boundary effect on the actual distribution of stress and displacements that exist around the footing.

This problem can be solved more efficiently by GLFEM without sacrifice of modeling capability. By St. Venant's principle, note that the far field displacements and stresses should behave according to Boussinesq's solution (6), i.e., the problem of a point load acting on an otherwise stress free surface of a semi-infinite, homogeneous, isotropic medium. The radial and axial displacements (u,w) in Boussinesq's solution for a point load with magnitude P have the form:

$$u(r,z) = \frac{P}{4\pi\mu}\left[\frac{rz}{R^3} - (1-2\nu)\frac{r}{R(R+z)}\right]$$
$$w(r,z) = \frac{P}{4\pi\mu}\left[\frac{z^2}{R^3} + 2(1-\nu)\frac{1}{R}\right] \qquad (9)$$

where μ, ν are the shear modulus and Poisson's ratio, respectively, and

$$R^2 = r^2 + z^2 \qquad (10)$$

Observe that the displacements decay in the order of $O(1/R)$. In the GLFEM scheme, Boussinesq's displacement field (9) is taken as the global function and a coefficient a_1 is introduced as the global generalized coordinate, i.e., it is used as the multiplier of this solution form. Appropriate continuity conditions between the interface of the finite element mesh and the far field must be

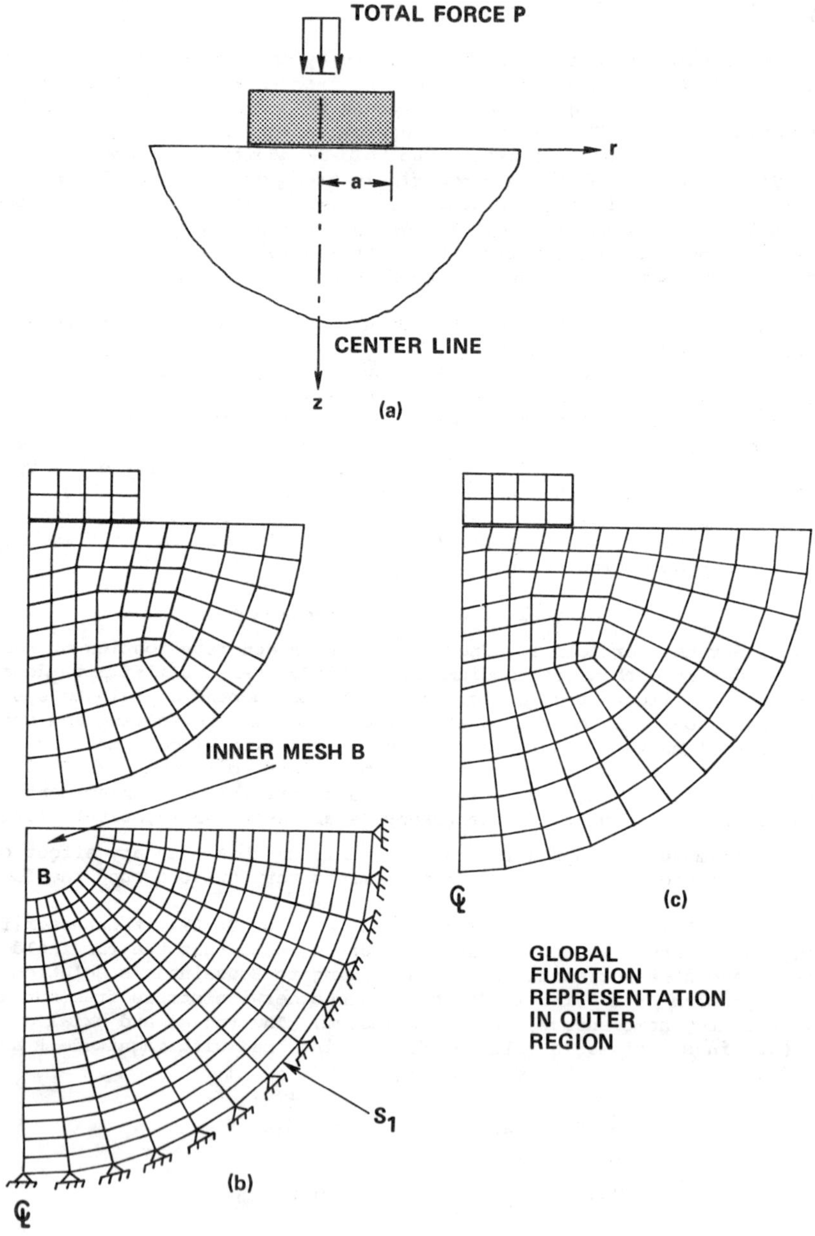

FIG. 3 Circular Concrete Footing in Smooth Contact with Soil
(a) Diagram of Footing and Soil; (b) Finite Element Model
(c) Global-Local Finite Element Model

prescribed which relates the nodal displacements to generalized coordinate a_1. The GLFEM solution, which is based on a minimization process, will then yield the values of the finite element degrees of freedom and a_1 simultaneously. Even though the accuracy of the GLFEM solution remains dependent upon the finite element mesh size, the soil region modeling can be abbreviated substantially in comparison to that for a conventional finite element analysis (see Fig. 3c).

Intuitively, one would anticipate that the solution of a rigid circular punch acting on a half-space, due to Harding and Sneddon (7), would be a better far field approximation. Typical ratio of elastic moduli of concrete to soil would justify the far field equivalence with this punch problem. The displacements have the form:

$$u(r,z) = -\frac{P}{4\pi\mu a}\left[(1-2\nu)J_o^1(r,z) - \frac{z}{a}J_1^1(r,z)\right]$$

$$w(r,z) = \frac{P}{4\pi\mu a}\left[2(1-\nu)J_o^o(r,z) + \frac{z}{a}J_1^o(r,z)\right] \tag{11}$$

where

$$J_m^n(r,z) = \int_o^\infty p^{m-1}\sin(p)e^{-pz/a}J_n(pr/a)dp$$

$$(m,n = 0,1) \tag{12}$$

Except for J_o^o which cannot be reduced further, the other three integrals have simpler closed form representations:

$$J_o^1 = \frac{a}{r}[1-R_1^{\frac{1}{2}}\sin(\psi/2)]$$

$$J_1^o = R_1^{-\frac{1}{2}}\sin(\psi/2)$$

$$J_1^1 = aR_1^{-\frac{1}{2}}\sin(\theta-\psi/2) \tag{13}$$

with

$$R_1^2 = [(r/a)^2 + (z/a)^2 -1]^2 + 4(z/a)^2$$

$$z\tan(\theta) = a \quad ; \quad [(r/a)^2 + (z/a)^2 -1]\tan(\psi) = 2z/a$$

Although Eq. (11) with formulas (12) and (13) appear to be a better choice, it is cumbersome to employ as a global function in GLFEM. This is due to the integral representation of J_o^o, which needs to be evaluated at many points of the finite element mesh-far field interface. Also, the somewhat inconvenient manner in which ψ and θ appear adds to the unattractiveness of this choice as a global function.

Desirable attributes for candidate global functions are that they are relatively simple in form and amenable to direct evaluation. Also, the ease with which they can be coded as function subprograms for implementation in a GLFEM code is an important consideration. A more simplified set of global functions for the far field behavior based on asymptotic solutions will be discussed.

Stress Singularities

Consider a planar isotropic structure containing a crack and adopt an x-y rectangular Cartesian coordinate system with origin at crack tip. Using complex variable notation, the stresses ($\tau_{xx}, \tau_{yy}, \tau_{xy}$) and displacements (u,v) in a crack tip's vicinity are given by

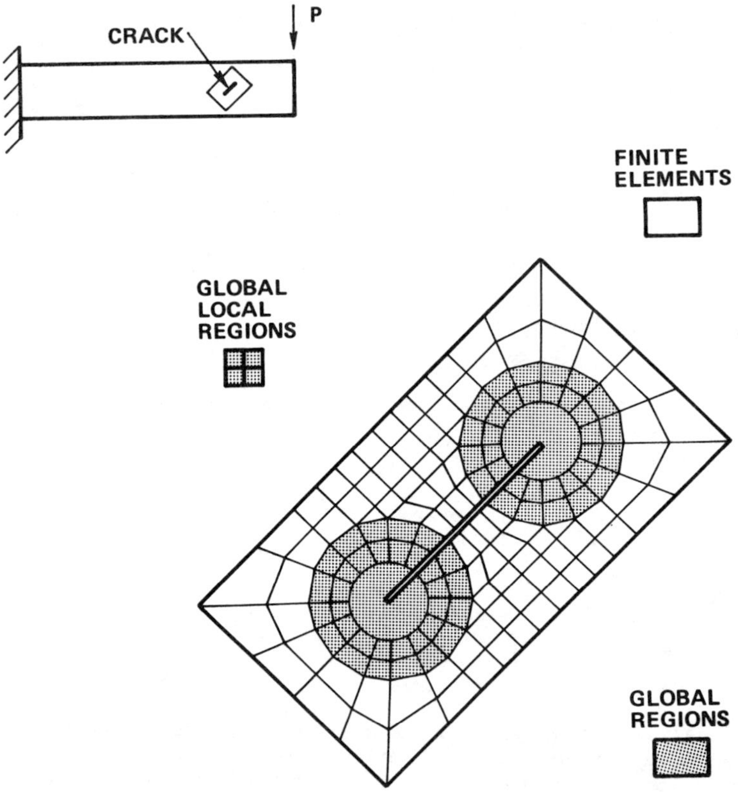

FIG. 4 Cantilever Beam with Diagonal Crack

$$\tau_{xx} + \tau_{yy} = 2[\Phi(z) + \overline{\Phi(z)}] \tag{14}$$

$$\tau_{yy} - i\tau_{xy} = \Phi(z) + \Omega(\bar{z}) + (z-\bar{z})\Phi'(z) \tag{15}$$

$$2\mu(u + iv) = \kappa\phi(z) - \omega(\bar{z}) - (z-\bar{z})\overline{\phi(z)} + a_o + ib_o z \tag{16}$$

where $z = x + iy$, a superior bar denotes complex conjugation, a prime represents differentiation with respect to z, and $\kappa = 3-4\nu$ or $\kappa = (3-\nu)/(1+\nu)$ for plane strain or plane stress. The constants a_0, b_0 represent rigid body translation and rotation, and functions $\phi(z)$, $\omega(z)$ are related to $\Phi(z)$, $\Omega(z)$ by

$$\phi(z) = \int \Phi(z)dz \quad ; \quad \omega(z) = \int \Omega(z)dz \tag{17}$$

For a crack tip singularity, $\Phi(z)$ and $\Omega(z)$ have the forms:

$$\Phi(z) = z^{-\frac{1}{2}} \sum_{n=0}^{N} a_{1,n} z^n + \sum_{n=0}^{N} a_{2,n} z^n \tag{18}$$

$$\Omega(z) = z^{-\frac{1}{2}} \sum_{n=0}^{N} a_{1,n} z^n - \sum_{n=0}^{N} a_{2,n} z^n \tag{19}$$

where coefficients $a_{1,0}$ in the leading terms are related to stress intensity factors K_I and K_{II} for the opening and sliding modes.

Finite element analysis using a special crack tip element based on Eqs. (18) and (19) is available in the literature and is discussed in Chapter 4. Two important considerations are critical to the analysis: (1) the size of the element; and (2) the number of terms in expansions (18) and (19). If the element is too small, it is effectively not present. On the other hand, making the element too large results in poor accuracy if an insufficient number of terms are used to represent the mechanical field. Tong and Pian (8) pointed out these considerations in connection with the convergence of the finite element method for problems with singularity. Thus, experience and judgment are needed to select the element size and the attendant number of terms in the series expansion.

GLFEM with overlapping regions may be employed to temper these considerations. As an illustration, consider a planar cantilever beam with a crack that is oriented diagonally relative to the beam's axis. The beam is subjected to a point load at its free end. Its finite element discretization is shown in Fig. 4. Let the immediate vicinity of each crack tip be modeled by global regions. In each global region, adopt series solutions (18) and (19), and the global functions with an $a_{1,n}$ and $a_{2,n}$ as the global generalized coordinates. Immediately beyond a global region, a region with overlapping of the global functions with the finite element representations may be used. No restriction is placed on the size of the overlap region, but preferably it should not encroach onto the other crack tip or any surrounding boundary. In selecting the global functions for the overlap region, be cognizant that the terms in them are not duplicates of any finite element approximating functions, otherwise linear dependence in the stiffness relations will result. Outside the overlap region, regular finite elements can be employed for the remainder of the model.

BASIC EQUATIONS IN GLOBAL-LOCAL FINITE ELEMENTS

The development of global-local finite element matrices and load vectors is based on Hamilton's principle:

$$\delta \int_{t_1}^{t_2} \left\{ \frac{1}{2} \int_{vol} \left[\rho \{\dot{\underline{u}}\}^T \{\dot{\underline{u}}\} - \{\underline{\varepsilon}\}^T [\underline{C}] \{\underline{\varepsilon}\} \right] d(vol) \right.$$

$$+ \int_{vol} \left[\{\underline{\varepsilon}\}^T [\underline{C}] \{\underline{\varepsilon}_o\} + \{\underline{\varepsilon}\}^T [\underline{C}] \{\underline{\alpha}\} \Delta T + \{\underline{\varepsilon}\}^T \{\underline{P}\} \right] d(vol)$$

$$\left. + \int_{surf} \{\underline{u}_s\}^T \{\underline{\tau}_s\} \, d(surf) \right\} dt = 0 \tag{20}$$

where the terms in the three integrals are consecutively the kinetic energy, strain energy, potential energies due to initial strains $\{\underline{\varepsilon}_o\}$, temperature change ΔT, body force densities $\{\underline{P}\}$, and prescribed surface tractions $\{\underline{\tau}_s\}$.

Consider an element where both finite element approximating functions and global (Rayleigh-Ritz) functions are employed. Let $\{\underline{\delta}\}$ denote the discrete coordinates at the nodes and let $\{\underline{S}\}$ be the set of generalized coordinates associated with the global functions. The interpolation of the displacement field $\{\underline{u}\}$ over an element can be stated as

$$\{\underline{u}\} = [\underline{N}_\ell]\{\underline{\delta}\} + [\underline{N}_g]\{\underline{S}\} \tag{21}$$

where $[\underline{N}_\ell]$ contains the finite element interpolating polynomials and $[\underline{N}_g]$ represents the global functions. Throughout our discussion, the subscripts ℓ and g will refer to local and global quantities, respectively. The strain displacement relations have the general form

$$\{\underline{\varepsilon}\} = [L]\{\underline{u}\} \tag{22}$$

where [L] is a differential operator describing the geometry of deformation. The form and size of [L] is dependent upon the adopted coordinate system and dimensionality of the element. Substituting Eq. (21) into Eq. (22) gives

$$\{\underline{\varepsilon}\} = [\underline{B}_\ell]\{\underline{\delta}\} + [\underline{B}_g]\{\underline{S}\} \tag{23}$$

where the local and global strain-transformation matrices are defined as

$$[\underline{B}_\ell] = [L][\underline{N}_\ell] \quad ; \quad [\underline{B}_g] = [L][\underline{N}_g] \tag{24}$$

Substituting Eqs. (21) and (23) into Eq. (20) yields all the global-local element matrices and consistent load vectors:

(1) Kinetic Energy

$$T = \frac{1}{2} \left[\{\dot{\underline{\delta}}\}^T \ \{\dot{\underline{S}}\}^T \right] \begin{bmatrix} [\underline{M}_{\ell\ell}] & [\underline{M}_{\ell g}] \\ [\underline{M}_{g\ell}] & [\underline{M}_{gg}] \end{bmatrix} \begin{bmatrix} \{\dot{\underline{\delta}}\} \\ \{\dot{\underline{S}}\} \end{bmatrix} \tag{25}$$

where

$$[\underline{M}_{\ell\ell}] = \int_{vol} \rho [\underline{N}_\ell]^T [\underline{N}_\ell] \, d(vol) \tag{25a}$$

$$[\underline{M}_{\ell g}] = [\underline{M}_{g\ell}]^T = \int_{vol} \rho [\underline{N}_\ell]^T [\underline{N}_g] \, d(vol) \tag{25b}$$

$$[\underline{M}_{gg}] = \int_{vol} \rho [\underline{N}_g]^T [\underline{N}_g] \, d(vol) \tag{25c}$$

(2) Strain Energy

$$V_e = \frac{1}{2}\left[\{\underline{\delta}\}^T \; \{\underline{S}\}\right] \begin{bmatrix} [\underline{K}_{\ell\ell}] & [\underline{K}_{\ell g}] \\ [\underline{K}_{g\ell}] & [\underline{K}_{gg}] \end{bmatrix} \begin{bmatrix} \{\underline{\delta}\} \\ \{\underline{S}\} \end{bmatrix} \tag{26}$$

where

$$[\underline{K}_{\ell\ell}] = \int_{vol} [\underline{B}_\ell]^T \, [\underline{C}] \, [\underline{B}_\ell] \, d(vol) \tag{26a}$$

$$[\underline{K}_{\ell g}] = [\underline{K}_{g\ell}]^T = \int_{vol} [\underline{B}_\ell]^T \, [\underline{C}] \, [\underline{B}_g] \, d(vol) \tag{26b}$$

$$[\underline{K}_{gg}] = \int_{vol} [\underline{B}_g]^T \, [\underline{C}] \, [\underline{B}_g] \, d(vol) \tag{26c}$$

(3) Potential Energies of Initial Strain and Thermal Deformation, Body Forces, and Surface Tractions

$$W = W_t + W_b + W_s = \left[\{\underline{\delta}\}^T \{\underline{S}\}^T\right]\left[\{\underline{F}_t\} + \{\underline{F}_b\} + \{\underline{F}_s\}\right] \tag{27}$$

where

$$\{\underline{F}_t\} = \begin{bmatrix} \{\underline{F}_{t\ell}\} \\ \{\underline{F}_{tg}\} \end{bmatrix} ; \quad \{\underline{F}_b\} = \begin{bmatrix} \{\underline{F}_{b\ell}\} \\ \{\underline{F}_{bg}\} \end{bmatrix} ; \quad \{\underline{F}_s\} = \begin{bmatrix} \{\underline{F}_{s\ell}\} \\ \{\underline{F}_{sg}\} \end{bmatrix} \tag{28}$$

with

$$\{\underline{F}_{t\ell}\} = \int_{vol} [\underline{B}_\ell]^T \, [\underline{C}] \left[\{\underline{\varepsilon}_0\} + \{\underline{\alpha}\}\Delta T\right] d(vol) \tag{29a}$$

$$\{\underline{F}_{tg}\} = \int_{vol} [\underline{B}_g]^T \, [\underline{C}] \left[\{\underline{\varepsilon}_0\} + \{\underline{\alpha}\}\Delta T\right] d(vol) \tag{29b}$$

$$\{\underline{F}_{b\ell}\} = \int_{vol} [\underline{N}_\ell]^T \, \{\underline{P}\} \, d(vol) \tag{30a}$$

$$\{\underline{F}_{bg}\} = \int_{vol} [\underline{N}_g]^T \, \{\underline{P}\} \, d(vol) \tag{30b}$$

$$\{\underline{F}_{s\ell}\} = \int_{surf_s} [\underline{N}_{\ell s}]^T \{\underline{\tau}_s\} \, d(surf) \tag{31a}$$

$$\{\underline{F}_{sg}\} = \int_{surf_s} [\underline{N}_{gs}]^T \{\underline{\tau}_s\} \, d(surf) \tag{31b}$$

The generation of element matrices and consistent load vectors for any type of element can be carried out by adopting these general formulas. To accommodate a wide variety of global function forms in the general purpose computer code, it is suggested that numerical integration such as Gaussian quadrature with the appropriate order be the most feasible approach.

Global-local element matrices and consistent load vectors for axisymmetric element, three-dimensional solid, and plate bending element may be found in

Ref. (9). The axisymmetric and planar elements described therein can accommodate general loading conditions (i.e., three dimensional) that is expressible in terms of a Fourier series expansion.

In elastostatic problem with subregions utilizing only global functions, only the global part of the stiffness matrix is required. This can be carried out according to Eq. (26c). However, in certain problems such as those dealing with stress singularities or with infinite volumns, there are sources of potential inaccuracies in the numerical volume integration. Such difficulties may be obviated by transforming the volume integrals into surface integrals by means of Green's theorem or Clapeyron's theorem. For example, for the global stiffness matrix, the internal strain energy V_e can be expressed as the external work W_e of the boundary tractions acting over their corresponding displacements:

$$V_e = W_e = \frac{1}{2} \int_{surf} \left[\tau_{nn} u_n + \tau_{ns} u_s + \tau_{nt} u_t\right] d(surf) \tag{32}$$

where both displacement and stress field in Eq. (32) are evaluated from the global approximating functions.

CONSTRAINT EQUATIONS

The various types of global/local configurations are illustrated in Fig. 5. In a given problem, the modeling may take the form of any one of these configurations. Also, the modeling in an analysis may require the catenation of two or more configurations. In order for this global/local modeling versatility, displacement continuity between dissimilar subregions must be enforced by means of constraint equations.

To formulate the constraint equations, consider a given node (say node n where $\underline{x} = \underline{x}_n$) and focus on a particular displacement component. The total displacement u can be written as

$$u(\underline{x}_n) = u_{FEM} + \sum_{i=1}^{N} S_i N_{g_i}(\underline{x}_n) \tag{33}$$

where u_{FEM} denotes the finite element degree of freedom and S_i are the global coordinates corresponding to global functions $N_{g_i}(x)$ evaluated at $\underline{x} = \underline{x}_n$. The summation over N represents the N global functions arising from the elements adjoining this node. Note that each element contiguous with this node may have a distinct subset of global functions which may be different from all the other elements.

Now, consider an element whose displacement u at node n may be written as

$$u(\underline{x}_n) = u^e_{FEM} + \sum_{i=1}^{M} S_i N_{g_i}(\underline{x}_n) \tag{34}$$

where u^e_{FEM} denotes the finite element displacement and the summation over M represents the M global functions that are operative in this element. The constraint equation expressing displacement continuity is obtained by equating Eqs. (33) to Eq. (34). If u^e_{FEM} is considered as the dependent variable, then the displacement continuity takes the form

$$u^e_{FEM} = u_{FEM} + \sum_{i=M+1}^{N} S_i N_{g_i}(\underline{x}_n) \tag{35}$$

where the global functions are ordered such that the summation over M+1 to N

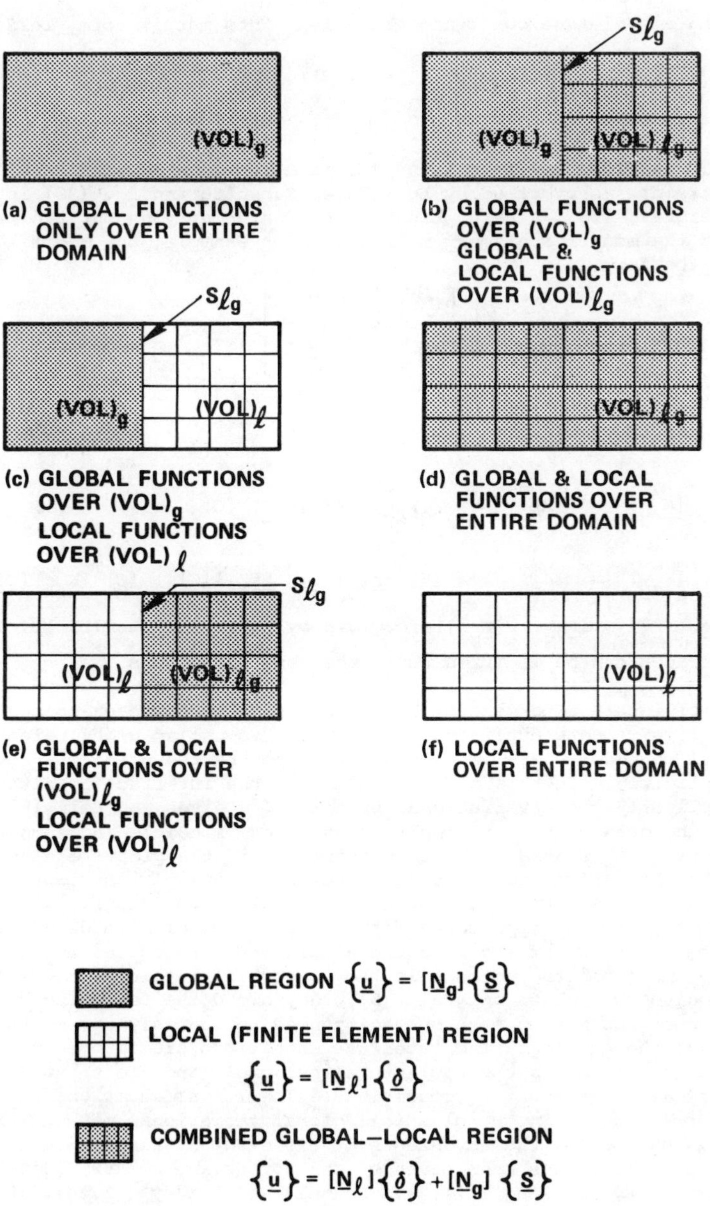

FIG. 5 Basic Global-Local Configurations

represents the complement between the global functions of the node and the global functions operative within the element. Continuity of other displacement components for the element will lead to a similar constraint equation.

Casting all element constraint equations into matrix form yields:

$$\begin{bmatrix} \{\underset{\sim}{\delta}\} \\ \hline \{\underset{\sim}{s}\} \end{bmatrix} = \left[\begin{array}{c|c} [I] & [C] \\ \hline 0 & [I] \end{array}\right] \begin{bmatrix} \{\underset{\sim}{\delta}\} \\ \hline \{\underset{\sim}{s}\} \end{bmatrix} \tag{36}$$

where [I] is the identity matrix and [C] is a matrix which expresses the global-local constraints as typified by Eq. (36). Substituting Eq. (36) into the element energies, i.e., strain, kinetic, etc., and carrying out the matrix products yield the modified element matrices. For example, the modified stiffness matrix has the form:

$$[\underline{K}^M] = \left[\begin{array}{c|c} [\underline{K}^M] & [\underline{K}^M{}_g] \\ \hline [\underline{K}^M_g] & [\underline{K}^M_{gg}] \end{array}\right] \tag{37}$$

where

$$[\underline{K}^M_{\ell\ell}] = [\underline{K}_{\ell\ell}]$$

$$[\underline{K}^M_{\ell g}] = [\underline{K}^M_{g\ell}]^T = [\underline{K}_{\ell g}] + [\underline{K}_{\ell\ell}]\,[C]$$

$$[\underline{K}^M_{gg}] = [\underline{K}_{gg}] + [C]^T[\underline{K}_{\ell g}] + [\underline{K}_{g\ell}][C] + [C]^T[\underline{K}_{\ell\ell}][C] \tag{38}$$

The matrices $[\underline{K}_{\ell\ell}]$, $[\underline{K}_{\ell g}]$, $[\underline{K}_{gg}]$ are given by Eqs. (25a) to (25c). The other element matrices can be modified using the same operations.

It is of interest to mention here a contrasting approach to the GLFEM continuity requirements outlined above. In the so-called global element methods and regional methods, there is no need for imposing the essential boundary conditions explicitly. In this class of methods, the interface conditions are imposed implicitly via a variational principle. Delves and Hall (5) gave the details on the essence of this implicit matching principle and summarized the previous work in this area. The discretization in the global element methods occurs with subdivision into a small number of relatively substantial size subregions (as opposed to a much greater discretization effort in finite elements). In the various approaches within this class of methods, differences exist in the treatment of the modeling within each subregion, however, the commonality among all the methods is the concept of implicit matching. In the discussion given by Delves and Hall (5), they cited the following advantages. The trial functions within each subregion need not satisfy any of the boundary conditions of the problem. The interface conditions are imposed only implicitly through the functional in the variational principle and are treated in exactly the same way as other boundary conditions. The linear equations that arise have the same form as those in the classical global variational method for simple domains and thus enjoy the advantages of efficient matrix set-up and solutions. Similar applications have been given by Wachspress and Becker (10), Yasinsky and Kaplan (11), Henry and Yang (12), and Hennell and Hendry (13,14). More recently, Hendry (15) applied Delves and Hall's approach to the solution of two-dimensional regions containing a singularity.

COMPUTER CONSIDERATIONS AND EQUATION SOLVER

A GLFEM system matrix, such as the system stiffness, in normal form has an "arrowhead" appearance as shown in Fig. 6a. Because of the sparsity of this matrix, it is stored within the computer as shown in Fig. 6b. Note that only the finite element portion has skew storage, with the global-local coupling

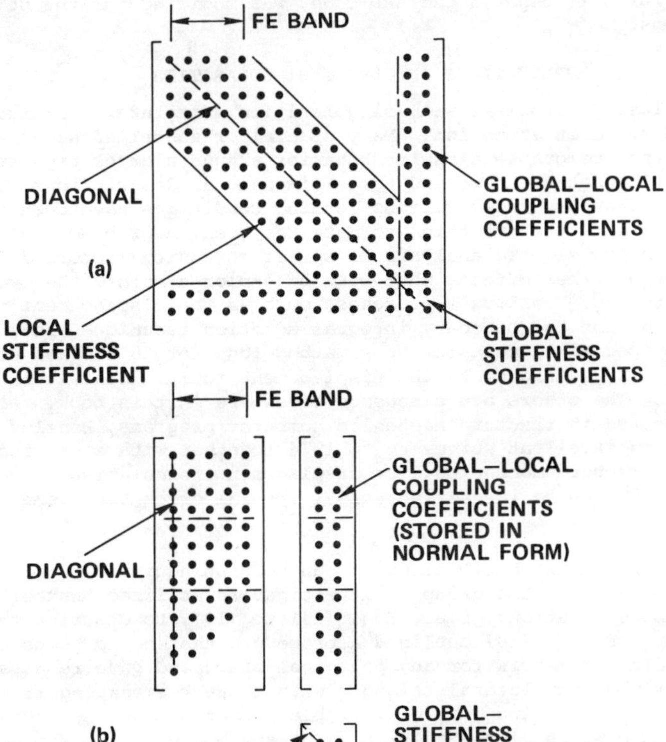

FIG. 6 Forms of Assembled Stiffness Matrix
(a) Normal Form
(b) Skew Storage Form in Computer

coefficients remaining in normal (rectangular) form. The dotted horizontal lines in Fig. 6b indicate the blocking of the stiffness coefficients for an out-of-core solution. The global stiffness coefficients reside in core continuously because they are needed in the solution reduction of the global-local coupling coefficients. Although the global stiffness is shown in normal form, it could also be placed in skew storage if its size requirement is a consideration. With the advent of virtual memory computers, the need to consider blocking strategies may be obviated.

For solution of a problem, any existing band-type equation solver can be easily adapted to include numerical operations on the global-local coupling and stiffness coefficients, i.e., the arrowhead. In Ref. (9), the SESOL equation solver (16), which is used in the SAP code, was modified for the solution of GLFEM equations.

APPLICATIONS INVOLVING SINGULARITIES

Of the class of problems with singularities, fracture mechanics applications have received the most attention. Many special or so-called super elements embodying the non-removable singular behavior around a crack tip have been reported in the literature. Two-and three-dimensional descriptions of elastic and inelastic behaviors under various loading conditions have been studied. However, the bulk of the attention to date has been on problems based on two-dimensional linear, elastic analysis of stress intensity factors and there remains a number of other effects that must be explored before the overall problem is fully understood. Various approaches, such as the displacement method, hybrid formulation and the boundary integral equation technique, have been used to construct the special elements or as a methodology for this class of problems. Our discussion is restricted to the displacement formulation within the framework of GLFEM. The others are discussed elsewhere in this book. Also, for readers interested in fracture mechanics computer programs, Benzley and Park (17) have provided an excellent survey up to 1974 together with a critical review of computational fracture mechanics. On displacement formulations, two distinct variants of GLFEM can be identified, viz., special crack tip elements and the superposition method.

Two-dimensional crack tip elements can be distinguished according to their method of formulation. One group of investigators utilized Muskhelishvili's complex variables equations, i.e., Eqs. (14) to (19), to describe the near field behavior. Byskov (18) outlined a procedure that could be used to develop the global stiffness matrix for any polygonal shape and gave results for the case of a four node equilateral triangle with a crack emanating from one of the vertices. Those also using complex variable equations as the basis for their formulations were Walsh (19), Rao et al (20), and Morley (21), who developed stiffness relations for rectangular and triangular elements. Another group of investigators adopted appropriate asymptotic equations around the crack tip:

$$
\begin{aligned}
2\mu u(r,\theta) &= K_I\sqrt{\frac{r}{2\pi}}\left[(\kappa-1)\cos(\theta/2) + \sin(\theta)\sin(\theta/2)\right] \\
&\quad + K_{II}\sqrt{\frac{r}{2\pi}}\sin(\theta/2)\left[(\kappa+1) + 2\cos^2(\theta/2)\right] \\
2\mu v(r,\theta) &= K_I\sqrt{\frac{r}{2\pi}}\left[(\kappa+1)\sin(\theta/2) - \sin(\theta)\cos(\theta/2)\right] \\
&\quad + K_{II}\sqrt{\frac{r}{2\pi}}\cos(\theta/2)\left[(\kappa-1) + 2\sin^2(\theta/2)\right] \qquad (39)
\end{aligned}
$$

where the origin of coordinates coincides with the crack tip with the negative x-axis running along the crack face, and the angle θ is measured counterclockwise from the x-axis. Hilton and Hutchinson (22), Hilton and Sih (23), and Wilson (24,25,26), developed elements with the near field behavior given by Eq. (39).

Moreover, Hilton et al, in addition to a near field global region with Eq. (39), used a far field global region wherein the displacement field was taken as a Laurent series. A third group can be identified by enriching their conventional finite element displacement field with known singular solutions, which can be interpreted as a global-local element. Strang and Fix (27) proposed a global displacement field in the form:

$$u(r,\theta) = \sum_{j=1} a_j r^{\nu_j} \sin \nu_j \theta \tag{40}$$

in the derivation of a square element. Benzley (28) developed a global-local isoparametric quadrilateral crack tip element with the singular behavior given by Eq. (39), and gave a method which utilizes an intermediate global-local region wherein the global function is adjusted to allow complete interelement continuity and therefore monotonic convergence. Lastly, another group can be identified by their employment of an approximate $\sqrt{r}$ displacement field assumption around the crack tip. Tracey (29) proposed a "centered fan" element, which can be used to surround the entire crack tip. Interelement compatibility is preserved with this centered fan element. Blackburn (30) suggested a more elaborate approximate field in the form:

$$u = a + b\sqrt{\zeta} + c\zeta \tag{41}$$

where ζ is the distance from the crack tip and developed triangular and tetrahedronal elements for two and three-dimensional analyses. However, Blackburn resorted to a J-integral calculation for the stress intensity factors.

Mention should also be made of the following miscellaneous GLFEM-type displacement formulations: Blackburn and Hellen (31) for their three-dimensional calculation of stress intensity factors; Admad and Loo (32) for their analysis of plate bending problems using the Williams series to describe the singular field in calculating bending and shear stress intensity factors; and Bradford et al (33) for the development of a two-dimensional center crack element, which automatically includes the tip to tip interaction.

Special convergence considerations must be applied to the singular finite element solutions using special crack elements. As mentioned earlier, Tong and Pian (8) discussed the necessity for a finite size global singular region. Moreover, as in the case with conventional finite elements, monotronic convergence under the theorem of minimum potential energy is possible only when interelement compatibility is maintained. In examining a particular approach for an application, an awareness of these considerations is essential in order to interpret the results meaningfully.

In the superposition method in fracture mechanics, analytical solution and finite element representations extend over the entire domain, i.e., Fig. (5d). This method appeared to have been first suggested by Yamamoto (34), who together with his co-workers, gave a number of results for two-dimensional plane and axisymmetrical problems (35,36,37,38,39). Yagawa, Nishioka, Ando and Ogura (40) have also discussed the superposition method for calculation of stress intensity factors. A series of papers have emerged from these two Japanese groups on extension of the superposition method to elastic-plastic behavior around holes (41), treatment of stress intensity factors for plate bending including transverse shear deformation (42,43), transient and steady-state creep analyses (44,45), and three-dimensional crack analyses (46,47).

Some examples of global-local modeling of singularities outside of fracture mechanics include Fix's vibration analysis of L-shaped membranes (48), and Wait and Mitchell's consideration of corner singularities in elliptic boundary value problems (49).

APPLICATIONS INVOLVING A FAR FIELD

Numerous problems in engineering require the consideration of an unbounded region. Examples can be easily drawn from solid and fluid mechanics, acoustics, transfer processes and electromagnetics. As pointed out earlier, finite element modeling, which employs the artifice of truncating the unbounded region by an entirely arbitrarily selected boundary, presents two principal drawbacks. First, the resulting solution offers no clue to the error involved in the geometric truncation except by repeated solutions using various size meshes. Secondly, computational inflation is inherent because of a need for a sufficiently large model in order to minimize the interaction between the artificial boundary and the regions of primary interest. For dynamic problems, geometric truncation is either not acceptable or greatly inhibitive in terms of the types of problems that can be properly modeled. GLFEM appears to be a natural approach for overcoming many difficulties associated with the conventional FEM.

One of the first analytical treatments of the far field in conjunction with a conventional finite element model occurred in electrostatics. Silvester and Hsieh (50) developed an "exterior" element for problems governed by Laplace's equation. They derived the equivalent of a global stiffness matrix using projection methods (51), which appear to be closely akin to techniques of the boundary integral method. More in the GLFEM modus operandi was Wood's (52) comparison of a steady-state seepage analysis (also governed by Laplace's equation) using three approaches for the far field: (1) geometric truncation, (2) introduction of a global function for the far field, but restricting it to a large but finite exterior region, and (3) using the same global function and allowing its influence to extend to infinity. As would be intuitively expected, the third approach provided for faster convergence with fewer equations than the other two. Dynamic soil foundation interaction models which reflect far field considerations have been proposed by a number of investigators. Lysmer and Kuhlemeyer (53) suggested the use of a "standard viscous boundary" as a frequency independent energy absorbing mechanism in which lumped dashpots are employed. The parameters of this boundary were determined by a trial and error evaluation to give the most "efficient" absorption. White et al (54) offered another approach for establishing these parameters based on a minimization procedure. This technique does not have theoretical appeal because it lacks the ability to model the physical behavior at the finite element boundary realistically over a broad range of frequencies. In Lysmer and Waas's approach (55,56), a dynamic stiffness matrix for the far field in the form of a layered region of infinite horizontal extent was proposed. This stiffness was linked to that for the conventional finite element model of the soil-structure interaction region. In their study, only horizontally polarized motions were considered. This stiffness matrix for the infinite region required data from a frequency domain analysis and is, therefore, frequency dependent. Liang (57) and Kausel (58) extended Lysmer and Waas's method to other soil-structure interaction problems involving vertically polarized motions and axisymmetric motions. The construction of dynamic stiffness matrices for a viscoelastic half plane was considered by Chopra et al (59) and Dasgupta and Chopra (60). Although all of these investigators used some analytical means to represent the far field, none embraced the GLFEM spirit as it is described herein in terms of the basis and techniques upon which the global-local equations are established.

Additional examples in other disciplines can be cited. Chen and Mei (61) and Berkhoff (62) studied tidal and surface wave problems using a series solution to represent the outer field. A similar approach was employed by Hunt et al (63,64) for acoustic radiation and scattering from elastic structures. Recently, Yeh et al (65) used an analytical expression embodying the far field decay in the finite element analysis of electromagnetic wave propagation. The fan-like appearance of this far field element is reminiscent of the complement of Tracey's element (29) in fracture mechanics. Bettess (66) proposed an infinite element using an exponential decay multiplied by Lagrangian polynomials as the interpolation functions. Parametric infinite elements were also discussed and applications in viscous flow were given. Viscous flow problems using a special element extending to infinity have also been discussed by Gartling and Becker (67). Bettess and Zienkiewicz (68) employed these infinite elements in the study of surface wave refraction and diffraction. The critical parameter in these infinite elements is the characteristic decay length which must be assigned. Therefore, sound physical insight is required.

In our earlier example of a footing resting on a smooth infinite medium, it was explained that although a more accurate solution was available for the far field, it was not feasible in the GLFEM scheme because of the considerable effort necessary to evaluate it. A similar criticism may be leveled at many of the far field models cited in the previous two paragraphs. Candidate global functions should have simple forms in order for straight-forward GLFEM implementation. For elastostatic problems involving a half space, the classical singular solutions due to Boussinesq, Cerruti and Mindlin (see Love (69), for example, for the Boussinesq and Cerruti solutions and Mindlin (70)) together with directional derivatives of these solutions constitute a vast basis for representing any conceivable far field behavior. These analytical solutions are algebraic in nature and are, therefore, easily evaluated for any field point. Their asymptotic behavior as the field points tend to infinity can be immediately seen from inspection. Moreover, it is relatively easy to sense which global functions will be effective by resolving the surface or interior distributed forces into resultant forces, moments, etc. These far field interpretations are direct results of St. Venant's principle. Details concerning these aspects were explained by Muki and Dong (71). For a more precise representation of the far field due to distributed loads, it is possible to integrate these singular solutions to obtain the appropriate results. However, these solutions usually appear as integral representations, which are not convenient to work with as noted previously. Another means of establishing global functions that contain the essence of the far field behavior is to extract asymptotic solutions from these integral representations and use only the leading terms of such expansions. Such asymptotic expansions for homogeneous, isotropic half space and layered half space have been given by Muki and Dong (71,72), who also demonstrated their effectiveness in some GLFEM analyses.

Some Other Global-Local Approaches

The discussion to this point has been confined to a particular methodology for establishing global-local equations based on simultaneous use of conventional finite element and classical Rayleigh-Ritz modeling. Mention is made here of another method of using global functions, but for a coordinate reduction. This alternate approach has already shown its effectiveness on geometrically nonlinear beam, arch and shell problems. The general scheme begins with the conventional finite element modeling of the nonlinear system. Then, this system of equations is reduced by means of a limited number of suitably chosen Rayleigh-Ritz functions, which may be called the basis vectors. The nonlinear analysis required strategies for computation as well as for selection of the Rayleigh-Ritz approximations and their automatic updating during the solution process. These computational strategies greatly influence the total solution effort, and hence, its viability as an effective approach. This method has been referred to as the reduced basis technique. The use of suitably chosen approximation vectors spanning the entire domain of consideration for the coordinate transformation is reminiscent of linear eigensolution techniques under various names: simultaneous iteration, Block-Stodola and subspace iteration (73, 74, 75, 76). Besseling (77, 78) and Nagy (79) applied this method to problems where mild nonlinearities existed and used the linear bifurcation buckling modes as the basis vectors. Almroth et al (80) devised a computational scheme that employed the linear solutions as the initial set of basis vectors and monitored the corrections to these during the analysis. Examples of beams and shallow circular arches where the behavior went well into the geometrically nonlinear range were given to illustrate their approach. Noor et al (81, 82, 83) used a nonlinear solution together with various order path derivatives of the nonlinear solution as the basis vectors and demonstrated relatively high accuracy using only a few vectors (five was the maximum). Examples were given for beams, arches, cylindrical shells and shallow spherical shells.

It should also be mentioned that a class of methods called multigrid methods (84, 85, 86) can be viewed as another version of global-local methods. The principal idea here is the solution of a problem for a particular grid by refinement of another solution using a coarser grid. A commonly used technique for this "smoothing" operation is the Gauss-Seidel method. In this case, the global functions are obviously the solution to the coarser mesh.

CONCLUDING REMARKS

GLFEM methodology has been discussed in this chapter and some important applications utilizing this approach were surveyed. The attractiveness of this method lies in the case in which known physical behavior can be incorporated into a numerical analysis in order for better modeling with substantially fewer degrees of freedom. Although it was Mote (4), who coined the phrase "Global Local Finite Elements" in 1971, the concept of supplementing conventional finite element modeling with global functions was applied in various forms by others around the same time period. Liberty was taken herein to cite all these applications within the general framework of GLFEM if they exhibit any analytical essence resembling some rudiment of this technique. That many applications could be found testifies to the wide appeal of the GLFEM approach. In the future, GLFEM will undoubtedly find considerably more applications as its full potential has not yet been completely explored.

A forecase of future developments in GLFEM may be summarized in three areas as follows: (1) problem areas where GLFEM may be advantageous, (2) numerical and algorithmic innovations, and (3) software development. A major problem area is dynamic analysis involving a far field. Diffraction and scattering problems and computations for the temporal evolution of physical phenomena remain high on the priority list of topics to be studied. Associated with far field problems, a continued development of a greater library of asymptotic results is needed to facilitate a wider range of applications. In the area of numerical and algorithmic innovations, mention is made of particular structures of global-local systems of equations that arise which afford special numerical treatment. For example, if the global function essentially captures the behavior except for a minor part, then the finite element degrees of freedom may be regarded as perturbation variables. Such problems may be more efficiently handled by Gauss-Siedel iteration rather than Gaussian elimination or Cholesky factorization such as in the multigrid methods. Details of an example of such is given by Wilson (87). In the third area, it is noted that most applications to date relied on special purpose computer codes. An attempt for a general purpose GLFEM computer problem is that called GLASS II (9), which would be regarded as primitive in terms of current day standards in its evaluation of usability. Substantially more work is needed here to encourage more natural uses of the GLFEM concept. This is a difficult task, and recognizing that special features exist in given problems, the extent to which a general purpose GLFEM code can be formulated will more than likely fall short of any utopian expectation.

Finally, from a philosophical viewpoint, the Global-Local Finite Element Method is appealing in that it offers a means to unite the efforts of theoretical and applied (numerical) analysts for solution of problems. In the past, more often than not, these two groups have been engaged either in friendly competition with or completely independent of one another for solutions of common problems.

ACKNOWLEDGMENTS

Sincere appreciation is expressed to Professor R. Muki of UCLA for his many discussions on this subject. A portion of the work was funded by the Electric Power Research Institute, Palo Alto, California. The support and guidance of Drs. C. Chan and H.T. Tang of EPRI are greatly appreciated.

REFERENCES

1 Ritz, W.,"Über eine neue Methode zur Lösung gewisser Variationsprobleme der mathematischen Physik," Journ. f.d. reine u. angew. Math., Vol. 135, 1909, pp. 1-61.

2 Lord Rayleigh, The Theory of Sound, (1st ed.), 1877, (2nd ed.), 1894. Republished by Dover Publications, Inc., New York, 1945.

3 Courant, R. and Hilbert, D., Methods of Mathematical Physics, Vol. 1, Interscience Publishers, Inc. New York, 1953, p. 174.

4 Mote, Jr., C. D., "Global-Local Finite Element," Int. J. Num. Meth. Engng., Vol. 3, 1971, pp. 565-574.

5 Delves, L. M. and Hall, C. A., "An Implicit Matching Principle for Global Element Calculations," J. Inst. Maths. Applics., Vol. 23, 1979, pp. 223-234.

6 Boussinesq, J., Applications des Potentials a l'Etude de l'Equilibre et du Movement des Solides Elastique, Paris, Gauthier-Villars, 1885.

7 Harding, J. W. and Sneddon, I. N., "The Elastic Stresses Produced by the Indentation of the Plane Surface of a Semi-Infinite Elastic Solid by a Rigid Punch," Proc. Cambridge Phil Soc., Vol. 41, 1945, pp. 16-26.

8 Tong, P. and Pian, T. H. H., "On the Convergence of the Finite Element Method for Problems with Singularity," Int. J. Solids Struct., Vol. 9, 1973, pp. 313-321.

9 Bradford, L. G., Dong, S. B., Tessler, A. and Westmann, R. A., "GLASS II - Global-Local Finite Element Analysis of Structural Systems," Electric Power Research Institute NP-1089, Research Project 299-1, Report, June, 1979.

10 Wachspress, E. L. and Becker, M., "Variational Synthesis with Discontinuous Trial Functions," Proc. Conf. Appl. Comp. Methods in Reactor Problems, ANL-7050, Argonne National Laboratory, 1965, p. 191.

11 Yasinsky, J. B. and Kaplan, S., "Synthesis of Three-Dimensional Flux Shapes Using Discontinuous Sets of Trial Functions," Nucl. Sci. Engng., Vol. 28, 1967, pp. 426-437.

12 Henry, A. F. and Yang, S. T., "The Finite Element Synthesis Method," Nucl. Sci. Engng., Vol. 59, 1976, pp. 63-67.

13 Hennell, M. A. and Hendry, J. A., "Variational Methods with Trial Functions Not Satisfying Prescribed Boundary Conditions," Journal of Physics A, Vol. 8, 1975, pp. 299-312.

14 Hendry, J. A. and Hennell, M. A., "The Global Element Method Applied to a Discontinuous Nuclear Potential," J. Comp. Phys., Vol. 28, 1978, pp. 376-394.

15 Hendry, J. A., "Singular Problems and the Global Element Method," Comp. Meth. Appl. Mech. Engng., Vol. 21, 1980, pp. 1-15.

16 Wilson, E. L., Bathe, K. J. and Doherty, W. P., "Direct Solution of Large Systems of Linear Equations," Comp. Struct., Vol. 4, 1974, pp. 363-372.

17 Benzley, S. E. and Parks, D. M., "Fracture Mechanics," Structural Mechanics Computer Programs - Surveys, Assessments and Availability, Eds. W. Pilkey, K. Saczalski and H. Schaeffer, University Press of Virginia, 1974, pp. 81-102.

18 Byskov, E., "The Calculation of Stress Intensity Factors Using the Finite Element Method with Cracked Elements," Int. J. Fract. Mech., Vol. 6, 1970, pp. 159-167.

19 Walsh, P. F., "The Computation of Stress Intensity Factors by a Special Finite Element Technique," Int. J. Solids Struct., Vol. 7, 1971, pp. 1333-1342.

20 Rao, A. K., Raju, I. S. and Krisna Murty, A. V., "A Powerful Hybrid Method in Finite Element Analysis," Int. J. Num. Meth. Engng., Vol. 3, 1971, pp. 389-403.

21 Morley, L. S. D., "Finite Element Solution of Boundary Value Problems with Non-Removable Singularities," Philosophical Transactions - Royal Soc. of London, Series A, Vol. 275, No. 1252, 1973, pp. 463-488.

22 Hilton, P. D. and Hutchinson, J. W., "Plastic Intensity Factors for Cracked Plates," Engng. Fract. Mech., Vol. 3, 1971, pp. 435-451.

23 Hilton, P. D. and Sih, G. C., "Applications of the Finite Element Method to the Calculations of Stress Intensity Factors," Mechanics of Fracture, Vol. 1, Methods of Analysis and Solutions of Crack Problems, Ed. G. C. Sih, Noordhoff, Leyden, The Netherlands, 1973, pp. 426-483.

24 Wilson, W. K., "Combined Mode Fracture Mechanics," Ph.D. Dissertation, University of Pittsburgh, 1969.

25 Wilson, W. K., "Some Crack Tip Finite Elements for Plane Elasticity," Stress Analysis and Growth of Cracks, Proceedings of the 1971 National Symposium on Fracture Mechanics, Part 1, ASTM Special Publication 513, 1972, pp. 90-105.

26 Wilson W. K., "Finite Element Methods for Elastic Bodies Containing Cracks," Mechanics of Fracture, Vol. 1, Methods of Analysis and Solutions of Crack Problems, Ed. G. C. Sih, Noordhoff, Leyden, The Netherlands, 1973, pp. 484-515.

27 Strang, G. and Fix, G.J., An Analysis of the Finite Element Method, Prentice-Hall, Englewood Cliff, N.J., 1973, Chap. 8, Singularities, pp. 257-280.

28 Benzley, S.E., "Representation of Singularities with Isoparametric Finite Elements," Int. J. Num. Meth. Engng., Vol. 8, 1974, pp. 537-545.

29 Tracey, D. M., "Finite Elements for the Determination of Crack Tip Elastic Stress Intensity Factors," Engr. Fract. Mech., Vol. 3, 1971, pp. 255-265.

30 Blackburn, W. S., "Calculation of Stress Intensity Factors at Crack Tips Using Special Finite Elements," The Mathematics of Finite Element, Ed. J. Whitman, Academic Press, 1973, pp. 327-336.

31 Blackburn, W. S. and Hellen, T. K., "Calculation of Stress Intensity Factors in Three Dimensions by Finite Element Methods," Int. J. Num. Meth. Engng., Vol. 11, 1977, pp. 211-229.

32 Ahmad, J. and Loo, F. T. C., "Solution of Plate Bending Problems in Fracture Mechanics Using a Specialized Finite Element Technique," Eng. Fract. Mech., Vol. 11, 1979, pp. 661-673.

33 Bradford, L. G., Dong, S. B., Nicol, D. A. C. and Westmann, R. A., "Application of Global-Local Finite Element Method to Fracture Mechanics," Electric Power Research Institute NP-239, Research Project 299-1, Report, Sept. 1976.

34 Yamamoto, Y., "Finite Element Approach with the Aid of Analytical Solutions," Recent Advances on Matrix Methods of Structural Analysis and Design, University of Alabama Press, 1971, pp. 85-103.

35 Yamamoto, Y. and Tokuda, N., "Determination of Stress Intensity Factors in Cracked Plates by the Finite Element Method," Int. J. Num. Meth. Engng., Vol. 6, 1973, pp. 427-439.

36 Yamamoto, Y., Tokuda, N. and Sumi, Y., "Finite Element Treatment of Singularities of Boundary Value Problems and Its Applications of Stress Intensity Factors," Theory and Practice in Finite Element Structural Analysis, University of Tokyo Press, 1973, pp. 75-90.

37 Yamamoto, Y. and Sumi, Y., "Stress Intensity Factors of a Twisted Round Bar with a Circumferential Crack," Int. J. Fract., Vol. 10, 1974, pp. 269-271.

38 Yamamoto, Y., Sumi, Y. and Ao, K., "Stress Intensity Factors of Cracks Emanating From Semi-Elliptical Side Notches in Plates," Int. J. Fract., Vol. 10, 1974, pp. 593-595.

39 Yamamoto, Y. and Ao, K., "Stress Intensity Factors for Cracks in Notch Bend Specimens for Three-Point Bending," Int. J. Fract., Vol. 12, 1976, pp. 495-498.

40 Yagawa, G., Nishioka, T., Ando, Y. and Ogura, N., "The Finite Element Calculation of Stress Intensity Factors Using Superposition," Computational Fracture Mechanics, Eds. E. Rybicki and S. Benzley, ASME Special Publ., 1975, pp. 21-34.

41 Yagawa, G., Nishioka, T. and Ando, Y., "Elastic-Plastic Finite Element Analysis Using Superposition," Nucl. Engng. Des., Vol. 34, 1975, pp. 247-254.

42 Nishioka, T. and Yagawa, G., "The Finite Element Analysis of Stress Intensity Factors for Plate Bending Problems Including the Effect of Transverse Shear Deformation," Proc. Japanese Society of Mech. Engrs., 760-1, 1976, pp. 37-40 (in Japanese).

43 Yagawa, G. and Nishioka, T., "Finite Element Analysis of Stress Intensity Factors for Plane Extension and Plate Bending," Int. J. Num. Meth. Engng., Vol. 14, 1979, pp. 727-740.

44 Yagawa, G., Miyazaki, N. and Ando, Y., "Superposition Method of Finite Element and Analytical Solutions for Transient Creep Analysis," Int. J. Num. Meth. Engng., Vol. 11, 1977, pp. 1107-1115.

45 Yagawa, G. and Miyazaki, N., "Steady State Creep Analysis of a Cracked Body Using the Superposition Method," Nucl. Engng. Des., Vol. 54, 1979, pp. 79-89.

46 Yamamoto, Y. and Sumi, Y., "Stress Intensity Factors for Three-Dimensional Cracks," Int. J. Fract., Vol. 14, 1978, pp. 17-35.

47 Yagawa, G., Miyazaki, N. and Ando, Y., "Three-Dimensional Finite Element Analysis for Through-Wall Crack in Thick Plate," Int. J. Num. Meth. Engng., Vol. 12, 1978, pp. 1295-1310.

48 Fix, G., "Higher Order Rayleigh-Ritz Approximations," J. Math. Mech., Vol. 18, 1969, pp. 645-658.

49 Wait, R. and Mitchell, A.R., "Corner Singularities in Elliptic Problems by Finite Element Methods," J. Comp. Phys., Vol. 8, 1971, pp. 42-52.

50 Silvester, P., and Hseih, M.S., "Finite-Element Solution of 2-Dimensional Exterior Field Problems", Proc, IEE, Vol. 118, 1971, pp. 1743-1747.

51 Silvester, P., and Hseih, M.S., "Projective Solution of Integral Equations Arising in Electric and Magnetic Field Problems," J. Comp. Phys., Vol. 8, 1971, pp. 73-82.

52 Wood, W. L., "On the Finite Element Solution of an Exterior Boundary Value Problem," Int. J. Num. Engng., Vol. 10, 1976, pp. 885-891.

53 Lysmer, J. and Kuhlemeyer, R. L., "Finite Dynamic Model for Infinite Media," J. Engng. Mech. Div., ASCE, Vol. 95, 1969, pp. 859-877.

54 White, W., Valliappan, S. and Lee, I. K., "Unified Boundary for Finite Dynamic Models," J. Engng. Mech. Div., ASCE, Vol. 103, 1977, pp. 949-964.

55 Lysmer, J. and Waas, G., "Shear Waves in Plane Infinite Structures," J. Engng. Mech. Div., ASCE, Vol. 98, 1972, pp. 85-105.

56 Waas, G., "Linear Two-Dimensional Analysis of Soil Dynamics Problems in Semi-Infinite Layer Media," Ph.D. Dissertation, University of California, Berkeley, 1972.

57 Liang, V. C., "Dynamic Response of Structures in Layered Soils," Dept. Civ. Engng., MIT Res. Rep. R74-10, 1974.

58 Kausel, E., "Forced Vibrations of Circular Foundations on Layered Media," Dept. Civ. Engng., MIT Res. Rep. R74-11, 1974.

59 Chopra, A. K., Chakrabarti, P. and Dasgupta, G., "Dynamic Stiffness Matrices for Viscoelastic Half-Plane Foundations," J. Engng. Mech. Div., ASCE, Vol. 102, 1976, pp. 497-514.

60 Dasgupta, G. and Chopra, A. K., "Dynamic Stiffness Matrices for Viscoelastic Half Planes," J. Engng. Mech. Div., ASCE, Vol. 105, 1979, pp. 729-745.

61 Chen, H. S. and Mei, C. C., "Oscillations and Wave Forces in an Offshore Harbor," Ralph M. Parsons Laboratory for Water Resources and Hydrodynamics Dept. No. 190, Dept. Civ. Engng., M.I.T., 1974.

62 Berkhoff, J. C. W., "Linear Wave Propagation Problems and the Finite Element Method," Finite Elements in Fluids, Eds. R. H. Gallagher et al, John Wiley, London, Vol. 1, 1975, pp. 251-264.

63 Hunt, J. T., Knittel, M. R. and Barach, D., "Finite Element Approach to Acoustic Radiation from Elastic Structures," J. Acoust. Soc. Am., Vol. 55, 1974, pp. 269-280.

64 Hunt, J. T., Knittel M. R., Nichols, C. S. and Barach, D., "Finite Element Approach to Acoustic Scattering from Elastic Structures," J. Acoust. Soc. Am., Vol. 57, 1975, pp. 287-299.

65 Yeh, C., Ha, K., Dong, S. B. and Brown, W. P., "Single-Mode Optical Waveguides," Appl. Optics, Vol. 18, 1979, pp. 1490-1504.

66 Bettess, P., "Infinite Elements," Int. J. Num. Meth. Engng., Vol. 11, 1977, pp. 53-64.

67 Gartling, D. K. and Becker, E. B., "Finite Element Analysis of Viscous Incompressible Fluid Flow," Comp. Meth. Appl. Mech. Engng., Vol. 8, 1976, pp. 51-60.

68 Bettess, P. and Zienkiewicz, O. C., "Diffraction and Refraction of Surface Waves Using Finite and Infinite Elements," Int. J. Num. Meth. Engng., Vol. 11, 1977, pp. 1271-1290.

69 Love, A. E. H., A Treatise on the Mathematical Theory of Elasticity, 4th Ed, Cambridge, 1927.

70 Mindlin, R. D., "Forces at a Point in the Interior of a Semi-Infinite Solid," Physics, Vol. 7, 1936, pp. 195-202.

71 Muki, R. and Dong, S. B., "Some Remarks on the Use of Asymptotic Solutions in Global Local Finite Element Analysis for an Elastic Half Space," Recent Research on Mechanical Behavior of Solids, Tokyo University, 1979.

72 Muki, R. and Dong, S. B., "Elastrostatic For Field Behavior in a Layered Half-Space Under Surface Pressure," J. Appl. Mech., Vol. 47, 1980, pp. 504-512.

73 Jennings, A. and Orr, D. R. L., "Application of Simultaneous Iteration Method to Undamped Vibration Problems," Int. J. Num. Meth. Engng., Vol. 3, 1971, pp. 13-24.

74 Dong, S. B., Wolf, Jr., J. A. and Peterson, F. E., "On a Direct-Iteration Eigensolution Technique," Int. J. Num. Meth. Engng., Vol. 4, 1972, pp. 151-161.

75 Bathe, K. J. and Wilson, E. L., "Large Eigenvalue Problems in Dynamic Analysis," J. Engng. Mech. Div., ASCE, Vol. 98, 1972, pp. 1471-1485.

76 Dong, S. B., "A Block-Stodola Eigensolution Technique for Large Algebraic System with Non-symmetrical Matrices," Int. J. Num. Meth. Engng., Vol. 11, 1977, pp. 247-267.

77 Besseling, J. F., "Nonlinear Analysis of Structures by the Finite Element Method as a Supplement to a Linear Analysis," Comp. Meth. Appl. Mech. Engng., Vol. 3, 1974, pp. 173-194.

78 Besseling, J. F., "Post-buckling and Nonlinear Analysis by the Finite Element Method as a Supplement to a Linear Analysis," ZAMM, Vol. 55, 1975, pp. 13-16.

79 Nagy, D. A., "Modal Representation of Geometrically Nonlinear Behavior by the Finite Element Method," Comp. Struct., Vol. 10, 1979, pp. 683-688.

80 Almroth, B. O., Stern, P. and Brogan, F. A., "Automatic Choice of Global Shape Functions in Structural Analysis," AIAA J., Vol. 16, 1978, pp. 525-528.

81 Noor, A. K. and Peters, J. M., "Reduced Basis Technique for Nonlinear Analysis of Structures," Proc. 20th AIAA/ASME/ASCE/AMS Struct. Structural Dyn. and Mat. Conf., St. Louis, Missouri, 1979, pp. 116-126.

82 Noor, A. K., Andersen, C. M. and Peters, J. M., "Global-Local Approach for Nonlinear Shell Analysis," Proc. 7th ASCE Conf. Electronic Comp., St. Louis, Missouri, 1979, pp. 634-657.

83 Noor, A. K. and Peters, J. M., "Nonlinear Analysis Via Global-Local Mixed Finite Element Approach," Int. J. Num. Meth. Engng., Vol. 15, 1980, pp. 1363-1380.

84 Nicolaides, R. A., "On Some Theoretical and Practical Aspects of Multigrid Methods," Math. Compnt., Vol. 33, No. 147, 1979, pp. 933-952.

85 Brandt, A., "Multi-Level Adaptive Techniques (MLAT): Ideas and Software," Proc. Symp. Mathematical Software III, MRC, Madison, Wisconsin, 1977.

86 Wachpress, E. L., "Two-Level Finite Element Computation," Formulation and Computational Algorithms in Finite Element Analysis - U.S. - Germany Symposium, edited by K. J. Bathe, J. T. Oden and W. Wunderlich, M.I.T. Press, 1976, pp. 877-913.

87 Wilson, E. L., "Special Numerical and Computer Techniques for the Analysis of Finite Element Systems," Formulation and Computational Algorithms in Finite Element Analysis - U.S. - Germany Symposium, edited by K. J. Bathe, J. T. Oden and W. Wunderlich, M.I.T. Press, 1976, pp. 3-25.

CHAPTER FIFTEEN

FINITE ELEMENT AND BOUNDARY ELEMENT

C. A. Brebbia
University of Southampton, England

ABSTRACT

The fundamentals of boundary element techniques are presented with an explanation of how the external surface of the region under consideration can be divided into a series of elements over which the unknown functions are assumed to vary in much the same way as in finite elements. The chapter then discusses two different approaches to combine the two techniques. The chapter presents examples illustrating the advantages of boundary element solutions when used on their own or coupled with finite elements.

INTRODUCTION

In recent years, engineers have shown a preference for the applications of boundary solutions rather than domain type techniques such as finite elements. Domain techniques have been known under different names such as integral equations (1), boundary integral methods, and singular integral techniques. The classical approach has been to use constant values for the unknowns on part of the boundary, but, more recently, the unknowns have been allowed to vary along part of the boundary surface or "element," and hence, the term Boundary Elements has been adopted as the name for the technique (2).

In this chapter the fundamentals of the boundary elements are presented with an explanation of how the external surface of the body can be divided into a series of elements over which the functions under consideration are assumed to vary in much the same way as in finite elements. This produces a series of nodal unknowns on the surface of the body only, which are then related through influence functions. The capability of using different types of surface elements is important, as it permits the combination of boundary and finite element regions without loss of compatibility.

The technique is now being re-examined, using weighted residual type statements (3), which allow for the method to be more easily extended to nonlinear, time-dependent and other complex problems. The case of time-dependent problems is considered in detail together with future trends of the technique.

The idea of combining finite elements with boundary element techniques can be attributed to Wexler (4), who started to use integral equation solutions to represent the unbounded field problem early in the 1970s. The advantage of this method is that it allowed for the use of appropriate conditions to represent the infinite domain. The integral equation technique is also of interest where regions of high stress or potential gradients exist, but finite elements are adequate for other parts of the body and may be simple to use in cases such as layered continuum, and anisotropic and certain nonlinear materials. Hence, it is important for the analyst to be able to represent a body using finite or boundary element techniques which depend on the particular geometry, boundary conditions, and other parameters.

Another way of combining the two techniques in potential problems was presented in 1977 by Zienkiewicz et al (5). The approach was based on energy considerations. Mei (6) explained in 1975 the way to combine both solutions for wave propagation problems using variational techniques.

The first combination of the two methods for elastostatics appears to be by Osias (7) in 1977. Brebbia and Georgiou (8) presented two different approaches in 1979, both based on weighted residual considerations.

This chapter examines the combination of the two techniques and illustrates how the combination can be effected.

POTENTIAL PROBLEMS

Let us first consider a potential function u over a domain where the following governing equation is to be satisfied.

$$\nabla^2 u - p = 0 \text{ in } \Omega \tag{1}$$

The boundary conditions corresponding to this problem are of two types: essential conditions, such as $u=\bar{u}$ on $\Gamma_1 = \Gamma_1 + \Gamma_2$, and natural conditions $q=\bar{q}$ or Γ_2. The total boundary is $\Gamma = \Gamma_1 + \Gamma_2$.

For our numerical solution u will be approximated, and we can minimize the error thus introduced by weighting the governing equation by a new function u*. This gives:

$$\int_\Omega (\nabla^2 u - p) u^* d\Omega = \int_{\Gamma_2} (q-\bar{q}) u^* d\Gamma - \int_{\Gamma_1} (u-\bar{u}) q^* d\Gamma \tag{2}$$

where $q^* = \partial u^*/\partial n$.

After integrating by parts twice the terms in the Laplacian equation (2) become:

$$\int_\Omega (\nabla^2 u^*) u d\Omega - \int_\Omega p u^* d\Omega = -\int_{\Gamma_2} \bar{q} u^* d\Gamma - \int_{\Gamma_1} q u^* d\Gamma + \int_{\Gamma_2} u q^* d\Gamma + \int_{\Gamma_1} \bar{u} q^* d \tag{3}$$

The function u* is now assumed to the fundamental solution of the equation, representing a concentrated source at a point i, i.e., the solution of:

$$\nabla^2 u^* + \delta_i = 0 \tag{4}$$

where δ_i is the Dirac delta function. Hence, equation (3) can be written as:

$$u_i + \int_{\Gamma_2} u q^* d\Gamma + \int_{\Gamma_1} \bar{u} q^* d\Omega = \int_\Omega p u^* d\Omega + \int_{\Gamma_2} \bar{q} u^* d\Gamma + \int_{\Gamma_1} q u^* d\Gamma \tag{5}$$

For an isotropic three-dimensional medium the fundamental solution of equation (4) is:

$$u^* = \frac{1}{4\Pi r} \tag{6}$$

where r is the distance from the point of application of the concentrated potential to the point under consideration. For two dimensions, the solution is:

$$u^* = \frac{1}{2\Pi} \ln \frac{1}{r} \tag{7}$$

Other fundamental solutions for potential and elasticity problems are given in Table 1 (8).

TABLE 1 - SOME FUNDAMENTAL SOLUTIONS (Ref. 8)

	Equation	Fundamental Solution
(i) One-Dimensional Equations		
Laplace	$\frac{d^2u^*}{dx^2} = \delta_o$	$u^* = -r/2 \quad r = \|x\|$
Helmholtz	$\frac{d^2u^*}{dx^2} + \lambda^2 u^* = \delta_o$	$u^* = \frac{1}{2\lambda} \sin(\lambda r)$
Wave Equation	$c^2 \frac{\partial^2 u^*}{\partial x^2} - \frac{\partial^2 u^*}{\partial t^2} = \delta_o \delta(t)$	$u^* = -\frac{1}{2c} H(ct-r)$ where H is the Heaviside or unit step function
Diffusion Equation	$\frac{\partial^2 u^*}{\partial x^2} - \frac{1}{k}\frac{\partial u^*}{\partial t} = \delta_o \delta(t)$	$u^* = \frac{H(t)}{\sqrt{4\pi k t}} \exp\left(-\frac{r^2}{4kt}\right)$
Convection/ Decay Equation	$\frac{\partial u^*}{\partial t} + \bar{u}\frac{\partial u^*}{\partial x} + \beta u^* = \delta_o \delta(t)$	$u^* = c^{-\beta r/\bar{u}} \delta\left(t - \frac{r}{\bar{u}}\right)$
(ii) Two-Dimensional Equations		$r = \sqrt{x_1^2 + x_2^2}$
Laplace	$\frac{\partial^2 u^*}{\partial x_1^2} + \frac{\partial^2 u^*}{\partial x_2^2} = \delta_o$	$u^* = -\frac{1}{2\pi} \ln\left(\frac{1}{r}\right)$
Helmholtz	$\frac{\partial^2 u^*}{\partial x_1^2} + \frac{\partial^2 u^*}{\partial x_2^2} + \lambda^2 u^* = \delta_o$	$u^* = -\frac{1}{4i} H_o^{(2)}(\lambda r)$ where H is a Hankel function
D'Arcy	$k_1 \frac{\partial^2 u^*}{\partial x_1^2} + k_2 \frac{\partial^2 u^*}{\partial x_2^2} = \delta_o$ (orthotropic case)	$u^* = -\frac{1}{\sqrt{k_1 k_2}} \frac{1}{2\pi} \ln\left(\frac{1}{r_o}\right)$ where $r_o = \left(\frac{x_1^2}{k_1} + \frac{x_2^2}{k_2}\right)^{1/2}$
Wave Equation	$c^2\left(\frac{\partial^2 u^*}{\partial x_1^2} + \frac{\partial^2 u^*}{\partial x_2^2}\right) - \frac{\partial^2 u^*}{\partial t^2} = \delta_o \delta(t)$	$u^* \quad \frac{H(ct-r)}{2\pi c(c^2t^2 - r^2)}$
Plate Equation	$\left(\frac{\partial^2}{\partial t^2} - \mu^2 \nabla^4\right) u^* = \delta_o \delta(t)$ $\nabla^4 = (\nabla^2)^2$ in two dimensions	$u^* = -\frac{H(t)}{4\pi\mu} S_i \left(\frac{r}{4\mu t}\right)$ S_i is the integral sine function $S_i(u) = -\int_u^\infty \frac{\sin v}{v} dv$

Equation		Fundamental Solution
(ii) Two-Dimensional Equations (Cont'd.)		
Reduced Plate Equation	$k_p = w/\mu$ $(\nabla^4 - k_p^4)u^* = \delta_o$	$u^* = \frac{1}{8ik_p^2}(H_o(k_p r)\frac{2i}{\pi} K_o(k_p r))$
Navier's Equation (Kelvin Solution)	$\frac{\partial\sigma^*_{jk}}{\partial x_j} = \delta_\ell$ (point load in direction 1)	Displacement in direction k $u^*_k = U^*_{\ell k}\varepsilon_k$ $= -\frac{[(3-4\nu)\log(1/r)\delta_{k\ell} + r_{2k}r_{2\ell}]\varepsilon_1}{8\pi G(1-\nu)}$ Traction in direction k $T^*_k = T^*_{k\ell}\varepsilon_\ell$ $= \frac{1}{r}(\frac{dr}{dn}[(1-2\nu)\delta_{\ell k}$ $+ 2r,_\ell 2r,_k$ $- (1-2\nu)(n_\ell r_{2k} - n_k r_{2\ell})$ $\frac{\varepsilon_\ell}{4\pi(1-\nu)}$
(iii) Three-Dimensional Equations		$r = \sqrt{x_1^2 + x_2^2 + x_3^2}$
Laplace	$\frac{\partial^2 u^*}{\partial x_1^2} + \frac{\partial^2 u^*}{\partial x_2^2} + \frac{\partial^2 u^*}{\partial x_3^2} = \delta_o$	$u^* = -1/4\pi r$
Helmholtz	$\frac{\partial^2 u^*}{\partial x_1^2} + \frac{\partial^2 u^*}{\partial x_2^2} + \frac{\partial^2 u^*}{\partial x_3^2}$ $+ \lambda^2 u^* = \delta_o$	$u^* = \frac{1}{4\pi r}\exp(-i\lambda r)$
D'Arcy	$k_1 \frac{\partial^2 u^*}{\partial x_1^2} + k_2 \frac{\partial^2 u^*}{\partial x_2^2}$	$u^* = \frac{1}{\sqrt{k_1 k_2 k_3}} \frac{1}{4\pi} \frac{1}{r_o}$ where $r_o = \sqrt{\frac{x_1^2}{k_1} + \frac{x_2^2}{k_2} + \frac{x_3^2}{k_3}}$
Wave Equation	$c^2\nabla^2 u^* - \frac{\partial^2 u^*}{\partial t^2} = \delta_o \delta(t)$	$u^* = -\frac{\delta(t-(r/c))}{4\pi r}$
Navier's Equation (Isotropic, Homogeneous, Kelvin Solution)	$\frac{\partial\sigma^*_{jk}}{\partial x_j} = \delta_\ell$	Displacement in direction k $u^*_k = U^*_{\ell k}\varepsilon_\ell$

Equation	Fundamental Solution
(iii) Three-Dimensional Equations (Cont'd.)	
	$u^*_{\ell k} = \frac{1}{16\pi G(1-\nu)} \left(\frac{3-4\nu}{r}\delta_{\ell k} + \frac{\partial r}{\partial x}\frac{\partial r}{\partial x_k}\right)$
(point load in direction ℓ)	Traction in direction K
	$T^*_i = T^*_{ji}\varepsilon_j$
	$T^*_j = T^*_{ij}\varepsilon_i$
	$= \frac{1}{8\pi(1-\nu^2)r^2}\left(\frac{\partial r}{\partial n}[(1-2\nu)\delta_{ij}\right.$
	$+ 3r,_i r,_j]$
	$+ (1-2\nu)(n_j r,_i - n_i r,_j)\varepsilon_j$

Equation (5) is valid for any point inside the domain, but in order to formulate the problem using boundary techniques, one needs to take this point to the boundary. For this case, equation (5) can be written as:

$$c_i u_i + \int_\Gamma uq^* d\Gamma + \int_\Omega pu^* d\Omega = \int_\Gamma qu^* d\Gamma \tag{8}$$

We have written the integrals for the whole $\Gamma=\Gamma_1+\Gamma_2$ boundary but, depending on which part of the boundary we consider, the $\bar{u}$ or $\bar{q}$ values will be known. We can introduce these boundary conditions at a later stage.

The value of c is 1 for an internal point, 0 for an external point and 1/2 for a boundary point on a smooth boundary.

Boundary Elements

Equation (8) can now be applied on the boundary of the domain under consideration. This boundary can be divided into N elements. The points where the unknown values are considered are called nodes and are similar to those of finite elements. The main difference is that now elements and nodes are defined only on the Γ boundary. The functions u and q over each boundary element are given by:

$$u = \tilde{\phi}^T \tilde{u} \qquad q = \tilde{\Psi}^T \tilde{q} \tag{9}$$

and equation (8) is discretized as follows:

$$c_i u_i + \sum_{j=1}^{n} \int_{\Gamma_j} uq^* d\Gamma + \sum_{k=1}^{m} \int_{\Omega_k} pu^* d\Omega = \sum_{j=1}^{n} \int_{\Gamma_j} qu^* d\Gamma \tag{10}$$

Note that m internal elements or cells need to be defined to compute the integrals in Ω, but these elements do not introduce any further unknowns, and hence, the problem is still a boundary problem.

We can substitute the u and q values given by equation (9) into (10) and carry out the integrations (usually numerically). This gives for each node, after assembling, the following equation:

$$c_i u_i + \sum_{j=1}^{n} \hat{H}_{ij} u_j + B_i = \sum_{j=1}^{n} G_{ij} Q_j \tag{11}$$

$$\sum_{j=1}^{n} H_{ij} u_j + B_i = \sum_{j=1}^{n} G_{ij} q_j \tag{12}$$

where the B_i term is the result of having integrated the domain term and $H_{ij}=\hat{H}_{ij}$ for $i \neq j$ and $H_{ij} = \hat{H}_{ij} + c_i$ for $i=j$. n is the total number of nodes.

The whole set can be written in matrix form as follows:

$$HU + B = GQ \tag{13}$$

Note that n_1 values of u and n_2 values of q are known on the boundary; hence, equation (13) can be reordered so that all the unknowns are on the left hand side, i.e.,

$$AX = F \tag{14}$$

where X is the vector of unknowns u and q.

When the surface is not smooth at the point 'i', the $c_i=1/2$ value is no longer valid. However, we can always calculate the diagonal terms of H by the fact that when a uniform potential is applied over the whole boundary, the normal derivatives must be zero. Hence, equation (13) in the absence of the vector B becomes:

$$HU = 0 \tag{15}$$

where U is a uniform potential. Thus, the sum of all the elements of H in any row ought to be zero, and the value of the coefficients on the diagonal can be calculated once the off-diagonal coefficients are all known, i.e.,

$$H_{ii} = - \sum_{\substack{j=1 \\ (i \neq j)}}^{n} H_{ij} \tag{16}$$

Once the values of the boundary unknowns are found, the values of u and q anywhere can be calculated using equation (8).

Example 1 - Flow Under A Dam With Sheet Piles

The impermeable dam is resting on permeable isotropic soil with an impermeable stratum underneath. Both the horizontal and vertical coefficients of permeability are equal to 0.03048 m/min. The base width is 79 m, and the total hydraulic head is 30 m.

The pressure distribution on the dam base was obtained by employing the relation $h=p/\gamma$ where γ is the unit weight of water.

This problem has been solved analytically. Here it is analyzed using both the boundary element method and finite element method. Note that the boundary element solution has been found by subdividing the soil into three regions.

The pressure distributions on the base of the dam obtained by the three different methods are plotted (Fig. 1) for comparison. It is clear from the plot that the accuracy of the boundary element method is high in comparison to the finite element results.

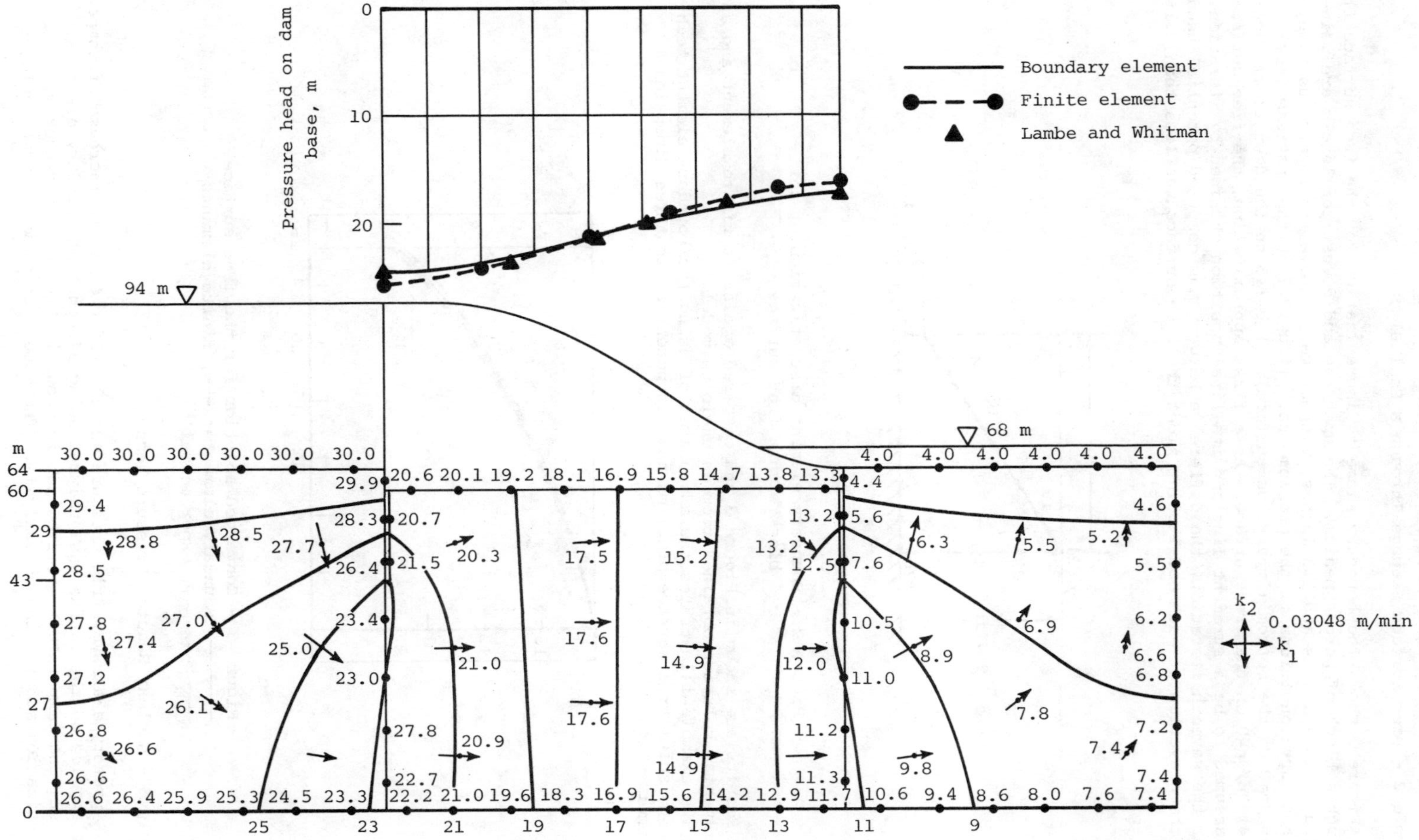

Figure 1 - Pressure distribution and flow under two-piled dam.

Example 2 - Free Surface Seepage Through a Soil Block

Figure 2 shows the boundary element discretization for the free surface flow through a block of porous medium. The upstream and downstream levels are maintained at 19.7 inches and 1.3 inches, respectively, above the impervious base. The boundary conditions of the problem are: 1) u=19.7 on the upstream face; 2) $\partial u/\partial n=0$ on the bottom (impervious surface); 3) u=1.3 on the downstream face; and 4) $\partial u/\partial n=0$ on the free surface. As a first approximation, the free surface was assumed to be a straight line and its final position obtained by iteration. After the seventh iteration, the difference between the computed potential head and the elevation of each nodal point along the free surface was less than 0.1%.

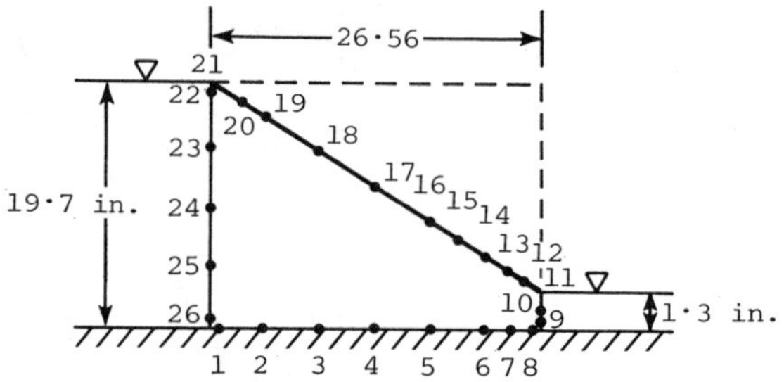

Figure 2 - Boundary element discretization of soil block with a free surface

Results are shown in Figure 3 and compared against a finite element and an experimental solution obtained from an analogue model.

The example illustrates the advantages of using the boundary element technique to solve free surface problems and its potential in three-dimensional problems.

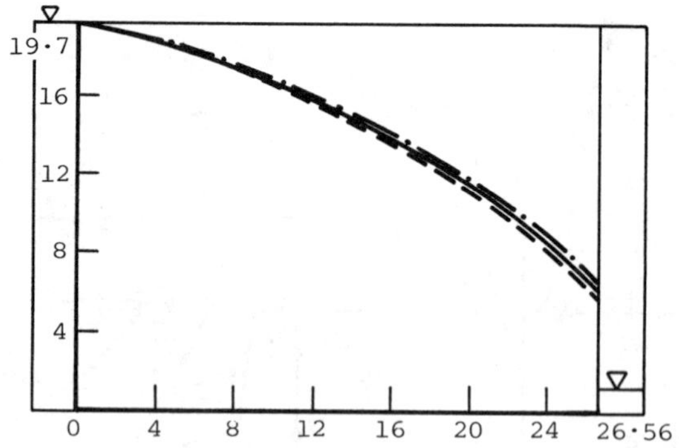

Figure 3 - Converged solution for the free surface. ———, Boundary elements; ---, finite elements; — - — - —, experimental

Example 3 - Nuclear Reactor Pressure Vessel

A prototype axisymmetric pressure vessel subjected to an increase of temperature applied on the inside was analyzed using 31 constant boundary elements. The resulting temperature distribution is shown in Figure 4, together with the discretization adopted in the analysis. The same problem was studied using 96 triangular finite elements (14) and the results as well as the mesh employed are shown in Figure 5 for comparison.

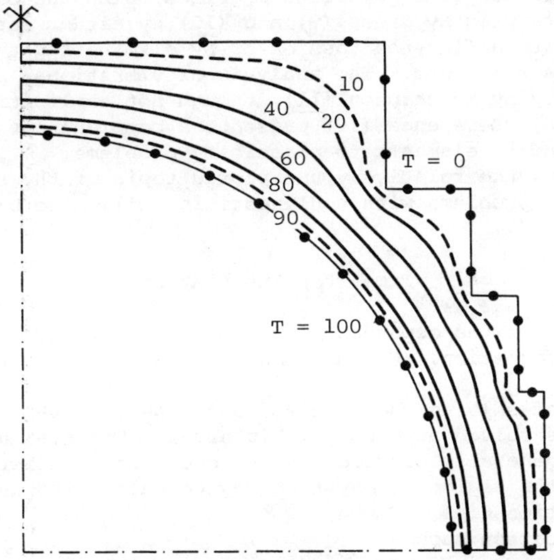

Figure 4 - Axisymmetric pressure vessel. BEM discretization and isothermals.

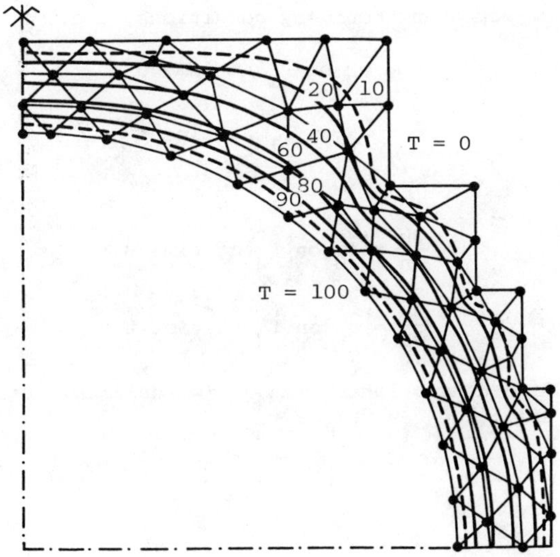

Figure 5 - Axisymmetric pressure vessel. FEM mesh and isothermals.

TIME-DEPENDENT AND NONLINEAR PROBLEMS

Up to now, we have considered time-independent problems. Many situations of physical interest involve the solution of problems with some time component, such as vibration problems where a steady-state solution is sought, a problem where the response to some transient effect is required, or the case where the properties of the material itself are time-dependent.

Previous analyses of time-dependent problems using the boundary element method have been attempted by Cruse (9) and (10) by either integrating numerically in time in some finite difference fashion or by eliminating the time variation by the use of a Laplace transform. The analysis of vibrational problems has been presented effectively by Hutchinson (11), though not explicitly, using the Fourier decomposition method. Reference (12) presents a comprehensive review of the applications of boundary elements to plasticity problems.

In this section, the relatively unexplored topic of the application of boundary elements to problems with nonlinearities will also be discussed.

Time-Step Integration

Let us assume that the dependence on the governing equation cannot be removed using a transformation. We can then integrate in time a parabolic or hyperbolic system.

The usual way of solving the problem is to use a time-stepping type technique where the problem is solved at each time interval. The evaluation of the time-dependent terms is generally carried out in some finite difference way. Values at the interior of the region at any time may be calculated using the boundary element method relationships.

Consider an equation such as:

$$\nabla^2 u = \frac{\partial u}{\partial t} \tag{17}$$

To solve the problems we require some initial values over the whole of Ω at time $t=0$, defined by $\Omega(0)$. Say

$$u(\bar{x},0) = u_0 \tag{18}$$

We may also have time-dependent boundary conditions, i.e.,

$$\begin{aligned} u &= \bar{u}_0 \text{ on } \Gamma_1 \text{ at time } 0 \\ u &= \bar{u}_t \text{ on } \Gamma_1 \text{ at time } t \end{aligned} \tag{19}$$

and

$$\begin{aligned} \frac{\partial u}{\partial n} &= \bar{q}_0 \text{ on } \Gamma_2 \text{ at time } 0 \\ \frac{\partial u}{\partial n} &= \bar{q}_t \text{ on } \Gamma_2 \text{ at time } t \end{aligned} \tag{20}$$

If we wish to find u at a later time Δt (we call this value of u, u_t) where Δt is sufficiently small, we can write:

$$\nabla^2 u_t = \frac{u_t - u_0}{\Delta t} \tag{21}$$

or

$$\nabla^2 u_t - \frac{u_t}{\Delta t} = -\frac{u_0}{\Delta t} \tag{22}$$

The fundamental solution corresponding to equation (22) in two dimensions can be chosen from Table 1 and satisfies:

$$\nabla^2 u_t^* - \frac{1}{\Delta t} u_t^* = \delta \tag{23}$$

The weighted residual expression for u_t becomes:

$$\int_\Omega (\nabla^2 u_t^* - \frac{1}{\Delta t} u_t^*) u_t d\Omega = \int_\Gamma q^*{}_t u_t d\Gamma - \int_\Gamma u_t^* q_t d\Gamma + \frac{1}{\Delta t}\int_\Omega u_0 d\Omega \tag{24}$$

For our boundary values of u_t this gives the usual integral relationship:

$$c_i u_t^i = \int_\Gamma q_t^* u_t d\Gamma - \int_\Gamma q_t u_t^* d\Gamma + \frac{1}{\Delta t}\int_\Omega u_0 d\Omega \tag{25}$$

which is the starting point for our boundary element formulation.

The process can be repeated for each Δt. The technique is similar to the one usually employed in finite elements or finite differences to analyze time-dependent problems.

Time-Dependent Fundamental Solution

Let us return to equation (17), plus the corresponding initial and boundary conditions, equations (18) to (20). One can use weighted residuals, and also integrate with respect to time. Weighting equation (17), we have (13):

$$\int_0^t \int_\Omega (\nabla^2 u - \frac{\partial u}{\partial t}) u^* d\Omega d\tau = \int_0^t \int_{\Gamma_2} (q-\bar{q}) u^* d\Gamma d\tau - \int_0^t \int_{\Gamma_1} (u-\bar{u}) q^* d\Gamma d\tau \tag{26}$$

where $0<\tau<t$.

Integrating by parts twice, we find:

$$\int_0^t \int_\Omega (\nabla^2 u^* + \frac{\partial u^*}{\partial t}) u d\Omega d\tau - \left[\int_\Omega u u^* d\Omega\right]_{\tau=0} + \int_0^t \int_\Gamma q u^* d\Gamma d\tau = \int_0^t \int_\Gamma u q^* d\Gamma d\tau \tag{27}$$

where the $\partial u^*/\partial t$ term was obtained by integrating by parts with respect to time.

The corresponding fundamental solution for this equation is:

$$u^* = \frac{1}{(4\Pi\xi)^{d/2}} \exp\left(\frac{-r^2}{4\xi}\right) \tag{28}$$

where $\xi = t-\tau$ and d is the number of spatial dimensionality, i.e., d=3 for three-dimensional problems, etc. The fundamental solution possesses the properties:

$$\nabla^2 u^* + \frac{\partial u^*}{\partial t} = 0 \text{ in } \Omega \text{ for all } \tau \tag{29}$$

and for $\tau = t$:

$$\int_\Omega u^* d\Omega = \begin{cases} 0 \text{ for } r \neq 0 \\ 1 \text{ for } r = 0 \end{cases} \tag{30}$$

Substituting this solution into equation (27), one obtains for a point 'i':

$$u_i + \int_0^t \int_\Gamma u q^* d\Gamma d\tau = \int_0^t \int_\Gamma q u^* d\Gamma d\tau + \left[\int_\Omega u u^* d\Omega\right]_{\tau=0} \tag{31}$$

The last term in the above formula corresponds to the initial conditions at $\tau=0$. Since the fundamental solution itself is time-dependent, one does not need to propose the type of iterative scheme used in finite elements or finite differences to solve time-dependent problems.

Nonlinear Problems

The boundary element method may seem at first sight to be inapplicable to nonlinear problems as the source type solutions depend on superposition for their usefulness. We shall, however, indicate an iterative method which may supply a solution to some fairly well behaved weakly nonlinear problems.

The nonlinear terms can be treated as forcing functions, i.e., we transfer these terms to the right hand side and treat them as known functions.

Consider the nonlinear equation:

$$\nabla^2 u + \left(\frac{\partial u}{\partial x}\right)^2 = p \text{ in } \Omega \tag{32}$$

and the fundamental solution

$$\nabla^2 u^* = \delta_i \tag{33}$$

The iterative procedure required to solve equation (32) may consist of writing it as:

$$\nabla^2 u = p - \left(\frac{\partial u}{\partial x}\right)^2 \tag{34}$$

Making some realistic guess for the initial value of u and u_0, and substituting this into the nonlinear terms on the right hand side gives:

$$\nabla^2 u_1 = p - \left(\frac{\partial u_0}{\partial x}\right)^2 \tag{35}$$

Let us start by writing the integral statement corresponding to equation (32) and the solution given by equation (33):

$$c_i u_i = -\int_\Gamma u^* q \, d\Gamma + \int_\Gamma q^* u \, d\Gamma + \int_\Omega p u^* \, d\Omega - \int_\Omega u^* \left(\frac{\partial u}{\partial x}\right)^2 d\Omega \tag{36}$$

Equation (36) has been obtained using weighted residuals and integrating twice by parts.

The last term of equation (36) involves the integration of the unknown functions, so we cannot apply the boundary element method directly to this equation. Notice that if u_0=constant, we can find a new value of u:

$$c_i u_1^i = - \;{}_{\Gamma} u^* q_1 \, d\Gamma + \;{}_{\Gamma} q^* u \, d\Gamma + \;{}_{\Omega} p u^* \, d\Omega \tag{37}$$

The next iteration will be given by:

$$c_i u_2^i = -\int_\Gamma u^* q_2 \, d\Gamma + \int_\Gamma q^* u_2 \, d\Gamma + \int_\Omega p u^* \, d\Omega - \int_\Omega u^* \left(\frac{\partial u_1}{\partial x}\right)^2 d\Omega \tag{38}$$

and so on. For convergence we may require that the difference between two successive values of u, or their norms, be small.

Example 4 - Fuel Element for Nuclear Reactor

This application considers the problem of a transient heat flow in a fuel element for a nuclear reactor. Figure 6 shows the general configuration of the problem as well as the symmetric portion of the cross-section that was analyzed. A constant heat flux of $1W/cm^2$ is applied at time t=0 along the interface A-C between fuel and canning. The numerical values assured for the material constants are $k=0.1W/cm^2\ ^{\circ}C$; $\rho=100\ kg/cm^3$ and $c=0.01\ J/kg\ ^{\circ}C$. The temperature of the coolant material is $0^{\circ}C$ and the surface heat transfer coefficient on the interface D-E is equal to $1\ W/cm^2\ ^{\circ}C$.

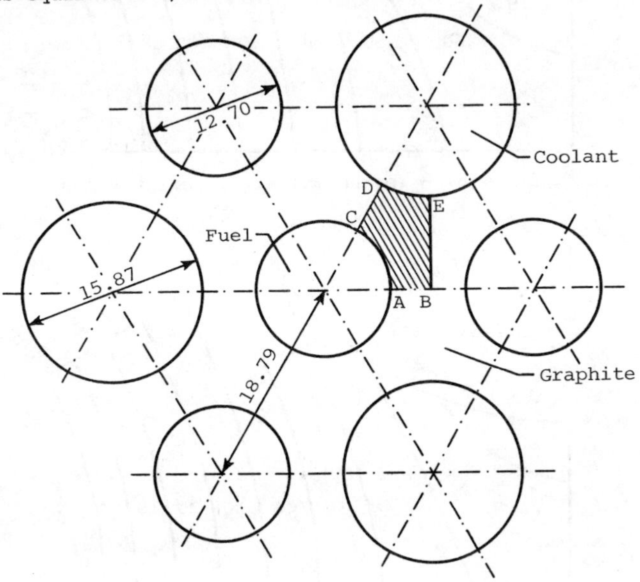

Figure 6 - Fuel element for a nuclear reactor

Isothermals at various times are plotted in Figure 7, together with the results obtained with a steady-state analysis. The boundary was divided into 33 linear elements and the domain into 94 cells with 34 internal nodes. The problem was also studied using finite elements (16), but no results of this kind were presented.

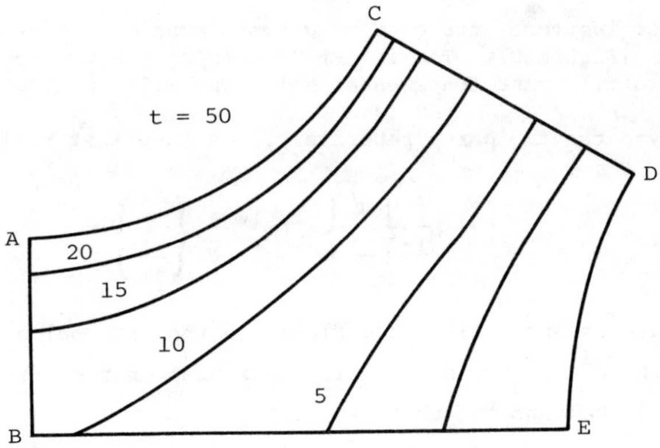

Figure 7(a) - Isothermal at different times

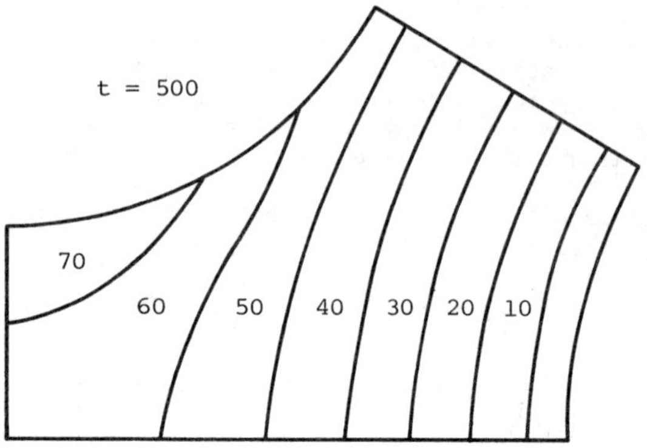

Figure 7(b) - Isothermal at different times

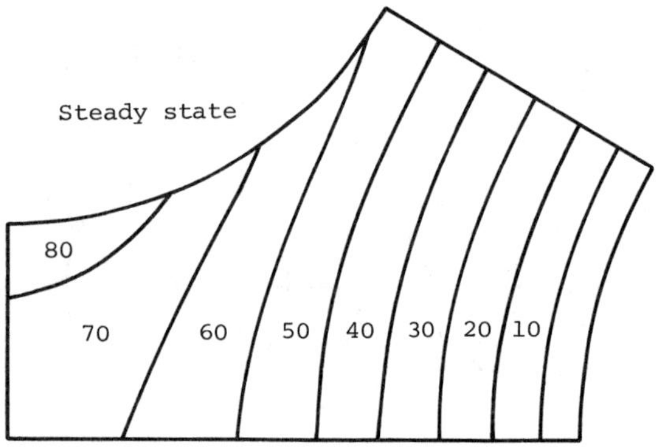

Figure 7(c) - Isothermal at different times

COMBINATION OF REGIONS

In many practical applications it is necessary to divide the body into several regions. This may be because a body is nonhomogeneous or because the dimensions of the body are not regular. Long bodies, for instance, produce numerical accuracy problems as the influence of some nodes over others becomes very weak.

Consider, for instance, the case of a two-dimensional body divided into two different regions (Figure 8). The interface between the two regions will be called Γ_I, and two different fundamental solutions will apply over parts 1 and 2 of the domain.

Let us analyze the two parts separately. On the first region we have:

$$[H^1 \; H_I^1] \begin{Bmatrix} U^1 \\ U_I^1 \end{Bmatrix} = [G^1 \; G_I^1] \begin{Bmatrix} Q^1 \\ Q_I^1 \end{Bmatrix} \tag{39}$$

where U^1 and Q^1 are the potentials and fluxes on the external surface of subdomain 1 and U_I^1 and Q_I^1 are the potentials and fluxes on the interface Γ_I, considering that it belongs to subdomain 1.

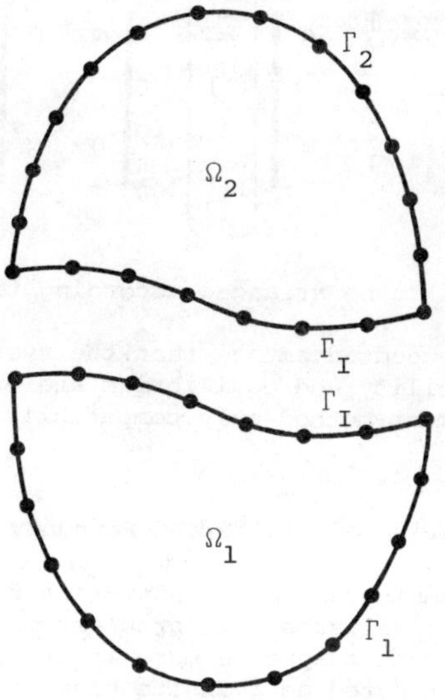

Figure 8 - Body divided into two regions

For the second region we have:

$$[H^{I} \; H_{I}^{2}] \begin{Bmatrix} U^{2} \\ U_{I}^{2} \end{Bmatrix} = [G^{2} \; G_{I}^{2}] \begin{Bmatrix} Q^{2} \\ Q_{I}^{2} \end{Bmatrix} \tag{40}$$

where U^2 and Q^2 are the potentials and fluxes on the external surface of subdomain 2 and U_I^2 are the potentials and fluxes on the interface Γ_I, considering that it belongs to subdomain 2.

If we call U_I and Q_I the potentials and fluxes on the interface Γ_I, we can write the following conditions:

i) Compatibility: $U_I = U_I^1 = U_I^2$ (41)

ii) Equilibrium: $Q_I = Q_I^1 = -Q_I^2$ (42)

Hence, equations (39) and (40) can be rewritten as:

$$[H^{1} \; H_{I}^{1} \; -G_{I}^{1}] \begin{Bmatrix} U^{1} \\ U_{I} \\ Q_{I} \end{Bmatrix} = G^{1} \, Q^{1} \tag{43}$$

$$[H^{2} \; H_{I}^{2} \; G_{I}^{2}] \begin{Bmatrix} U^{2} \\ U_{I} \\ Q_{I} \end{Bmatrix} = G^{2} \, Q^{2} \tag{44}$$

Equations (43) and (44) can be written together as follows:

$$\begin{bmatrix} H^1 & H_I^1 & -G_I^1 & 0 \\ 0 & H_I^2 & G_I^2 & H^2 \end{bmatrix} \begin{Bmatrix} U^1_I \\ \hline U_I \\ Q_I \\ \hline U^2 \end{Bmatrix} = \begin{bmatrix} G^1 & 0 \\ 0 & G^2 \end{bmatrix} \begin{Bmatrix} Q^1 \\ Q^2 \end{Bmatrix} \tag{45}$$

The system needs still to be arranged according to the prescribed displacements and tractions.

The solution has the added advantage that the system of equations is now banded. Note that compatibility and equilibrium are explicitly satisfied between regions (in the finite element method only compatibility is identically satisfied).

Combination of Finite and Boundary Elements

In this section the combination of boundary and finite element methods is attempted for two-dimensional elastostatic problems and two different approaches are discussed here. The one that appears more interesting is that for which the boundary element region is treated as a finite element and can thus be easily incorporated into existing finite element computer packages.

The starting expression for a finite element potential formulation is:

$$\int_\Omega \left(\frac{\partial u}{\partial x_k}\right)\left(\frac{\partial u^*}{\partial x_k}\right) d\Omega = \int_\Omega p u^* d\Omega + \int_{\Gamma_2} \bar{q} u^* d\Gamma \tag{46}$$

where u^* is the virtual increment δu.

The corresponding boundary element expression (equation (18)) is:

$$c_i u_i + \int_\Gamma u q^* d\Gamma + \int_\Omega p u^* d\Omega = \int_\Gamma q u^* d\Gamma \tag{47}$$

where $\Gamma = \Gamma_1 + \Gamma_2$, and u^* repeats the fundamental solution.

The standard finite element system can be written as:

$$KU = F + D \tag{48}$$

where K is the stiffness matrix for the system, F the equivalent nodal actions vector and D the vector due to the right hand side term p.

The vector F is obtained by weighting the applied fluxes $\bar{q}$ on Γ_2 by the interpolation functions used for the displacements:

$$u^{*n,T} F = \Sigma \int_{\Gamma_2} \bar{q} u^* d\Gamma \tag{49}$$

where $u^{*n,T}$ is the vector of nodal virtual potentials for the complete system. The summation applies over the element sides on the boundary. Under these conditions we can write F as:

$$F = MQ \tag{50}$$

where Q is a vector of applied nodal fluxes and where M is a matrix due to the weighting of the boundary tractions by the interpolation functions for the displacements. The exact nature of M can be simply explained by considering the term:

$$\int_{\Gamma_2} \bar{q}u^*d\Gamma \qquad (51)$$

For the case of $\bar{q}$ being discontinuous at a node (such as a corner node) care should be taken to define two different values of $\bar{q}$ at the same node, in much the same way as is done for corner nodes in the boundary-element-only solution. In equation (46) the term (51) represents the boundary fluxes weighted by the virtual displacements, or it may be interpreted as the external energy expended due to a virtual displacement u*. For a particular element, $\bar{q}$ is a function of the nodal value of the fluxes and u* is a function of the nodal arbitrary virtual potentials. The term (51) may now be written as:

$$\int_{\Gamma} u^*q d\Gamma \qquad (52)$$

Assuming the interpolation functions for u and q are:

$$u^* = \underset{\sim}{\phi}^T \underset{\sim}{u}^* \qquad q = \underset{\sim}{\psi}^T \underset{\sim}{q} \qquad (53)$$

the above term reduces to:

$$u^{*,T} \int_{\Gamma} \phi\psi^T d\Gamma \; \underset{\sim}{q} \qquad (54)$$

The matrix M may then be expressed as defined in equation (54). Hence, we can write equation (48) as:

$$KU = MQ + D \qquad (55)$$

which is similar in form to the boundary element equation resulting from (47), i.e.

$$HU = GQ + B \qquad (56)$$

Consider a problem consisting of two domains Ω^1 and Ω^2 joined by an interface and which makes use of a finite element formulation in Ω^2 and a boundary element formulation in Ω^1 (Figure 9).

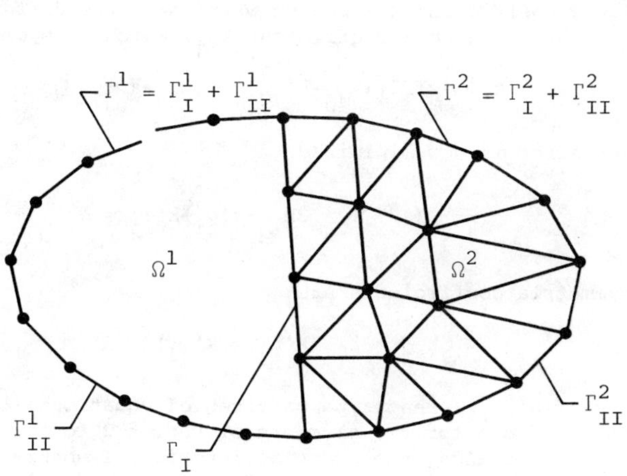

Figure 9 - Domain divided into finite elements and boundary elements

In order to join the two parts we apply compatibility and equilibrium conditions along the interface Γ^1:

$$U_I^1 = U_I^2 \qquad Q_I^1 + Q_I^2 = 0 \tag{57}$$

where U_I and Q_I refer to the potentials and fluxes on the interface Γ_I for the region under consideration.

We now have two alternative ways to approach the problem. We can develop the boundary element region Ω^2 as an equivalent finite element stiffness matrix, such as that of the finite elements of region Ω^2, and solve the overall system as a stiffness problem, or we can consider Ω^1 and Ω^2 as if they were both boundary element regions.

Using the first approach, we can transform equation (56) by inverting $\bar{G}$, such that:

$$G^{-1}(HU-B) = Q \tag{58}$$

and pre-multiply them by the matrix M defined by equation (50), giving:

$$(MG^{-1}H)U-(MG^{-1}B) = MQ \tag{59}$$

The matrix G will be singular for the case of having defined two different values of q at the same node. In this case G^{-1} cannot be performed and we need to define only one fictitious and continuous boundary value as an approximation.

We can now define

$$K' = MG^{-1}\,H \quad ; \quad D' = MG^{-1} \quad ; \quad F' = MQ \tag{60}$$

Hence, equation (59) has the following finite element form:

$$K'U = F' + D' \tag{61}$$

The main discrepancy which arises with the above formulation is the fact that the matrix K' is generally asymmetric although we know from superposition principles that a stiffness matrix should be symmetric. The asymmetry arises due to the approximations involved in the discretization process and the choice of the assumed solution. The matrix can be made symmetric by minimizing the square of the errors in the nonsymmetric off-diagonal terms.

The error for a coefficient k_{ij} can be written as the difference between k_{ij} and k_{ji} and the still unknown coefficient k_{ij}, which is symmetric:

$$\varepsilon_{ij} = 1/2[(k_{ij}-k'_{ij}) + (k_{ij}-k'_{ji})] \tag{62}$$

The square of this error is now minimized

$$\frac{\partial}{\partial k_{ij}}(\varepsilon^2_{ij}) = 2k_{ij}-k'_{ji}-k'_{ij} = 0 \tag{62}$$

Hence, the new symmetric coefficients are:

$$k_{ij} = 1/2(k'_{ij} + k'_{ji}) \tag{63}$$

The equivalent finite element type matrices of equations (61) may now be assembled with the matrices for the elements of region 2 to form a global system of equations. Assembling along the nodes of interface I ensures the conditions (57); as the matrix M transforms the vector Q into the equivalent consistent nodal vector F, by having zeros in the vector F corresponding to the nodes u^1, condition (57) is satisfied.

Using the second approach, mentioned above, for combining the two methods, we can consider region 2 as a boundary element type region.

For region 1 we can write:

$$[H^1 \ H_I^1] \begin{Bmatrix} U^1 \\ U_I^1 \end{Bmatrix} = [G^1 \ G_I^1] \begin{Bmatrix} Q^1 \\ Q_I^1 \end{Bmatrix} + B^1 \tag{64}$$

and for region 2

$$[K^2 \ K_I^2] \begin{Bmatrix} U^2 \\ U_I^2 \end{Bmatrix} = [M^2 \ M_I^2] \begin{Bmatrix} Q^2 \\ Q_I^2 \end{Bmatrix} + D^2 \tag{65}$$

By writing $Q_I = Q_I^1 = -Q_I^2$ and $U_I = U_I^1 = U_I^2$ we automatically satisfy conditions (57), and equations (65) and (66) can be rearranged as follows:

$$[H^1 \ H_I^1 \ \ -G_I^1] \begin{Bmatrix} U^1 \\ U_I \\ Q_I \end{Bmatrix} = [G^1]\{Q^1\} + B^1 \tag{67}$$

and

$$[K^2 \ K_I^2 \ M_I^2] \begin{Bmatrix} U^2 \\ U_I \\ Q_I \end{Bmatrix} = [M^2]\{Q^2\} + D^2 \tag{68}$$

Writing these two equations together as a single matrix equation, we have:

$$\begin{bmatrix} H^1 & H_I^1 & -G_I^1 & 0 \\ & & & \\ 0 & K_I^2 & M_I^2 & K^2 \end{bmatrix} \begin{Bmatrix} U^1 \\ U_I \\ Q_I \\ U^2 \end{Bmatrix} = \begin{bmatrix} G^1 & 0 \\ & \\ 0 & M^2 \end{bmatrix} \begin{Bmatrix} Q^1 \\ \\ Q^2 \end{Bmatrix} + \begin{Bmatrix} B^1 \\ \\ D^2 \end{Bmatrix} \tag{69}$$

region 1   interface   region 2

Note that on the boundary of the finite element region Ω^2, only the displacements on Γ_1 have to be prescribed, while on the boundary of Ω^2 we prescribe the displacements on tractions and consequently need to reorder the equations.

The advantage of the second approach is that it does not require an inversion.

Example 5

A test problem used for the combination of finite and boundary element techniques is shown in Figure 10. The domain has been divided into two regions, the first of which is decentralized into finite elements and the second using boundary elements. The problem studied is a two-dimensional elasticity problem and two loads were considered. Load 1 is a uniformly distributed load at the top and Load 2 a horizontal concentrated load. Note that concentrated forces cannot be applied with boundary elements.

Finally the problem was analyzed using only finite elements (Figure 11a).

The program developed combines constant boundary elements with quadratic finite elements and, although this combination is not fully compatible, it gives good results in practice and also has the advantage of avoiding the corners (Figure 11b).

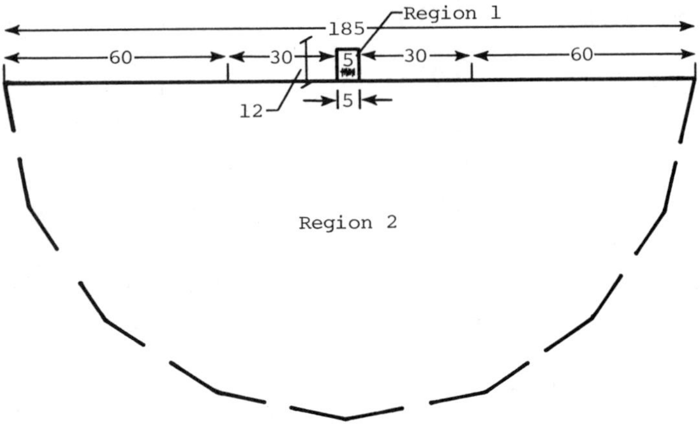

Figure 10 - Two Regions Problem

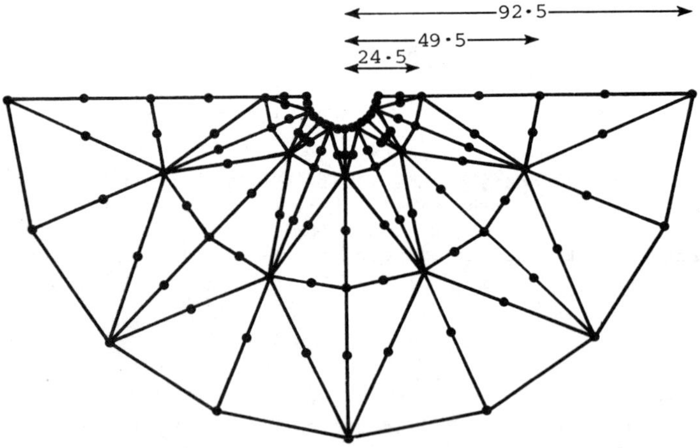

i) Finite element mesh for part of Region 2

Figure 11a - Finite element mesh

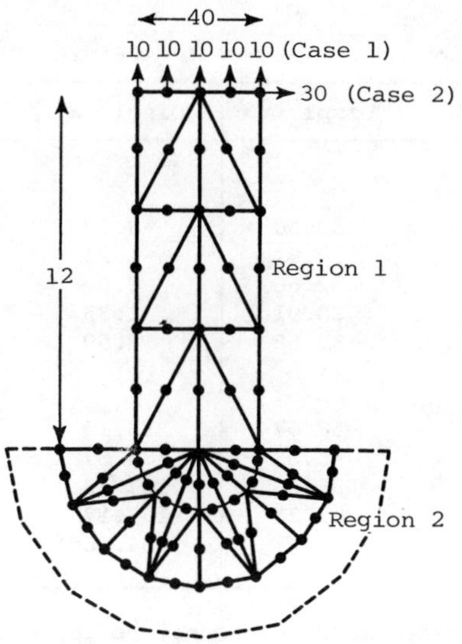

ii) Finite element mesh for Region 1 and part of 2

Figure 11a - Finite element mesh

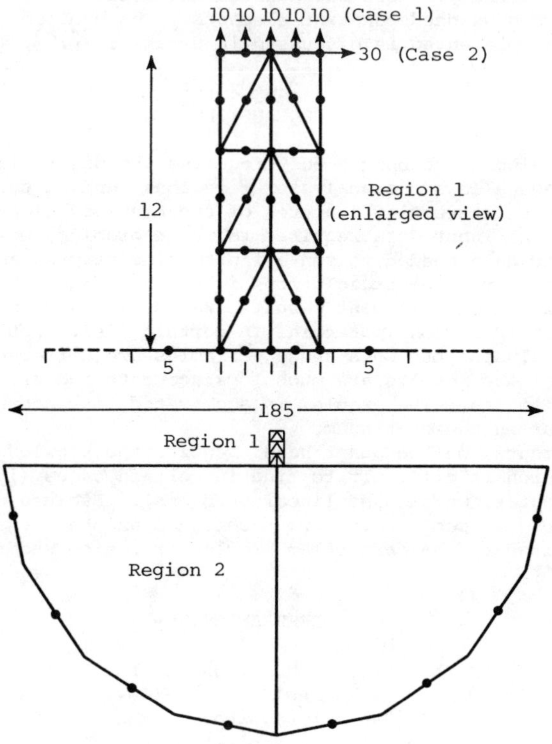

Figure 11b - Finite and boundary element combination mesh

TABLE 2

	Combination		Finite Elements Only	
	Displ. X	Displ. Y	Displ. X	Displ. Y
Case 1				
	-3.59	33.50	-3.50	33.40
	-1.35	30.91	-1.35	30.84
	0.00	32.66	0.00	32.62
	1.35	30.91	1.35	30.84
	3.59	33.50	3.59	33.40
Case 2				
	211.55	-58.67	213.19	-58.58
	183.05	-0.83	184.67	-0.79
	165.85	36.36	167.43	36.27
	161.48	62.33	163.17	62.12
	162.32	97.41	164.06	97.20

Note: The concentrated load, H, cannot be represented accurately as a nodal force in the boundary element method.

Results for displacements along the top five nodes are compared in Table 2. Notice that there is close agreement between the combination solution obtained using equation (61) and the finite element results which are usually good for displacements. This example does not address the issue of corner behavior in the interface as we have used constant elements. The problem of how the corner behavior could be implemented is discussed in detail in [17].

CONCLUSIONS

The boundary element technique only requires the discretization of the surface of the body and allows the analysis of regions tending to infinity.

One of the most interesting features of the boundary element technique is the simplicity of the input data required to run a problem, which contrasts with the large amount of data needed to run a finite element program. In addition, the accuracy of boundary element solutions is often greater than that of finite element techniques. Finite element results are usually accurate for the original variables under consideration (potential in certain field problems or displacements in stress analysis) but when these variables are differentiated (to obtain fluxes or stresses) the results are much less accurate and are usually discontinuous between elements. The problem is aggravated if regions of flux or stress concentration occur in the continuum.

Boundary elements, on the other hand, require the knowledge of the fundamental solution which is difficult to find in certain cases (i.e., inhomogeneous and anisotropic median, certain nonlinear problems). Because of this it is important to be able to combine the two techniques and have the possibility of using the best suited to the particular problem or region under consideration.

REFERENCES

1 Cruse, T. A., "Mathematical Foundations of the Boundary-Integral Equation Method in Solid Mechanics," AFOSR-TR-77-1002, July 1977.

2 Brebbia, C. A. (Ed.), "Recent Advances in Boundary Element Methods," Proceedings of the First International Seminar on Recent Advances in Boundary Element Methods, Southampton University, July 1978, Pentech Press, London, 1978.

3 Brebbia, C. A., The Boundary Element Method for Engineers, Halsted Press, New York, 1978.

4 McDonald, B. H., and Wexler, A., "Finite Element Solution of Unbounded Field Problems," IEEE Trans. Microwave Theory Techniques, MIT-20, No. 12, December 1972, pp. 841-847.

5 Zienkiewicz, O. C., Kelly, D. W., and Bettess, P., "The Coupling of the Finite Element Method and Boundary Solution Procedures," International Journal for Numerical Methods in Engineering, Vol. 11, 1977, p. 355.

6 Chen, H. S. and Mei, C. C., "Oscillations and Wave Forces in a Man-Made Harbor in the Open Sea," Proceedings of the Tenth Symposium on Naval Hydrodynamics, Cambridge, Massachusetts, June 24-28, 1974, Office of Naval Research (ACR-204), pp. 573-596.

7 Oasias, J. R., Wilson, R. B., and Seitelman, L. A., "Combined Boundary Integral Equation Finite Element Analysis of Solids," Proceedings of the First Symposium on Innovative Numerical Analysis in Applied Engineering Science, Versailles, France, May 23-27, 1977.

8 Brebbia, C. A., and Walker, S., Boundary Element Techniques in Engineering, Butterworths, London, 1979.

9 Cruse, T. A., and Rizzo, F. J., "A Direct Formulation and Numerical Solution of the General Transient Elastodynamic Problem I," Journal of Mathematical Analysis and Applications, Vol. 22, No. 1, 1968, pp. 244-259.

10 Cruse, T. A., "A Direct Formulation and Numerical Solution of the General Transient Elastodynamic Problem II," Journal of Mathematical Analysis and Applications, Vol. 22, No. 2, 1968, pp. 341-355.

11 Hutchinson, J. R., "Determination of Membrane Vibrational Characteristics by the Boundary-Integral Equation Method," Proceedings of the First International Seminar on Recent Advances in Boundary Element Methods, edited by C. A. Brebbia, Pentech Press, London, 1978.

12 Telles, J. C. F., and Brebbia, C. A., "On the Application of the Boundary Element Method to Plasticity," Applied Mathematical Modeling Journal, Vol. 3, No. 6, December 1979, pp. 466-470.

13 Brebbia, C. A., and Wrobel, L. C., "Steady and Unsteady Potential Problems Using the Boundary Element Method," in Recent Advances in Numerical Methods in Fluids, edited by C. Taylor and K. Morgan, Pineridge Press, London, 1980.

14 France, P. W., Parekh, C. J., Peters, J. C., and Taylor, C., "Numerical Analysis of Free Surface Seepage Problems," Journal of the Irrigation of Drainage Division, ASCE, Vol. 97, IR 1, March 1971, pp. 165-179.

15 Zienkiewicz, O. C., and Cheung, Y. K., "Finite Elements in the Solution of Field Problems," The Engineer, Vol. 220, 1965, pp. 507-510.

16 Donea, J., "On the Accuracy of Finite Element Solutions to the Transient Heat Conduction Equation," International Journal for Numerical Methods in Engineering, Vol. 8, 1974, pp. 103-110.

17 Georgiu, P., "Combination of Finite Element and Boundary Element Solutions," Ph.D. Dissertation, Southampton University, England, 1982.

ADDITIONAL BIBLIOGRAPHY

1 Brebbia, C. A. (Ed.), New Developments in Boundary Element Methods, Proceedings of the Second International Conference on Boundary Element Methods, Southampton University, 1980, CML Publications.

2 Brebbia, C. A. (Ed.), Boundary Element Methods, Proceedings of the Third International Conference on Boundary Element Methods, Irvine, California, 1981, Springer-Verlag, Berlin, 1981.

3 Brebbia, C. A. (Ed.), Boundary Elements, Proceedings of the Fourth International Conference on Boundary Element Methods, Southampton University, England, 1982, Springer-Verlag, Berlin, 1982.

4 Brebbia, C. A., Telles, J., and L. Wrobel, Boundary Elements - Theory and Application in Engineering, Springer-Verlag, New York, 1983.

CHAPTER SIXTEEN

IMPACT OF NEW COMPUTING SYSTEMS ON FINITE ELEMENT COMPUTATIONS

A. K. Noor, O. O. Storaasli and R. E. Fulton
NASA Langley Research Center
Hampton, Virginia

ABSTRACT

Recent advances in computer technology that are likely to impact finite element computations are reviewed. The characteristics of supersystems, highly parallel systems, and small systems (mini and microcomputers) are summarized. The interrelations of numerical algorithms and software with parallel architectures are discussed. A scenario is presented for future hardware/software environment and finite element systems. A number of research areas which have high potential for improving the effectiveness of finite element analysis in the new environment are identified.

1. INTRODUCTION

The last two decades have witnessed an explosive growth in computer technology. This growth shows no sign of abating; all the indications are that the changes during the next decades will prove to be even greater, particularly with the introduction of novel forms of machine architecture (e.g., vector, array, and multiprocessor systems). The computer hardware developments are most noticeable at the two extremes of the spectrum. At one end, the large expensive computer systems, usually referred to as supersystems, such as CRAY-1S, CDC CYBER 205 and Denelcor HEP1 have radically different and novel architectures resulting in very high performance (computational speed of the order of 100 million floating-point operations per second (100 MFLOPS) or more). At the other end of the spectrum are the various types of minicomputers, desktop (or micro) computers, microprocessors and hand-held computers.

The introduction of these new computing systems has made a strong impact on finite element technology. The large supersystems have made possible new levels of sophistication in finite element modeling as well as in problem depth and scope which were not possible before. More importantly, however, the new supersystems have opened up a view of the next steps to be taken in the development of finite element analysis software/hardware systems. In order to realize the full potential of the supersystems in finite element computation special parallel numerical algorithms, programming strategies and programming languages need to be developed.

The small, low-cost computer systems (mini and microcomputers) provided a high degree of interactivity and freed the finite element analysts from the constraints that are often imposed on them by large centralized computation centers.

However, the effectiveness of the small computers for solving large-scale finite element problems is limited. The combination of a fast attached processor with a mini (or micro) computer into a dual-processor system can extend the range of finite element problems that can effectively be solved by the minicomputer. In recent years several general-purpose finite element programs have been made operational on the minicomputers and new finite element software is currently being developed for microcomputers.

The objectives of the present chapter are: a) to discuss key finite element requirements placed on evolving computer technology; b) to summarize some of the developments in computing systems during recent past and near-term future and relate these developments to finite element technology; and c) to outline the likely directions of finite element software/hardware systems over the next five to ten years.

A number of previous attempts have been made to predict the characteristics of future finite element systems and the impact of the advances in computing systems on finite element analysis (see, for example, Refs. 1 to 7). The discussion presented herein is much more detailed than that given in the cited references because the authors feel that engineers need to become familiar with the characteristics of the new computing systems in order to realize their full potential in advanced analysis methods in general, and in finite element computations in particular.

2. TECHNICAL NEEDS FOR ENGINEERING COMPUTATIONS

The driving force for future developments in engineering computations will continue to be the need for improved productivity and cost-effective engineering systems. To achieve this goal, the following sets of technical needs can be identified:

1) Expanding the scope of engineering problems considered. This includes examination of more complex physical phenomena (e.g., progressive failure of fibrous composite structures); study of interaction phenomena (as would be required in the hydrodynamic/structural coupling in deep sea mining and the thermal/control/structural coupling in space exploration); and the prediction of the reliability of the model's performance to uncertainties in its input parameters. Such reliability-based analysis can help in making rational design decisions and in achieving realistic cost/performance trade-offs.

2) Development of a hierarchy of models, algorithms and procedures for engineering systems. Simplified and specialized models and algorithms are appropriate for use in the preliminary and conceptual design phases and more sophisticated models are used in the detailed design phase.

3) Development of effective integrated design, synthesis and evaluation tools to support all phases of product development including the design, management and manufacturing cycle.

4) Continued reduction of cost and/or time for obtaining solutions to engineering design/analysis problems.

The hardware and software requirements to meet the aforementioned technical needs include:

a) a spectrum of available computer capabilities ranging from high-performance computing systems for large complex problems to low-cost workstations which provide convenient computer capabilities at the engineer's desk.

b) distributed asynchronous processors which carry out several different calculations in parallel using the same or different code and referencing the same or different databases.

c) user-friendly hardware interface or engineering workstation with the following capabilities: high-speed graphics; high-speed long distance communication; and verbal (audio) as well as visual interfaces.

d) artificial intelligence-based expert systems, incorporating the experience and expertise of practitioners, to aid in the modeling of the engineering system, the adaptive refinement of the model, and the selection of the appropriate algorithm and procedure used in the solution.

e) powerful engineering database management system.

Beginning in 1960, the number of components on a chip has increased, more or less, exponentially with time. For the case when no differentiation is made between logic and memory the progression is shown in Fig. 2.

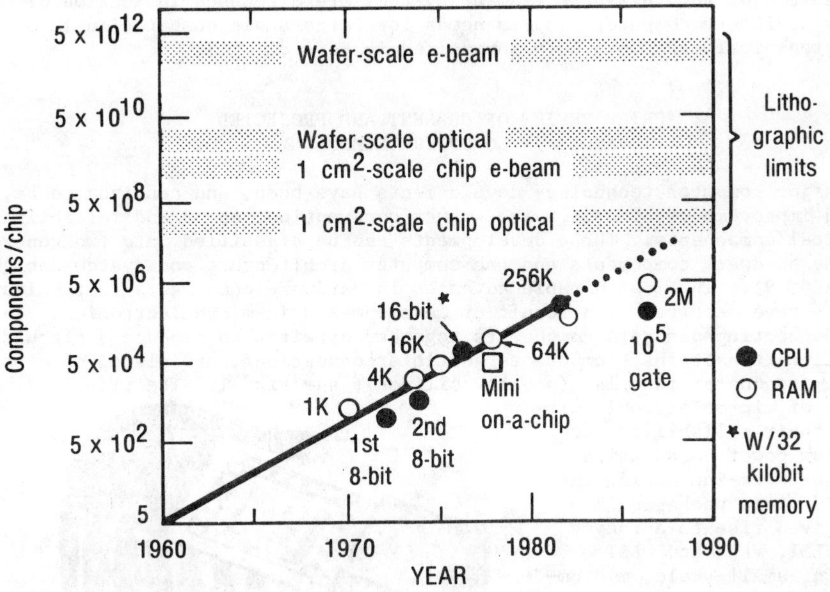

Figure 2 - Digital logic capability commercially available on a single chip (based on a report by A. C. Haussmann, Lawrence Livermore National Lab.).

The full range of hardware components (computer building blocks) are now available on microelectronic chips; these include memory units, addressing units (i.e., counters and decoders) and complete central processing units (CPU) called microprocessors; and even complete microcomputers (which include the CPU, memory, and input/output functions all residing on a single chip). Significant architectural advances resulted from imaginative ways of configuring these basic blocks.

The net effect of the aforementioned developments has been a significant decrease in the cost of performing computations. This is illustrated in Fig. 3

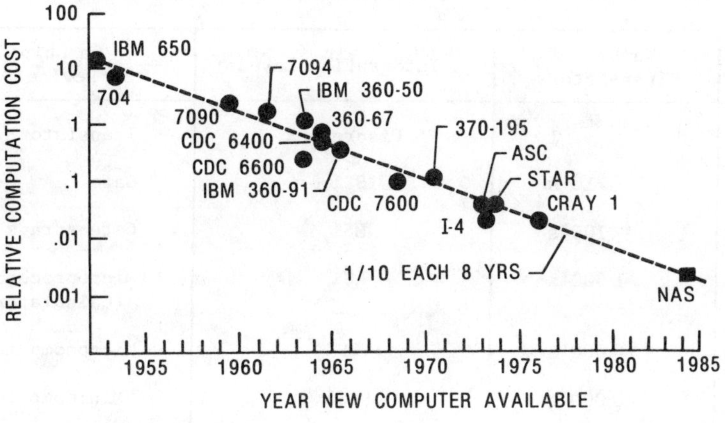

Figure 3 - Trend of relative computation cost (Ref. 10).

f) turnkey engineering-application software systems which have advanced modeling and analysis capabilities and are easy to learn and use.

The implication of these requirements on finite element technology along with a scenario of future finite element systems are discussed in Section 6. An assessment of future computer-systems needs for large-scale computation in a number of technical areas has been summarized in Ref. 8.

3. BRIEF REVIEW OF CURRENT AND PROJECTED ADVANCES IN COMPUTER TECHNOLOGY

The major computer technology developments have been, and continue to be, focused on improvements of cost, size, power consumption, speed and reliability of electrical components. These developments can be classified into two general areas: the hardware components and the computer architecture and system design methods (Ref. 9). The most notable advances in hardware components in the last two decades have occurred as a result of developments in microelectronics. Instead of connecting discrete components together by wires to produce a circuit, complete circuit patterns, components and interconnections, are placed on a small chip of semiconductor material (usually silicon); see Fig. 1. The principal advantages of microelectronic circuits are their reliability, low cost and low power consumption. The trend of ever-increasing the number of devices packaged on a chip has given rise to acronyms SSI, MSI, LSI, VLSI and ULSI standing for small-scale, medium-scale, large-scale, very large-scale and ultra large-scale integration, respectively. The beginning time frame for each of these technologies along with the chip density ranges are listed in Table 1.

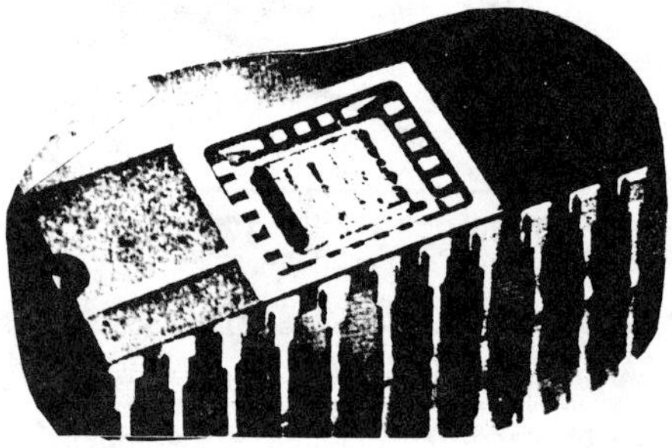

Figure 1 - Silicon chip.

Table 1 - Semiconductor developments (based on copyright information by Integrated Computer Systems - Santa Monica, California)

Date	Number of Transistors	Integration Level	On Chip Device
1960	1	Discrete	Transistor
1964	10's	SSI	Gate
1968	100's	MSI	Gate Arrays
1972	1 000's	LSI	Microprocessors (Calculators)
1976	10 000's	VLSI	Microcomputers
1980	100 000's	ULSI	"Minicomputers"
1984	1 000 000's	ULSI	"Computers"

where it can be seen that the cost of performing a given calculation has decreased by a factor of ten every eight years (Ref. 10).

In the present and succeeding section the major advances in hardware components are reviewed and some of the new computing systems are briefly described. The survey given here is by no means complete or exhaustive; the intention is to concentrate primarily on those developments which have had, or promise to have, the greatest impact on the manner in which finite element computations are performed. Discussion is focused on semiconductor technology; processor speed; memory organization, secondary storage devices; access facilities and user interface; and networking.

3.1 Semiconductor Technology

The predominant semiconductor material in use to date is silicon. Better understanding of this material as well as better processing, tooling and packaging techniques enabled the design of fast dense circuitry. Current semiconductor technologies fall into two categories (Ref. 11):

a. Logic made from bipolar transistors which are current controlled. Three classes of Logic can be identified in this category; namely, Transistor-Transistor Logic (TTL); Emitter Coupled Logic (ECL); and Integrated Injection Logic (I^2L). The first is used in SSI and MSI. The second is suitable for LSI and the third is good for VLSI.

b. Logic made from field effect transistors (FET) which are voltage controlled. A number of classes can be distinguished within this group including metal-oxide semiconductor (MOS); complementary MOS usually referred to as CMOS; and MOS devices fabricated in silicon grown on sapphire SOS/MOS. The logic circuit integration level attainable by each of the aforementioned technologies is depicted in Fig. 4.

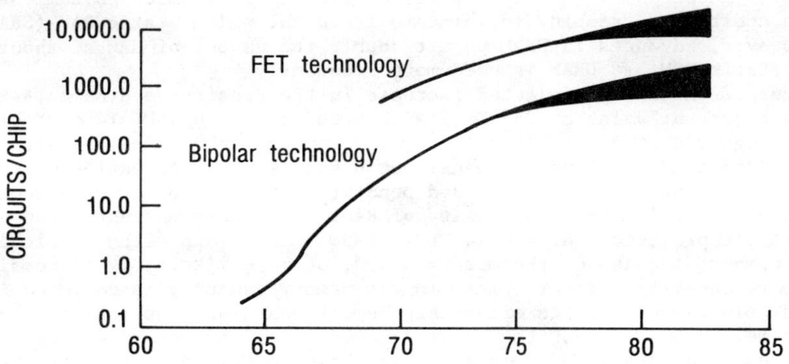

Figure 4 - Logic circuits integration level (Ref. 9).

Current research is directed towards: a) shrinking of conductor and device dimensions (scaling) to micron and submicron dimensions (Ref. 12); and b) increasing the speed of logic circuits (to achieve a machine cycle time of the order of one nanosecond (1×10^{-9} second) - Ref. 13).

The first objective can be accomplished by using recent and improved lithography tools (including optical, electron beams, UV optics, direct-write electron beam, X-ray, and ion beam techniques). Two candidate technologies are likely to achieve the second objective of ultra-fast logic circuits. These technologies are: a) FET technology using gallium arsenide (GaAs), a component semiconductor material instead of silicon; and b) using Josephson Junction devices which consist of sandwiches of insulating oxides between two strips of superconducting metals. Heat dissipation is still an important limitation with gallium arsenide. Josephson Junctions, with several orders of magnitude less power dissipation, essentially remove this limitation. However, their drawback is the intense cryostatic environment (4^oK above absolute zero) required for the operation of these devices.

3.2 Memory

Memory is the most advancing technology in microelectronics. Recent progress include developments of an entire hierarchy of addressable memories, and of high-speed, random access chips with many bits of data. Each level in the hierarchy represents an order of magnitude decrease in access speed, and several orders of magnitude increase in capacity, for the same cost. The techniques of splitting and interleaving among various types of memory hierarchies in individual systems have changed some of the basic concepts of computing itself. Instead of just a few registers in the central processing unit (CPU) and a single-level memory, a typical machine may now have:

a) a number of high-speed, general-purpose registers
b) a cache memory for very rapid access to small amounts of data or instructions
c) standard central or equivalent memory
d) extended memory, directly addressable, but at a lower speed
e) hardware-implemented virtual memory, extending the amount of addressable space.

Initially, memories were based on bipolar transistor technology. However, by 1980 MOS technology accounted for over 80 percent of the semiconductor memory market. CMOS devices are becoming increasingly important because of their lower power requirements.

There are several types of semiconductor memories. These include Random Access and Read Only memories. In Random Access Memory (RAM), data can be written into or read out of any storage location in random fashion without regard to its physical location relative to other storage locations. Read Only Memory (ROM), contains a permanent data pattern stored during the manufacture of the semiconductor chip in the form of transistors at each storage location that are either operable or inoperable. RAM can be either static or dynamic. Dynamic RAM (DRAM) requires constant refreshing to maintain its data, which static RAM (SRAM) does not. However, advances in DRAM permit double the amount of RAM at about the same cost as static RAM, so DRAM is used more frequently.

Figure 2 shows the projected increase in the density of dynamic RAM chips from their current value of 256 K bits (256,000 bits) to 4 MB (4×10^6 bits) in 1990 on roughly a linear scale. These improvements take place by factors of four merely by reducing the linear dimensions in half in each direction which results in one quarter the area with an added benefit of reduced power requirements.

The increase in the chip density of RAM, from their current value of 256 K bits to their projected value of 4 MB in 1990, can be exploited by either reducing the number of chips on the memory board, or more likely, by increasing the user-memory capacity. The increase in the memory capacity is depicted in Fig. 5 for hand-held computers with eight-chip memory board and desktop computers with 128-chip memory board. For the sake of comparison, the memory capacity of the current and planned supersystems are also shown in Fig. 5. The data presented in Fig. 5 is based on projections made in the current electronics literature. The impact of increased memory for finite element analysis in the future is quite significant since memory capacity directly translates to increased problem size capability. Developments with low power complementary metal oxide semiconductor (CMOS) memory and higher speed gallium arsenide instead of silicon, promise additional benefits for specialized applications. However, for most applications, dynamic RAM in high densities is expected to be of major benefit to finite element analysts since it will permit larger problems to be solved at reduced cost.

3.3 Processor Speed and New Architectures

The advances in microprocessor miniaturization allow several dozen layers (miniature buildings) in a single microprocessor CPU chip with hundreds of thousands of equivalent transistors on each layer. In addition to more compact CPU chips, the speed at which they are capable of operating will continue to increase. This is important to finite element computations since the clock speed at which microprocessors can operate is directly proportional to the number of floating point operations possible per second (the speed of computation). Early

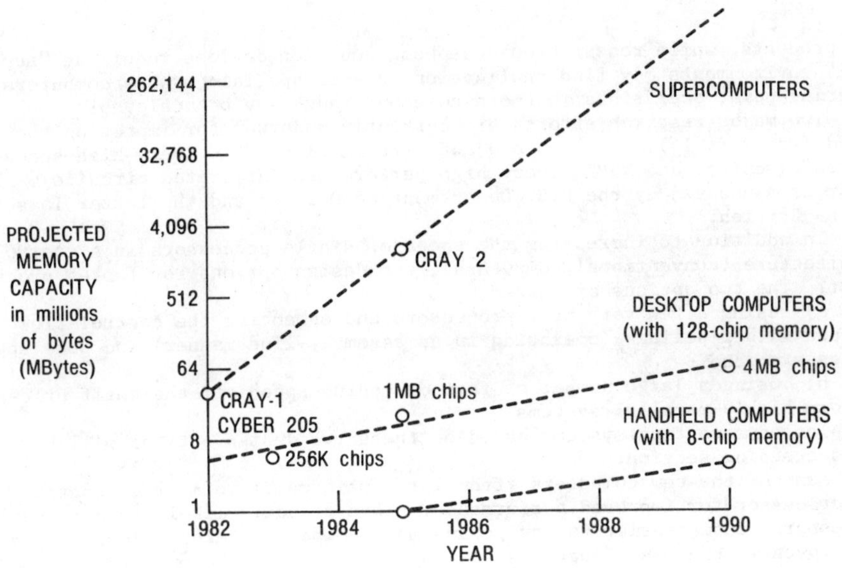

Figure 5 - Projected computer memory based on chip density increases.

microprocessors had a clock speed of 1 MHz, which increased to 12 MHz in current microprocessors and, based on current projections in the electronics literature, future speeds of over 50 MHz are expected (Fig. 6). The increase in the clock

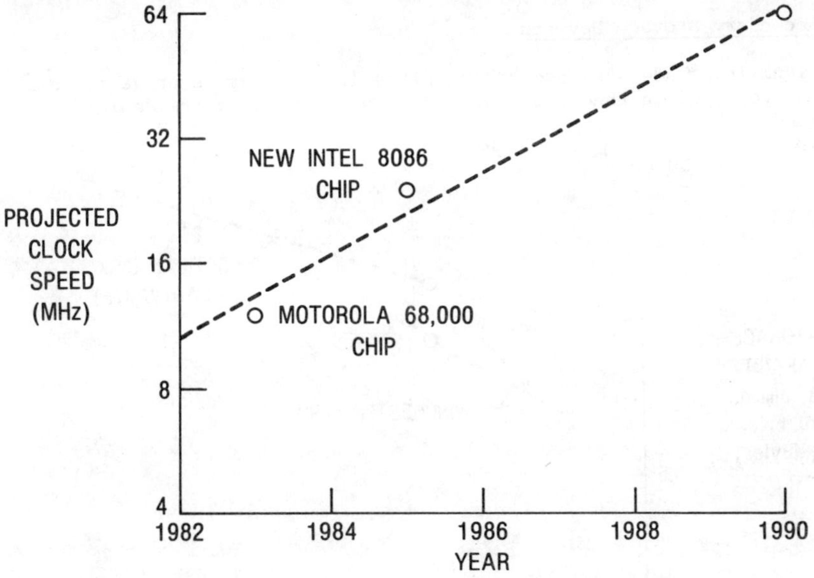

Figure 6 - Projected clock speed of CPU chips.

speed, measured in MHz, directly affects the throughput of engineering calculations measured in terms of the number of floating-point operations per second (FLOPS). The use of new materials such as gallium arsenide circuits in CPU chips is also expected to increase the CPU speed significantly. The impact of VLSI is likely to continue to play the most dominant role for immediate application in new products, while research on Josephson Junction devices requiring "super-cool" environments may find application to some special-purpose computers where floating-point operations in the nanosecond range may be achievable.

Two major research efforts are currently underway for improving the processor speed (see Ref. 14). The two projects are labeled VHSIC (very high-speed integrated circuits) and VHPIC (very high-performance integrated circuits). The first is sponsored by the U.S. Department of Defense and the latter is supported by the British.

In addition to increasing the speed of single processors in a control-flow architecture (conventional computers), two design options for faster processing exist. The two options are based on:

a) using a few very fast processors and enhancing the control-flow architecture with pipelines (operating in an assembly-line manner) and some specialized processors; and

b) using a large number of fast or medium-speed off-the-shelf processors to form highly-parallel systems.

Examples of computing systems based on these two design options will be given in the succeeding section.

Many of the new computers (from large mainframes to micros) contain more than one processor for improved performance. This trend is likely to continue as processors become easier to design and more compact. Before microprocessor CPUs were invented the most laborious part of developing new computers was the signal, backplane and digital component wiring of a multiboard CPU. Now that the CPU is on a VLSI chip and associated chips are available for memory management, input/output and other functions formerly taking up one or more boards, the entire CPU and associated functions are being condensed to one board with additional boards for memory. In the case of microcomputers, all functions including memory are reduced to a single board. It is expected that the majority of computers in the future will be single-board computers or if additional boards are required they will be for memory or peripheral controller functions only.

3.4 Secondary Storage Devices

Significant advances are taking place in secondary storage technology. The advances reported in the literature for disk technology are depicted in Fig. 7.

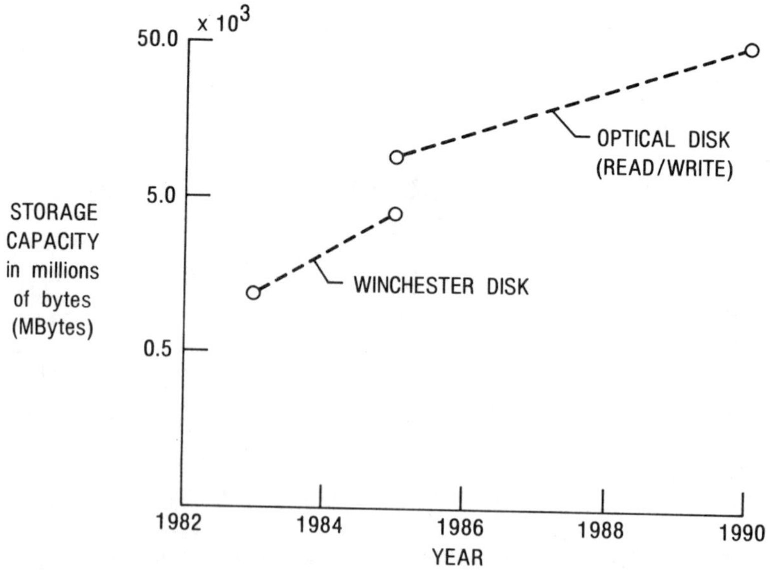

Figure 7 - Projected disk storage capacity.

While the conventional hard disks (Winchester disks) are increasing in density of storage (currently in excess of 1 Gigabyte (1×10^9 bytes)) and floppy disks are approaching 1 MByte, the optical disk promises to make the most dramatic impact on computer secondary storage. For example, the capability to read and write rapidly and inexpensively 20 Gigabytes (i.e., 20 billion characters) of data (equivalent to the contents of the Encyclopedia Britanica) promises to provide an attractive and cost-effective storage for large volumes of data in relatively long-term project files typically used for multidisciplinary design projects. The future architectures promise to offer specialized hardware (e.g., chips) for fast floating-point calculations, interactive graphics, algebraic manipulation, input/output processing, and most other standard procedures, eventually including finite element analysis on silicon or gallium arsenide chips.

3.5 User-Interface Hardware and Software

A great deal of effort is currently taking place to improve the productivity of the analyst by developing user-friendly software and hardware interfaces. More finite element software systems are becoming "turnkey" with defaults built-in, and with simple menu options. Future menu options are likely to be controlled by lightpen, voice or mouse (which is an advanced user-friendly capability for accessing the system - first introduced for the Apple Lisa microcomputer). The finite element model can be generated by using either one of the geometric modeling software packages or a CAD system. The model data can be changed whenever desired via voice or mouse.

3.6 Distributed Computing and Networking

The first large-scale computer network, the ARPANET, was initiated in the mid-sixties. The major objective of this network was to explore the possibilities and implications of large-scale distributed computing, where the analyst at one location could have direct access to computing facilities and/or databases at another, remote location. This initial work has pointed the way to the feasibility and practicality of distributed computing. However, a tremendous amount of work remains to be done in developing uniform protocols, standard control structures and uniform data description standards before distributed computing can be done routinely on a large scale. When these problems are solved, as they undoubtedly will be, many applications and extensions of distributed computing will take place. For example, distributed computing can be recursively applied to component subtasks according to a number of criteria.

Two recent developments will greatly enhance distributed computing. The first is the widescale availability of engineering workstations (personal and desktop computers), and the second is new communication technology based on packet switching, which has already emerged. In this technology information is transmitted in packets, typically a few hundred bytes. This is the first communication technology geared to data transmission and is likely to permit economic implementation of distributed computing. The coupling of digital networking with the existing telephone and PBX exchange systems promises to offer access to a wide range of data and central computers via desktop workstations.

4. MAJOR FEATURES OF NEW COMPUTING SYSTEMS

Because of the rapid progress made in recent years in semiconductor technology, a number of novel forms of computer architectures have emerged. In order to put the new computer architectures in proper perspective, a classification of computing systems is needed. Several classifications have been proposed in the literature based on the mode of processing instructions and data; and the mode of interaction between different processors (see, for example, Ref. 11). One of the earliest and most commonly-used classifications is that introduced by Flynn (Ref. 15), and is based on how the machine relates its instructions to the data being processed. A stream is defined as a sequence of items (instructions or data) as executed or operated on by a processor.

Four broad classes can be identified according to whether the instruction or data streams are single or multiple (Fig. 8):

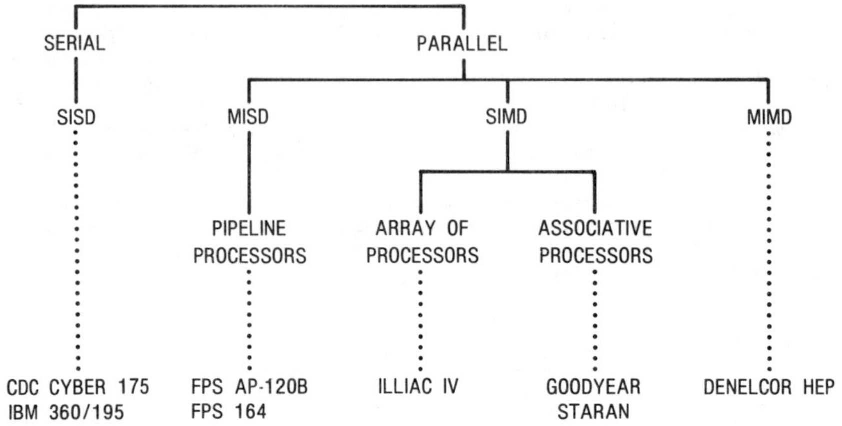

Figure 8 - Classification of computing systems.

1. Single instruction stream/single data stream (SISD) machines. These include the conventional serial computers which execute instructions sequentially, one at a time.

2. Single instruction stream/multiple data stream (SIMD) machines. These are computers that have a single control unit, a collection of identical processors (or processing elements), a memory or memories, and an interconnection network which allows processors to exchange data. An example of an SIMD machine is depicted in Fig. 9. During execution of a program the central control unit (CU) fetches and decodes the instructions and then broadcasts control to the processing elements. Each processor performs the same instruction sequences, but uses different data. These operations are usually referred to as *lockstep operations*.

3. Multiple instruction stream/single data stream (MISD) machines. There is some disagreement on the computers belonging to this classification. The various pipeline (or vector) processors, which segment computations into consecutive stations, are possible candidates of this class (Ref. 17). However, in many computer science publications pipeline processors are classified as SIMD machines. In pipeline processors, the basic arithmetic operations are broken up into a set of elementary steps which, when performed in series, achieve the desired operation. Each elementary step is then implemented into hardware and the resulting arithmetic unit operates as a production (or assembly) line called the pipeline.

4. Multiple instruction stream/multiple data stream (MIMD) machines. These are computers which contain a number of *interconnected processors*, each of which is programmable and can execute its own instructions. The instructions for each processor can be the same or different. The processors operate on a shared memory (or memories), generally in an asynchronous manner. The interconnection between processors distinguishes an MIMD machine from a set of independent computers (see Fig. 9). The computers of the MIMD class are the most general of all new computers and include all forms of multiprocessor configurations, from linked mainframe computers to large arrays of microprocessors. However, the increased flexibility is at the cost of increased synchronization, overhead, and programming complexity.

Examples of computing systems which belong to each of the four classes are given in Fig. 8.

In this section, the major features of some of the new computing systems which can have a strong impact on finite element computations are reviewed. For convenience, the computing systems considered are divided into five groups:

a) supersystems;
b) highly-parallel systems;
c) finite element machines;
d) small systems; and,
e) attached processors.

The first group consists of the general-purpose machines with very-high throughput performance. The machines of the second group achieve high performance through extensive use of LSI, VLSI and ULSI memory chip technology. Finite element machines are a subclass of the highly parallel systems and are discussed separately because of their high potential for cost-effective, large-scale finite element computations. The small systems considered include the various minicomputers, engineering workstations, microcomputers (e.g., desktop and hand-held personal computers). The attached processors are fast backend computers which, when combined with the minicomputers (or the micros), can extend the range of the finite element problems that are solved effectively on these small systems. Some of the computing systems considered herein are commercially available, others are still research tools aimed at achieving high performance and/or low-cost computations.

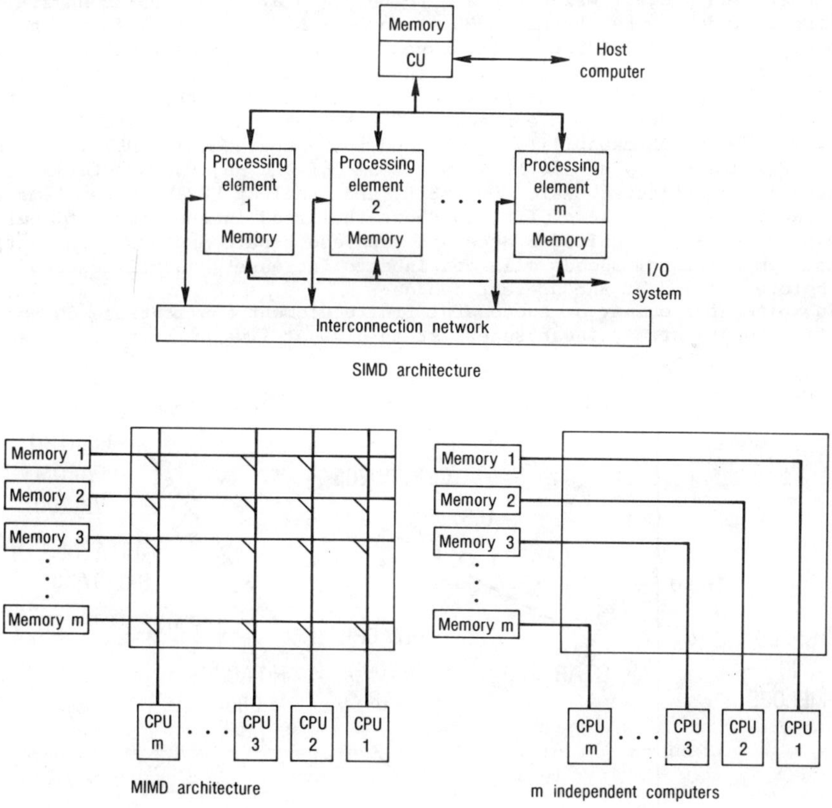

Figure 9 - Block diagrams for SIMD, MIMD architectures and m independent computers (Ref. 16).

4.1 Supersystems

Supersystems are a class of general-purpose computers designed for extremely high throughput performance. The three major characteristics of supersystems are (see Ref. 18):

a) high computational speeds (or the order of 50 MFLOPS or more);

b) large main (or central) memory (with a capacity of 8 MBytes or more); and,

c) fast and large secondary memory with a sophisticated memory management system.

The development of supersystems now spans two generations. The first generation included the array of processors ILLIAC IV (SIMD machine); and the pipeline (or vector) computers CDC STAR-100 and Texas Instruments Advanced Scientific Computer (ASC). The second generation supersystems used a hybrid combination of pipeline and array processors to achieve computational speeds in excess of 100 MFLOPS. Examples of these supersystems are the CRAY-1S; the CRAY X-MP; the CDC CYBER 205; and the Denelcor Heterogeneous Element Processor (HEP1). The latter is the only general-purpose commercial MIMD machine built. As of July 1983, there are 51 CRAY-1, 2 CRAY X-MP, 18 CYBER 205 and 7 Denelcor HEP1 installed. The next generation of supersystems currently under design include CRAY 2 (successor to CRAY 1 with planned delivery in 1985); CDC CYBER 2XX (1986), Denelcor HEP2 (1986); the Japanese supersystems: Hitachi S-810/20 (1984), FUJITSU FACOM VP-200 (1985); the Japanese Super-Speed Computer Project aimed at developing a machine with peak performance of 10 GigaFLOPS (1989); the Japanese fifth generation project which appears to be aimed at establishing an artificial intelligence industry by the mid 1990's; and the NASA Numerical Aerodynamic Simulation capability (NAS). The latter's goal is to perform most calculations required for new aircraft, thereby improving technical insight and significantly reducing wind tunnel and flight testing. It is estimated that by 1984 a NAS capability will be built with a speed of 250 MFLOPS and a high-speed memory of 64 M. words. The NAS capability is planned to be upgraded in 1987 to a speed of 1 GigaFLOP and a memory of 256 M. words. Some of the major characteristics of the current and projected CRAY, CDC CYBER, and Denelcor HEP1 supersystems are summarized in Table 2. Also, Fig. 10 shows the trend in the computational speeds provided by the United States and Japanese supercomputers. Indications are that computational speeds will continue to increase, and will exceed 10 GigaFLOPS before the end of the present decade.

In spite of a number of successful finite element applications on the first-generation supersystems, these supersystems did not live up to their expectations

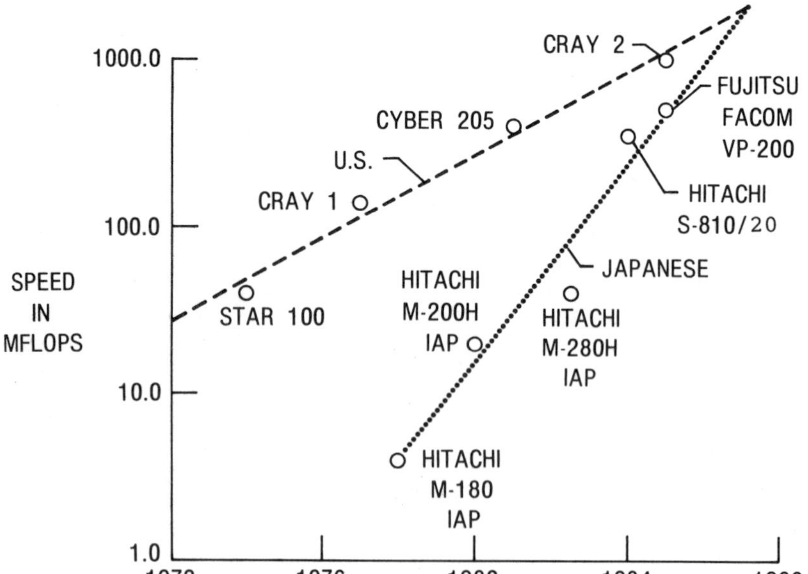

Figure 10 - Trends in computing speeds for U.S. and Japanese supercomputers.

Table 2 - Architectural features of some of the current and projected supercomputers

	CRAY			CDC CYBER*		Denelcor** HEP1
	1 S	X-MP	2	203	205-444	
Maximum memory capacity (words)	4 M.	4 M.	256 M.	2 M.	4 M.	16 M. program memory 128 M. data memory
Maximum high-speed auxiliary memory capacity (words)	32 M.	32 M.	?	-	-	-
Virtual memory	No	No	No	Yes up to 4×10^{12} words	Yes up to 2×10^{12} words	-
Memory word length (bits)	64	64	64	64/32 (half word)	64/32 (half word)	64
Clock period (ns)	12.5	9.5	4.0	40.0 for vectors 20.0 for scalars	20.0	100/16
Estimated speed (MFLOPS)	150	400	1000	50	400	160 (10 MFLOPS per processor)
Technology chip type	4 chip types	1 chip type	?	40 chip types	29 chip types	
Logic family	SSI/ECL with 1 ns gate delay	SSI/ECL with 750 p.sec. gate delay	SSI/ECL with 650 p.sec. gate delay	LSI/ECL bipolar circuitry for the scalar unit	LSI/ECL bipolar circuitry	SSI/ECL MOS memory
Other features	1 CPU (dedicated for arithmetic operations)	2 CPU's	4 CPU's	2 vector pipelines	1-4 vector pipelines	up to 16 PEMS

*CDC CYBER 2XX (1986) will use very high density CMOS circuitry and multiple pipelines.
**Denelcor HEP2 (1986) is expected to have a speed of 1 GigaFLOP.

in large-scale finite element computations. This is because the ILLIAC IV operated efficiently *only* when performing an identical operation over an entire array, and the STAR-100 operated efficiently *only on long vectors*.

On the other hand, the second generation supersystems achieve reasonable performance with scalar and short-vector computations. Nonetheless, the efficient use of these supersystems in large-scale finite element calculations requires new ways of structuring the finite element procedure, new algorithms, and new software tools. Direct conversion of finite element programs from sequential computers does not realize the full potential of these supersystems (Ref. 19). A number of large-scale finite element programs have already been installed on the CRAY-1 computer. These include ANSYS, ASAS, ASKA, EISI-EAL, MARC, MSC/NASTRAN, PAFEC 75, and STAGS.

4.2 Highly Parallel Systems

The demand for greater performance than can be provided by circuit speed alone, coupled with the advances made in the design and fabrication of VLSI circuits have led to the introduction of parallelism in a number of new computing systems. Parallelism refers to the ability to overlap or perform simultaneously many of the tasks performed by the computer (e.g., memory fetch or store, arithmetic or logical operation and I/O operation). There are four principal ways of introducing parallelism into the architecture of computers, namely (Ref. 11):

a) Pipelining. Based on the application of assembly-line techniques to improve the performance of an arithmetic or control unit.

b) Functional. Through providing several independent units or performing different operations such as logic, addition or multiplication, and allowing these units to operate simultaneously on different data.

c) Array. By using an array of identical processors under common control, all performing the same operation simultaneously on different data.

d) Multiprocessing. Based on the use of several asynchronous processors, each obeying its own instructions, with some mechanisms for interprocessor communication, and local and global control.

Highly-parallel systems composed of a large number of computing elements can be classified into the following groups (Ref. 20):

- o Multiple special-purpose functional units;
- o Associative processors;
- o Array of processors
- o Multiprocessors (with multiple CPUs); and,
- o Data flow processors.

For their specific tasks, multiple special-purpose functional units are the fastest, but they are the least general. They can be designed for almost 100 percent hardware efficiency (in the sense that a large percentage of the hardware is in use at any given time) and require little or no software to perform their unique tasks. In comparison with the multiple special-purpose functional units, the other machines are more general. However, the more general the machine is, the lower the hardware efficiency (in the sense described above), and the more complicated the software needed is likely to get.

Examples of the aforementioned machine types are given subsequently. Note that to date there is no truly general-purpose parallel architecture to which all algorithms can be effectively mapped.

a. Multiple Special-Purpose Functional Units. These are useful for performing computationally intensive basic mathematical operations such as matrix multiplication and solution of linear algebraic equations. An example of these machines is provided by *systolic arrays* in which high-level computations are directly mapped into hardware structures. Systolic arrays are based on the principle of replacing a single processing element (cell) by an array of processing elements (cells), in order to achieve a high computational throughput without having to increase the memory bandwidth (Ref. 21). This is depicted in Fig. 11.

In a systolic system data flows from the computer memory in a regular fashion, passing through many processing elements with built-in hardware instructions before it returns to memory. Currently available systolic arrays have four basic characteristics, namely:

- o They involve only few types of simple cells.
- o Data and control flows are simple and regular.
- o Algorithms used support high degrees of pipelining and parallelism.
- o Each input data item is used in a multiplicative and effective manner.

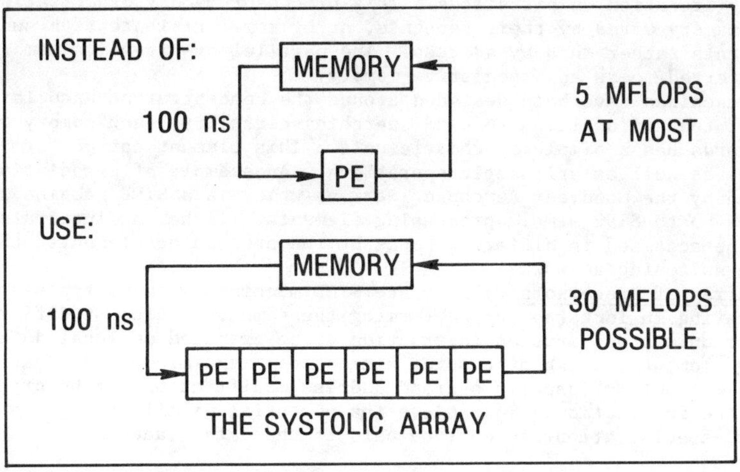

Figure 11 - Basic principle of a systolic system (Ref. 21).

A list of prototype realizations of systolic arrays for various algorithms is given in Ref. 22. Potential applications of systolic arrays for finite element computations are discussed in Refs. 23 and 24.

b. Associative Processors. In these processors parallelism is introduced in the memory organization by using the bit-slice scheme. This is depicted in Fig. 12 for a w word memory with word width b. In conventional computers, access

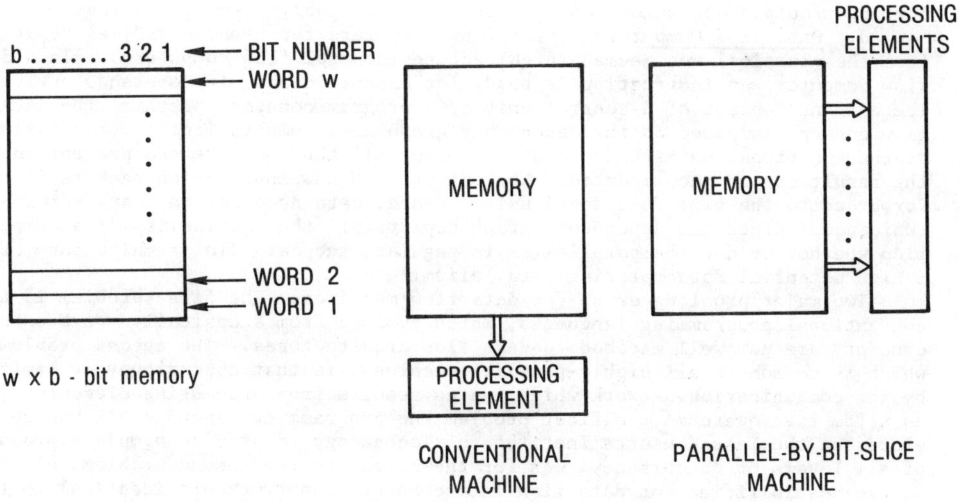

Figure 12 - Conventional and parallel-by-bit-slice machines.

is restricted to sets of b bits which form a word, no other set of b bits can usually be accessed in parallel. On the other hand, in the bit-slice parallel computers, the memory slice accessed consists of s bits, with only one bit from each word (Ref. 11). This structure is orthogonal to that of the conventional machines, or would be if s were equal to w. In general, s will be very large, measured in thousands. Since one bit of any memory word is available on one access, it is possible to search the whole memory simultaneously for specified contents by iteration on bit slices. This processor-memory organization is used to select memory words by their contents, or by some attribute of a subfield of their contents rather than by address. The parallel by-bit-slice memory is usually referred to as an associative memory.

Many machines have been designed around the concept of an associative memory, except that in addition to data searching circuitry, each memory word or group of words has a simple arithmetic unit. This element can perform numerical comparisons as well as arithmetic operations. An example of associative machines is provided by the Goodyear Aerospace Staran, which is a SIMD machine which can accommodate up to 8192 simple processing elements. It has an integrated memory which may be accessed in different modes by the processing elements, through a multistage switching network.

c. Array of Processors. These are SIMD machines with multiple arithmetic units operating in lockstep and performing the same operation on different data. The control unit broadcasts an instruction to be executed on local data by all processing elements. Each processing element can make minor modifications to the broadcast instruction (usually operand address modification) or be programmed to ignore the instruction. To achieve the potential parallelism of an array of processors, special attention must be paid to the data placement and algorithm design.

Machines built of array of processors can be distinguished by the following characteristics:

- Number of processors;
- Number of memory banks;
- Form of communication network; and,
- Form of local and global control.

Examples of machines built of array of processors are provided by ILLIAC IV and Goodyear Aerospace Massively Parallel Processor (MPP). The latter contains 16,384 single bit-serial processing elements connected in a square array (128 x 128) with strictly nearest-neighbor connections. It has a speed of 430 MFLOPS for 32-bit floating-point addition and 216 MFLOPS for multiplication. The input/output operations can be done simultaneously with processing.

d. Data Flow Computers. Data flow computers represent a radical departure from the classical von Neumann architecture (control flow computers). In a data flow computer, an instruction is ready for execution when its operands arrive. There is no concept of a control unit or a program counter. Rather, the data flow concept is based on the dependency graph of a computation. Operands flow to the functional units and operate whenever all the operands are present and the result can be accommodated. The output with new instruction packets is then forwarded to the next functional unit. Hence, data need not have any permanent residence. Since the dependency graph depicts all the parallelism of a computation whether or not the parallelism is regular, the data flow architecture offers a high potential for capturing parallelism.

Two major problems arise for data flow machines. The first problem is that conventional programming languages, which evolved from a basically von Neumann concept, are not well matched to data flow architectures. The second problem which is common to all highly-parallel machines, is that concurrency is limited by the communication network which routes results from processing elements. In an attempt to overcome the first problem the programming language VAL was developed at the Massachusetts Institute of Technology to provide simple expression of all levels of concurrency. As for the remedy to the second problem, all the viable possibilities for data flow interconnection network are identical to those of conventional multiprocessor structures.

Despite the aforementioned problems, data flow structures have high potential for use as attached processors to general-purpose computers.

e. Multiple Processors. Multiple processors are MIMD machines in which each processor is fully programmable and can execute its own program. Various classifications exist for these machines according to interprocessor communication (including the data transfer mode and the interconnection topology), and control (see Ref. 17). Multiprocessor systems can provide, at most, a linear speedup factor over single processors. That is, n processors, at best, can perform the same task as a single processor in 1/nth the time. However, there are a number of factors that can prevent the realization of linear speedup. They include the following:

o *Synchronization.* Performance can be lost if the algorithm requires the processors to be periodically coordinated.

o *Algorithm.* An algorithm designed for a serial computer might not expose all the parallelism present in the problem. Also, a parallel algorithm might require more computations than its serial counterpart to solve the same problem.

o *Contention.* Multiple processors vying for the same resource (e.g., shared variable) can slow down the execution of individual processors.

o *Input/Output Operations.* Traditional I/O structures cannot feed a high performance processor fast enough to avoid processor idle time.

Examples of multiple processor machines are provided by the NASA Langley finite element machine and the Cm* machine designed and built at Carnegie-Mellon University. The first will be discussed in the next section. The basic building block of the Cm* machine is a processor-memory pair called a computer module, or Cm. The memory local to a processor is also the shared memory in the system. Up to 14 Cm's are connected to a cluster. The cluster processors share a single bus and memory mapping processor. Clusters are connected via intercluster buses.

f. Other Highly-Parallel Architectures. Several highly-parallel architectures which do not fall in the previous categories have been designed and/or built. Most of these machines are research tools for advanced parallel architectures. A partial list of these machines is given subsequently (Ref. 14):

The Texas Reconfigurable Array Computer (TRAC) built at the University of Texas in Austin. It currently has four processors and nine memories. However, the design can be easily scaled up to many processors and memories. Because it is based on dynamically coupled processors, input/output units, and memories in a variety of configurations, TRAC can implement many different models of advanced architectures, i.e., the configuration can be changed to suit the structure of the problem.

The Blue CHiP (Configurable Highly-Parallel Computer) designed and built at Purdue University in West Lafayette, Indiana. It consists of a collection of homogeneous processing elements (PEs) placed at regular intervals in a lattice of programmable switches. Each PE is a computer with its own local memory. This architecture is targeted at wafer-scale implementation.

The Ultracomputer is a project at New York University which has, as yet, not been built. The highly-parallel MIMD machine aims to combine hundreds of thousands of small, relatively conventional processing elements, all using a large shared memory. Processors communicate with memory through a very high-bandwidth switching network which executes a few operations vital to very highly-parallel interprocess synchronization, in addition to its basic data-routing function.

g. Potential of Highly-Parallel Architectures for Finite Element Computations. In evaluating the impact of highly-parallel machines on finite element computations, it is useful to define two classes of problems and two distinct approaches to bringing the power of highly parallel machines to bear. The two classes of problems are:

o *Large-Scale Complicated Problems.* These are problems that are much too large to fit on any commercially available computer (e.g., number of unknowns in excess of one billion). Examples of these problems are large, three-dimensional turbulent eddy simulations of aerodynamic flows and large nonlinear interaction problems.

o *Medium-Scale Problems.* These are problems that can be solved on current supersystems (e.g., nonlinear problems with tens of thousands of unknowns). However, the cost of running them can be fairly high and, therefore, parametric studies cannot be made. Examples are provided by aerodynamic simulations of compressor- or turbine-blade flow fields and large nonlinear structural dynamic problems.

The most suitable approach for the first class of problems is based on using multiple processor machines with many processors. The interconnection between the processors must reflect both the geometry of the problem and the nature of the algorithms employed. A square grid of processors with only nearest-neighbor connections is the most obvious first choice.

The spatial allocation of processors involves mapping the different activities to be performed onto the processors of the system. With static mapping, the spatial allocation is fixed before the program execution begins. A variety of mapping schemes can be used such as one zone and/or one node per processor, or one row of nodes per processor. Adjacent zone computations can be mapped onto adjacent processors. As long as the size of the problem matches the size of the system, and the amount of computation per processor can be reasonably well equalized, this approach is quite attractive.

If, on the other hand, the program size and structure do not match the system size and structure, complete locality cannot be maintained. If resources are allocated dynamically, the assignment function must map operations which are likely to communicate onto nearby processors. This would greatly complicate the resourse allocation problem. The practical application of multiprocessor machines to large-scale problems requires the development of semiautomatic procedures to program a large amount of processors to perform similar but different tasks.

For the second class of problems, high throughput performance can be obtained by attaching multiple special-purpose functional units to a mainframe (or a supermini computer) through the use of a fast bus (or buses). These special-purpose functional units can be thought of as replacing many of the subroutines in a scientific software library. They could include linear algebra systolic array modules, a sparse matrix processor, and an inner product chip.

The major problem in the effective use of this approach is communication between the different devices. Much numerical analysis must be rethought in this architectural context. For example, higher-order temporal integration schemes and higher-order techniques for solution of nonlinear equations, requiring less data to drive them (at a cost of increased arithmetic), might be more attractive than lower-order methods.

4.3 The Finite Element Machine

The Finite Element Machine (FEM) is an MIMD computer being developed at NASA Langley Research Center as an experimental research tool with the goal of demonstrating the potential of using highly-parallel architectures for high-speed, yet low-cost solutions of finite element problems. Many aspects of finite element calculations are well suited to parallel computation (e.g., generation of elemental arrays, and iterative solution of global equations).

The NASA Langley Finite Element Machine, shown in Fig. 13, is designed to have 36 processors operating asynchronously in parallel and communicating via a local and a global bus. Currently, eight of the processors on the machine are operational. Each of the processors contain a 16-bit CPU, a special floating-point unit, 32K bytes of local RAM and 32K bytes of ROM. The ROM contains a special parallel operating system, termed NODAL EXEC together with a library of frequently-used Pascal-callable routines, termed PASLIB. Figure 13 shows that the FEM will house the 36 processors and a typical 16-bit CPU board (one of 108 boards). The controller of the array of processors is a minicomputer with 116 MBytes of disk storage, tape drive, and printer. The controller is accessed via terminals (both text and graphics) and can transfer data to and from a DEC VAX 11/780 supermini computer. Two strategies for exploiting parallelism are currently being explored using the eight-processor FEM (see Ref. 25): performing all the computations in parallel on the array of processors; and distributing the computations between the array of processors and the controller. In Ref. 26 the application of iterative algorithms to the solution of large sparse finite element equations on the finite element machine is examined.

The architecture of the FEM provides for nearest-neighbor connection as well as global connection which appears to have high potential for large-scale finite element applications including steady-state and transient response problems.

Recently other studies based on the Finite Element Machine concept have been made (see Refs. 27 and 28). In Ref. 27 the application of a Finite Element Machine concept to the generation and assembly of finite element stiffness

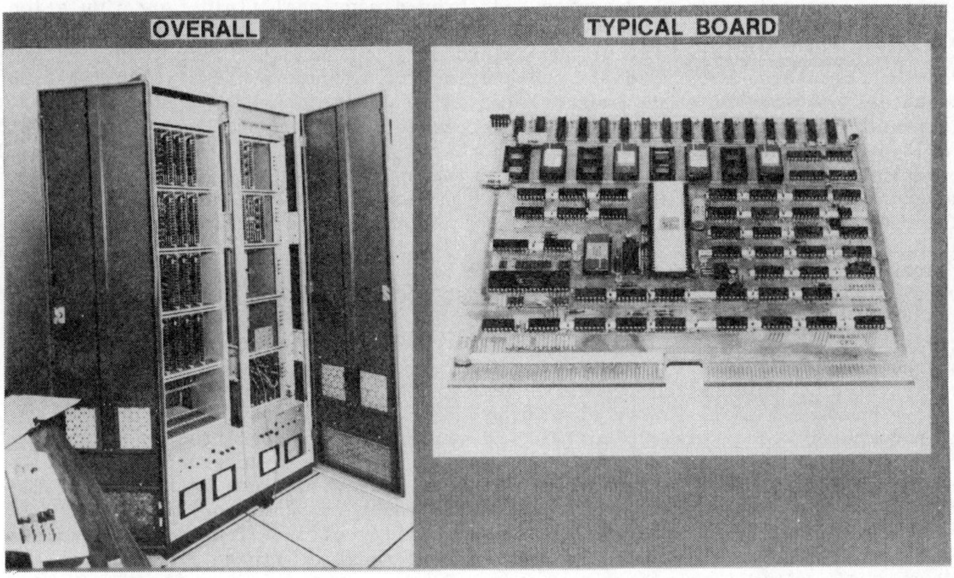

Figure 13 - Prototype NASA Langley FEM hardware.

matrices is described. The hardware used consisted of an IEEE-696 S-100 bus microcomputer with a 16-bit CPU and a master processor which controls and coordinates the activities of 8086/8087 VLSI chip set processors working in parallel. In Ref. 28 several parallel algorithms for the solution of the finite element equations are examined. On the basis of the results shown in Ref. 28, it appears that for computers with unlimited number of processors, the direct cyclic reduction algorithm is best suited, and for machines with limited number of parallel processors, both the direct Gauss factorization and the Jacobi-like iterative methods rank favorably.

4.4 Small Systems

To date a broad spectrum of low-cost small systems exist including hand-held computers (the micro micros - see Ref. 29), desktop computers, minicomputers and superminis. Several classifications have been attempted for these systems based on word length (8-bit, 16-bit and 32-bit machines), cost, amount of directly addressable memory, and computing speed (see, for example, Ref. 30). However, the dramatic increase in hardware capabilities of small systems coupled with the rapid reduction in cost make these classifications of questionable value. Herein, a brief discussion is given of the impact of minicomputers and microcomputers on finite element computations.

a. Minicomputers and Superminis. Minicomputers were introduced in the late 1960's as a new concept in decentralized computing. At first minicomputers were used only for pre- and postprocessing of finite element calculations. However, as minicomputers with larger address spaces and faster arithmetic appeared, a migration of finite element software to minicomputers started to take place, and with the emergence of the superminis having 32-bit word length, very large address spaces, and fast hardware or firmware for floating-point operations (e.g., the DEC VAX 11/780 and the PRIME 750), many of the large-scale finite element programs (e.g., ASKA, ANSYS, MARC, MSC/NASTRAN, and SPAR (predecessor of EISI-EAL)), were installed on the minicomputer (see, for example, Ref. 31).

Minicomputers provide user-friendly operational characteristics including interactive operating systems, local control over resources and turnaround, and high-speed graphics. However, currently available minicomputers (including the superminis) are considerably slower than mainframes, and therefore, their effectiveness is limited in solving large-scale finite element problems such as those encountered in crash dynamics and three-dimensional fluid-flow simulations (see Refs. 32 and 33).

b. Microcomputers. There now exists a large number of microcomputers and desktop computers, both portable and stationary. A partial list of the desktop computers and some of their characteristics is given in Ref. 34. The first generation of microcomputers had 8-bit processor chips and 64K bytes of RAM (a few 8-bit designs have increased the addressable RAM to 256K bytes). The second-generation machines are 16-bit machines with up to 1 Mbyte of RAM. They generally use one of three CPU chips (Ref. 35): the Intel 8088, Intel 8086, or the Motorola 68000. The Intel 8088 uses 16-bit architecture internally, but handles data on an 8-bit bus. By contrast, the 8086 is a 16-bit processor and, therefore, it is more powerful and faster because it transfers more data at one time. The Motorola 68000 which is the most powerful of the three, takes data on a 16-bit bus but does its processing internally 32 bits at a time. The third-generation microcomputers are likely to have 32-bit processor chips and over 16 Mbytes of addressable memory, and replace current superminis as engineering workstations. An example of such systems is the Apollo computer.

A number of small finite element programs have been developed for the microcomputers (see Refs. 36 to 40). If the program is segmented in order to reduce high-speed memory requirements, fairly large finite element problems can be solved on the microcomputer (see Ref. 36). However, since many large problems require 64-bit accuracy, it could be slow to run them on microcomputers with 8-bit or even 16-bit processors. The availability of 32-bit microcomputers such as the Apollo computer is likely to extend the range of finite element problems that can be solved by the microcomputer.

4.5 Attached Processors

For cost-effective computing a fast backend computer can be attached to a slower host minicomputer to achieve computational speeds comparable to those of large mainframes at a fraction of the cost of the mainframes. The fast computer is referred to as the attached processor. The dual-processor system consisting of the minicomputer and the attached processor can be used to extend the range of problems that can be solved effectively on the minicomputer. The dual processor arrangement is particularly useful for a small user community. Examples of attached processors include the floating point systems FPS AP-120B, AP-190L, and FPS-164, the CSPI MAP-300 and MAP-6400 series, and the recently announced ST-100 attached processor of the Star Technologies, Inc. While the first two have synchronous architecture, the next two have asynchronous multiple-bus architecture. Each of the FPS attached processors has the following features (Ref. 11):

- It is designed and accessed as a peripheral (i.e., like a tape drive) for a conventional host minicomputer, and it is intended to enhance the performance of the host in specific numerical computing tasks.
- It achieves high performance through both parallelism and pipelining.
- It includes an arithmetic section containing one adder and one multiplier capable of operating in parallel.
- It is not hardwired. Rather, it can be programmed by the user in FORTRAN or assembler language to perform a variety of computational tasks.

Parallelism is a major feature of the FPS attached processors that allows high-speed vector and matrix processing. In addition, the parallel structure of the attached processors allows the overhead of loop indexing, array indexing, and data fetching to be performed in parallel with floating-point computations. Parallel operations include integer indexing, branch instructions, memory fetches, memory storage, I/O with the host, and floating-point arithmetic. These features make the FPS systems much faster processors than most general-purpose sequential computers. The peak processing rate of the FPS attached processors is 12 MFLOPS and a concurrent six-million integer and addressing operations per second. However, such performance is difficult to realize in practical applications.

The ST-100 attached processor with planned delivery in 1983 is advertised to have a peak performance of 100 MFLOPS. It has the following characteristics:

- Multiple programming internal processors and multiple arithmetic units.
- High-speed logic circuitry.

o Main memory of 512K 32-bit words which can be expanded to 8 M words.

o 48K words of cache memory.

Software for attached processors can be developed on three different levels:

o FORTRAN high-level language with many specialized functions;

o Assembly language macros using a library of routines provided by the manufacturer; and

o Pure micro-assembly language at the machine level.

Recently, the software support capabilities of the attached processors have considerably improved. Such support software includes an ANSI FORTRAN-77 compiler, assembler, loader, object code linker, and simulator - all running on the host computer.

Recent studies (e.g., Refs. 41 and 42) have shown that the combination of a minicomputer and an attached processor in a dual-processor system can extend the range of finite element problems that can be solved effectively by the minicomputer. This capability is accomplished through efficient implementation of both the numerical algorithms used in the finite element solution and the communication protocol between the host minicomputer and the array processor. The question of synchronization between the different parts of the system to ensure correct and efficient function of the minicomputer/attached processor system is of paramount importance.

5. ADVANCES IN SPECIAL ALGORITHMS AND PROGRAMMING LANGUAGES FOR NEW COMPUTING SYSTEMS

The advent of new high-performance computing systems also introduces the problems of designing (a) numerical algorithms that execute efficiently on them, and (b) software with which these algorithms can be expressed. The development of parallel numerical algorithms for pipeline and parallel computers has received considerable attention since the early sixties even before the implementation of these architectures. A number of survey papers have been written on the subject (see, for example, Refs. 43 to 45). These studies have demonstrated that severalfold increases in speed over conventional sequential machines can be obtained if the calculations are arranged to take advantage of the specific hardware.

In this section a brief review is given of the recent progress made in special numerical algorithms and programming languages that are likely to impact finite element technology.

5.1 Parallel Numerical Algorithms

In parallel algorithms, independent computations are performed in parallel (i.e., executed simultaneously (or concurrently)). To achieve this parallelism, the algorithm is divided into a collection of independent tasks (or task modules) which can be executed in parallel and which communicate with each other during the execution of the algorithm. Parallel algorithms can be characterized by the following three factors (see Ref. 22):

a. Maximum amount of computation a typical task module can do before having to communicate with other modules;

b. Intermodule communication topology, which is the geometric layout of the network of task modules; and,

c. Executive control to schedule, enforce the interactions among the different task modules, and ensure the correctness of the parallel algorithm.

The three aforementioned factors have been used in Ref. 22 as a basis for classifying parallel algorithms on a conceptual level, and to relate each parallel algorithm to the parallel (or pipeline) architecture to which it naturally corresponds.

The design of a parallel algorithm must deal with a host of complex problems, including data manipulation, storage allocation, memory interference, and in the case of parallel processors, interprocessor communication.

5.2 Matching Numerical Algorithms with Computer Architectures

In order to obtain the optimum performance from any computing system it is necessary to tailor the numerical algorithm to suit the architecture of the computer, or to select the architecture which will effectively execute the numerical algorithm. The numerical algorithms developed for synchronous, asynchronous parallel computers and systolic machines are discussed subsequently.

a. Algorithms for Synchronous Parallel Computers (MISD and SIMD Machines). The introduction of parallelism in the numerical algorithm used on synchronous parallel computers is usually referred to as *vectorization*. The vectorization of any mathematical operation is dependent on the particular hardware. As an example, for a task to be vectorizable on pipeline computers, it should contain three characteristics: 1) repeated operations; 2) independence of each result from the others; and 3) the members of each operand are packed in either contiguous memory locations or at fixed intervals from each other (with some restrictions in certain hardware configurations). Efficiency and effectiveness of vectorized numerical algorithms on pipeline computers are affected by both the startup time and the average vector length.

Vectorized algorithms have been widely studied for a variety of applications and a variety of hardware configurations. Examples of successful vectorized algorithms that have been developed for synchronous computers include matrix operations, direct and iterative methods of solution of algebraic equations, eigenvalue extraction techniques, multigrid finite difference methods for solution of partial differential equations, and evaluation of elemental matrices for higher-order finite elements (see Refs. 46 to 49). Also, the development of parallel algorithms for the solution of partial differential equations on associative processors has been discussed in Ref. 50.

b. Algorithms for Asynchronous Parallel Computers (MIMD Machines). In comparison with the parallel algorithms for synchronous computers, only a few studies have been made on parallel algorithms for asynchronous computers. Of particular interest are the asynchronous parallel iterative methods in which processors are not synchronized at all. In a truly asynchronous iterative algorithm, a process keeps computing iterates by using whatever information is currently available and releases immediately its computed results to other processes. Thus, the actual iterates generated by the method depend on the relative speed of the processes. The philosophy of "not waiting for other processes to complete their tasks" has been found to be a useful criterion for developing efficient numerical algorithms for asynchronous multiprocessors (Ref. 22). A typical way to achieve this goal is to use copies. After a process completes its current task, it immediately starts working on a copy of the most recent global data.

c. Algorithms for Systolic Machines. Algorithms for systolic machines are designed for direct hardware implementation and, therefore, their task modules are simple and the interactions among them are frequent.

5.3 Performance Evaluation of Parallel Algorithms

It is important to make a distinction between two steps in evaluating the performance of new computing systems.

a. *Comparative Performance*. The ultimate cost-effective judgment that must be rendered in comparing new machines on a code can be a complicated function of architecture-related considerations. Moreover, the performance is so dependent on idiosyncrasies of the code and the compiler that such comparisons have a temporary value at best.

b. *Single Machine Performance*. The comparison of different algorithms and codings on a parallel machine is difficult to make when both parallel algorithm development (a general mathematical concept) and the control of data flow between parallel functional units and hierarchically-organized memories (a machine-dependent coding concept) are involved.

A number of measures have been proposed to quantify the performance of a computer program. One of the simplest, though inadequate measures is based on the CPU time consumed during the execution of the program (see Ref. 11). The two most commonly-used measures for the performance of parallel algorithms on multiple processor and array of processor type machines are based on: the ratio of the speedup over a single processor; and the ratio of the theoretical number of computation steps to the actual number of parallel steps. The first measure is suitable for machines with few processors. The second measure is used for machines with many processors and is strongly dependent on the complexity of the algorithm.

5.4 Software for Parallel Processing

The necessary software for supporting parallel processing includes special programming languages, data management systems and operating systems. Parallel programming is significantly more complicated than sequential programming because:

o It is difficult to keep track of several simultaneously occuring events.

o The potentially complex (time-dependent) interactions of the systems' components may result in elusive and nonrepeatable bugs.

There is a wide spectrum of language possibilities for improving the performance through parallel execution. Examples of the parallel processing languages are provided by Ada (Ref. 51) and Concurrent Pascal (Ref. 52). However, the suitability of these languages for multiple processor machines has not been investigated. Data management in highly-parallel systems can be a serious problem. The tasks performed by the data management system include supplying input to and analyzing output from the processors, and following a trace of the execution.

The operating sytems for highly-parallel machines must be considerably more sophisticated than those for conventional machines. In addition to the usual issues encountered with conventional machines, a number of new issues have to be addressed including physical distribution of tasks among different processors, resource sharing, and interprocessor communication. This is still a research area, and to-date no operating systems have been developed for highly-parallel machines.

The absence of software and languages for highly-parallel machines are severe barriers to progress, since without them assessment of the performance of these machines would be very difficult to make.

6. SCENARIO FOR FUTURE FINITE ELEMENT SYSTEMS

The changes in the computing environment and capabilities discussed in the previous sections suggest significant changes in finite element systems for the future. This section projects a scenario for a future finite element environment, the attendant computer hardware, software, and numerical algorithms together with implications for needed research.

6.1 Future Finite Element Method Environment

With the explosion in computer hardware alternatives as well as the maturing of the finite element method as a basic general-purpose numerical analysis tool competitive with other alternatives, the finite element environment in the next five to ten years should be quite different from today. The basic ingredients today evolve primarily around a standard finite element program/system implemented on a specific computer. The future environment should have several characteristics which are already becoming visible.

a. Comparable finite element capabilities will be available to the user on an array of different levels of processors from desktop (personal) computer to supercomputer. Each level will have features from which the user can select.

b. Finite element software and firmware (i.e., software on ROM) will exist which ranges from stand alone systems to major elements in large integrated CAD/CAM systems.

c. Hardware and software will be distributed and networked so that one can utilize combinations of functions distributed over different processors to maximize the advantages of each level of computation.

d. Arrays of user interface facilities will continue to grow to the level where modeling, mesh generation, user options, tutorials and other features will be so tailored that a user can be led through program use. Results will be readily presented in a variety of multicolored graphical displays. The simplified user interfaces typified by today's video games and cockpit simulations will begin to show up in finite element capabilities. Even some of the smart aids evolving from artificial intelligence and optimization theory will provide assistance to the user in decision making.

e. Algorithms will be expanded in scope and capability for finite element applications. The increased arrays of hardware available will require expansion of algorithm alternatives to exploit these hardware changes. Algorithms chosen will range from those appropriate for small SIMD hardware to those which exploit large highly-parallel MIMD architectures.

e. Specialized hardware/firmware devices will exist which are tailored to carrying out specific finite element tasks. Systolic machines, data flow machines, and chips will exist which generate elemental matrices, assemble these matrices, solve equations, or provide total finite element solutions. Thus the counterpart of electronic "blackboxes" which exist in applications of control theory (e.g., aircraft) will show up as finite element capabilities.

6.2 Future Computer Hardware Environment

The future computer hardware environment available to a user will be characterized by an array of computer hardware capabilities in an expanding level of facilities. Figure 14 shows one approach to visualizing these facilities. The hardware will range from a core capability of supercomputers to provide large-scale computations outward to a periphery which contains a wide variety of

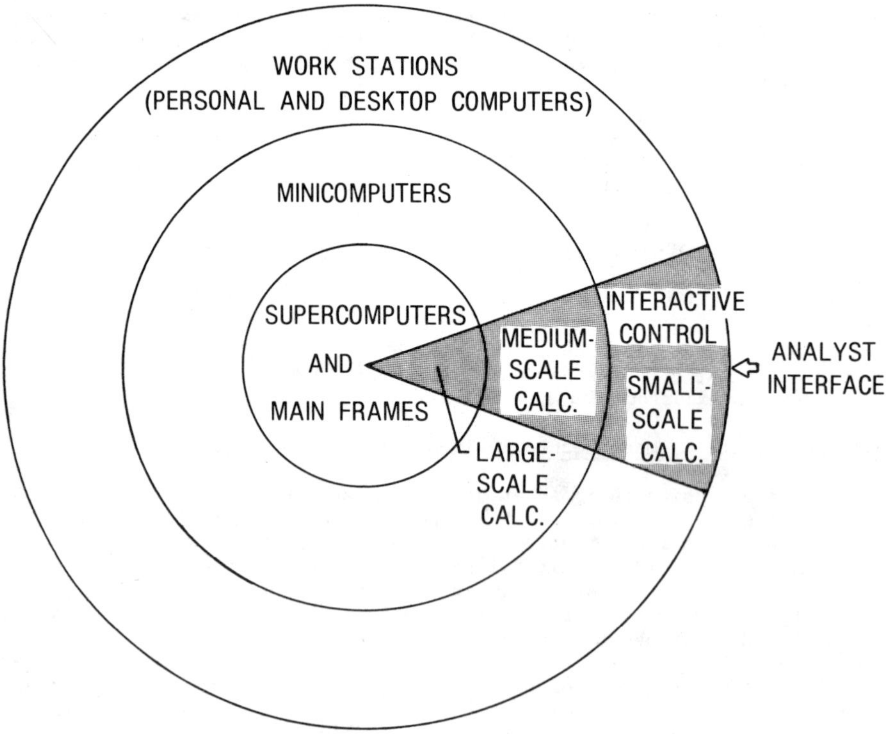

Figure 14 - Future hardware environment.

workstations (personal and desktop computers) well-suited for interactive user interface/control and moderate scale calculations. The number of alternatives for the central core computers will be relatively few whereas the workstation alternatives will be virtually unlimited. In some cases a computer facility may be just an array of networked workstations.

In the context of finite element applications, the interactive model generation and evaluation of results (in graphic form) can be done on the personal computers, and the solution of the global equations can be performed on the supercomputer. Intermediate calculations (e.g., element generation, assembly of elemental matrices, and computation of secondary fields) could be done on the minicomputers or on the personal computers, depending on the instantaneous load on the system.

The organization of this hardware will require:

a. Extensive facilities for local and long-range networking to make all hardware and attendant software readily available to each user.

b. Development of demand-sensitive load-sharing systems to allow programs to migrate from one hardware/operating environment to another. Figure 15 illustrates a typical arrangement of networked hardware composed of a loosely coupled very high-speed network to interface the minicomputers and the large-scale computers, and a moderate-speed local area network to connect workstations. Local networking can facilitate cooperative multidisciplinary investigations and design projects among team members interacting through shared databases. Inexpensive long-range networking can have several significant effects. Issues

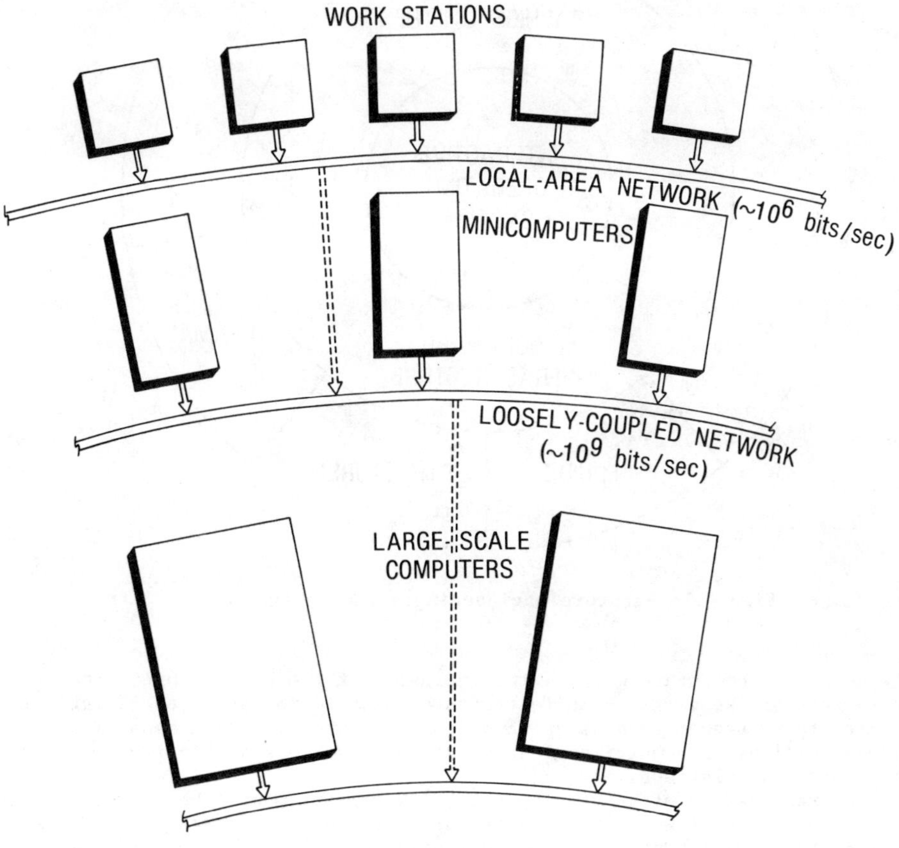

Figure 15 - Future hardware configuration.

of proprietary data can be reduced by sending the program to the location of the owner of the proprietary data, performing the computations there, and receiving only the processed nonproprietary results.

6.3 Future Engineering Software System

The organization of a future engineering software system will change as a result of the growing maturity of CAD/CAM systems and the recognition by computer vendors of the importance of supporting such software as a major business thrust. Instead of having an operating system and support software developed primarily for business applications, the vendor supported facilities will be tailored for CAD/CAM needs. The total engineering software system available to the user (see Fig. 16) can be conveniently visualized as an expanding level of capabilities and specializations emanating from a core containing a user-friendly operating system through a software "infrastructure" containing the engineering support software, and a periphery containing a large array of application programs. A

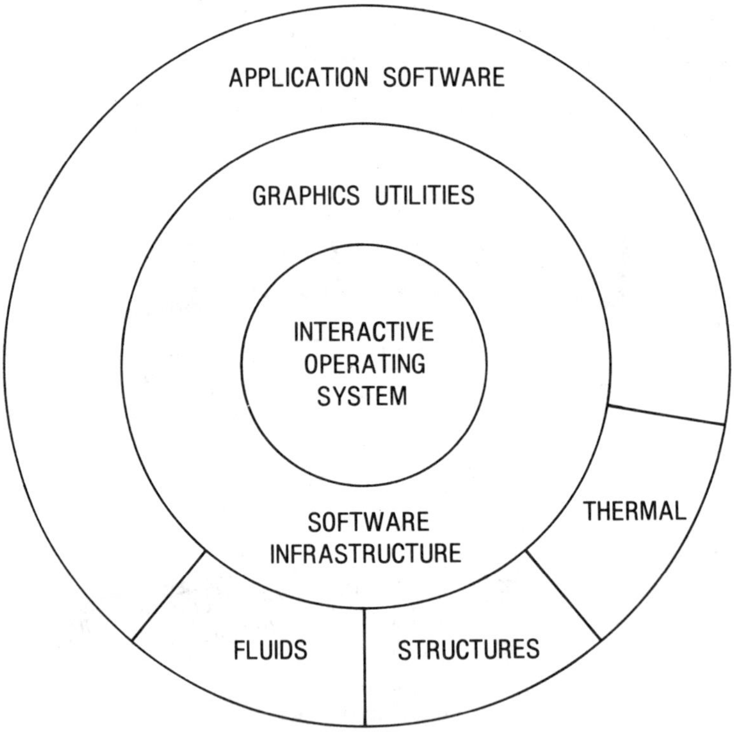

Figure 16 - Future engineering software system.

key element of the future will be the inclusion of the basic finite element software as part of the software infrastructure which is incorporated as part of system software rather than as application programs. The data management and utilities will provide multilevel integration of various applications for multidisciplinary calculations.

The organization of a future finite element system will be compatible with this concept and will exploit the data management and other features of the infrastructure. One approach to the organization of a future finite element system is shown in Fig. 17. This figure shows the basic finite element software (such as data management, control, equation solving, etc.) as part of the software infrastructure and the discipline specifics (such as element properties) as

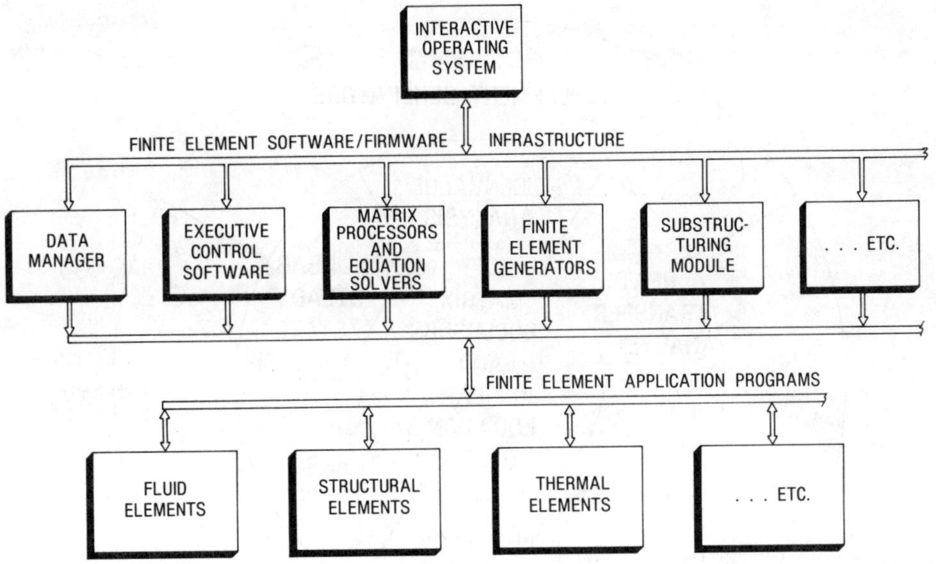

Figure 17 - Organization of future finite element software/firmware

part of the application software. Thus, the infrastructure provides the information manipulation and handling capabilities, and the applications layer contains the fundamental engineering theory and assumptions.

Of the major database models, the relational database management system (see, for example, Ref. 53) appears to be the most suitable for integration with finite element databases because of its formalism and higher level of physical and logical data independence. Research towards more advanced engineering database concepts such as the IPAD multischema approach (Ref. 54) should continue to expand the information management facilities available to support engineering analysis and design.

6.4 Future Finite Element Numerical Algorithms

Numerical algorithms available in the software for solution to finite element problems will expand significantly beyond today's relatively stable set. This expansion will be due to the many available alternatives in hardware as well as the expanding capabilities of the software infrastructure. The core of the numerical algorithms available to the finite element analyst will continue to be the strategy used to solve simultaneous linear algebraic equations and manipulate matrices (see Fig. 18 for one visualization). The next layer will be the specific classes of applications and the outer periphery will contain a wide variety of support algorithms and techniques to provide such functions as modeling, accuracy improvement and computational speedup.

One hierarchical approach to organization of finite element algorithms is shown in Fig. 19. At the top level are the matrix processors and the linear equation solver. The second level contains the specific applications such as linear and nonlinear steady-state analysis, eigenvalue analysis and transient response analysis. The third level contains the wide array of algorithms for specific tasks (e.g., generation of finite element arrays for a variety of applications). In the application of the total set of algorithms, control software provides the user with facilities for automatic or user-directed selection of appropriate combinations of algorithms for the specific application.

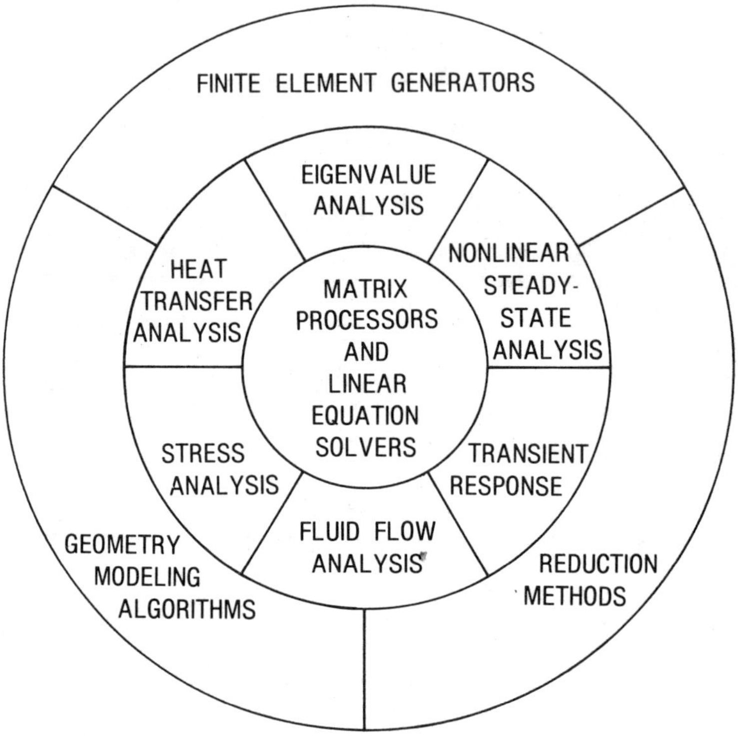

Figure 18 - Future numerical algorithms.

6.6 Future Research Areas

Research is needed in a number of areas to support effective extensions of today's finite element capabilities into the future environment (next five to ten years) characterized here. The two key elements of the future are *explosion of alternatives* and *planning for changes*. Research needs include:

Engineering Research

- o Identification of requirements for a future finite element system
- o Modeling strategies for various disciplines and physical problems
- o Continued advancements in analytical capabilities to simulate the response of complex engineering systems

Engineering/Computer Science Research Tailored to Finite Element Requirements

- o Distributed processing
- o High-speed communications and networking
- o Control of distributed activities
- o Information management
- o Three-dimensional geometry modeling and display
- o Software design of future finite element systems
- o Development/transfer of algorithms to microprocessor implementation

Engineering/Management Research

- o Managing strategies for finite element hardware/software capabilities
- o Matching hardware/software alternatives to achieve cost-effective results
- o Standards for integrating distributed finite element systems
- o Selection/management/control of finite element capabilities to solve new complex problems

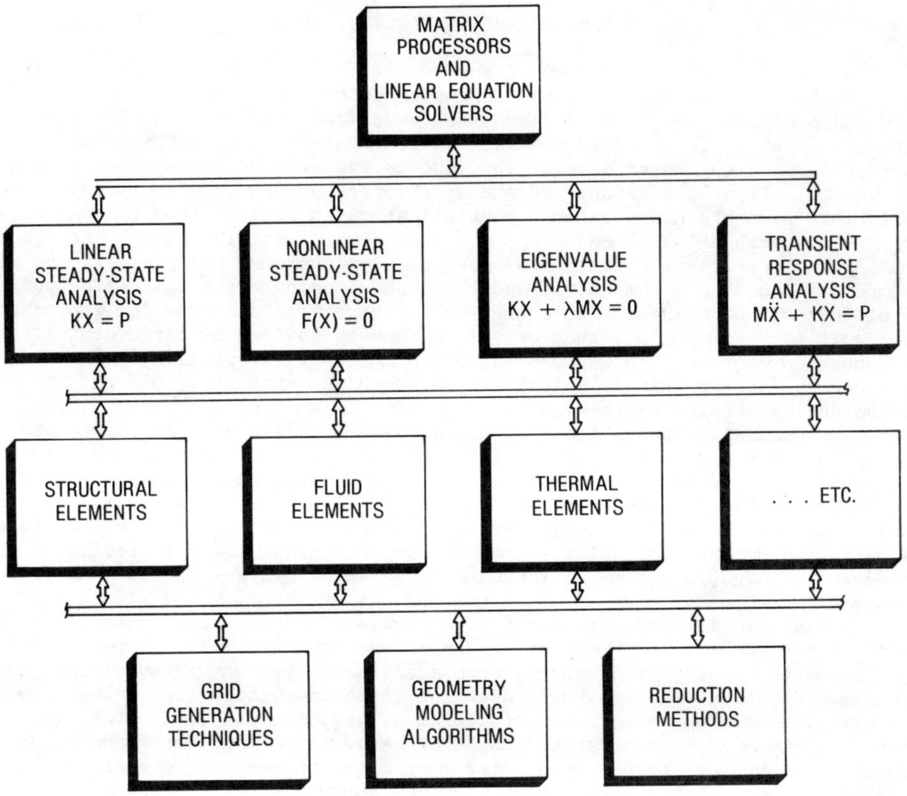

Figure 19 - Hierarchy of numerical methods and algorithms.

Numerical Algorithms

- o Identification of and methods for parallelism in finite element calculations
- o Distribution of finite element calculations
- o Methods for decomposition of calculations into arrays of different processors
- o Development of firmware algorithms for special tasks.

6.6 Summary of Changes for Future Finite Element Methods

In summary, the scenario of the future finite element systems will encompass more choices and options for finite element solution strategies using hardware, software and algorithms. There will be arrays of hardware, different levels of computational capabilities, large arrays of software packages, work distributed across many processors and packages of capability on specific processors. Software and applications interface standards, information management and control procedures will become increasingly important. Finite element research and development must become multidisciplinary, blending the combined technologies of computer hardware/software, engineering, mathematics and even management. Finite element applications will require better management strategies together with increased standardization to maximize efficiency and minimize cost. Key ingredients of finite element technical work of the future will be management of change and considerations of alternatives rather than the current approach of addressing technical advances in a relatively structured hardware/software environment.

7. SUMMARY AND CONCLUDING REMARKS

A detailed review is given of the recent advances in computer technology that are likely to impact finite element computations. The characteristics of new and projected computing systems are summarized. At one end of the spectrum there are the large supersystems such as the CRAY-1S and the CDC CYBER 205. The performance of supersystems will continue to improve and their speed is likely to reach 10 GigaFLOPS before the end of the present decade. These supersystems will make possible new levels of sophistication in finite element modeling as well as in problem depth and scope which were not possible before. At the other end of the spectrum the small low-cost computer systems, particularly the microcomputers (hand-held computers) and the desktop computers (engineering workstations) will provide a high degree of interactivity and free the finite element analysts from constraints that are often imposed on them by large centralized computation centers. To improve the performance of the small systems, attached processors (some on single chips) will be combined with them to form high-performance dual-processor systems.

The special-purpose highly-parallel systems will occupy an intermediate position between the two extremes (the supersystems and the small systems). Special-purpose processors such as the Finite Element Machine, Navier-Stokes machines and Partial Differential Equation (PDE) machines will continue to be built for fast solution of engineering problems. However, their effectiveness will depend on the availability of software to exploit the parallelism in these processors (e.g., programming languages, operating systems and data management systems).

A scenario is presented for future hardware/software environment and finite element systems. In this scenario a broad spectrum of finite element software and firmware is projected ranging from stand-alone systems to modules in large integrated CAD/CAM systems. The user interface facilities (including geometric modeling, mesh generation, input facilities, graphics displays, etc.) will continue to improve. The networked computer hardware/software environment of the future will be more complex and offer many more choices to the user than are available today. This environment provides an opportunity for some very creative research on management-type methods for selecting the best combinations of hardware and software for cost-effective solutions to problems. It is likely that the selection of the appropriate finite element software, firmware and hardware for the solution of an engineering problem will be done with the aid of artificial intelligence-based expert systems.

The discussion of the new computing systems presented herein is intended to give finite element analysts some insight into the potential of these systems for providing cost-effective solutions of complex engineering problems, and to stimulate research and development of the necessary numerical algorithms, firmware and software to realize this potential.

REFERENCES

1 Schrem, E., "Finite Element Software in the Next Decade," Proceedings of the World Congress on Finite Element Methods in Structural Mechanics, Bournemouth, Oct. 12-17, 1975.

2 Fenves, S. J., "Future Directions of Structural Engineering Applications," Computers and Structures, Vol. 10, Nos. 1/2, April 1979, pp. 3-5.

3 MacNeal, R. H., "One Man's View of Trends in Finite Element Analysis," in Computational Aspects of the Finite Element Method, ed. by J. F. Gloudeman and R. E. Rosanoff, Bundesanstalt für Materialprüfung, Berlin, 1979, pp. 1-19.

4 Swanson, J. A., "Present Trends in Computerized Structural Analysis," Computers and Structures, Vol. 10, Nos. 1/2, 1979, pp. 33-37.

5 Stevenson, D., "New Computing Systems and Their Impact on Computation," Supplement to NASA CP-2147, 1981, pp. 1-6.

6 Swanson, J. A., "Opportunities Provided by Large Computers," in New and Future Developments in Commercial Finite Element Methods, ed. by J. Robinson, Robinson and Associates, Dorset, England, 1981, pp. 436-450.

7 MacNeal, R. H., "Trends in Finite Element Structural Analysis," presented at the AIAA/ASME/ASCE/AHS 23rd Structures, Structural Dynamics and Materials Conference, New Orleans, Louisiana, May 10-12, 1982.

8 Lykos, P. and White, J., "An Assessment of Future Computer System Needs for Large-Scale Computation," NASA TM-78613, 1980.

9 Bloch, E. and Galage, D. J., "Component Progress: Its Effect on High Speed Computer Architecture and Machine Organization," in High Speed Computer and Algorithm Organization, ed. by D. J. Kuck, D. H. Lawrie, and A. H. Sameh, Academic Press, New York, 1977, pp. 13-39.

10 Chapman, D. R., "Computational Aerodynamics Development and Outlook," AIAA Journal, Vol. 17, No. 12, Dec. 1979, pp. 1293-1313.

11 Hockney, R. W. and Jesshope, C. R., Parallel Computing, Adam Hilger, Inc., Bristol, 1981.

12 Reisman, A., "Device, Circuit and Technology Scaling to Micron and Submicron Dimensions," Proceedings of the IEEE, Vol. 71, No. 5, May 1983, pp. 550-565.

13 Swartzlander, E. E. and Gilbert, B. K., "Supersystems: Technology and Architecture," IEEE Transactions on Computers, Vol. C-31, No. 5, May 1982, pp. 399-409.

14 Manuel, T., "Parallel Processing," Electronics, June 16, 1983, pp. 105-114.

15 Flynn, M. J., "Some Computer Organizations and Their Effectiveness," IEEE Transactions on Computers, Vol. C-21, 1972, pp. 948-960.

16 Ostlund, N. S., Hibbard, P. G., and Whiteside, R. A., "A Case Study in the Application of a Tightly Coupled Multiprocessor to Scientific Computations," in Parallel Computations, ed. by G. Rodrigue, Academic Press, 1982, pp. 315-364.

17 Fathi, E. T. and Krieger, M., "Multiple Microprocessor Systems: What, Why and When," Computer, Vol. 16, No. 3, March 1983, pp. 23-32.

18 Infotech State of the Art Report "Supercomputers," Vols. 1 and 2, Infotech International, Ltd., Maidenhead, Berkshire, England, 1979.

19 Oakes, W. R. and Browning, R. V., "Experiences Running ADINA on CRAY-1," Proceedings of the ADINA Conference, Aug. 1979, Report 82448-9, Massachusetts Institute of Technology, Cambridge, Massachusetts, pp. 27-42.

20 Haynes, L. S., Lau, R. L., Siewiorek, D. P., and Mizell, D. W., "A Survey of Highly-Parallel Computing," Computer, Jan. 1982, pp. 9-24.

21 Kung, H. T., "Why Systolic Architectures," Computer, Jan. 1982, pp. 37-46.

22 Kung, H. T., "The Structure of Parallel Algorithms," Advances in Computers, Vol. 19, Academic Press, 1980, pp. 65-112.

23 Law, K. H., "Systolic Schemas for Finite Element Methods," Report R-82-139, Department of Civil Engineering, Carnegie-Mellon University, July 29, 1982.

24 Melhem, R., "Formal Verification of a Systolic System for Finite Element Stiffness Matrices," Technical Report ICMA-83-56, Institute for Computational Mathematics and Applications, University of Pittsburgh, Pennsylvania, 1983.

25 Storaasli, O. O., Peebles, S. W., Crockett, T. W., Knott, J. D., and Adams, L., "The Finite Element Machine: An Experiment in Parallel Processing," NASA TM-84514, NASA Langley Research Center, Hampton, Virginia, July 1982.

26 Adams, L. M., "Iterative Algorithms for Large Sparse Linear Systems on Parallel Computers," NASA CR-166027, NASA Langley Research Center, Hampton, Virginia, Nov. 1982.

27 Salama, M., Utku, S., and Melosh, R., "Parallel Solution of Finite Element Equations," Proceedings of the Eighth ASCE Conference on Electronic Computation, University of Houston, Houston, Texas, Feb. 21-23, 1983, pp. 526-539.

28 McGregor, J. and Salama, M., "Finite Element Computation with Parallel VLSI," Proceedings of the Eighth ASCE Conference on Electronic Computation, University of Houston, Houston, Texas, Feb. 21-23, 1983, pp. 540-553.

29 Tyler, M., "The Micro Micros," Datamation, Vol. 28, No. 13, Dec. 1982, pp. 34-42.

30 Conaway, J. H., "Structural Engineering Software on Small Computers," American Society of Mechanical Engineers, Paper 80-C2/Aero-7, Aug. 1980.

31 Foster, E. P. and Storaasli, O. O., "Structural Analysis on a Minicomputer," Engineering Software, ed. by R. A. Adey, Pentech Press, London, 1979, pp. 43-54.

32 Storaasli, O. O. and Murphy, R. C., "Finite Element Analysis in a Minicomputer/Mainframe Environment," in Research in Computerized Structural Analysis and Design, NASA CP-2059, 1978, pp. 77-83.

33 Wilson, E. L., "The Use of Minicomputers in Structural Analysis," Proceedings of the ADINA Conference, Aug. 1979, Report 82448-9, Massachusetts Institute of Technology, Cambridge, Massachusetts, pp. 293-303.

34 Edwards, J., "The Desktop Buyer's Guide to Small Computers," Desktop Computing, April 1983, pp. 52-69.

35 Lu, C., "Microcomputers: The Second Wave," High Technology, Vol. 2, No. 5, Sept./Oct. 1982, pp. 36-52.

36 Backx, E., Rammant, J. P., and Schymkowitz, "Case Study on Desk Computer: Finite Element Analysis in BASIC," Finite Element Methods in the Commercial Environment, ed. by J. Robinson and published by Robinson and Associates, Dorset, England, 1978, Vol. 2, pp. 670-680.

37 Firmin, A., "FESDEC - A Finite Element System for Desktop Computers," Finite Element News, Jan. 1980, pp. 22-23.

38 Wilson, E. L., "SAP-80 - Structural Analysis Programs for Small or Large Computer Systems," presented at CEPA 1980 Fall Conference and Annual Meeting, Newport Beach, California, Oct. 13-15, 1980.

39 Kelly, P. and Watson, A. S., "Structural Analysis Using Desktop Computers," in Engineering Software II - Proceedings of the Second International Conference on Engineering Software, held at Imperial College of Science and Technology, London, March 1981, CML Publications, Ltd., Southampton, 1981, pp. 346-359.

40 Griffen, O. H. and Wilson, C. R., "Finite Element Analysis on A Microprocessor-Based Personal Workstation," Technical Note, Computers and Structures, Vol. 17, No. 4, 1983, pp. 617-619.

41 Strohkorb, G. A. and Noor, A. K., "Potential of Minicomputer/Array-Processor System for Nonlinear Finite-Element Analysis," NASA TM 84566, June 1983.

42 Swanson, J. A., Cameron, G. R., and Haberland, J. C., "Adapting the ANSYS Finite-Element Analysis Program to an Attached Processor," Computer, Vol. 16, No. 6, June 1983, pp. 85-91.

43 Miranker, W. L., "A Survey of Parallelism in Numerical Analysis," SIAM Review, Vol. 13, No. 4, Oct. 1971, pp. 524-547.

44 Sameh, A. H., "Numerical Parallel Algorithms - A Survey," in High-Speed Computer and Algorithm Organization, Academic Press, 1977, pp. 207-228.

45 Heller, D., "A Survey of Parallel Algorithms in Numerical Linear Algebra," SIAM Review, Vol. 20, No. 4, Oct. 1978, pp. 740-777.

46 Voigt, R. G., "The Influence of Vector Computer Architecture on Numerical Algorithms," in High-Speed Computer and Algorithm Organization, Academic Press, 1977, pp. 229-244.

47 Ortega, J. M. and Voigt, R. G., "Solution of Partial Differential Equations on Vector Computers," Proceedings of the 1977 Army Numerical Analysis and Computers Conference, ARO Report 77-3, pp. 475-525.

48 Rodrigue, G. (ed.), Parallel Computations, Academic Press, 1982.

49 Noor, A. K. and Hartley, S. J., "Evaluation of Element Stiffness Matrices on CDC STAR-100 Computer," Computers and Structures, Vol. 9, No. 2, 1978, pp. 151-161.

50 Gilmore, P. A., "Numerical Solution of Partial Differential Equations by Associative Processing," Proceedings of the 1971 Fall Joint Computer Conference, AFIPS, Vol. 39, pp. 411-418.

51 Brender, R. F. and Massi, I. R., "What is Ada?," Computer, Vol. 14, No. 6, June 1981, pp. 17-22, 24.

52 Coleman, D., Gallimore, R. M., Hughes, J. W., and Powell, M. S., "An Assessment of Concurrent Pascal," Software - Practice and Experiment, Vol. 9, No. 10, Oct. 1979, pp. 827-837.

53 RIM User's Guide, Academic Computer Center, University of Washington, W33, Jan. 1980.

54 Fulton, R. E., "CAD/CAM Approach to Improving Industry Productivity Gathers Momentum," Astronautics and Aeronautics, Vol. 20, Feb. 1982, pp. 64-70.